Lory Ramos

Diabetic Meal Prep Cookbook for Beginners

New Edition

850+ Delicious Recipes. A 4-Week Meal Plan to Manage Newly Diagnosed Type 2 And Prediabetes. With an Easy Guide to Understand and Living Better with Diabetes

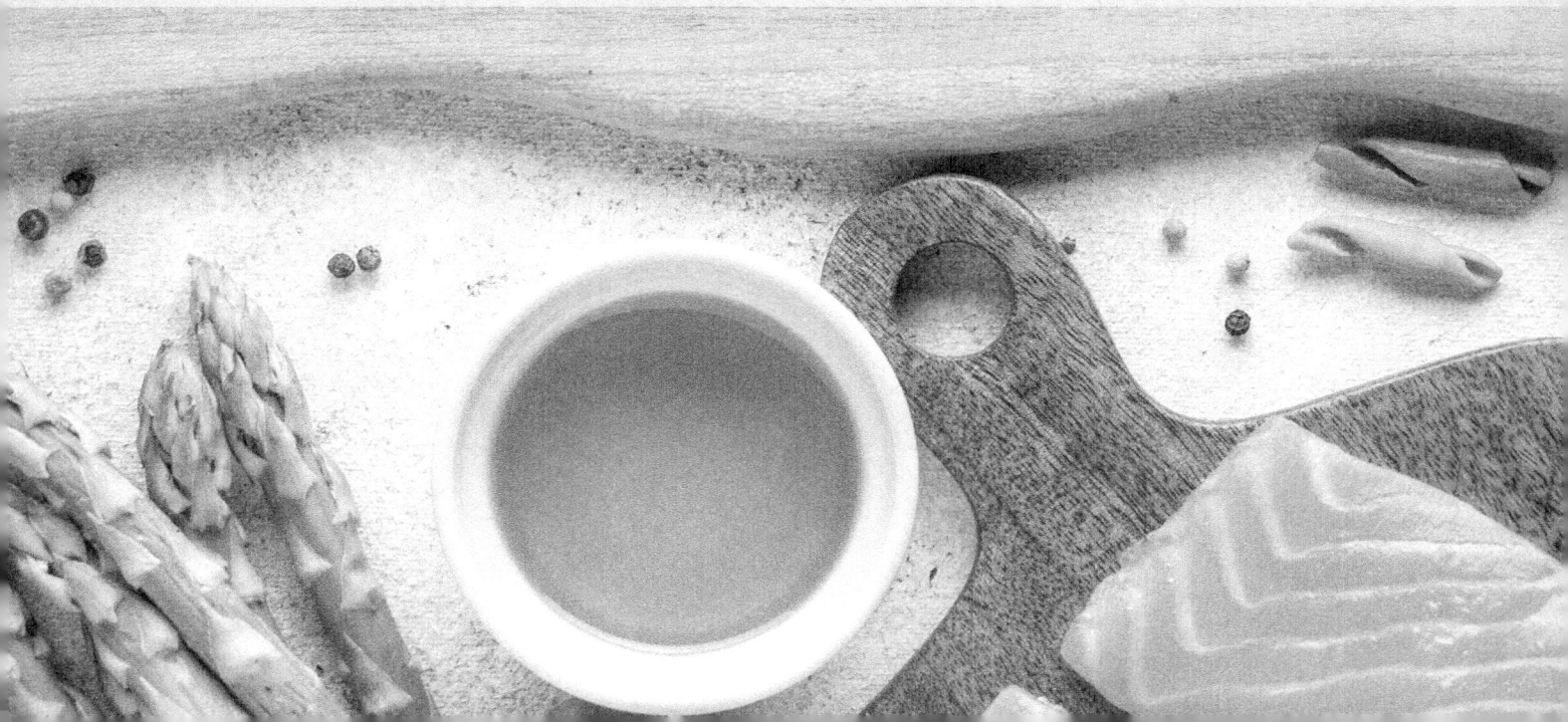

Table of Contents

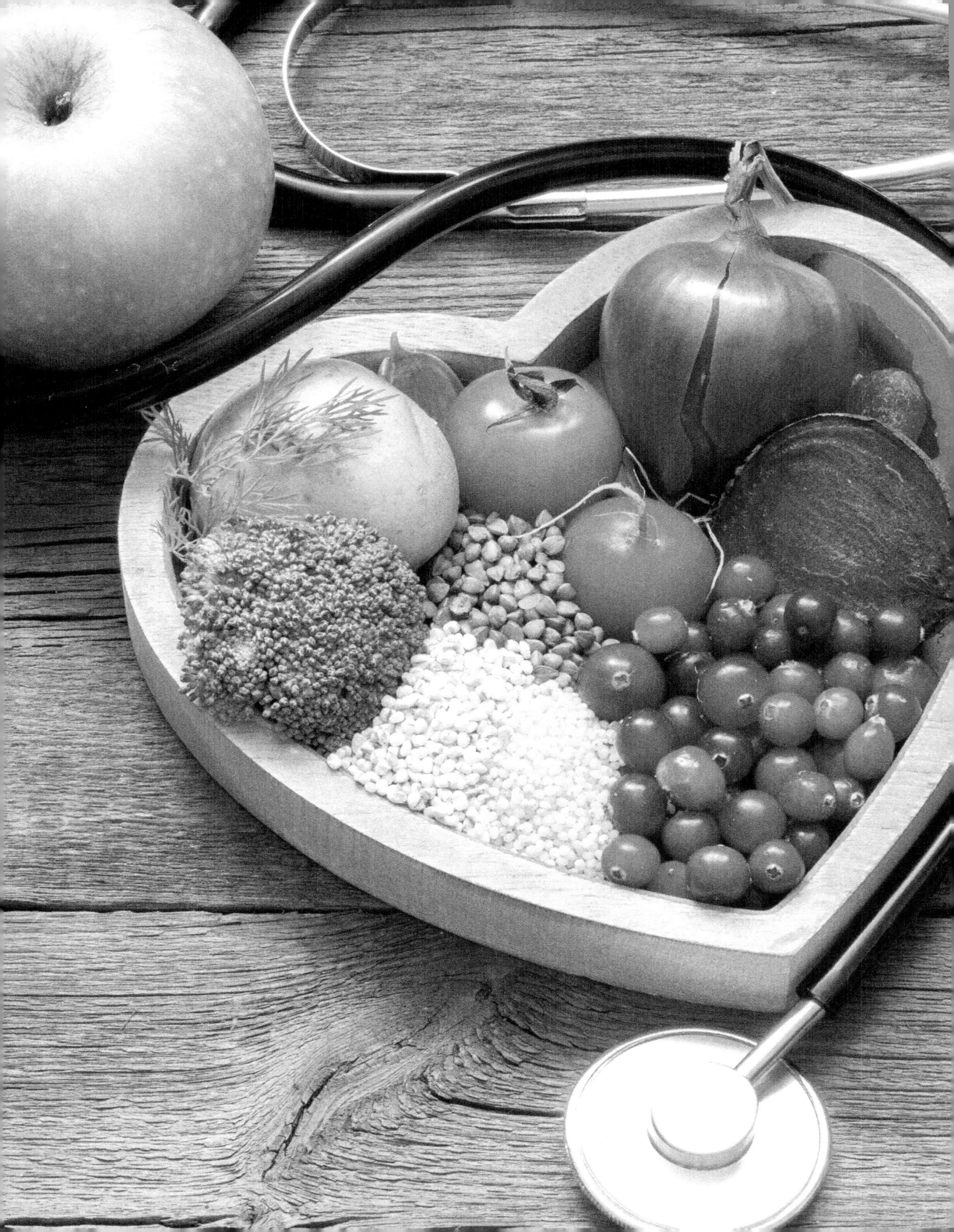

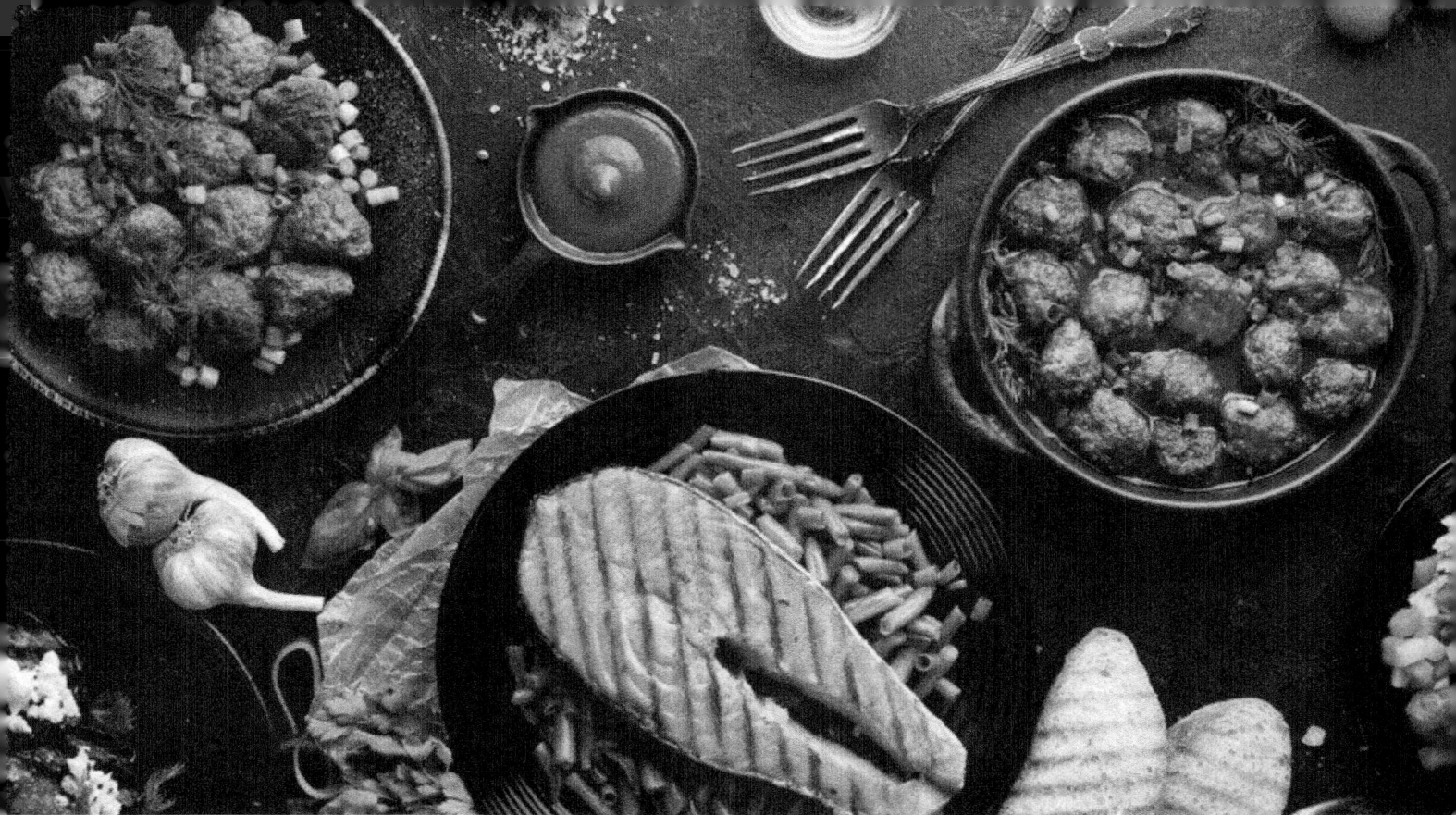

Introduction

The Benefits of the Diabetes Meal Prep ●● ●

Meal planning is extremely helpful in many practical ways, but one of its greatest benefits is on a person's health, particularly if it combines healthy balanced food and proper portion control.

Benefit # 1 - It helps improve your general health

Whether or not you have a medical condition, meal planning can help you improve your overall health when the meals provide all the macro and micronutrients your body needs. It also helps you avoid saturated fats and processed sugars, which is what most people would reach for if they're hungry and just want something satisfying.

Benefit # 2 - It ensures that you can eat on time

Preparing your meals in advance helps manage hunger pains. Missing a meal or delaying it can cause your blood sugar level to drop too low, a condition otherwise known as hypoglycemia.

Hypoglycemia can cause shaking, disorientation, and irritability. You may even have a seizure if your blood sugar level gets any lower. Having your meal already prepared ensures that you can always eat on time and, therefore, decrease the risk of low blood glucose.

Benefit # 3 - It lowers your risk of heart disease

Diabetes increases the risk of heart disease. With the help of a dietician, planning your meals can help you reduce this risk. Because meal prep reduces the time you need to spend in the kitchen, you'll have more opportunities to exercise and do other activities that promote a healthier lifestyle.

Benefit # 4 - It lowers your risk of cancer

Diabetes also increases the risk of all forms of cancer. While experts are still unable to identify the exact link between these two conditions, they expect that it has something to do with insulin resistance and obesity. Cancer patients are advised to pursue a healthy lifestyle, which includes eating a balanced diet and getting adequate exercise. Because these activities are also encouraged among diabetics, the risk of cancer is lowered.

Benefit # 5 - It helps you maintain healthy body weight

Again, portion control plays a part in this area. Even if you eat healthy food, overindulging can lead to an unhealthy weight gain, which can make it harder to control your blood sugar level.

If left unchecked, this could lead to high blood sugar levels or hyperglycemia, which can cause various complications that include heart and liver damage as well as the loss of kidney function.

It's important to note that while meal planning can help keep the effects of diabetes under control, you and your dietician still need to conduct a periodic review of its effectiveness and make changes whenever necessary.

How to identify if you have Diabetes

The early signs of diabetes include:

- **Hunger and fatigue**
  When your body consumes food, it converts it into glucose so that the cells can use it for energy. The body needs insulin so that the cells can take in the glucose. Without enough insulin or if the cells are unable to use insulin, the body does not get any energy, making you feel tired as well as hungry all the time.
- **Excessive thirst and urination**
  Usually, a person pees from four to seven times a day. But with people who suffer from diabetes pee a lot more. This also makes you thirsty more frequently.
- **Dry mouth and itchy skin**
  When the body uses fluids to create urine, it has less moisture to keep the mouth and skin from drying.
- **Blurry vision**
  Changes in the body's fluid levels can inflame the lens of the eyes, making it more difficult for the eyes to focus.

Symptoms of type-2 diabetes include:

- Yeast infections
- Slow-healing wounds
- Pain in the muscles
- Numbness of legs and feet

Symptoms of type-1 diabetes are the following:

- Unexplained weight loss
- Nausea and vomiting

As for gestational diabetes, there are no symptoms. The condition is only determined during prenatal screening.

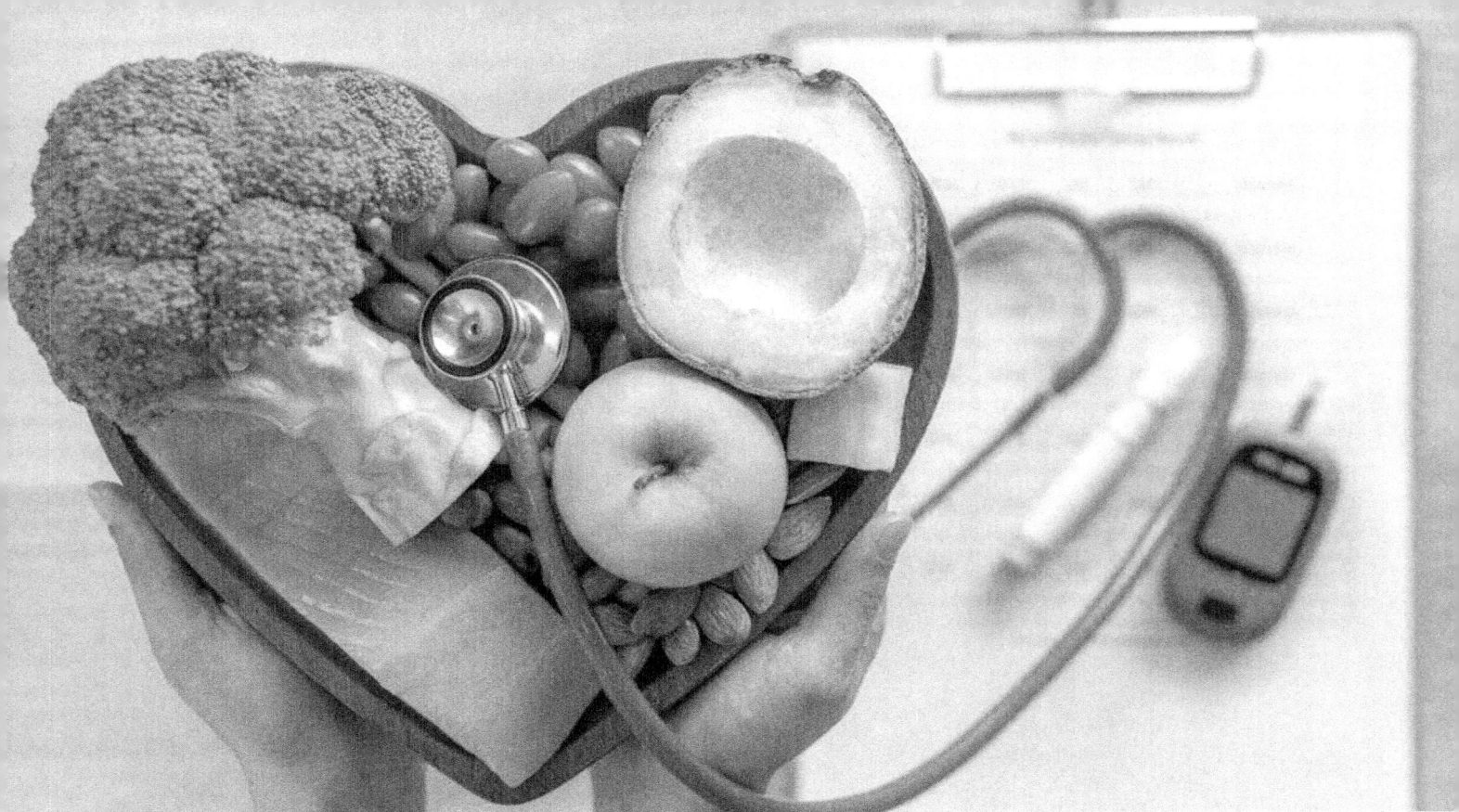

How to Manage Diabetes If You Have Just Been Diagnosed

Recommendations for Type 1 Diabetes ● ● ●

If you have type 1 diabetes, there are certain methods of treatment that you can use that will help you to manage yourself better. You will have very specific goals that are put out for you to help with the management of your disease. You will be expected to, for example, make sure that you are managing your blood sugar and pressure. According to the experts at Kaiser Permanent, an American nationwide healthcare provider and the largest nonprofit health plan throughout the US, blood sugar should follow these guidelines to be considered well controlled:

Timing	Target
Before meals	80-130 mg/dL
2 hours after meals	160 mg/dL
Bedtime	80-130 mg/dL
3 a.m.	80-130 mg/dL

When diagnosed with type 1 diabetes, you will find that a lot changes. You need to be able to change how you are living your life. In particular, you must change up your diet, make sure that exercise is a priority, and make sure that you are consuming the highest amounts of healthy foods possible. You will be recommended to make sure that you are providing yourself with as much good, healthy foods as possible, and you will want to keep your weight healthy. Keep in mind that type 1 diabetes is permanent—there is no way to cure it. However, you will need to treat yourself with insulin on a regular basis. You must make sure that you are giving yourself insulin, either through injections or pumps, to make sure that your body is able to function regardless of what you eat. Without providing your body that insulin, you will not be able to regulate that blood sugar. Your doctor will focus mostly on teaching you what it will take for you to know what it is that your body needs at any given time based on the foods that you are eating. If you know that blood sugar rises after eating, you know that you need to also inject yourself with insulin.

However, the amount of insulin that you inject varies greatly from person to person, as well as based on the carbs that you consumed.

Recommendations for Type 2 Diabetes ● ● ●

As with type 1 diabetes, type 2 comes with very similar recommendations. You will need to make sure that you are managing your health in general, but you will also be recommended to be more mindful of the foods that you are eating. You may also be recommended to work to lose weight. This is because type 2 diabetes is entirely controllable through just diet and exercise. You will be able to treat yourself without the need for insulin because the problem is not that you don't have insulin at all—the problem is that your body isn't responding to it.

Your diet will be more strictly monitored on type 2 diabetes, and it will be harder to keep it in line if you are not treating yourself carefully. However, because you can effectively reverse this disease over time with the right diet, it is one that is highly favored over other options.

How to Break Free of Your Sugar Habit ● ● ●

So, maybe you're at risk of diabetes, or maybe you already have it but don't know what you can do to lessen your sugar consumption habits. The good news is it isn't that bad to break these habits. It can take a while, and you need willpower, but if you have that, you should be able to fight off the habits as well. All you have to do is be willing to make some significant changes to your diet.

Ultimately, people are hardwired to desire sugar—when we didn't have easy access to sugar, we needed to want as many carbs as possible to keep ourselves healthy and alive; the carbs would help us to create fats. They would also help to keep us full. However, nowadays, because we don't have to forage or hunt and gather for food, we have our own problems. Nowadays, the problem is that food is too easy to find. Because it is so readily available, you run into the problem of potentially storing up too much fat as a direct result. However, you can learn to prevent this from being a problem.

We are hardwired to want to go for those sugary choices. Most animals are—studies have shown that animals will go out of their way to choose sugar over cocaine in lab tests. However, sugar is not good for us in excess, as we have established thus far. This means that you will need to be mindful of what you are doing to prevent yourself from getting ill. You will need to figure out how you can make sure that you do not unintentionally poison yourself with too much sugar. Now, let's look at what goes into breaking that habit—or even that addiction in some cases.

A Brief Guide to Eliminating Sugar ● ● ●

First, before we begin, consider the fact that sugar comes in all sorts of forms. It comes in the form of sucrose and fructose. Lactose and maltose are two others. Sucrose can be found, as well. As you can see, hover, they all end in "-ose." That is the sign that you are looking at a sugar if you don't see the actual word written in front of you. Because sugars come in so many different forms, it can be difficult to truly eliminate them. It can be impossible for you to figure out what you will need to do to prevent yourself from getting ill from these effects—you will need to make sure that you are working hard to ensure that your diet is well-managed. Ultimately, if you are able to recognize these different forms of sugar, you will be able to prevent yourself from eating things that aren't going to help you.

As an additional note before we begin, consider the fact that you don't need to cut out all forms of sugar—you just want to cut it out when it is added to your diet. This means that it is okay to eat whole food that breaks down into carbs—but you don't want to eat something that is laden with high fructose corn syrup. Eating foods that are loaded up with sugars can be a huge problem, and most people don't even realize that they are doing it—they just do so because they think that since the word sugar isn't on the ingredient list, they are safe to eat it without a concern.

If you are ready to cut out sugar from your diet, there are a few steps that you should follow to help yourself do so. These aren't necessarily difficult to do, but many people find that it is hard to stick to it. They get caught up in the cravings, or they give into the withdrawals that they feel when they do cut them out. Your body gets used to those higher levels of sugar in your diet and comes to rely on them; when you cut them out, you are likely to run into some symptoms as your body has to develop and adjust to its new normal.

Cutting sugar by tossing out added sugar sources the first step to making sure that you can eliminate sugar is to take the time to genuinely cut it out in the first place. If you have added sugar options in your home, such as white and brown sugars, or also eliminating the honey. If you are going to make yourself coffee or tea, you want to make sure that you aren't adding these. At first, make sure that you do so gradually. You want to start out by cutting the amounts of sugar in half and slowly weaning down over the period of a couple of weeks. This is what is best for you.

Cut out liquid sugars ● ● ●

All too often, people drink sugars that they don't even realize. Soda is one of the biggest sources of sugar that we get. Additionally, you can see that adding honey or sugar to coffees and teas is another common source, as is drinking juice. None of these are very healthy options; you need to make sure that you are cutting out those sugars over time. Coffee and tea are fine, so long as you are mindful of the sugars that you put into them.

Choose fresh fruits ● ● ●

If you want something sweet, go for fruit, but still, be mindful. Fresh fruit is usually the best for you, but you can also go for unsweetened frozen fruit or even canned fruit if it is in water or natural juices. Make sure that you avoid the fruit that is canned in heavy syrups; this is a common source of sugars that people don't realize that they are using. You can also use fruit as a natural sweetener. If you are going to use a sweetener of some sort for yogurt, cereals, or oatmeal, this is a great option for you. Fruit is a great option to flavor your teas or water as well if you are someone that's used to sweetened and flavored drinks.

Always compare food labels ● ● ●

When you look at your food labels, make sure that you choose those that have the lowest amounts of added sugars. Many foods are naturally going to have carbohydrates in them—and that's okay in moderation. You must make sure that you are cutting out those high added sugar foods to keep yourself healthy. This means that if you have a food with 22 grams of sugar and 18 are added, and you can also choose a food that has 25 grams of sugar with just 4 or 5 added the second food is going to be the healthier choice because it doesn't involve adding any natural sugars.

Extracts for flavor ● ● ●

Instead of relying on sweeteners like sugar, you can use extracts like vanilla or lemon to add some richness and flavor without the calories.

Non-nutritive sweeteners ● ● ●

If you just can't cut the sugar entirely, you can make it a point to limit the sugar that you do consume, switching it out with non-nutritive sweeteners. However, treat this as a crutch rather than a permanent option. It is better for you to just keep things natural and avoid adding any sweeteners entirely.

Substitute or replace it ● ● ●

If you are cooking something, there are several options that you can use as a way of avoiding the sugar entirely. You could use spices to enhance the foods instead of using sweeteners. You can also use ingredients such as applesauce to replace sugar and fats in many baking dishes as a nice way to cut out the added sugars.

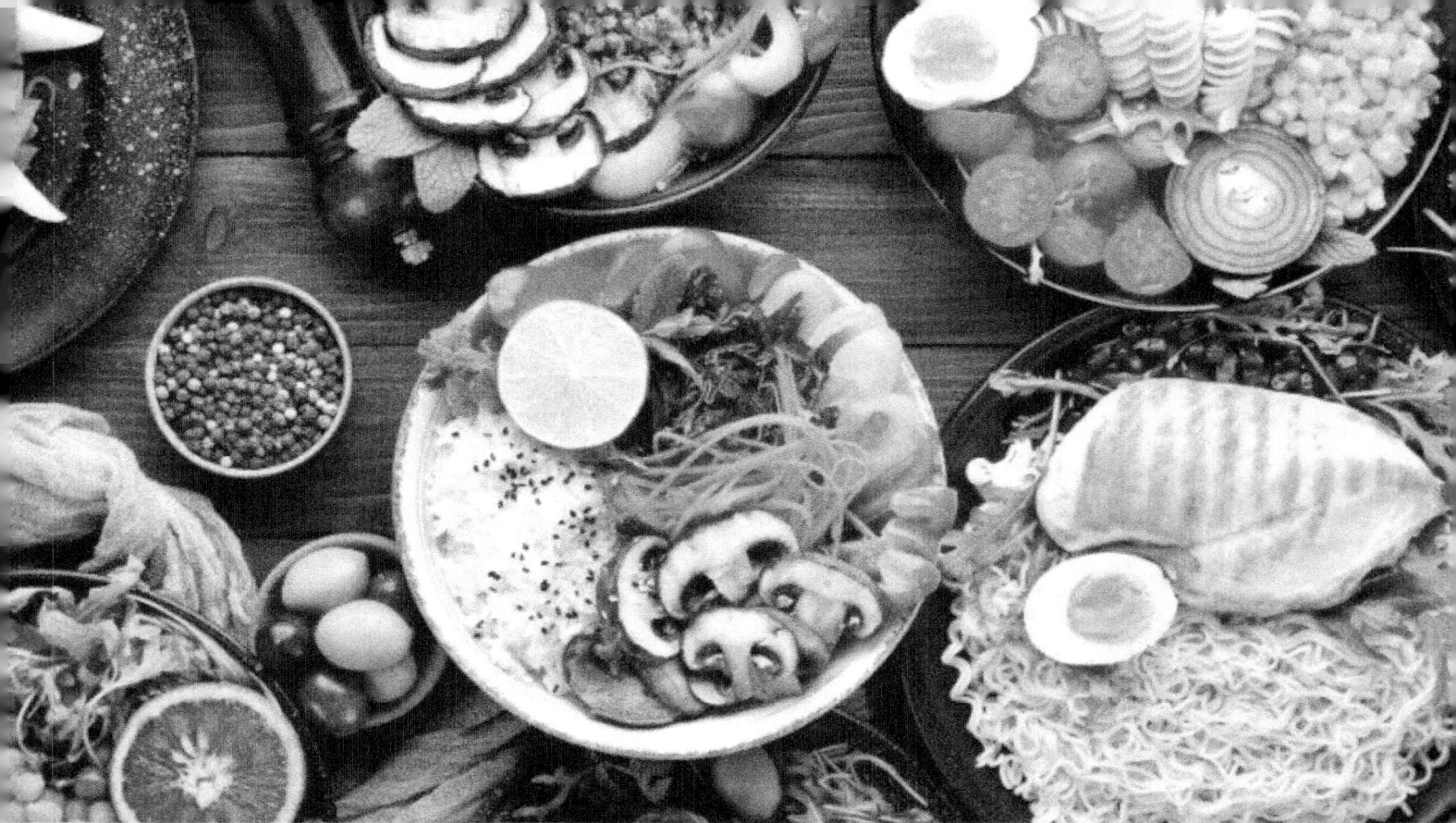

A Healthy Meal Can Help Reduce the Effects of Diabetes

Relationship between Meals and Your Blood Sugar ●●

Your daily meals have a direct effect on your body's blood glucose levels. Some foods raise blood glucose more than others while some other foods do not (have minimal effects on blood sugar levels. Therefore, managing what you eat, knowing their calorie content, knowing what they contain and how they affect your glucose levels and your body is very important. Basically, three major classes of food appear in most of our meals or diets. They include carbohydrates, fats and proteins. Vegetables, fruits and fiber appear much less in meals and diets. An understanding of these food classes and their effects on the body is very important.

Proteins

Proteins are important parts of our diet. In an experiment where Protein of the same quantity and carbohydrate of the same quantity is taking by two individuals at the same time, the individual who took the carbohydrate would most likely get hungry first. This shows how important they are. They help to create satiety. Proteins mildly contribute to the glucose (sugar levels) in the body, and are usually increased in most diabetes meal plans. Proteins are equally the building blocks of the body, and generally help the body to recover from stress and ailments.

Generally, to create a balanced diet (in relation to diabetes). These three classes should be included, albeit in differing quantities.

Vegetables and fruit

Vegetables and fruits are very helpful in the creation of balanced diabetes meal plans. They help in flushing and cleansing the body. They equally contain many vitamins and minerals that help in regulating blood sugar levels in the body. They can equally be used as snacks, because most of them contain fibers. Hence, they can easily cause satiety. Fruits equally contain natural sugars that are less harmful to the body.

Artificial Sweeteners and Weight

As a diabetic, it is generally recommended that you avoid artificial sweeteners or drinks that have artificial sweeteners. They might seem insignificant, but over time they can cause serious harm to the body.

Recent research has shown that despite the fact sweeteners are very low in kilojoules; they can actually make you gain weight. A standardized review studied all published randomized controlled trials and investigative studies on body weight. The review discovered that the use of artificial sweeteners led to a significant increase in body weight.

Generally, sweeteners are divided into two. They are nutritive and non- nutritive. Ongoing research from scientists indicates that non- nutritive sweeteners might be inconsequential, especially when the user does not take additional processed food. It is however advised that sweeteners should be avoided, as much as possible.

Some sweetener protagonists argue that the quantity used is usually set aside. They believe that some of these findings are biased. That most of them based their calculations on doses that are never used. They believe that the quantity of sweeteners used is negligible.

Whether these findings are true or not, it is generally advised that individuals (especially diabetics), should avoid diabetes as much as possible.

Check What You Drink

Drinks are equally an important part of our diet. For good health and optimum fitness, the body requires between thirty-five and forty-five milliliters of fluid for each kilo of weight every day.

There might be alterations based on gender, level of physical activity, body composition and the weather. For example, the common Australian lady weighs about 70 kg on average, while an Australian man weighs an average of 80 kg. Therefore, a typical lady needs 2.5 to 3.2 liters, and a man about 3.0 to 3.9 liters of fluid every day. All fluids don't have to come from drinks; however, as around 750 milliliter comes from our food and an extra 250 milliliter comes from the metabolism of food. So, on average, girls ought to aim to drink 1.5 to 2.2 liters and men ought to aim to drink 2.0 to 2.9 liters every day.

With such a large amount of drinks available now, it is understandable if you get confused (on what to drink. Your choice depends on your personal circumstances and health status.

Water

Plain water is the best drink to quench your thirst: it's refreshing and provides zero kilojoules, and a number of minerals. Pure water doesn't have any taste, though the minerals that are generally found in water naturally (for example, fluoride), will have an effect on its flavor. If water flavor is a problem for you, attempt using a water apparatus or adding a slice or 2 of lemon or lime.

Depending on the supply, drinking water typically contains little amounts of metallic element, potassium, metal and metal, and is appropriate for individuals with polygenic disease (diabetes)

Diet soft drinks

People with diabetes will benefit from a diet or low sugar and soft drinks, however they ought to not consume them on a routine. This is often as a result of sugar-based beverages which are acidic and frequent consumption could increase the danger of developing high sugar levels. There's proof that subbing regular soft drinks with a proper diet or low-joule varieties can facilitate health recovery in some individuals.

Fruit juices and fruit drinks

Fruit juices and fruit drinks may be enjoyed often, however ideally not on a routine. They supply kilojoules, vitamin C, dietary fiber and sugar. Fruit juices and drinks are acidic and also are a supply of possible sugar for the cariogenic bacterium; therefore, frequent consumption of those drinks could increase the danger of developing diseases...

Fruit juices and drinks raise glucose levels in individuals with diabetes. On average, they supply twenty-two g of sugar per 250 milliliters serve. Fruit juices made of low-GI fruit and most fruit drinks have a reduced glycemic index (GI), whereas a 250-milliliter serve of most varieties features a medium glycemic load (GL).

Fruit juices are related to an increased risk of type 2 diabetes in empirical studies. This association is also thanks to their kilojoules content, which can contribute to weight gain, and glycemic load, which can contribute to duct gland stress. Higher-quality analysis is additionally needed to prove this association.

Regular sugar-sweetened soft drink

Sugar-sweetened soft drinks are related to associate to magnified increase in the occurrence of diabetes empirical studies. Like fruit juices and drinks, this association is also thanks to the sugar content of those drinks, which can contribute to weight gain, and their glycemic load, which can contribute to duct gland stress.

Alcohol

While alcohol isn't a necessary nutrient, it's however enjoyed by the bulk of adults living in the world today. Alcohol provides twenty-nine kJ of energy for each gram consumed — second solely to fats in energy density. Once consumed, alcohol is then absorbed into the blood from the abdomen and bowel. It doesn't need any digestion, and may consequently induce the acquainted feelings of high spirits among minutes if it's consumed on an empty abdomen.

Alcohol is metabolized within the liver, however there's a limit to what quantity it will handle — about (or 11/2 normal drinks) per hour. Therefore, excess amounts will cause a buildup of sugar within the blood if you drink over one or two normal drinks per hour.

Other Food Tips:

• **Take your meals at regular time intervals**

Taking meals at regular intervals helps the body to regulate blood sugar. Our bodies are adaptive and intelligent. Over time they learn to expertly manage and process these foods, because they already know what to expect. Hence food processing (in the body) becomes faster and efficient.

• **Monitor your food portions**

The quantity of food you eat is an important part of diabetes management. Portion sizes are usually dependent on the level of a patient's diabetes (blood sugar level). Equally portions are directly related to an individual's weight. Heavier persons tend to eat more. Any decrease in food portions should be done gradually.

Canada's Food Guide suggests one way to plan your portions. Half of your plate should be filled with vegetables and fruits. It should be more vegetables than fruit because, vegetables have less sugar. The other half of your plate should be between proteins and carbohydrates. Portion control is very important in diabetes control. For overweight diabetes patients, this might be the fastest way to lose weight and regulate blood sugar.

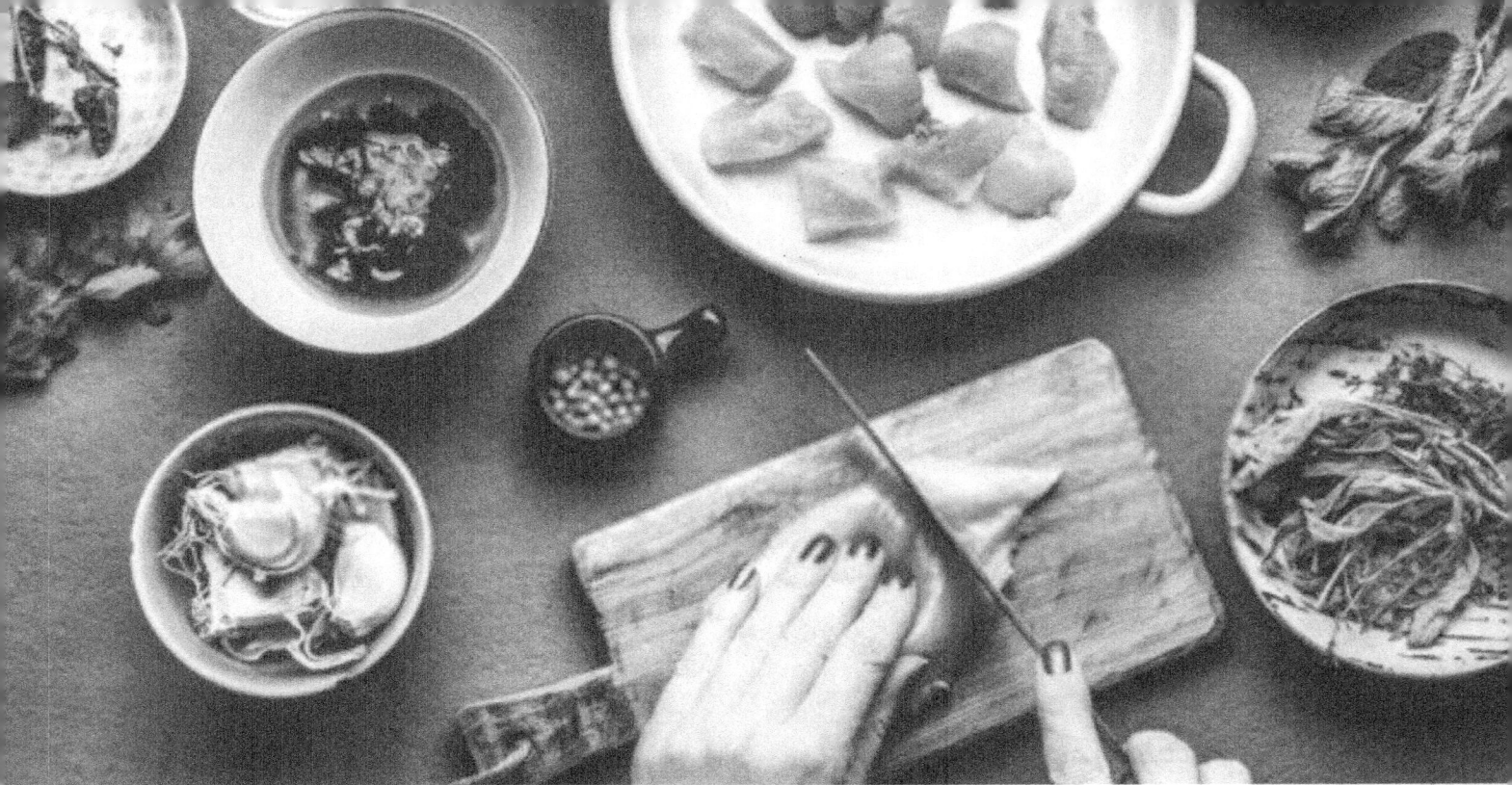

The Basics of Meal Prep

It is time for us first to look into the basics of being able to prep and plan your meals to help keep your diet on track. Being able to prep and plan your meals can help you greatly with making sure that you stay healthy and to ensure that your food is nourishing your body the right way. We are going to address topics such as how to choose healthy foods at the store and how you should be working to stock your kitchen. You will also see what goes into planning a diet, how you can determine what the right foods for your meal plan will be, and you will be introduced to meal prepping—the idea that you can create your meals and even start with parts of your meals in advance so that you can cut down the cooking time when it's time to eat.

The Foods to Choose at the Store ● ● ●

It's easy for you to think that you are making a good choice for your food, only to realize that the choice that you did make is actually not very practical or healthy at all. In particular, when we see all of these different foods that claim on their packaging that they are healthy or complete, we can run into a very simple problem—we buy things without actually knowing what is in them.

However, you can avoid that problem just by learning what you should be looking for when you are shopping. Consider these points when you are making your shopping plans:

- Always read the nutrition label: No matter what the front box says, make sure that you always take the time to figure out what is actually inside the foods that you pick up. Double-check how healthy the food that you are looking at actually is. Make sure that you check the label—and compare it to other options as well. Take the time to compare the ingredients and choose those that have the lowest amounts of sodium, unhealthy fats, and sugars.

- Avoid tricky Ingredients a lot of ingredients that are in your food are hidden under other names. You might not see sugar on the top three ingredients—but is high fructose corn syrup up there? Or any other of the —ose ingredients? That ending is specific to sugars, and if you know that it is high in one of the other —ose endings, you know that it is actually high in sugar, even if it doesn't say sugar.
- If fresh produce isn't available, always choose frozen: When you have to choose between no produce and frozen produce, you should choose the frozen. If you can't get frozen, choose canned, but make sure that you choose options that are lower in sodium and added sugars or syrups.
- Opt for whole-grain Ingredients when you go shopping; make sure that you choose those whole-grain options. Pasta, bread, crackers, and all sorts of other foods all come in whole-grain forms that will help you enjoy them without getting those high blood sugar spikes.
- If you can't pronounce the ingredients, avoid it: Take a look at the ingredient names. You need to make sure that you are eating mostly healthy whole foods, and that means making sure that you should actually recognize the names of what you are eating.

Stocking Your Kitchen ● ● ●

Of course, any good meal plan is only as good as the kitchen that it is cooked in, and that means that you need to make sure that you are giving yourself plenty of good foods that will keep you full for longer. We're going to take a look at several of the essential food items that you can keep in your kitchen at all times. Consider these the basics that you should keep constantly stocked on top of anything else that you may decide that you want to eat based on your meal plan.

Whole grains to keep on hand

- Whole wheat flours and oats
- Brown rice
- Whole wheat bread, cereals, and pasta
- Quinoa

Beans and legumes to keep on hand

- Variety of canned beans (red, pinto, garbanzo, etc.)
- Dried lentils and peas

Healthy fats to keep on hand

- No sugar added nut butter
- Olive oil
- Coconut oil
- Canola oil
- Avocado oil

Canned fruits and veggies to keep on hand

- Tomatoes (diced and sauced)
- Green beans
- Artichokes

Fresh produce to keep on hand

- In-season produce
- Citrus fruits of choice
- Avocados
- Onions
- Sweet potatoes
- Spinach
- Kale
- Broccoli

- Zucchini
- Squash

- Tomatoes

Protein sources to keep on hand

- Canned salmon or tuna in water, not oil
- Chicken breast

- Fresh meats of choice
- Eggs

Snacks to keep on hand

- Whole-grain crackers (low-carb)
- Multi-grain chips

- Seeds and nuts (unsalted)
- Popcorn

Seasonings to keep on hand

- Garlic
- Herbs and spices to limit salt content

How to Meal Plan ● ● ●

Now consider that you will need to plan out your meals to make sure that you stick to the right tasks at hand. Making your shopping list and avoiding the frustration of figuring out what you are going to eat is all simplified with one simple task: Meal planning.

When you meal plan, you make yourself a menu for the week. You make it so that you are able to find the meals that will work for you to make sure that you are eating foods that will be healthy, but also so that you don't unnecessarily buy foods that you don't actually need. To meal plan, all you need to do, then, is writing down what you will eat that week.

Breakfasts, lunches, dinners, and snacks should all be planned out. When you do that and make sure that you know what it is that you want to eat, you can then assemble your shopping list. When you have that shopping list, you buy only what you need, meaning that you save money and avoid waste! Your meal plan should incorporate meals with similar ingredients so that you can either reuse the same bunch of ingredients, or it may contain leftovers intentionally to slow down how much you have to cook. We will look at how to create a 30-day meal plan.

When you have your meal plan, you have a few simple benefits—you are able to meal prep, for example. You can make sure that you prepare ingredients in advance if it works better for your schedule. When you do this, you can make meals that might have a lot of prep actually work better during days that are actually quite busy. Say you want to eat enchiladas for dinner, for example, but you are going to be busy. The best way to make that work is to prep what you can before that. When you know what you will be eating, you know that you can prep the foods that you want in advance and know that you aren't just taking a shot in the dark.

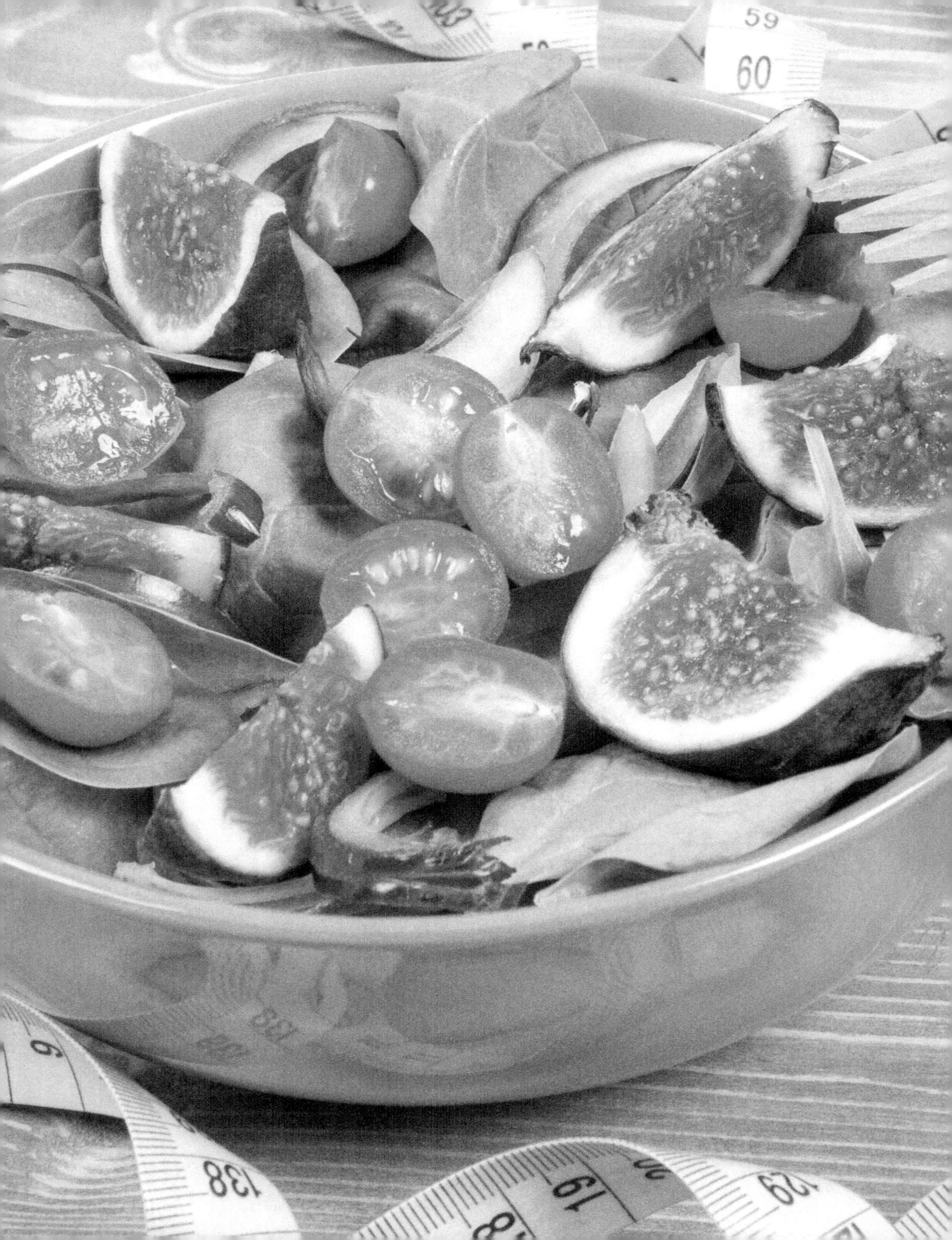

Recipes

BREAKFAST

1) *Berry-Oat Breakfast Bars*

Ingredients:

- 2 cups fresh raspberries or blueberries
- 2 tablespoons sugar
- 2 tablespoons freshly squeezed lemon juice
- 1 tablespoon cornstarch
- 1/2 cups rolled oats
- 1/2 cup whole-wheat flour
- 1/2 cup walnuts
- ¼ cup chia seeds
- ¼ cup extra-virgin olive oil
- ¼ cup honey
- 1 large egg

Direction: Preparation Time: 10 minutes Cooking Time: 25 minutes Servings: 12

- ✓ Preheat the oven to 350F.
- ✓ In a small saucepan over medium heat, stir together the berries, sugar, lemon juice, and cornstarch. Bring to a simmer. Reduce the heat and simmer for 2 to 3 minutes, until the mixture thickens.
- ✓ In a food processor or high-speed blender, combine the oats, flour, walnuts, and chia seeds. Process until powdered. Add the olive oil, honey, and egg. Pulse a few more times, until well combined. Press half of the mixture into a 9-inch square baking dish.
- ✓ Spread the berry filling over the oat mixture. Add the remaining oat mixture on top of the berries. Bake for 25 minutes, until browned.
- ✓ Let cool completely, cut into 12 pieces, and serve. Store in a covered container for up to 5 days.

Nutrition: Calories: 201; Total fat: 10g; Saturated fat: 1g; Protein: 5g; Carbs: 26g; Sugar: 9g; Fiber: 5g; Cholesterol: 16mg; Sodium: 8mg

2) *Whole-Grain Breakfast Cookies*

Ingredients:

- 2 cups rolled oats
- 1/2 cup whole-wheat flour
- ¼ cup ground flaxseed
- 1 teaspoon baking powder
- 1 cup unsweetened applesauce
- 2 large eggs
- 2 tablespoons vegetable oil
- 2 teaspoons vanilla extract
- 1 teaspoon ground cinnamon
- 1/2 cup dried cherries
- ¼ cup unsweetened shredded coconut

- 2 ounces dark chocolate, chopped

Direction: Preparation time: 20 minutes

Cooking time: 10 minutes Servings: 18 cookies

- ✓ 1. Preheat the oven to 350F.
- ✓ 2. In a large bowl, combine the oats, flour, flaxseed, and baking powder. Stir well to mix.
- ✓ 3. In a medium bowl, whisk the applesauce, eggs, vegetable oil, vanilla, and cinnamon. Pour the wet mixture into the dry mixture, and stir until just combined.
- ✓ 4. Fold in the cherries, coconut, and chocolate. Drop tablespoon-size balls of dough onto a baking sheet. Bake for 10 to 12 minutes, until browned and cooked through.
- ✓ 5. Let cool for about 3 minutes, remove from the baking sheet, and cool completely before serving. Store in an airtight container for up to 1 week.

Nutrition: Calories: 136; Total fat: 7g; Saturated fat: 3g; Protein: 4g; Carbs: 14g; Sugar: 4g; Fiber: 3g; Cholesterol: 21mg; Sodium: 11mg

3) *Blueberry Breakfast Cake*

Ingredients:

FOR THE TOPPING

- ¼ cup finely chopped walnuts
- 1/2 teaspoon ground cinnamon
- 2 tablespoons butter, chopped into small pieces
- 2 tablespoons sugar

FOR THE CAKE

- Nonstick cooking spray
- 1 cup whole-wheat pastry flour
- 1 cup oat flour
- ¼ cup sugar
- 2 teaspoons baking powder
- 1 large egg, beaten
- 1/2 cup skim milk
- 2 tablespoons butter, melted
- 1 teaspoon grated lemon peel
- 2 cups fresh or frozen blueberries

Direction: Preparation time: 15 minutes Cooking time: 45 minutes Servings: 12

TO MAKE THE TOPPING

- ✓ In a small bowl, stir together the walnuts, cinnamon, butter, and sugar. Set aside.

TO MAKE THE CAKE

✓ Preheat the oven to 350F. Spray a 9-inch square pan with cooking spray. Set aside.

✓ In a large bowl, stir together the pastry flour, oat flour, sugar, and baking powder.

✓ Add the egg, milk, butter, and lemon peel, and stir until there are no dry spots.

✓ Stir in the blueberries, and gently mix until incorporated. Press the batter into the prepared pan, using a spoon to flatten it into the dish.

✓ Sprinkle the topping over the cake.

✓ Bake for 40 to 45 minutes, until a toothpick inserted into the cake comes out clean, and serve.

Nutrition: Calories: 177; Total fat: 7g; Saturated fat: 3g; Protein: 4g; Carbs: 26g; Sugar: 9g; Fiber: 3g; Cholesterol: 26mg; Sodium: 39mg

4) Whole-Grain Pancakes

Ingredients:

- 2 cups whole-wheat pastry flour
- 4 teaspoons baking powder
- 2 teaspoons ground cinnamon
- 1/2 teaspoon salt
- 2 cups skim milk, plus more as needed
- 2 large eggs
- 1 tablespoon honey
- Nonstick cooking spray
- Maple syrup, for serving
- Fresh fruit, for serving

Direction: Preparation time: 10 minutes Cooking time: 15 minutes Servings: 4 to 6

✓ In a large bowl, stir together the flour, baking powder, cinnamon, and salt.

✓ Add the milk, eggs, and honey, and stir well to combine. If needed, add more milk, 1 tablespoon at a time, until there are no dry spots and you has a pourable batter.

✓ Heat a large skillet over medium-high heat, and spray it with cooking spray. ✓ Using a ¼-cup measuring cup, scoop 2 or 3 pancakes into the skillet at a time. Cook for a couple of minutes, until bubbles form on the surface of the pancakes, flip, and cook for 1 to 2 minutes more, until golden brown and cooked through. Repeat with the remaining batter.

✓ Serve topped with maple syrup or fresh fruit.

Nutrition: Calories: 392; Total fat: 4g; Saturated fat: 1g; Protein: 15g; Carbs: 71g; Sugar: 11g; Fiber: 9g; Cholesterol: 95mg; Sodium: 396mg

5) Buckwheat Grouts Breakfast Bowl

Ingredients:

- 3 cups skim milk
- 1 cup buckwheat grouts
- ¼ cup chia seeds
- 2 teaspoons vanilla extract
- 1/2 teaspoon ground cinnamon
- Pinch salt
- 1 cup water
- 1/2 cup unsalted pistachios
- 2 cups sliced fresh strawberries
- ¼ cup cacao nibs (optional)

Direction: Preparation time: 5 minutes, plus overnight to soak Cooking time: 10 to 12 minutes Servings: 4

✓ In a large bowl, stir together the milk, groats, chia seeds, vanilla, cinnamon, and salt. Cover and refrigerate overnight.

✓ The next morning, transfer the soaked mixture to a medium pot and add the water. Bring to a boil over medium-high heat, reduce the heat to maintain a simmer, and cook for 10 to 12 minutes, until the buckwheat is tender and thickened.

✓ Transfer to bowls and serve, topped with the pistachios, strawberries, and cacao nibs (if using).

Nutrition: Calories: 340; Total fat: 8g; Saturated fat: 1g; Protein: 15g; Carbs: 52g; Sugar: 14g; Fiber: 10g; Cholesterol: 4mg; Sodium: 140mg

6) Peach Muesli Bake

Ingredients:

- Nonstick cooking spray
- 2 cups skim milk
- 11/2 cups rolled oats
- 1/2 cup chopped walnuts
- 1 large egg
- 2 tablespoons maple syrup
- 1 teaspoon ground cinnamon
- 1 teaspoon baking powder
- 1/2 teaspoon salt
- 2 to 3 peaches, sliced

Direction: Preparation time: 10 minutes Cooking time: 40 minutes Servings: 8

✓ Preheat the oven to 375F. Spray a 9-inch square baking dish with cooking spray. Set aside.

✓ In a large bowl, stir together the milk, oats, walnuts, egg, maple syrup, cinnamon, baking powder, and salt. Spread half the mixture in the prepared baking dish.

✓ Place half the peaches in a single layer across the oat mixture.

✓ Spread the remaining oat mixture over the top. Add the remaining peaches in a thin layer over the oats. Bake for 35 to 40 minutes, uncovered, until thickened and browned.

✓ Cut into 8 squares and serve warm.

Nutrition: Calories: 138; Total fat: 3g; Saturated fat: 1g; Protein: 6g; Carbs: 22g; Sugar: 10g; Fiber: 3g; Cholesterol: 24mg; Sodium: 191mg

7) *Steel-Cut Oatmeal Bowl with Fruit and Nuts*

Ingredients:

- 1 cup steel-cut oats
- 2 cups almond milk
- ¾ cup water
- 1 teaspoon ground cinnamon
- ¼ teaspoon salt
- 2 cups chopped fresh fruit, such as blueberries, strawberries, raspberries, or peaches
- 1/2 cup chopped walnuts
- ¼ cup chia seeds

Direction: Preparation time: 5 minutes

Cooking time: 20 minutes Servings: 4

✓ In a medium saucepan over medium-high heat, combine the oats, almond milk, water, cinnamon, and salt. Bring to a boil, reduce the heat to low, and simmer for 15 to 20 minutes, until the oats are softened and thickened.

✓ Top each bowl with 1/2 cup of fresh fruit, 2 tablespoons of walnuts, and 1 tablespoon of chia seeds before serving.

Nutrition: Calories: 288; Total fat: 11g; Saturated fat: 1g; Protein: 10g; Carbs: 38g; Sugar: 7g; Fiber: 10g; Cholesterol: 0mg; Sodium: 329mg

8) *Whole-Grain Dutch Baby Pancake*

Ingredients:

- 2 tablespoons coconut oil
- 1/2 cup whole-wheat flour
- ¼ cup skim milk
- 3 large eggs
- 1 teaspoon vanilla extract
- 1/2 teaspoon baking powder
- ¼ teaspoon salt
- ¼ teaspoon ground cinnamon
- Powdered sugar, for dusting

Direction: Preparation time: 5 minutes Cooking time: 25 minutes Servings: 4

✓ Preheat the oven to 400F.

✓ Put the coconut oil in a medium oven-safe skillet, and place the skillet in the oven to melt the oil while it preheats.

✓ In a blender, combine the flour, milk, eggs, vanilla, baking powder, salt, and cinnamon. Process until smooth.

✓ Carefully remove the skillet from the oven and tilt to spread the oil around evenly.

✓ Pour the batter into the skillet and return it to the oven for 23 to 25 minutes, until the pancake puffs and lightly browns.

✓ Remove, dust lightly with powdered sugar, cut into 4 wedges, and serve.

Nutrition: Calories: 195; Total fat: 11g; Saturated fat: 7g; Protein: 8g; Carbs: 16g; Sugar: 1g; Fiber: 2g; Cholesterol: 140mg; Sodium: 209mg

9) *Mushroom, Zucchini, and Onion Frittata*

Ingredients:

- 1 tablespoon extra-virgin olive oil
- 1/2 onion, chopped
- 1 medium zucchini, chopped
- 11/2 cups sliced mushrooms
- 6 large eggs, beaten
- 2 tablespoons skim milk
- Salt
- Freshly ground black pepper
- 1 ounce feta cheese, crumbled

Direction: Preparation time: 10 minutes

Cooking time: 20 minutes Servings: 4

✓ Preheat the oven to 400F.

✓ In a medium oven-safe skillet over medium-high heat, heat the olive oil.

✓ Add the onion and sauté for 3 to 5 minutes, until translucent.

✓ Add the zucchini and mushrooms, and cook for 3 to 5 more minutes, until the vegetables are tender.

✓ Meanwhile, in a small bowl, whisk the eggs, milk, salt, and pepper. Pour the mixture into the skillet, stirring to combine, and transfer the skillet to the oven. Cook for 7 to 9 minutes, until set.

✓ Sprinkle with the feta cheese, and cook for 1 to 2 minutes more, until heated through.

✓ Remove, cut into 4 wedges, and serve.

Nutrition: Calories: 178; Total fat: 13g; Saturated fat: 4g; Protein: 12g; Carbs: 5g; Sugar: 3g; Fiber: 1g; Cholesterol: 285mg; Sodium: 234mg

10) *Spinach and Cheese Quiche*

Ingredients:

- Nonstick cooking spray
- 8 ounces Yukon Gold potatoes, shredded
- 1 tablespoon plus 2 teaspoons extra-virgin olive oil, divided
- 1 teaspoon salt, divided
- Freshly ground black pepper
- 1 onion, finely chopped
- 1 (10-ounce) bag fresh spinach
- 4 large eggs
- 1/2 cup skim milk
- 1 ounce Gruyere cheese, shredded

Direction: Preparation time: 10 minutes, plus 10 minutes to rest Cooking time: 50 minutes Servings: 4 to 6

✓ Preheat the oven to 350F. Spray a 9-inch pie dish with cooking spray. Set aside.

✓ In a small bowl, toss the potatoes with 2 teaspoons of olive oil, 1/2 teaspoon of salt, and season with pepper. Press the potatoes into the bottom and sides of the pie dish to form a thin, even layer. Bake for 20 minutes, until golden brown. Remove from the oven and set aside to cool.

✓ In a large skillet over medium-high heat, heat the remaining 1 tablespoon of olive oil.

✓ Add the onion and sauté for 3 to 5 minutes, until softened.

✓ By handfuls, add the spinach, stirring between each addition, until it just starts to wilt before adding more. Cook for about 1 minute, until it cooks down.

✓ In a medium bowl, whisk the eggs and milk. Add the Gruyère, and season with the remaining 1/2 teaspoon of salt and some pepper. Fold the eggs into the spinach. Pour the mixture into the pie dish and bake for 25 minutes, until the eggs are set.

✓ Let rest for 10 minutes before serving.

Nutrition: Calories: 445; Total fat: 14g; Saturated fat: 4g; Protein: 19g; Carbs: 68g; Sugar: 6g; Fiber: 7g; Cholesterol: 193mg; Sodium: 773mg

11) *Spicy Jalapeno Popper Deviled Eggs*

Ingredients:

- 4 large whole eggs, hardboiled
- 2 tablespoons Keto-Friendly mayonnaise
- ¼ cup cheddar cheese, grated
- 2 slices bacon, cooked and crumbled
- 1 jalapeno, sliced

Direction: Preparation Time: 5 minutes

Cooking Time: 5 minutes Servings: 4

✓ Cut eggs in half, remove the yolk and put them in bowl

✓ Lay egg whites on a platter

✓ Mix in remaining ingredients and mash them with the egg yolks

✓ Transfer yolk mix back to the egg whites

✓ Serve and enjoy!

Nutrition: Calories: 176; Fat: 14g; Carbohydrates: 0.7g; Protein: 10g

12) *Lovely Porridge*

Ingredients:

- 2 tablespoons coconut flour
- 2 tablespoons vanilla protein powder
- 3 tablespoons Golden Flaxseed meal
- 1 and 1/2 cups almond milk, unsweetened
- Powdered erythritol

Direction: Preparation Time: 15 minutes

Cooking Time: Nil Servings: 2

✓ Take a bowl and mix in flaxseed meal, protein powder, coconut flour and mix well

✓ Add mix to the saucepan (placed over medium heat)

✓ Add almond milk and stir, let the mixture thicken

✓ Add your desired amount of sweetener and serve

Nutrition: Calories: 259; Fat: 13g; Carbohydrates: 5g; Protein: 16g

13) *Salty Macadamia Chocolate Smoothie*

Ingredients:

- 2 tablespoons macadamia nuts, salted
- 1/3 cup chocolate whey protein powder, low carb
- 1 cup almond milk, unsweetened

Direction: Preparation Time: 5 minutes Cooking

Time: Nil Servings: 1

✓ Add the listed ingredients to your blender and blend until you have a smooth mixture
✓ Chill and enjoy it!

Nutrition: Calories: 165; Fat: 2g; Carbohydrates: 1g; Protein: 12g

14) *Basil and Tomato Baked Eggs*

Ingredients:

- 1 garlic clove, minced
- 1 cup canned tomatoes
- ¼ cup fresh basil leaves, roughly chopped
- 1/2 teaspoon chili powder
- 1 tablespoon olive oil
- 4 whole eggs
- Salt and pepper to taste

Direction: Preparation Time: 10 minutes

Cooking Time: 15 minutes Servings: 4

✓ Preheat your oven to 375 degrees F
✓ Take a small baking dish and grease with olive oil
✓ Add garlic, basil, tomatoes chili, olive oil into a dish and stir
✓ Crackdown eggs into a dish, keeping space between the two
✓ Sprinkle the whole dish with salt and pepper
✓ Place in oven and cook for 12 minutes until eggs are set and tomatoes are bubbling
✓ Serve with basil on top
✓ Enjoy!

Nutrition: Calories: 235; Fat: 16g; Carbohydrates: 7g; Protein: 14g

15) *Cinnamon and Coconut Porridge*

Ingredients:

- 2 cups of water
- 1 cup 36% heavy cream
- 1/2 cup unsweetened dried coconut, shredded
- 2 tablespoons flaxseed meal
- 1 tablespoon butter
- 1 and 1/2 teaspoon stevia
- 1 teaspoon cinnamon
- Salt to taste
- Toppings as blueberries

Direction: Preparation Time: 5 minutes Cooking

Time: 5 minutes Servings: 4

✓ Add the listed ingredients to a small pot, mix well
✓ Transfer pot to stove and place it over medium-low heat
✓ Bring to mix to a slow boil
✓ Stir well and remove the heat
✓ Divide the mix into equal servings and let them sit for 10 minutes
✓ Top with your desired toppings and enjoy!

Nutrition: Calories: 171; Fat: 16g; Carbohydrates: 6g; Protein: 2g

16) *An Omelet of Swiss chard*

Ingredients:

- 4 eggs, lightly beaten
- 4 cups Swiss chard, sliced
- 2 tablespoons butter
- 1/2 teaspoon garlic salt
- Fresh pepper

Direction: Preparation Time: 5 minutes

Cooking Time: 5 minutes Servings: 4

✓ Take a non-stick frying pan and place it over medium-low heat
✓ Once the butter melts, add Swiss chard and stir cook for 2 minutes
✓ Pour egg into the pan and gently stir them into Swiss chard
✓ Season with garlic salt and pepper
✓ Cook for 2 minutes
✓ Serve and enjoy!

Nutrition: Calories: 260; Fat: 21g; Carbohydrates: 4g; Protein: 14g

17) *Cheesy Low-Carb Omelet*

Ingredients:

- 2 whole eggs
- 1 tablespoon water
- 1 tablespoon butter
- 3 thin slices salami
- 5 fresh basil leaves
- 5 thin slices, fresh ripe tomatoes
- 2 ounces fresh mozzarella cheese
- Salt and pepper as needed

Direction: Preparation Time: 5 minutes Cooking Time: 5 minutes Servings: 5

✓ Take a small bowl and whisk in eggs and water
✓ Take a non-stick Sauté pan and place it over medium heat, add butter and let it melt
✓ Pour egg mixture and cook for 30 seconds
✓ Spread salami slices on half of egg mix and top with cheese, tomatoes, basil slices
✓ Season with salt and pepper according to your taste
✓ Cook for 2 minutes and fold the egg with the empty half
✓ Cover and cook on LOW for 1 minute
✓ Serve and enjoy!

Nutrition: Calories: 451; Fat: 36g; Carbohydrates: 3g; Protein:33g

18) *Yogurt And Kale Smoothie*

Ingredients:

• 1 cup whole milk yogurt
• 1 cup baby kale greens
• 1 pack stevia
• 1 tablespoon MCT oil
• 1 tablespoon sunflower seeds
• 1 cup of water

Direction: Servings: 1 Preparation Time: 10 minutes

✓ Add listed ingredients to the blender
✓ Blend until you have a smooth and creamy texture
✓ Serve chilled and enjoy!

Nutrition: Calories: 329; Fat: 26g; Carbohydrates: 15g; Protein: 11g

19) *Bacon and Chicken Garlic Wrap*

Ingredients:

• 1 chicken fillet, cut into small cubes
• 8-9 thin slices bacon, cut to fit cubes
• 6 garlic cloves, minced

Direction: Preparation Time: 15 minutes

Cooking Time: 10 minutes Servings: 4

✓ Preheat your oven to 400 degrees F
✓ Line a baking tray with aluminum foil
✓ Add minced garlic to a bowl and rub each chicken piece with it
✓ Wrap bacon piece around each garlic chicken bite
✓ Secure with toothpick
✓ Transfer bites to the baking sheet, keeping a little bit of space between them
✓ Bake for about 15-20 minutes until crispy
✓ Serve and enjoy!

Nutrition: Calories: 260; Fat: 19g; Carbohydrates: 5g; Protein: 22g

20) *Grilled Chicken Platter*

Ingredients:

• 1/2 a cup of roasted red peppers, cut in long strips
• 1 teaspoon of olive oil
• 2 garlic cloves, minced
• Salt and pepper as needed

Direction: Preparation Time: 5 minutes

Cooking Time: 10 minutes Servings: 6

✓ Preheat your oven to 400 degrees Fahrenheit
✓ Slice 3 chicken breast lengthwise
✓ Take a non-stick pan and grease with cooking spray
✓ Bake for 2-3 minutes each side
✓ Take another skillet and cook spinach and garlic in oil for 3 minutes
✓ Place chicken on an oven pan and top with spinach, roasted peppers, and mozzarella
✓ Bake until the cheese melted
✓ Enjoy!

Nutrition: Calories: 195; Fat: 7g; Carbohydrates: 3g; Protein: 30g

21) *Parsley Chicken Breast*

Ingredients:

• 1 tablespoon dry parsley
• 1 tablespoon dry basil
• 4 chicken breast halves, boneless and skinless
• 1/2 teaspoon salt
• 1/2 teaspoon red pepper flakes, crushed
• 2 tomatoes, sliced

Direction: Preparation Time: 10 minutes

Cooking Time: 40 minutes Servings: 4

✓ Preheat your oven to 350 degrees F
✓ Take a 9x13 inch baking dish and grease it up with cooking spray
✓ Sprinkle 1 tablespoon of parsley, 1 teaspoon of basil and spread the mixture over your baking dish
✓ Arrange the chicken breast halves over the dish and sprinkle garlic slices on top
✓ Take a small bowl and add 1 teaspoon parsley, 1 teaspoon of basil, salt, basil, red pepper and mix well. Pour the mixture over the chicken breast
✓ Top with tomato slices and cover, bake for 25 minutes

✓ Remove the cover and bake for 15 minutes more
✓ Serve and enjoy!

Nutrition: Calories: 150; Fat: 4g; Carbohydrates: 4g; Protein: 25g

22) *Mustard Chicken*

Ingredients:

- 4 chicken breasts
- 1/2 cup chicken broth
- 3-4 tablespoons mustard
- 3 tablespoons olive oil
- 1 teaspoon paprika
- 1 teaspoon chili powder
- 1 teaspoon garlic powder

Direction: Preparation Time: 10 minutes

Cooking Time: 40 minutes Servings: 4

✓ Take a small bowl and mix mustard, olive oil, paprika, chicken broth, garlic powder, chicken broth, and chili
✓ Add chicken breast and marinate for 30 minutes
✓ Take a lined baking sheet and arrange the chicken
✓ Bake for 35 minutes at 375 degrees Fahrenheit
✓ Serve and enjoy!

Nutrition: Calories: 531; Fat: 23g; Carbohydrates: 10g; Protein: 64g

23) *Balsamic Chicken 1*

Ingredients:

- 6 chicken breast halves, skinless and boneless
- 1 teaspoon garlic salt
- Ground black pepper
- 2 tablespoons olive oil
- 1 onion, thinly sliced
- 14 and 1/2 ounces tomatoes, diced
- 1/2 cup balsamic vinegar
- 1 teaspoon dried basil
- 1 teaspoon dried oregano
- 1 teaspoon dried rosemary
- 1/2 teaspoon dried thyme

Direction: Preparation Time: 10 minutes
Cooking Time: 25 minutes Servings: 6

✓ Season both sides of your chicken breasts thoroughly with pepper and garlic salt
✓ Take a skillet and place it over medium heat

✓ Add some oil and cook your seasoned chicken for 3-4 minutes per side until the breasts are nicely browned
✓ Add some onion and cook for another 3-4 minutes until the onions are browned
✓ Pour the diced up tomatoes and balsamic vinegar over your chicken and season with some rosemary, basil, thyme, and rosemary
✓ Simmer the chicken for about 15 minutes until they are no longer pink
✓ Take an instant-read thermometer and check if the internal temperature gives a reading of 165 degrees Fahrenheit
✓ If yes, then you are good to go!

Nutrition: Calories: 196; Fat: 7g; Carbohydrates: 7g; Protein: 23g

24) *Greek Chicken Breast*

Ingredients:

- 4 chicken breast halves, skinless and boneless
- 1 cup extra virgin olive oil
- 1 lemon, juiced
- 2 teaspoons garlic, crushed
- 1 and 1/2 teaspoons black pepper
- 1/3 teaspoon paprika

Direction: Preparation Time: 10 minutes
Cooking Time: 25 minutes Servings: 4

✓ Cut 3 slits in the chicken breast
✓ Take a small bowl and whisk in olive oil, salt, lemon juice, garlic, paprika, pepper and whisk for 30 seconds
✓ Place chicken in a large bowl and pour marinade
✓ Rub the marinade all over using your hand
✓ Refrigerate overnight
✓ Pre-heat grill to medium heat and oil the grate
✓ Cook chicken in the grill until center is no longer pink
✓ Serve and enjoy!

Nutrition: Calories: 644; Fat: 57g; Carbohydrates: 2g; Protein: 27g

25) *Chipotle Lettuce Chicken*

Ingredients:

- 1 pound chicken breast, cut into strips
- Splash of olive oil
- 1 red onion, finely sliced
- 14 ounces tomatoes

- 1 teaspoon chipotle, chopped
- 1/2 teaspoon cumin
- Pinch of sugar
- Lettuce as needed
- Fresh coriander leaves
- Jalapeno chilies, sliced
- Fresh tomato slices for garnish
- Lime wedges

Direction: Preparation Time: 10 minutes

Cooking Time: 25 minutes Servings: 6

✓ Take a non-stick frying pan and place it over medium heat
✓ Add oil and heat it up
✓ Add chicken and cook until brown
✓ Keep the chicken on the side
✓ Add tomatoes, sugar, chipotle, cumin to the same pan and simmer for 25 minutes until you have a nice sauce
✓ Add chicken into the sauce and cook for 5 minutes
✓ Transfer the mix to another place
✓ Use lettuce wraps to take a portion of the mixture and serve with a squeeze of lemon
✓ Enjoy!

Nutrition: Calories: 332; Fat: 15g; Carbohydrates: 13g; Protein: 34g

26) *Stylish Chicken-Bacon Wrap*

Ingredients:

- 8 ounces lean chicken breast
- 6 bacon slices
- 3 ounces shredded cheese
- 4 slices ham

Direction: Preparation Time: 5 minutes

Cooking Time: 50 minutes Servings: 3

✓ Cut chicken breast into bite-sized portions
✓ Transfer shredded cheese onto ham slices
✓ Roll up chicken breast and ham slices in bacon slices
✓ Take a skillet and place it over medium heat
✓ Add olive oil and brown bacon for a while
✓ Remove rolls and transfer to your oven
✓ Bake for 45 minutes at 325 degrees F
✓ Serve and enjoy!

Nutrition: Calories: 275; Fat: 11g; Carbohydrates: 0.5g; Protein: 40g

27) *Healthy Cottage Cheese Pancakes*

Ingredients:

- 1/2 cup of Cottage cheese (low-fat)
- 1/3 cup (approx. 2 egg whites) Egg whites
- ¼ cup of Oats
- 1 teaspoon of Vanilla extract
- Olive oil cooking spray
- 1 tablespoon of Stevia (raw)
- Berries or sugar-free jam (optional)

Direction: Preparation Time: 10 minutes

Cooking Time: 15 Servings: 1

✓ Begin by taking a food blender and adding in the egg whites and cottage cheese. Also add in the vanilla extract, a pinch of stevia, and oats. Palpitate until the consistency is well smooth.
✓ Get a nonstick pan and oil it nicely with the cooking spray. Position the pan on low heat.
✓ After it has been heated, scoop out half of the batter and pour it on the pan. Cook for about 2 1/2 minutes on each side.
✓ Position the cooked pancakes on a serving plate and cover with sugar-free jam or berries.

Nutrition: Calories: 205 calories per serving Fat – 1.5 g, Protein – 24.5 g, Carbs– 19 g

28) *Avocado Lemon Toast*

Ingredients:

- Whole-grain bread – 2 slices
- Fresh cilantro (chopped) – 2 tablespoons
- Lemon zest – ¼ teaspoon
- Fine sea salt – 1 pinch
- Cayenne pepper – 1 pinch
- Chia seeds – ¼ teaspoon
- Avocado – 1/2
- Fresh lemon juice – 1 teaspoon

Direction: Preparation Time: 10 minutes

Cooking Time: 13 minutes Servings: 2

✓ Begin by getting a medium-sized mixing bowl and adding in the avocado. Make use of a fork to crush it properly.
✓ Then, add in the cilantro, lemon zest, lemon juice, sea salt, and cayenne pepper. Mix well until combined.
✓ Toast the bread slices in a toaster until golden brown. It should take about 3 minutes.
✓ Top the toasted bread slices with the avocado

mixture and finalize by drizzling with chia seeds.

Nutrition: Calories: 72 calories per serving; Protein – 3.6 g; Fat – 1.2 g; Carbs – 11.6 g

29) *Healthy Baked Eggs*

Ingredients:

- Olive oil – 1 tablespoon
- Garlic – 2 cloves
- Eggs – 8 large
- Sea salt – 1/2 teaspoon
- Shredded mozzarella cheese (medium-fat) – 3 cups
- Olive oil spray
- Onion (chopped) – 1 medium
- Spinach leaves – 8 ounces
- Half-and-half – 1 cup
- Black pepper – 1 teaspoon
- Feta cheese – 1/2 cup

Direction: Preparation Time: 10 minutes

Cooking Time: 1 hour Servings: 6

- ✓ Begin by heating the oven to 375F.
- ✓ Get a glass baking dish and grease it with olive oil spray. Arrange aside.
- ✓ Now take a nonstick pan and pour in the olive oil. Position the pan on allows heat and allows it heat.
- ✓ Immediately you are done, toss in the garlic, spinach, and onion. Prepare for about 5 minutes. Arrange aside.
- ✓ You can now Get a large mixing bowl and add in the half, eggs, pepper, and salt. Whisk thoroughly to combine.
- ✓ Put in the feta cheese and chopped mozzarella cheese (reserve 1/2 cup of mozzarella cheese for later).
- ✓ Put the egg mixture and prepared spinach to the prepared glass baking dish. Blend well to combine. Drizzle the reserved cheese over the top.
- ✓ Bake the egg mix for about 45 minutes.
- ✓ Extract the baking dish from the oven and allow it to stand for 10 minutes.
- ✓ Dice and serve!

Nutrition: Calories: 323 calories per serving; Fat 22.3 g; Protein 22.6 g; Carbs 7.9 g

30) *Quick Low-Carb Oatmeal*

Ingredients:

- Almond flour – 1/2 cup

- Flax meal – 2 tablespoons
- Cinnamon (ground) – 1 teaspoon
- Almond milk (unsweetened) – 11/2 cups
- Salt – as per taste
- Chia seeds – 2 tablespoons
- Liquid stevia – 10 – 15 drops
- Vanilla extract – 1 teaspoon

Direction: Preparation Time: 10 minutes

Cooking Time: 15 minutes Servings: 2

- ✓ Begin by taking a large mixing bowl and adding in the coconut flour, almond flour, ground cinnamon, flax seed powder, and chia seeds. Mix properly to combine.
- ✓ Position a stockpot on a low heat and add in the dry ingredients. Also add in the liquid stevia, vanilla extract, and almond milk. Mix well to combine.
- ✓ Prepare the flour and almond milk for about 4 minutes. Add salt if needed.
- ✓ Move the oatmeal to a serving bowl and top with nuts, seeds, and pure and neat berries.

Nutrition: Calories: calories per serving; Protein – 11.7 g;
Fat – 24.3 g; Carbs – 16.7 g

31) *Tofu and Vegetable Scramble*

Ingredients:

- Firm tofu (drained) – 16 ounces
- Sea salt – 1/2 teaspoon
- Garlic powder – 1 teaspoon
- Fresh coriander – for garnishing
- Red onion – 1/2 medium
- Cumin powder – 1 teaspoon
- Lemon juice – for topping
- Green bell pepper – 1 medium
- Garlic powder – 1 teaspoon
- Fresh coriander – for garnishing
- Red onion – 1/2 medium
- Cumin powder – 1 teaspoon
- Lemon juice – for topping

Direction: Preparation Time: 10 minutes

Cooking Time: 15 minutes Servings: 2

- ✓ Begin by preparing the ingredients. For this, you are to extract the seeds of the tomato and green bell pepper. Shred the onion, bell pepper, and tomato into small cubes.
- ✓ Get a small mixing bowl and position the fairly hard tofu inside it. Make use of your hands to break the

fairly hard tofu. Arrange aside.
- ✓ Get a nonstick pan and add in the onion, tomato, and bell pepper. Mix and cook for about 3 minutes.
- ✓ Put the somewhat hard crumbled tofu to the pan and combine well.
- ✓ Get a small bowl and put in the water, turmeric, garlic powder, cumin powder, and chili powder. Combine well and stream it over the tofu and vegetable mixture.
- ✓ Allow the tofu and vegetable crumble cook with seasoning for 5 minutes. Continuously stir so that the pan is not holding the ingredients.
- ✓ Drizzle the tofu scramble with chili flakes and salt. Combine well.
- ✓ Transfer the prepared scramble to a serving bowl and give it a proper spray of lemon juice.
- ✓ Finalize by garnishing with pure and neat coriander. Serve while hot!

Nutrition: Calories: 238 calories per serving; Carbohydrates – 16.6 g; Fat – 11 g

32) *Breakfast Smoothie Bowl with Fresh Berries*

Ingredients:

- Almond milk (unsweetened) – 1/2 cup
- Psyllium husk powder – 1/2 teaspoon
- Strawberries (chopped) – 2 ounces
- Coconut oil – 1 tablespoon
- Crushed ice – 3 cups
- Liquid stevia – 5 to 10 drops
- Pea protein powder – 1/3 cup

Direction: Preparation Time: 10 minutes Cooking Time: 5 minutes Servings: 2

- ✓ Begin by taking a blender and adding in the mashed ice cubes. Allow them to rest for about 30 seconds.
- ✓ Then put in the almond milk, shredded strawberries, pea protein powder, psyllium husk powder, coconut oil, and liquid stevia. Blend well until it turns into a smooth and creamy puree.
- ✓ Vacant the prepared smoothie into 2 glasses.
- ✓ Cover with coconut flakes and pure and neat strawberries.

Nutrition: Calories: 166 calories per serving; Fat – 9.2 g; Carbs – 4.1 g; Protein – 17.6 g

33) *Chia and Coconut Pudding*

Ingredients:

- Light coconut milk – 7 ounces
- Liquid stevia – 3 to 4 drops
- Kiwi – 1

- Chia seeds – ¼ cup
- Clementine – 1
- Shredded coconut (unsweetened)

Direction: Preparation Time: 10 minutes

Cooking Time: 5 minutes Servings: 2

- ✓ Begin by getting a mixing bowl and putting in the light coconut milk. Set in the liquid stevia to sweeten the milk. Combine well.
- ✓ Put the chia seeds to the milk and whisk until well-combined. Arrange aside.
- ✓ Scrape the clementine and carefully extract the skin from the wedges. Leave aside.
- ✓ Also, scrape the kiwi and dice it into small pieces.
- ✓ Get a glass vessel and gather the pudding. For this, position the fruits at the bottom of the jar; then put a dollop of chia pudding. Then spray the fruits and then put another layer of chia pudding.
- ✓ Finalize by garnishing with the rest of the fruits and chopped coconut.

Nutrition: Calories: 201 calories per serving; Protein – 5.4 g; Fat – 10 g; Carbs – 22.8 g

34) *Tomato and Zucchini Sauté*

Ingredients:

- Vegetable oil – 1 tablespoon
- Tomatoes (chopped) – 2
- Green bell pepper (chopped)
- Black pepper (freshly ground) – as per taste
- Onion (sliced)
- 1 Zucchini (peeled) – 2 pounds and cut into 1-inch-thick slices
- Salt – as per taste
- Uncooked white rice – ¼ cup

Direction: Preparation Time: 10 minutes

Cooking Time: 43 minutes Servings: 6

- ✓ Begin by getting a nonstick pan and putting it over low heat. Stream in the oil and allow it to heat through.
- ✓ Put in the onions and sauté for about 3 minutes.
- ✓ Then pour in the zucchini and green peppers. Mix well and spice with black pepper and salt.
- ✓ Reduce the heat and cover the pan with a lid. Allow the veggies cook on low for 5 minutes.
- ✓ While you're done, put in the water and rice. Place the lid back on and cook on low for 20 minutes.

Nutrition: Calories: 94 calories per serving; Fat – 2.8 g; Protein – 3.2 g; Carbs – 16.1 g

35) *Steamed Kale with Mediterranean Dressing*

Ingredients:

- Kale (chopped) – 12 cups
- Olive oil – 1 tablespoon
- Soy sauce – 1 teaspoon
- Pepper (freshly ground) – as per taste
- Lemon juice – 2 tablespoons
- Garlic (minced) – 1 tablespoon
- Salt – as per taste

Direction: Preparation Time: 10 minutes Cooking Time: 25 minutes Servings: 6

✓ Get a gas steamer or an electric steamer and fill the bottom pan with water. If making use of a gas steamer, position it on high heat. Making use of an electric steamer, place it on the highest setting.
✓ Immediately the water comes to a boil, put in the shredded kale and cover with a lid. Boil for about 8 minutes. The kale should be tender by now.
✓ During the kale is boiling, take a big mixing bowl and put in the olive oil, lemon juice, soy sauce, garlic, pepper, and salt. Whisk well to mix.
✓ Now toss in the steamed kale and carefully enclose into the dressing. Be assured the kale is well-coated.
✓ Serve while it's hot!

Nutrition: Calories: 91 calories per serving; Fat – 3.5 g; Protein – 4.6 g; Carbs – 14.5 g

36) *Vegetable Noodles Stir-Fry*

Ingredients:

- White sweet potato – 1 pound
- Zucchini – 8 ounces
- Garlic cloves (finely chopped) – 2 large
- Vegetable broth – 2 tablespoons
- Salt – as per taste
- Carrots – 8 ounces
- Shallot (finely chopped) – 1
- Red chili (finely chopped) – 1
- Olive oil – 1 tablespoon
- Pepper – as per taste

Direction: Preparation Time: 10 minutes

Cooking Time: 40 minutes Servings: 4

✓ Begin by scrapping the carrots and sweet potato. Make Use a spiralizer to make noodles out of the sweet potato and carrots.
✓ Rinse the zucchini thoroughly and spiralize it as well.

✓ Get a large skillet and position it on a high flame. Stream in the vegetable broth and allow it to come to a boil.
✓ Toss in the spiralized sweet potato and carrots. Then put in the chili, garlic, and shallots. Stir everything using tongs and cook for some minutes.
✓ Transfer the vegetable noodles into a serving platter and generously spice with pepper and salt.
✓ Finalize by sprinkling olive oil over the noodles. Serve while hot!

Nutrition: Calories: 169 calories per serving; Fat 3.7 g; Protein 3.6 g; Carbs – 31.2 g

37) *Millet Porridge*

Ingredients:

- 1 cup millet, rinsed and drained
- Pinch of salt
- 3 cups water
- 2 tablespoons almonds, chopped finely
- 6-8 drops liquid stevia
- 1 cup unsweetened almond milk
- 2 tablespoons fresh blueberries

Direction: Preparation Time: 10 minutes Cooking Time: 25 minutes Servings: 4

✓ In a nonstick pan, add the millet over medium-low heat and cook for about 3 minutes, stirring continuously.
✓ Add the salt and water and stir to combine Increase the heat to medium and bring to a boil.
✓ Cook for about 15 minutes.
✓ Stir in the almonds, stevia and almond milk and cook for 5 minutes.
✓ Top with the blueberries and serve. Meal Prep Tip:
✓ Transfer the cooled porridge in an airtight container and preserve in the refrigerator for up to 2 days.
✓ Just before serving, reheat in the microwave.
✓ Serve with the topping of berries.

Nutrition: Calories 219 Total Fat 4.5 g Saturated Fat 0.6 g Cholesterol 0 mg Total Carbs 38.2 g Sugar 0.6 g Fiber 5 g Sodium 92 mg Potassium 1721 mg Protein 6.4 g

38) *Sweet Potato Waffles*

Ingredients:

- 1 medium sweet potato, peeled, grated and squeezed
- 1 teaspoon fresh thyme, minced
- 1 teaspoon fresh rosemary, minced
- 1/8 teaspoon red pepper flakes, crushed
- Salt and ground black pepper, as required

Direction: Preparation Time: 10 minutes Cooking Time: 20 minutes Servings: 2

✓ Preheat the waffle iron and then grease it.

✓ In a large bowl, add all ingredients and mix till well combined.

✓ Place half of the sweet potato mixture into preheated waffle iron and cook for about 8-10 minutes or until golden brown.

✓ Repeat with the remaining mixture.

✓ Serve warm.

Meal Prep Tip:

✓ Store these cooled waffles into an airtight container by placing a piece of wax paper between each waffle.

✓ Refrigerate up to 5 days. Reheat in the microwave for about 1-2 minutes.

Nutrition: Calories 72 Total Fat 0.3 g Saturated Fat 0.1 g Cholesterol 0 mg Total Carbs 16.3 g Sugar 4.9 g Fiber 3 g Sodium 28 mg Potassium 369 mg Protein 1.6 g

39) *Quinoa Bread*

Ingredients:

- 1¾ cups uncooked quinoa, rinsed, soaked overnight and drained
- ¼ cup chia seeds, soaked in ½ cup of water overnight
- ½ teaspoon bicarbonate soda
- Pinch of sea salt
- ½ cup filtered water
- ¼ cup olive oil, melted
- 1 tablespoon fresh lemon juice

Direction: Preparation Time: 10 minutes Cooking Time: 1½ hours Servings: 12

✓ Preheat the oven to 320 degrees F. Line a loaf pan with a parchment paper.

✓ In a food processor, add all the ingredients and pulse for about 3 minutes.

✓ Transfer the mixture into prepared loaf pan evenly.

✓ Bake for about 1½ hours or until a wooden skewer inserted in the center of loaf comes out clean.

✓ Remove the pan from oven and place onto a wire rack to cool for about 10-15 minutes.

✓ Carefully, remove the bread from the loaf pan and place onto the wire rack to cool completely before slicing

✓ With a sharp knife, cut the bread loaf into desired sized slices and serve.

Meal Prep Tip:

✓ In a resealable plastic bag, place the bread and seal the bag after squeezing out the excess air.

✓ Set the bread away from direct sunlight and preserve in a cool and dry place for about 1-2 days.

Nutrition: Calories 137 Total Fat 6.5 g Saturated Fat 0.9 g Cholesterol 0 mg Total Carbs 16.9 g Sugar 0 g Fiber 2.6 g Sodium 203 mg Potassium 158 mg Protein 4 g

40) *Veggie Frittata*

Ingredients:

- 1 tablespoon olive oil
- 1 large sweet potato, peeled and cut into thin slices
- 1 yellow squash, sliced
- 1 zucchini, sliced
- ½ of red bell pepper, seeded and sliced
- ½ of yellow bell pepper, seeded and sliced
- 8 eggs
- Salt and ground black pepper, as required
- 2 tablespoons fresh cilantro, chopped finely

Direction: Preparation Time: 15 minutes Cooking Time: 25 minutes Servings: 6

✓ Preheat the oven to broiler.

✓ In a large oven proof skillet, heat the oil over medium-low heat and cook the sweet potato for about 6-7 minutes.

✓ Add the yellow squash, zucchini and bell peppers and cook for about 3-4 minutes.

✓ Meanwhile, in a bowl, add the eggs, salt and black pepper and beat until well combined.

✓ Pour egg mixture over vegetables mixture evenly.

✓ Immediately, reduce the heat to low and cook for about 8-10 minutes or until just done.

✓ Transfer the skillet in the oven and broil for about 3-4 minutes or until top becomes golden brown.

✓ With a sharp knife, cut the frittata in desired size slices and serve with the garnishing of cilantro.

Meal Prep Tip:

✓ In a resealable plastic bag, place the cooled frittata slices and seal the bag.

✓ Refrigerate for about 2-4 days.

✓ Reheat in the microwave on High for about 1 minute before serving.

Nutrition: Calories 143 Total Fat 8.4 g Saturated Fat 2.2 g Cholesterol 218 mg Total Carbs 9.3 g Sugar 4.2 g Fiber 1.1 g Sodium 98 mg Potassium 408 mg Protein 8.9 g

41) *Chicken & Sweet Potato Hash*

Ingredients:

- 2 tablespoons olive oil, divided
- 1½ pounds boneless, skinless chicken breasts, cubed

- Salt and ground black pepper, as required
- 2 celery stalks, chopped
- 1 medium white onion, chopped
- 4 garlic cloves, minced
- 1 tablespoon fresh oregano, chopped
- 1 tablespoon fresh thyme, chopped
- 2 large sweet potatoes, peeled and cubed
- 1 cup low-sodium chicken broth
- 1 cup scallion, chopped
- 2 tablespoons fresh lime juice

Direction: Preparation Time: 15 minutes Cooking Time: 35 minutes Servings: 8

✓ In a large skillet, heat 1 tablespoon of oil over medium heat and cook the chicken with a little salt and black pepper for about 4-5 minutes.
✓ Transfer the chicken into a bowl. In the same skillet, heat the remaining oil over medium heat and sauté celery and onion for about 3-4 minutes.
✓ Add the garlic and herbs and sauté for about 1 minute. Add the sweet potato and cook for about 8-10 minutes.
✓ Add the broth and cook for about 8-10 minutes.
✓ Add the cooked chicken and scallion and cook for about 5 minutes.
✓ Stir in lemon juice, salt and serve. Meal Prep Tip: Transfer the cooled hash in an airtight container and preserve in the refrigerator for up to 2 days. Just before serving, reheat in the microwave.

Nutrition: Calories 253 Total Fat 10 g Saturated Fat 2.3 g Cholesterol 76 mg Total Carbs 14 g Sugar 1.2 g Fiber 2.6 g Sodium 92 mg Potassium 597 mg Protein 26 g

42) *Strawberry & Spinach Smoothie*

Ingredients:

- 1½ cups fresh strawberries, hulled and sliced
- 2 cups fresh baby spinach
- ½ cup fat-free plain Greek yogurt
- 1 cup unsweetened almond milk
- ¼ cup ice cubes

Direction: Preparation Time: 10 minutes Servings: 2

✓ In a high-speed blender, add all the ingredients and pulse until smooth. Pour into serving glasses and serve immediately.

Meal Prep Tip:

✓ In 2 zip lock bags, divide the strawberries and spinach. Seal the bags and store in the freezer for about 2-3 days.
✓ Just before serving, remove from the freezer and transfer into a blender with yogurt, almond milk and

ice cubes and pulse until smooth.

Nutrition: Calories 96 Total Fat 2.3 g Saturated Fat 0.2 g Cholesterol 1 mg Total Carbs 12.3 g Sugar 7.7 g Fiber 3.9 g Sodium 144 mg Potassium 428 mg Protein 8.1 g

43) *Quinoa Porridge Recipe 1*

Ingredients:

- 2 cups water 1 cup dry quinoa, rinsed
- ½ teaspoon organic vanilla extract
- ½ cup unsweetened almond milk
- 10-12 drops liquid stevia
- ¼ teaspoon lemon peel, grated freshly
- ½ teaspoon ground cinnamon
- ½ teaspoon ground nutmeg
- Pinch of ground cloves
- 1 cup fresh mixed berries

Direction: Preparation Time: 10 minutes Cooking Time: 15 minutes Servings: 4

✓ In a pan, mix together the water, quinoa and vanilla essence over low heat and cook for about 15 minutes, stirring occasionally.
✓ Stir in the almond milk, stevia, lemon peel and spices and immediately, remove from the heat.
✓ Top with the berries and serve warm.

Meal Prep Tip:

✓ Transfer the cooled porridge in an airtight container and preserve in the refrigerator for up to 2 days.
✓ Just before serving, reheat in the microwave. Serve with the topping of berries.

Nutrition: Calories 186 Total Fat 3.3 g Saturated Fat 0.4 g Cholesterol 0 mg Total Carbs 32.3 g Sugar 2.7 g Fiber 4.6 g Sodium 25 mg Potassium 312 mg Protein 6.4 g

44) *Bell Pepper Pancakes*

Ingredients:

- ½ cup chickpea flour
- ¼ teaspoon baking powder
- Pinch of sea salt Pinch of red pepper flakes, crushed
- ½ cup plus
- 2 tablespoons filtered water
- ¼ cup green bell peppers, seeded and chopped finely
- ¼ cup scallion, chopped finely
- 2 teaspoons olive oil

Direction: Preparation Time: 15 minutes

Cooking Time: 8 minutes Servings: 2

✓ : In a bowl, mix together flour, baking powder, salt and red pepper flakes.

✓ Add the water and mix until well combined.

✓ Fold in bell pepper and scallion. In a large frying pan, heat the oil over low heat.

✓ Add half of the mixture and cook for about 1-2 minutes per side.

✓ Repeat with the remaining mixture.

✓ Serve warm.

Meal Prep Tip:

✓ Store these cooled pancakes into an airtight container by placing a piece of wax paper between each pancake.

✓ Refrigerate up to 4 days.

✓ Reheat in the microwave for about 1½-2 minutes.

Nutrition: Calories 232 Total Fat 7.8 g Saturated Fat 1 g Cholesterol 0 mg Total Carbs 32.7 g Sugar 6.4 g Fiber 9.3 g Sodium 132 mg Potassium 566 mg Protein 10 g

45) *Tofu Scramble*

Ingredients:

• ½ tablespoon olive oil

• 1 small onion, chopped finely

• 1 small red bell pepper, seeded and chopped finely

• 1 cup cherry tomatoes, chopped finely

• 1½ cups firm tofu, pressed and crumbled

• Pinch of ground turmeric

• Pinch of cayenne pepper

• 1 tablespoon fresh parsley, chopped

Direction: Preparation Time: 15 minutes Cooking Time: 15 minutes Servings: 2

✓ In a skillet, heat the oil over medium heat and sauté the onion and bell pepper for about 4-5 minute.

✓ Add the tomatoes and cook for about 1-2 minutes.

✓ Add the tofu, turmeric and cayenne pepper and cook for about 6-8 minutes.

✓ Garnish with parsley and serve. Meal Prep Tip:

✓ Transfer the cooled scramble into an airtight container and refrigerate for up to 3 days.

✓ Reheat in microwave before serving.

Nutrition: Calories 213 Total Fat 11.8 g Saturated Fat 2.2 g Cholesterol 0 mg Total Carbs 14.7 g Sugar 8 g Fiber 4.5 g Sodium 31 mg Potassium 872 mg Protein 17.3 g

46) *Apple Omelet*

Ingredients:

• 4 teaspoons olive oil, divided

• 2 small green apples, cored and sliced thinly

• ¼ teaspoon ground cinnamon

• Pinch of ground cloves

• Pinch of ground nutmeg

• 4 large eggs

• ¼ teaspoon organic vanilla extract

• Pinch of salt

Direction: Preparation Time: 10 minutes Cooking Time: 10 minutes Servings: 3

✓ In a large nonstick frying pan, heat 1 teaspoon of oil over medium-low heat. Place the apple slices and sprinkle with spices.

✓ Cook for about 4-5 minutes, flipping once halfway through.

✓ Meanwhile, in a bowl, add the eggs, vanilla extract and salt and beat until fluffy.

✓ Add the remaining oil in the pan and let it heat completely.

✓ Place the egg mixture over apple slices evenly and cook for about 3-5 minutes or until desired doneness.

✓ Carefully, turn the pan over a serving plate and immediately, fold the omelet.

✓ Serve immediately.

Meal Prep Tip:

✓ In a resealable plastic bag, place the cooled omelet slices and seal the bag.

✓ Refrigerate for about 2-4 days.

✓ Reheat in the microwave on High for about 1 minute before serving.

Nutrition: Calories 228 Total Fat 13.2 g Saturated Fat 3 g Cholesterol 248 mg Total Carbs 21.3 g Sugar 16.1 g Fiber 3.8 g Sodium 145 mg Potassium 251 mg Protein 8.8 g

47) *Spiced Overnight Oats*

Ingredients:

• 2 cups old-fashioned oats

• 1 cup fat-free milk

• 1 tablespoon vanilla extract

• 1 teaspoon liquid stevia extract

• 1 teaspoon ground cinnamon

• ¼ teaspoon ground nutmeg

• ½ cup toasted walnuts, chopped

Direction: Servings: 6 Cooking Time: None

✓ Stir together the oats, milk, vanilla extract, liquid stevia extract, cinnamon, and nutmeg in a large bowl. Cover and chill overnight until thick.

✓ Stir in the yogurt just before serving and spoon into cups.

✓ Top with chopped walnuts and fresh fruit to serve.

Nutrition: Calories 140, Total Fat 7.1g, Saturated Fat 0.5g, Total Carbs 12.7g, Net Carbs 10.4g, Protein 5.6g, Sugar 2.6g, Fiber 2.3g, Sodium 23mg

48) *Almond & Berry Smoothie*

Ingredients:

- : ⅔ cup frozen raspberries
- ½ cup frozen banana, sliced
- ½ cup almond milk (unsweetened)
- 3 tablespoons almonds, sliced flakes (unsweetened)
- ¼ teaspoon ground cinnamon
- ⅛ teaspoon vanilla extract
- ¼ cup blueberries
- 1 tablespoon coconut

Direction: Cooking Time: 0 Minute Servings: 1

✓ Put the Ingredients in a blender except coconut flakes. Pulse until smooth.

✓ Top with the coconut flakes before serving.

Nutrition: Calories 360 Total Fat 19 g Saturated Fat 3 g Cholesterol 0 mg Sodium 89 mg Carbohydrate 46 g Dietary Fiber 14 g Total Sugars 21 g Protein 9 g Potassium 736 mg

49) *Keto Low Carb Crepe*

Ingredients:

- 2 eggs 1 egg white
- 1 tbsp unsalted butter
- 1 1/3 tbsp cream cheese
- 2/3 tbsp psyllium husk

Direction: Servings: 2 Cooking Time: 4 Minutes

✓ Put all the ingredients in a bowl, except for butter, and then whisk by using a stick blender until smooth and very liquid.

✓ Bring out a skillet pan, put it over medium heat, add ½ tbsp butter and when it melts, pour in half of the batter, spread evenly, and cook until the top has firmed.

✓ Carefully flip the crepe, then continue cooking for 2 minutes until cooked and then move it to a plate.

✓ Add remaining butter and when it melts, cook another crepe in the same manner and then serve.

Nutrition: 118 Cal 9.4 g Fats 6.5 g Protein 1 g Net Carb 0.9 g Fiber

50) *Cinnamon Oat Pancakes*

Ingredients:

- 1 cup old-fashioned oats
- 1 cup whole-wheat flour
- 2 teaspoons baking powder
- 1 teaspoon salt
- 1 ½ cups fat-free milk
- ¼ cup canola oil
- 2 large eggs, whisked
- 1 teaspoon lemon juice
- ½ to 1 teaspoon liquid stevia extract

Direction: Servings: 6 Cooking Time: 15 Minutes

✓ Combine the oats, flour, baking powder, and salt in a medium mixing bowl. In a separate bowl, stir together the milk, canola oil, eggs, lemon juice, and stevia extract.

✓ Stir the wet ingredients into the dry until just combined.

✓ Heat a large skillet or griddle to medium-high heat and grease with cooking spray.

✓ Spoon the batter in ¼ cups into the skillet and cook until bubbles form on the surface.

✓ Flip the pancakes and cook to brown on the other side. Slide onto a plate and repeat with the remaining batter.

✓ Store the extra pancakes in an airtight container and reheat in the microwave or oven.

Nutrition: Calories 230, Total Fat 11.4g, Saturated Fat 1.3g, Total Carbs 24.3g, Net Carbs 23g, Protein 7.1g, Sugar 3.3g, Fiber 1.3g, Sodium 446mg

51) *Healthy Carrot Muffins*

Ingredients:

Dry ingredients
- Tapioca starch ¼ cup
- Baking soda – 1 teaspoon
- Cinnamon – 1 tablespoon
- Cloves – ¼ teaspoon

Wet ingredients
- Vanilla extract – 1 teaspoon
- Water – 1 1/2 cups
- Carrots (shredded) – 1 1/2
- Almond flour – 1¾ cups
- Granulated sweetener of choice – 1/2 cup
- Baking powder – 1 teaspoon
- Nutmeg – 1 teaspoon
- Salt – 1 teaspoon
- Coconut oil – 1/3 cup

- Flax meal – 4 tablespoons
- Banana (mashed) – 1 medium

Direction: Servings: 8 Cooking Time: 40 Minutes

✓ Begin by heating the oven to 350F. Get a muffin tray and position paper cups in all the moulds.

✓ Arrange aside. Get a small glass bowl and put half a cup of water and flax meal.

✓ Allow this rest for about 5 minutes. Your flax egg is prepared.

✓ Get a large mixing bowl and put in the almond flour, tapioca starch, granulated sugar, baking soda, baking powder, cinnamon, nutmeg, cloves, and salt.

✓ Mix well to combine. Conform a well in the middle of the flour mixture and stream in the coconut oil, vanilla extract, and flax egg.

✓ Mix well to conform a mushy dough. Then put in the chopped carrots and mashed banana.

✓ Mix until well-combined. Make use of a spoon to scoop out an equal amount of mixture into 8 muffin cups.

✓ Position the muffin tray in the oven and allow it to bake for about 40 minutes.

✓ Extract the tray from the microwave and allow the muffins to stand for about 10 minutes.

✓ Extract the muffin cups from the tray and allow them to chill until they reach room degree of hotness and coldness.

✓ Serve and enjoy!

Nutrition: Calories: 189 calories per serving; Fat 13.9 g; Protein 3.8 g; Carbs 17.3 g

52) *Keto Creamy Bacon Dish*

Ingredients:

- ½ tsp dried basil
- ½ tsp minced garlic
- ½ tsp tomato paste
- 2 oz unsalted butter, softened
- 3 slices of bacon, chopped

Direction: Servings: 2 Cooking Time: 5 Minutes

✓ Bring out a skillet pan, put it over medium heat, add 1 tbsp butter and when it starts to melts, add chopped bacon and cook for 5 minutes.

✓ Then remove the pan from heat, add remaining butter, along with basil and tomato paste, season with salt and black pepper and stir until well mixed.

✓ Move bacon butter into an airtight container, cover with the lid, and refrigerate for 1 hour until solid.

Nutrition: 150 Cal 16 g Fats 1 g Protein 0.5 g Net Carb 1 g Fiber

53) *Egg "dough" In A Pan*

Ingredients:

- ¼ tsp salt
- ½ of medium red bell pepper, chopped
- 1/8 tsp ground black pepper
- 2 eggs
- 2 tbsp chopped chives

Direction: Servings: 2 Cooking Time: 4 Minutes

✓ Turn on the oven, then set it to 350 degrees F and let it preheat. In the meantime, crack eggs in a bowl, add remaining ingredients and whisk until combined.

✓ Bring out a small heatproof dish, pour in egg mixture, and bake for 5 to 8 minutes until set. When done, cut it into two squares and then serve.

Nutrition: 87 Cal 5.4 g Fats 7.2 g Protein 1.7 g Net Carb 0.7 g Fiber

54) *Eggs Florentine*

Ingredients:

- 1 cup washed, fresh spinach leaves
- 2 tbsp freshly grated parmesan cheese
- Sea salt and pepper
- 1 tbsp white vinegar
- 2 eggs

Direction: Servings: 2 Cooking Time: 10 Minutes

✓ Cook the spinach the microwave or steam until wilted.

✓ Sprinkle with parmesan cheese and seasoning.

✓ Slice into bite-size pieces

✓ Simmer a pan of water and add the vinegar. Stir quickly with a spoon.

✓ Break an egg into the center.

✓ Turn off the heat and cover until set.

✓ Repeat with the second egg. Place the eggs on top of the spinach and serve.

Nutrition: 180 cal.10g fat 7g protein 5g carbs.

55) *Cucumber & Yogurt*

Ingredients:

- 1 cup low-fat yogurt
- ½ cup cucumber, diced
- ¼ teaspoon lemon zest
- ¼ teaspoon lemon juice
- ¼ teaspoon fresh mint, chopped Salt to taste

Direction: Servings: 1 Cooking Time: 0 Minute

✓ Mix all the Ingredients in a jar.
✓ Refrigerate and serve.

Nutrition: Calories 164 Total Fat 4 g Saturated Fat 2 g Cholesterol 15 mg Sodium 318 mg Total Carbohydrate 19 g Dietary Fiber 1 g Total Sugars 18 g Protein 13 g Potassium 683 mg

56) *Eggs Baked In Peppers*

Ingredients:

- 4 medium bell peppers, assorted
- 1 cup shredded low-fat cheddar cheese
- 8 large eggs Salt and pepper
- Fresh chopped parsley, to serve

Direction: Servings: 4 Cooking Time: 25 Minutes

✓ Preheat the oven to 400°F and slice the peppers in half.
✓ Remove the seeds and pith from each pepper and place them cut-side up in a baking dish large enough to fit them all.
✓ Divide the shredded cheese among the pepper halves and crack an egg into each.
✓ Season with salt and pepper then bake for 20 to 25 minutes until done to your liking.
✓ Garnish with fresh chopped parsley to serve.

Nutrition: Calories 260, Total Fat 16.3g, Saturated Fat 6.6g, Total Carbs 10.9g, Net Carbs 9.3g, Protein 20.8g, Sugar 6.8g, Fiber 1.6g, Sodium 374mg

57) *Easy Egg Scramble*

Ingredients:

- 2 large eggs
- 1 tablespoon fat-free milk Salt and pepper
- ¼ cup diced green pepper
- 2 tablespoons diced onion
- ¼ cup diced tomatoes

Direction: Servings: 1 Cooking Time: 10 Minutes

✓ Whisk together the eggs, milk, salt, and pepper in a small bowl. Heat a medium skillet over medium-high heat and grease with cooking spray.
✓ Add the green pepper and onion then cook for 2 to 3 minutes.
✓ Spoon the veggies into a bowl then reheat the skillet. Pour in the egg mixture and cook until the eggs start to thicken.
✓ Spoon in the cooked veggies and diced tomatoes. Stir the mixture and cook until the egg is set and scrambled. Serve hot.

Nutrition: Calories 170, Total Fat 10.1g, Saturated Fat 3.1g, Total Carbs 6.3g, Net Carbs 4.9g, Protein 13.9g, Sugar 4.1g, Fiber 1.4g, Sodium 152mg

58) *Strawberry Puff Pancake*

Ingredients:

- 3 eggs, large
- 1/8 teaspoon cinnamon, ground
- 1 cup strawberry, sliced
- 3/4 cup milk, fat-free What you will need from the store cupboard:
- 1 teaspoon vanilla extract
- ¾ cup of all-purpose flour
- 2 tablespoons of butter
- 1 tablespoon cornstarch
- ½ cup of water
- 1/8 teaspoon salt

Direction: Servings: 4 Cooking Time: 20 Minutes

✓ Keep the butter in a pie plate and keep in an oven for 4 to 5 minutes. In the meantime, whisk the vanilla, milk, and eggs in a bowl.
✓ Take another bowl and bring together the cinnamon, salt, and flour in it. Whisk this into the egg mix until it blends well. Pour this into the plate.
✓ Bake for 15 minutes. The sides should be golden brown and crisp. Add the cornstarch in your saucepan.
✓ Stir the water in until it turns smooth. Now add the strawberries.
✓ Cook while stirring till it thickens. Mash the strawberries coarsely and serve with the pancake.

Nutrition: Calories 277, Carbohydrates 38g, Fiber 2g, Cholesterol 175mg, Total Fat 10g, Protein 9g, Sodium 187mg

59) *Egg Porridge*

Ingredients:

- 2 organic free-range eggs
- 1/3 cup organic heavy cream without food additives
- 2 packages of your preferred sweetener
- 2 tbsp grass-fed butter ground organic cinnamon to taste

Direction: Servings: 1 Cooking Time: 10 Minutes

✓ In a bowl add the eggs, cream and sweetener, and mix together. Melt the butter in a saucepan over a medium heat.
✓ Lower the heat once the butter is melted. Combine together with the egg and cream mixture.

✓ While Cooking, mix until it thickens and curdles.

✓ When you see the first signs of curdling, remove the saucepan immediately from the heat.

✓ Pour the porridge into a bowl. Sprinkle cinnamon on top and serve immediately.

Nutrition: 604 cal 45g fat 8g protein 2.8g carbs.

60) *Breakfast Parfait*

Ingredients:

- 4 oz. unsweetened applesauce
- 6 oz. non-fat and sugar-free vanilla yogurt
- ¼ teaspoon pumpkin pie spice
- ¼ teaspoon honey
- 1 cup low-fat granola

Direction: Servings: 2 Cooking Time: 0 Minute

✓ Mix the Ingredients except the granola in a bowl..

✓ Layer the mixture with the granola in a cup. Refrigerate before serving

Nutrition: Calories 287 Total Fat 3 g Saturated Fat 1 g Cholesterol 28 mg Sodium 186 mg Total Carbohydrate 57 g Dietary Fiber 4 g Total Sugars2 g Protein 8 g

61) *Oatmeal Blueberry Pancakes*

Ingredients:

- ½ cup rolled oats
- ½ cup unsweetened almond milk
- ¼ cup unsweetened applesauce
- ¼ cup unsweetened vegan protein powder
- ½ tablespoon flax meal
- 1 teaspoon baking powder
- ½ teaspoon vanilla extract
- ¼ teaspoon baking soda
- ¼ teaspoon ground cinnamon
- 1/8 teaspoon salt
- ½ cup fresh blueberries

Direction: Servings: 4 Cooking Time: 40 Minutes

✓ Place all ingredients (except for blueberries) in a food processor and pulse until smooth.

✓ Transfer the mixture into a bowl and set aside for 5 minutes. Gently, fold in blueberries.

✓ Place a lightly greased medium skillet over medium heat until heated.

✓ Place desired amount of the mixture and cook for about 3–5 minutes per side.

✓ Repeat with the remaining mixture. Serve warm.

Nutrition: Calories 105 Total Fat 1.8 g Saturated Fat 0.2 g Cholesterol 0 mg Sodium 204 mg Total Carbs 15.4 g Fiber 2.2 g Sugar 5.2 g Protein 8 g

62) *Bulgur Porridge*

Ingredients:

- 2/3 cup unsweetened soy milk
- 1/3 cup bulgur, rinsed
- Pinch of salt
- 1 ripe banana, peeled and mashed
- 2 kiwis, peeled and sliced

Direction: Servings: 2 Cooking Time: 15 Minutes

✓ In a pan, add the soy milk, bulgur, and salt over medium-high heat and bring to a boil.

✓ Adjust the heat to low and simmer for about 10 minutes.

✓ Remove the pan of bulgur from heat and immediately, stir in the mashed banana.

✓ Serve warm with the topping of kiwi slices.

Nutrition: Calories 223 Total Fat 2.3 g Saturated Fat 0.3 g Cholesterol 0 mg Sodium 126 mg Total Carbs 47.5 g Fiber 8.6 g Sugar 17.4 g Protein 7.1 g

63) *Turkey-broccoli Brunch Casserole*

Ingredients:

- 2-1/2 cups turkey breast, cubed and cooked
- 16 oz. broccoli, chopped and drained
- 1-1/2 cups of milk, fat-free 1 cup cheddar cheese, low-fat, shredded
- 10 oz. cream of chicken soup. low sodium and low fat

What you will need from the store cupboard:

- 8 oz. egg substitute
- ¼ teaspoon of poultry seasoning
- ¼ cup of sour cream, low fat
- ½ teaspoon pepper
- 1/8 teaspoon salt 2 cups of seasoned stuffing cubes
- Cooking spray

Direction: Servings: 6 Cooking Time: 20 Minutes

✓ Bring together the egg substitute, soup, milk, pepper, sour cream, salt, and poultry seasoning in a big bowl.

✓ Now stir in the broccoli, turkey, ¾ cup of cheese and stuffing cubes.

✓ Transfer to a baking dish. Apply cooking spray.

✓ Bake for 10 minutes. Sprinkle the remaining cheese.

✓ Bake for another 5 minutes.

✓ Keep it aside for 5 minutes. Serve.

Nutrition: Calories 303, Carbohydrates 26g, Fiber 3g, Sugar 0.8g, Cholesterol 72mg, Total Fat 7g, Protein 33g Cheesy

64) *Low-carb Omelet*

Ingredients:

- 2 whole eggs
- 1 tablespoon water
- 1 tablespoon butter
- 3 thin slices salami
- 5 fresh basil leaves
- 5 thin slices, fresh ripe tomatoes
- 2 ounces fresh mozzarella cheese
- Salt and pepper as needed

Direction: Servings: 5 Cooking Time: 5 Minutes

✓ Take a small bowl and whisk in eggs and water

✓ Take a non-stick Sauté pan and place it over medium heat, add butter and let it melt

✓ Pour egg mixture and cook for 30 seconds Spread salami slices on half of egg mix and top with cheese, tomatoes, basil slices

✓ Season with salt and pepper according to your taste

✓ Cook for 2 minutes and fold the egg with the empty half

✓ Cover and cook on LOW for 1 minute Serve and enjoy!

Nutrition: Calories: 451; Fat: 36g; Carbohydrates: 3g; Protein:33g

65) *Apple & Cinnamon Pancake*

Ingredients:

- ¼ teaspoon ground cinnamon
- 1 ¾ cups Better Baking Mix
- 1 tablespoon oil
- 1 cup water
- 2 egg whites
- ½ cup sugar-free applesauce
- Cooking spray
- 1 cup plain yogurt
- Sugar substitute

Direction: Servings: 4 Cooking Time: 10 Minutes

✓ Blend the cinnamon and the baking mix in a bowl.

✓ Create a hole in the middle and add the oil, water, egg and applesauce.

✓ Mix well. Spray your pan with oil.

✓ Place it on medium heat. Pour ¼ cup of the batter.

✓ Flip the pancake and cook until golden.

✓ Serve with yogurt and sugar substitute.

Nutrition: Calories 231 Total Fat 6 g Saturated Fat 1 g Cholesterol 54 mg Sodium 545 mg Total Carbohydrate 37 g Dietary Fiber 4 g Total Sugars 1 g Protein 8 g Potassium 750 mg

66) *Guacamole Turkey Burgers*

Ingredients:

- 12 oz. turkey, ground
- 1-1/2 avocados
- 2 teaspoons of juice from a lime
- ½ teaspoon cumin
- 1 red chili, chopped

What you will need from the store cupboard:

- ½ teaspoon garlic powder
- ½ teaspoon onion powder
- 3 teaspoons of olive oil
- ½ teaspoon salt

Direction: Servings: 3 Cooking Time: 15 Minutes

✓ Mix the turkey with the cumin, chili, salt, garlic powder, and onion powder in a medium-sized bowl.

✓ Create 3 patties Pour 3 teaspoons olive oil in a skillet and heat over medium heat.

✓ Now cook your patties. Make sure that both sides are brown. Make the guacamole in the meantime.

✓ Mash together the garlic powder, juice from lime and avocados in a bowl.

✓ Add salt for seasoning. Serve the burgers with guacamole on the patties.

Nutrition: Calories 316, Carbohydrates 9g, Fiber 8g, Sugar 0g, Cholesterol 80mg, Total Fat 21g, Protein 24g

67) *Ham And Goat Cheese Omelet*

Ingredients:

- 1 slice of ham, chopped
- 4 egg whites
- 2 teaspoons of water
- 2 tablespoons onion, chopped
- 1 tablespoon parsley, minced

What you will need from the store cupboard:

- 2 tablespoons green pepper, chopped
- 1/8 teaspoon pepper
- 2 tablespoons goat cheese, crumbled Cooking spray

Direction: Servings: 1 Cooking Time: 10 Minutes

✓ Whisk together the water, pepper and egg whites in a bowl till everything blends well. Stir in the green pepper, ham, and onion.

✓ Now heat your skillet over medium heat after applying the cooking spray. Pour in the egg white mix towards the edge.

✓ As it sets, push the cooked parts to the center. Allow the uncooked portions to flow underneath.

✓ Sprinkle the goat cheese to one side when there is no liquid egg. Now fold your omelet into half.

✓ Sprinkle the parsley.

Nutrition: Calories 143, Carbohydrates 5g, Fiber 1g, Sugar 0.3g, Cholesterol 27mg, Total Fat 4g, Protein 21g

68) *Banana Matcha Breakfast Smoothie*

Ingredients:

- 1 cup fat-free milk
- 1 medium banana, sliced
- ¼ cup frozen chopped pineapple
- ½ cup ice cubes
- 1 tablespoon Matcha powder
- ¼ teaspoon ground cinnamon
- Liquid stevia extract, to taste

Direction: Servings: 1 Cooking Time: None

✓ Combine the ingredients in a blender.

✓ Pulse the mixture several times to chop the ingredients.

✓ Blend for 30 to 60 seconds until smooth and well combined. Sweeten to taste with liquid stevia extract, if desired.

✓ Pour into a glass and serve immediately.

Nutrition: Calories 230, Total Fat 0.4g, Saturated Fat 0.1g, Total Carbs 44.9g, Net Carbs 38g, Protein 12.6g, Sugar 30.9g, Fiber 6.9g, Sodium 135mg

69) *Basil And Tomato Baked Eggs*

Ingredients:

- 1 garlic clove, minced
- 1 cup canned tomatoes
- ¼ cup fresh basil leaves, roughly chopped
- 1/2 teaspoon chili powder
- 1 tablespoon olive oil
- 4 whole eggs
- Salt and pepper to taste

Direction: Servings: 4 Cooking Time: 15 Minutes

✓ Preheat your oven to 375 degrees F Take a small baking dish and grease with olive oil

✓ Add garlic, basil, tomatoes chili, olive oil into a dish and stir

✓ Crackdown eggs into a dish, keeping space between the two

✓ Sprinkle the whole dish with salt and pepper

✓ Place in oven and cook for 12 minutes until eggs are set and tomatoes are bubbling Serve with basil on top Enjoy!

Nutrition: Calories: 235; Fat: 16g; Carbohydrates: 7g;
Protein: 14g

70) *Cream Cheese Pancakes*

Ingredients:

- 2 oz cream cheese 2 eggs
- ½ tsp cinnamon
- 1 tbsp keto coconut flour
- ½ to 1 packet of Stevia

Direction: Servings: 1 Cooking Time: 5 Minutes

✓ Skillet with butter the pan or coconut oil on medium-high. Make them as you would normal pancakes.

✓ Cook and flip one side to cook the other side! Top with some butter and/or sugar-free syrup.

Nutrition: 340 cal.30g fat 7g protein 3g carbs

71) *Mashed Cauliflower*

Ingredients:

- 1 cauliflower head
- 1/8 cup plain yogurt, skim milk or butter 1 red chili, diced
- 1 tomato, sliced ½ chopped onion

What you will need from the store cupboard:

1 garlic clove, optional Salt and pepper Paprika to taste

Direction: Servings: 6 Cooking Time: 10 Minutes

✓ Steam the cauliflower till it becomes tender. You can steam with a garlic clove as well. Now cut your cauliflower into small pieces.

✓ Keep in your blender with yogurt, butter or milk.

✓ Season with pepper and salt. Whip until it gets smooth. Pour the cauliflower into a small baking dish.

✓ Sprinkle the paprika. Bake in the oven till it becomes bubbly.

Nutrition: Calories 57, Carbohydrates 12g, Total Fat 0g, Protein 4g, Fiber 5g, Sodium 91mg, Sugars 5g

72) *Quinoa Porridge Recipe2*

Ingredients:

- 1 cup dry quinoa, rinsed
- 1½ cups unsweetened almond milk
- 1 teaspoon vanilla extract
- 1 teaspoon ground cinnamon blueberries
- 2 tablespoons maple syrup
- 4 tablespoons peanut butter
- ¼ cup fresh strawberries, hulled and chopped
- ¼ cup fresh

Direction: Servings: 2 Cooking Time: 20 Minutes

- ✓ In a small pan, place quinoa, almond milk, vanilla extract, and cinnamon over medium heat and bring to a boil.
- ✓ Now, adjust the heat to low and simmer, covered for about 15 minutes or until all the liquid is absorbed.
- ✓ Remove the pan of quinoa from heat and stir in maple syrup and peanut butter.
- ✓ Serve warm with the topping of berries.

Nutrition: Calories 608 Total Fat 24 g Saturated Fat 4.2 g Cholesterol 0 mg Sodium 289 mg Total Carbs 81 g Fiber 10 g Sugar 17.9 g Protein 21.1 g

73) *Vanilla Mixed Berry Smoothie*

Ingredients:

- 1 cup fat-free milk
- ½ cup nonfat Greek yogurt, plain
- ½ cup frozen blueberries
- ¼ cup frozen strawberries
- 3 to 4 ice cubes
- 1 teaspoon fresh lemon juice
- Liquid stevia extract, to taste

Direction: Servings: 1 Cooking Time: None

- ✓ Combine the ingredients in a blender.
- ✓ Pulse the mixture several times to chop the ingredients.
- ✓ Blend for 30 to 60 seconds until smooth and well combined.
- ✓ Sweeten to taste with liquid stevia extract, if desired.
- ✓ Pour into a glass and serve immediately.

Nutrition: : Calories 220, Total Fat 0.3g, Saturated Fat 0g, Total Carbs 31.6g, Net Carbs 28.3g, Protein 21.6g, Sugar 27.3g, Fiber 3.3g, Sodium 204mg

74) *Granola With Fruits*

Ingredients:

- 3 cups quick cooking oats
- 1 cup almonds, sliced
- ½ cup wheat germ
- 3 tablespoons butter
- 1 teaspoon ground cinnamon
- 1 cup honey
- 3 cups whole grain cereal flakes
- ½ cup raisins
- ½ cup dried cranberries
- ½ cup dates, pitted and chopped

Direction: Servings: 6 Cooking Time: 35 Minutes

- ✓ Preheat your oven to 325 degrees F.
- ✓ Place the almonds on a baking sheet.
- ✓ Bake for 15 minutes.
- ✓ Mix the wheat germ, butter, cinnamon and honey in a bowl.
- ✓ Add the toasted almonds and oats. Mix well.
- ✓ Spread on the baking sheet.
- ✓ Bake for 20 minutes.
- ✓ Mix with the rest of the ingredients. Let cool and serve.

Nutrition: Calories 210 Total Fat 7 g Saturated Fat 2 g Cholesterol 5 mg Sodium 58 mg Total Carbohydrate 36 g Dietary Fiber 4 g Total Sugars 2 g Protein 5 g Potassium 250 mg

75) *Egg Muffins*

Ingredients:

- 1 tbsp green pesto
- 3 oz/75g shredded cheese
- 5 oz/150g cooked bacon
- 1 scallion, chopped
- 6 eggs

Direction: Servings: 6 Cooking Time: 20 Minutes

- ✓ You should set your oven to 350°F/175°C.
- ✓ Place liners in a regular cupcake tin.
- ✓ This will help with easy removal and storage.
- ✓ Beat the eggs with pepper, salt, and the pesto.
- ✓ Mix in the cheese.
- ✓ Pour the eggs into the cupcake tin and top with the bacon and scallion.
- ✓ Cook for 15-20 minutes

Nutrition: 190 cal.15g fat 7g protein 4g carbs.

76) *Eggs On TheGo*

Ingredients:

- 4 oz/110g bacon, cooked
- Pepper Salt
- 12 eggs

Direction: Servings: 4 Cooking Time: 5 Minutes

✓ You should set your oven to 200°C.
✓ Place liners in a regular cupcake tin.
✓ This will help with easy removal and storage.
✓ Crack an egg into each of the cups and sprinkle some bacon onto each of them.
✓ Season with some pepper and salt.
✓ Bake for 15 minutes, or until the eggs are set.

Nutrition: 75 cal. 6g fat 8g protein 1g carbs.

77) *Breakfast Mix*

Ingredients:

- 5 tbsp coconut flakes, unsweetened
- 7 tbsp hemp seeds
- 5 tbsp flaxseed, ground
- 2 tbsp sesame, ground
- 2 tbsp cocoa, dark, unsweetened

Direction: Servings: 1 Cooking Time: 5 Minutes

✓ Grind the sesame and flaxseed. only grind the sesame seeds for a small period.
✓ Mix all ingredients in a jar and shake it well. Keep refrigerated until ready to eat.
✓ Serve softened with black coffee or even with still water and add coconut oil if you want to increase the fat content.
✓ It also blends well with cream or with mascarpone cheese.

Nutrition: 150 cal.9g fat 8g protein 4g carbs.

78) *Vegetable Omelet*

Ingredients:

- ½ cup yellow summer squash, chopped
- ½ cup canned diced tomatoes with herbs, drained
- ½ ripe avocado, pitted and chopped
- ½ cup cucumber, chopped
- 2 eggs
- 2 tablespoons water
- Salt and pepper to taste
- 1 teaspoon dried basil, crushed
- Cooking spray ¼ cup low-fat

- Monterey Jack cheese, shredded
- Chives, chopped

Direction: Servings: 4 Cooking Time: 25 Minutes

✓ In a bowl, mix the squash, tomatoes, avocado and cucumber.
✓ In another bowl, mix the eggs, water, salt, pepper and basil.
✓ Spray oil on a pan over medium heat.
✓ Pour egg mixture on the pan. Put the vegetable mixture on top of the egg.
✓ Lift and fold.
✓ Cook until the egg has set.
✓ Sprinkle cheese and chives on top.

Nutrition: Calories 128 Total Fat 6 g Sodium 357mg Total Carbohydrate 7 g Dietary Fiber 3 g Total Sugars 4 g Protein 12 g Potassium 341 mg

79) *Vegetable Frittata*

Ingredients:

- 1 cup mushrooms, sliced
- 4 eggs, beaten lightly
- 2 tablespoons onion, chopped
- ½ cup broccoli, chopped
- ¼ cup cheddar cheese, shredded, low-fat

What you will need from the store cupboard:

- 2 tablespoons green pepper, chopped
- Dash of pepper
- 1/8 teaspoon of salt
- Cooking spray

Direction: Servings: 2 Cooking Time: 20 Minutes

✓ Bring together all the ingredients in your bowl.
✓ Coat your baking dish with cooking spray and pour everything into it.
✓ Bake for 20 minutes and serve immediately.

Nutrition: Calories 230, Carbohydrates 6g, Fiber 1g, Sugar 0.2g, Cholesterol 386mg, Total Fat 14g, Protein 20g

80) *Egg-veggie Scramble*

Ingredients:

- ¼ tsp salt
- 1 tbsp unsalted butter
- 1/8 tsp ground black pepper
- 3 eggs, beaten
- 4 oz spinach

Direction: Servings: 2 Cooking Time: 3 Minutes

✓ Bring out a frying pan, put it over medium heat, add butter and when it melts, add spinach and cook for 5 minutes until leaves have wilted.

✓ Then pour in eggs, season with salt and black pepper, and cook for 3 minutes until eggs have scramble to the desired level.

Nutrition: 90 Cal 7 g Fats 5.6 g Protein; 0.7 g Net Carb 0.6 g Fiber

81) *Veggie Fritters*

Ingredients:

- ½ tsp nutritional yeast
- 1 oz chopped broccoli
- 1 zucchini, grated, squeezed
- 2 eggs
- 2 tbsp almond flour

Direction: Servings: 2 Cooking Time: 3 Minutes

✓ Wrap grated zucchini in a cheesecloth, twist it well to remove excess moisture, and then

✓ Put zucchini in a bowl.

✓ Add remaining ingredients, except for oil, and then whisk well until combined.

✓ Bring out a skillet pan, put it over medium heat, add oil and when hot, drop zucchini mixture in four portions, shape them into flat patties and cook for 4 minutes per side until thoroughly cooked.

Nutrition: 191 Cal 16.6 g Fats 9.6 g Protein 0.8 g Net Carb 0.2 g Fiber

82) *Millet Porridge*

Ingredients:

- 1 cup millet, rinsed and drained
- Pinch of salt
- 3 cups water 2 tablespoons almonds, chopped finely
- 6-8 drops liquid stevia
- 1 cup unsweetened almond milk
- 2 tablespoons fresh blueberries

Direction: Servings: 4 Cooking Time: 25 Minutes

✓ In a nonstick pan, add the millet over medium-low heat and cook for about 3 minutes, stirring continuously.

✓ Add the salt and water and stir to combine

✓ Increase the heat to medium and bring to a boil. Cook for about 15 minutes.

✓ Stir in the almonds, stevia and almond milk and cook for 5 minutes.

✓ Top with the blueberries and serve.

Nutrition: Calories 219 Total Fat 4.5 g Saturated Fat

0.6 g Cholesterol 0 mg Total Carbs 38.2 g Sugar 0.6 g Fiber 5 g Sodium 92 mg Potassium 1721 mg Protein 6.4 g

83) *Tofu & Zucchini Muffins*

Ingredients:

- 12 ounces extra-firm silken tofu, drained and pressed
- ¾ cup unsweetened soy milk
- 2 tablespoons canola oil
- 1 tablespoon apple cider vinegar
- 1 cup whole-wheat pastry flour
- ½ cup chickpea flour
- 1 teaspoon baking powder
- ½ teaspoon baking soda
- 1 teaspoon smoked paprika
- 1 teaspoon onion powder
- 1 teaspoon salt
- ½ cup zucchini, chopped
- ¼ cup fresh chives, minced

Direction: Servings: 6 Cooking Time: 40 Minutes

✓ Preheat your oven to 400°F. Line a 12-cup muffin tin with paper liners.

✓ In a bowl, place tofu and with a fork, mash until smooth. In the bowl of tofu, add almond milk, oil, and vinegar, and mix until slightly smooth.

✓ In a separate large bowl, add flours, baking powder, baking soda, spices, and salt, and mix well.

✓ Transfer the mixture into muffin cups evenly.

✓ Bake for approximately 35–40 minutes or until a toothpick inserted in the center comes out clean.

✓ Remove the muffin tin from oven and place onto a wire rack to cool for about 10 minutes.

✓ Carefully invert the muffins onto a platter and serve warm.

Nutrition: Calories 237 Total Fat 9 g Saturated Fat 1 g Cholesterol 0 mg Sodium 520 mg Total Carbs 2293.3 g Fiber 5.9 g Sugar 3.7 g Protein 11.1 g

84) *Savory Keto Pancake*

Ingredients:

- ¼ cup almond flour
- 1 ½ tbsp unsalted butter
- 2 eggs
- 2 oz cream cheese, softened

Direction: Servings: 2 Cooking Time: 2 Minutes

✓ Bring out a bowl, crack eggs in it, whisk well until

fluffy, and then whisk in flour and cream cheese until well combined.

✓ Bring out a skillet pan, put it over medium heat, add butter and when it melts, drop pancake batter in four sections, spread it evenly, and cook for 2 minutes per side until brown.

Nutrition: 166.8 Cal 15 g Fats 5.8 g Protein 1.8 g Net Car 0.8 g Fiber

85) *Buckwheat Porridge*

Ingredients:

- 1½ cups water
- 1 cup buckwheat groats, rinsed
- ¾ teaspoon vanilla extract
- ½ teaspoon ground cinnamon
- ¼ teaspoon salt
- 2 tablespoons maple syrup
- 1 ripe banana, peeled and mashed
- 1½ cups unsweetened soy milk
- 1 tablespoon peanut butter
- 1/3 cup fresh strawberries, hulled and chopped

Direction: Servings: 2 Cooking Time: 15 Minutes

✓ Place the water, buckwheat, vanilla extract, cinnamon, and salt in a pan and bring to a boil.

✓ Now, adjust the heat to medium-low and simmer for about 6 minutes, stirring occasionally.

✓ Stir in maple syrup, banana, and soy milk, and simmer, covered for about 6 minutes.

✓ Remove the pan of porridge from heat and stir in peanut butter. Serve warm with the topping of strawberry pieces.

Nutrition: Calories 453 Total Fat 9.4 g Total Carbs 82.8 g Fiber 9.4 g Sugar 28.8 g Protein 16.2 g

86) *Breakfast Sandwich*

Ingredients:

- 2 oz/60g cheddar cheese
- 1/6 oz/30g smoked ham
- 2 tbsp butter 4 eggs

Direction: Servings: 2 Cooking Time: 0 Minutes

✓ Fry all the eggs and sprinkle the pepper and salt on them.

✓ Place an egg down as the sandwich base.

✓ Top with the ham and cheese and a drop or two of Tabasco.

✓ Place the other egg on top and enjoy.

Nutrition: 600 cal. 50g fat 12g protein 7g carbs.

87) *Eggplant Omelet*

Ingredients:

- 1 large eggplant
- 1 tbsp coconut oil, melted
- 1 tsp unsalted butter
- 2 eggs
- 2 tbsp chopped green onions

Direction: Servings: 2 Cooking Time: 5 Minutes

✓ Set the grill and let it preheat at the high setting.

✓ In the meantime, prepare the eggplant, and for this, cut two slices from eggplant, about 1-inch thick, and reserve the remaining eggplant for later use.

✓ Brush slices of eggplant with oil, season with salt on both sides, then put the slices on grill and cook for 3 to 4 minutes per side.

✓ Move grilled eggplant to a cutting board, let it cool for 5 minutes and then make a home in the center of each slice by using a cookie cutter.

✓ Bring out a frying pan, put it over medium heat, add butter and when it melts, add eggplant slices in it and crack an egg into its each hole.

✓ Let the eggs cook, then carefully flip the eggplant slice and continue cooking for 3 minutes until the egg has thoroughly cooked Season egg with salt and black pepper, move them to a plate, then garnish with green onions and serve.

Nutrition: 184 Cal 14.1 g Fats 7.8 g Protein 3 g Net Carb 3.5 g Fiber

88) *Breakfast Muffins*

Ingredients:

- 1 medium egg
- ¼ cup heavy cream
- 1 slice cooked bacon (cured, pan-fried, cooked)
- 1 oz cheddar cheese
- Salt and black pepper (to taste)

Direction: Servings: 1 Cooking Time: 5 Minutes

✓ Preheat the oven to 350°F.

✓ In a bowl, mix the eggs with the cream, salt and pepper.

✓ Spread into muffin tins and fill the cups half full.

✓ Place 1 slice of bacon into each muffin hole and half ounce of cheese on top of each muffin.

✓ Bake for around 15-20 minutes or until lightly browned. Add another ½ oz of cheese onto each muffin and broil until the cheese is slightly browned.

✓ Serve!

Nutrition: 150 cal 11g fat 7g protein 2g carbs

LUNCH

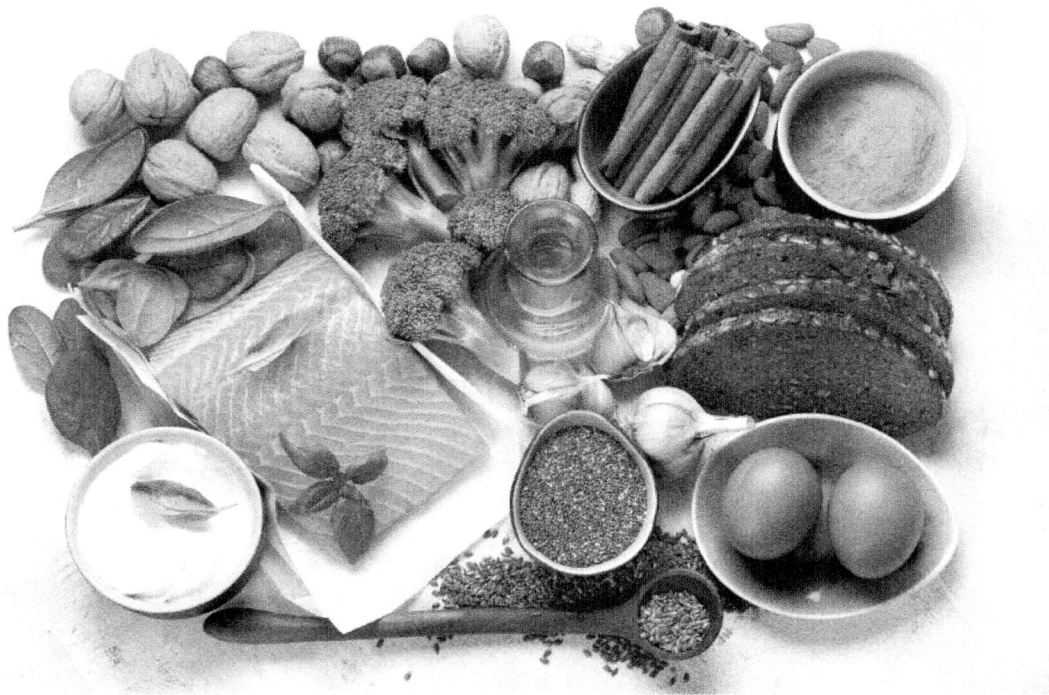

89) *Sweet Potato, Kale, and White Bean Stew*

Ingredients:

- 1 (15-ounce) can low-sodium cannellini beans, rinsed and drained, divided
- 1 tablespoon olive oil
- 1 medium onion, chopped
- 2 garlic cloves, minced
- 2 celery stalks, chopped
- 3 medium carrots, chopped
- 2 cups low-sodium vegetable broth
- 1 teaspoon apple cider vinegar
- 2 medium sweet potatoes (about 1¼ pounds)
- 2 cups chopped kale
- 1 cup shelled edamame
- ¼ cup quinoa
- 1 teaspoon dried thyme
- 1/2 teaspoon cayenne pepper
- 1/2 teaspoon salt
- ¼ teaspoon freshly ground black pepper

Direction: Preparation time: 15 minutes Cooking time: 25 minutes Servings: 4

- ✓ Put half the beans into a blender and blend until smooth. Set aside.
- ✓ In a large soup pot over medium heat, heat the oil. When the oil is shining, include the onion and garlic, and cook until the onion softens and the garlic is sweet, about 3 minutes. Add the celery and carrots, and continue cooking until the vegetables soften, about 5 minutes.
- ✓ Add the broth, vinegar, sweet potatoes, unblended beans, kale, edamame, and quinoa, and bring the mixture to a boil. Reduce the heat and simmer until the vegetables soften, about 10 minutes.
- ✓ Add the blended beans, thyme, cayenne, salt, and black pepper, increase the heat to medium-high, and bring the mixture to a boil. Reduce the heat and simmer, uncovered, until the flavors combine, about 5 minutes.
- ✓ Into each of 4 containers, scoop 1¾ cups of stew.

Nutrition: calories: 373; total fat: 7g; saturated fat: 1g; protein: 15g; total carbs: 65g; fiber: 15g; sugar: 13g; sodium: 540mg

90) *Slow Cooker Two-Bean Sloppy Joes*

Ingredients:

- 1 (15-ounce) can low-sodium black beans
- 1 (15-ounce) can low-sodium pinto beans
- 1 (15-ounce) can no-salt-added diced tomatoes
- 1 medium green bell pepper, cored, seeded, and chopped
- 1 medium yellow onion, chopped
- ¼ cup low-sodium vegetable broth
- 2 garlic cloves, minced
- 2 servings (¼ cup) meal prep barbecue sauce or bottled barbecue sauce
- ¼ teaspoon salt
- ¼ teaspoon freshly ground black pepper
- 4 whole-wheat buns

Direction: Preparation time: 10 minutes Cooking time: 6 hours Servings: 4

- ✓ In a slow cooker, combine the black beans, pinto beans, diced tomatoes, bell pepper, onion, broth, garlic, meal prep barbecue sauce, salt, and black pepper. Stir the ingredients, then cover and cook on low for 6 hours.
- ✓ Into each of 4 containers, spoon 1¼ cups of sloppy sloppy joe mix. Serve with 1 whole-wheat bun.
- ✓ Storage: place airtight containers in the refrigerator for up to 1 week. To freeze, place freezer-safe containers in the freezer for up to 2 months. To defrost, refrigerate overnight.
- ✓ Alternatively, reheat the entire dish in a saucepan on the stove top. Bring the sloppy joes to a boil, then reduce the heat and simmer until heated through, 10 to 15 minutes. Serve with a whole-wheat bun.
- ✓ To reheat individual portions, microwave uncovered on high for 2 to 21/2 minutes

Nutrition: calories: 392; total fat: 3g; saturated fat: 0g; protein: 17g; total carbs: 79g; fiber: 19g; sugar: 15g; sodium: 759mg

91) *Lighter Eggplant Parmesan*

Ingredients:

- Nonstick cooking spray
- 3 eggs, beaten, 1 tablespoon dried parsley
- 2 teaspoons ground oregano
- 1/8 teaspoon freshly ground black pepper
- 1 cup panko bread crumbs, preferably whole-wheat
- 1 large eggplant (about 2 pounds)
- 5 servings (21/2 cups) chunky tomato sauce or jarred low-sodium tomato sauce
- 1 cup part-skim mozzarella cheese
- ¼ cup grated parmesan cheese

Direction: Preparation time: 15 minutes Cooking time: 35 minutes Servings: 4

- ✓ Preheat the oven to 450f. Coat a baking sheet with cooking spray.

- In a medium bowl, whisk together the eggs, parsley, oregano, and pepper.
- Pour the panko into a separate medium bowl.
- Slice the eggplant into ¼-inch-thick slices. Dip each slice of eggplant into the egg mixture, shaking off the excess. Then dredge both sides of the eggplant in the panko bread crumbs. Place the coated eggplant on the prepared baking sheet, leaving a 1/2-inch space between each slice.
- Bake for about 15 minutes until soft and golden brown. Remove from the oven and set aside to slightly cool.
- Pour 1/2 cup of chunky tomato sauce on the bottom of an 8-by-15-inch baking dish. Using a spatula or the back of a spoon spread the tomato sauce evenly. Place half the slices of cooked eggplant, slightly overlapping, in the dish, and top with 1 cup of chunky tomato sauce, 1/2 cup of mozzarella and 2 tablespoons of grated parmesan. Repeat the layer, ending with the cheese.
- Bake uncovered for 20 minutes until the cheese is bubbling and slightly browned.
- Remove from the oven and allow cooling for 15 minutes before dividing the eggplant equally into 4 separate containers.

Nutrition: calories: 333; total fat: 14g; saturated fat: 6g; protein: 20g; total carbs: 35g; fiber: 11g; sugar: 15g

92) *Coconut-Lentil Curry*

Ingredients:

- 1 tablespoon olive oil
- 1 medium yellow onion, chopped, 1 garlic clove, minced
- 1 medium red bell pepper, diced
- 1 (15-ounce) can green or brown lentils, rinsed and drained
- 2 medium sweet potatoes, washed, peeled, and cut into bite-size chunks (about 1¼ pounds)
- 1 (15-ounce) can no-salt-added diced tomatoes
- 2 tablespoons tomato paste
- 4 teaspoons curry powder
- 1/8 teaspoon ground cloves
- 1 (15-ounce) can light coconut milk
- ¼ teaspoon salt
- 2 pieces whole-wheat naan bread, halved, or 4 slices crusty bread

Direction: Preparation time: 15 minutes Cooking time: 35 minutes Servings: 4

- In a large saucepan over medium heat, heat the olive oil. When the oil is shimmering, add both the onion and garlic and cook until the onion softens and the garlic is sweet, for about 3 minutes.
- Add the bell pepper and continue cooking until it softens, about 5 minutes more. Add the lentils, sweet potatoes, tomatoes, tomato paste, curry powder, and cloves, and bring the mixture to a boil. are softened, about 20 minutes.
- Reduce the heat to medium-low, cover, and simmer until the potatoes
- Add the coconut milk and salt, and return to a boil. Reduce the heat and simmer until the flavors combine, about 5 minutes.
- Into each of 4 containers, spoon 2 cups of curry.
- Enjoy each serving with half of a piece of naan bread or 1 slice of crusty bread.

Nutrition: calories: 559; total fat: 16g; saturated fat: 7g; protein: 16g; total carbs: 86g; fiber: 16g; sugar: 18g; sodium: 819mg

93) *Stuffed Portobello with Cheese*

Ingredients:

- 4 Portobello mushroom caps
- 1 tablespoon olive oil
- 1/2 teaspoon salt, divided
- ¼ teaspoon freshly ground black pepper, divided
- 1 cup baby spinach, chopped
- 11/2 cups part-skim ricotta cheese
- 1/2 cup part-skim shredded mozzarella cheese
- ¼ cup grated parmesan cheese
- 1 garlic clove, minced
- 1 tablespoon dried parsley
- 2 teaspoons dried oregano
- 4 teaspoons unseasoned bread crumbs, divided
- 4 servings (4 cups) roasted broccoli with shallots

Direction: Preparation time: 15 minutes Cooking time: 25 minutes Servings: 4

- Preheat the oven to 375f. Line a baking sheet with aluminum foil.
- Brush the mushroom caps with the olive oil, and sprinkle with ¼ teaspoon salt and 1/8 teaspoon pepper. Put the mushroom caps on the prepared baking sheet and bake until soft, about 12 minutes.
- In a medium bowl, mix together the spinach, ricotta, mozzarella, parmesan, garlic, parsley, oregano, and the remaining ¼ teaspoon of salt and 1/8 teaspoon of pepper.
- Spoon 1/2 cup of cheese mixture into each mushroom cap, and sprinkle each with 1 teaspoon of bread crumbs. Return the mushrooms to the oven for an additional 8 to 10 minutes until warmed through.

✓ Remove from the oven and allow the mushrooms to cool for about 10 minutes before placing each in an individual container. Add 1 cup of roasted broccoli with shallots to each container.

Nutrition: calories: 419; total fat: 30g; protein: 23g; total carbs: 19g; fiber: 2g; sugar: 3g; sodium: 790mg

94) *Lighter Shrimp Scampi*

Ingredients:

- 11/2 pounds large peeled and deveined shrimp
- ¼ teaspoon salt
- 1/8 teaspoon freshly ground black pepper
- 2 tablespoons olive oil
- 1 shallot, chopped
- 2 garlic cloves, minced
- ¼ cup cooking white wine
- Juice of 1/2 lemon (1 tablespoon)
- 1/2 teaspoon sriracha
- 2 tablespoons unsalted butter, at room temperature
- ¼ cup chopped fresh parsley
- 4 servings (6 cups) zucchini noodles with lemon vinaigrette

Direction: Preparation time: 15 minutes Cooking time: 15 minutes Servings: 4

✓ Season the shrimp with the salt and pepper.

✓ In a medium saucepan over medium heat, heat the oil. Add the shallot and garlic, and cook until the shallot softens and the garlic is fragrant, about 3 minutes. Add the shrimp, cover, and cook until opaque, 2 to 3 minutes on each side. Using a slotted spoon, transfer the shrimp to a large plate.

✓ Add the wine, lemon juice, and sriracha to the saucepan, and stir to combine. Bring the mixture to a boil, then reduce the heat and simmer until the liquid is reduced by about half, 3 minutes. Add the butter and stir until melted, about 3 minutes. Return the shrimp to the saucepan and toss to coat. Add the parsley and stir to combine.

✓ Into each of 4 containers, place 11/2 cups of zucchini noodles with lemon vinaigrette, and top with ¾ cup of scampi.

Nutrition: calories: 364; total fat: 21g; protein: 37g; total carbs: 10g; fiber: 2g; sugar: 6g; sodium: 557mg

95) *Maple-Mustard Salmon*

Ingredients:

- Nonstick cooking spray
- 1/2 cup 100% maple syrup
- 2 tablespoons Dijon mustard
- ¼ teaspoon salt
- 4 (5-ounce) salmon fillets
- 4 servings (4 cups) roasted broccoli with shallots
- 4 servings (2 cups) parsleyed whole-wheat couscous

Direction: Preparation time: 10 minutes, plus 30 minutes marinating time Cooking time: 20 minutes Servings: 4

✓ Preheat the oven to 400f. Line a baking sheet with aluminum foil and coat with cooking spray.

✓ In a medium bowl, whisk together the maple syrup, mustard, and salt until smooth.

✓ Put the salmon fillets into the bowl and toss to coat. Cover and place in the refrigerator to marinate for at least 30 minutes and up to overnight.

✓ Shake off excess marinade from the salmon fillets and place them on the prepared baking sheet, leaving a 1-inch space between each fillet. Discard the extra marinade.

✓ Bake for about 20 minutes until the salmon is opaque and a thermometer inserted in the thickest part of a fillet reads 145f.

✓ Into each of 4 resealable containers, place 1 salmon fillet, 1 cup of roasted broccoli with shallots, and 1/2 cup of parsleyed whole-wheat couscous.

Nutrition: calories: 601; total fat: 29g; saturated fat: 4g; protein: 36g; total carbs: 51g; fiber: 3g; sugar: 23g; sodium: 610mg

96) *Chicken Salad with Grapes and Pecans*

Ingredients:

- 1/3 cup unsalted pecans, chopped
- 10 ounces cooked skinless, boneless chicken breast or rotisserie chicken, finely chopped
- 1/2 medium yellow onion, finely chopped
- 1 celery stalk, finely chopped
- ¾ cup red or green seedless grapes, halved
- ¼ cup light mayonnaise
- ¼ cup nonfat plain Greek yogurt
- 1 tablespoon Dijon mustard
- 1 tablespoon dried parsley
- ¼ teaspoon salt
- 1/8 teaspoon freshly ground black pepper
- 1 cup shredded romaine lettuce
- 4 (8-inch) whole-wheat pitas

Direction: Preparation Time: 15 Minutes

Cooking Time: 5 Minutes Servings: 4

✓ Heat a small skillet over medium-low heat to toast the pecans. Cook the pecans until fragrant, about 3 minutes. Remove from the heat and set aside to cool.

- ✓ In a medium bowl, mix the chicken, onion, celery, pecans, and grapes.
- ✓ In a small bowl, whisk together the mayonnaise, yogurt, mustard, parsley, salt, and pepper. Spoon the sauce over the chicken mixture and stir until well combined.
- ✓ Into each of 4 containers, place ¼ cup of lettuce and top with 1 cup of chicken salad. Store the pitas separately until ready to serve.
- ✓ When ready to eat, stuff the serving of salad and lettuce into 1 pita.

Nutrition: Calories: 418; Total Fat: 14g; Saturated Fat: 2g; Protein: 31g; Total Carbs: 43g; Fiber: 6g;

97) *Lemony Salmon Burgers*

Ingredients:

- 2 (3-oz) cans boneless, skinless pink salmon
- 1/4 cup panko breadcrumbs
- 4 tsp. lemon juice
- 1/4 cup red bell pepper
- 1/4 cup sugar-free yogurt
- 1 egg
- 2 (1.5-oz) whole wheat hamburger toasted buns

Direction: Preparation Time: 10 Minutes

Cooking Time: 10 Minutes Servings: 4

- ✓ Mix drained and flaked salmon, finely-chopped bell pepper, panko breadcrumbs.
- ✓ Combine 2 tbsp. cup sugar-free yogurt, 3 tsp. fresh lemon juice, and egg in a bowl. Shape mixture into 2 (3-inch) patties, bake on the skillet over medium heat 4 to 5 Minutes per side.
- ✓ Stir together 2 tbsp. sugar-free yogurt and 1 tsp. lemon juice; spread over bottom halves of buns.
- ✓ Top each with 1 patty, and cover with bun tops.

This dish is very mouth-watering!

Nutrition: Calories 131 / Protein 12 / Fat 1 g / Carbs 19 g

98) *Caprese Turkey Burgers*

Ingredients:

- 1/2 lb. 93% lean ground turkey
- 2 (1,5-oz) whole wheat hamburger buns (toasted)
- 1/4 cup shredded mozzarella cheese (part-skim)
- 1 egg
- 1 small clove garlic
- 4 large basil leaves
- 1/8 tsp. salt
- 1/8 tsp. pepper
- 1 big tomato

Direction: •Preparation Time 10 Minutes Cooking Time: 10 Minutes Servings: 4

- ✓ Combine turkey, white egg, Minced garlic, salt, and pepper (mix until combined);
- ✓ Shape into 2 cutlets. Put cutlets into a skillet; cook 5 to 7 Minutes per side.
- ✓ Top cutlets properly with cheese and sliced tomato at the end of cooking.
- ✓ Put 1 cutlet on the bottom of each bun.
- ✓ Top each patty with 2 basil leaves. Cover with bun tops.

Nutrition: Calories 180 / Protein 7 g / Fat 4 g / Carbs 20 g

99) *Pasta Salad*

Ingredients:

- 8 oz. whole-wheat pasta
- 2 tomatoes
- 1 (5-oz) pkg spring mix
- 9 slices bacon
- 1/3 cup mayonnaise (reduced-fat)
- 1 tbsp. Dijon mustard
- 3 tbsp. apple cider vinegar
- 1/4 tsp. salt
- 1/2 tsp. pepper

Direction: Preparation Time: 15 Minutes Cooking Time: 15 Minutes Servings: 4

- ✓ Cook pasta.
- ✓ Chilled pasta, chopped tomatoes and spring mix in a bowl.
- ✓ Crumble cooked bacon over pasta.
- ✓ Combine mayonnaise, mustard, vinegar, salt and pepper in a small bowl.
- ✓ Pour dressing over pasta, stirring to coat.

Nutrition: Calories 200 / Protein 15 g / Fat 3 g / Carbs 6 g

100)   *Chicken, Strawberry, And Avocado Salad*

Ingredients:

- 1,5 cups chicken (skin removed)
- 1/4 cup almonds
- 2 (5-oz) pkg salad greens
- 1 (16-oz) pkg strawberries
- 1 avocado

- 1/4 cup green onion
- 1/4 cup lime juice
- 3 tbsp. extra virgin olive oil
- 2 tbsp. honey
- 1/4 tsp. salt
- 1/4 tsp. pepper

Direction: Preparation Time: 10 Minutes

Cooking Time: 5 Minutes

✓ Toast almonds until golden and fragrant.
✓ Mix lime juice, oil, honey, salt, and pepper.
✓ Mix greens, sliced strawberries, chicken, diced avocado, and sliced green onion and sliced almonds; drizzle with dressing. Toss to coat.

Nutrition: Calories 150 / Protein 15 g / Fat 10 g / Carbs 5 g

101)   *Lemon-Thyme Eggs*

Ingredients:

- 7 large eggs
- 1/4 cup mayonnaise (reduced-fat)
- 2 tsp. lemon juice
- 1 tsp. Dijon mustard
- 1 tsp. chopped fresh thyme
- 1/8 tsp. cayenne pepper

Direction: Preparation Time: 10 Minutes

Cooking Time: 5 Minutes Servings: 4

✓ Bring eggs to a boil.
✓ Peel and cut each egg in half lengthwise.
✓ Remove yolks to a bowl. Add mayonnaise, lemon juice, mustard, thyme, and cayenne to egg yolks; mash to blend. Fill egg white halves with yolk mixture.
✓ Chill until ready to serve.

Nutrition: Calories 40 / Protein 10 g / Fat 6 g / Carbs 2 g

102)   *Spinach Salad with Bacon*

Ingredients:

- 8 slices center-cut bacon
- 3 tbsp. extra virgin olive oil
- 1 (5-oz) pkg baby spinach
- 1 tbsp. apple cider vinegar
- 1 tsp. Dijon mustard
- 1/2 tsp. honey

- 1/4 tsp. salt
- 1/2 tsp. pepper

Direction: Preparation Time: 15 Minutes

Cooking Time: 0 Minutes Servings: 4

✓ Mix vinegar, mustard, honey, salt and pepper in a bowl.
✓ Whisk in oil. Place spinach in a serving bowl; drizzle with dressing, and toss to coat.
✓ Sprinkle with cooked and crumbled bacon.

Nutrition: Calories 110 / Protein 6 g / Fat 2 g / Carbs 1 g

103)   *Pea and Collards Soup*

Ingredients:

- 1/2 (16-oz) pkg black-eyed peas
- 1 onion
- 2 carrots
- 1,5 cups ham (low-sodium)
- 1 (1-lb) bunch collard greens (trimmed)
- 1 tbsp. extra virgin olive oil
- 2 cloves garlic
- 1/2 tsp. black pepper
- Hot sauce

Direction: Preparation Time: 10 Minutes

Cooking Time: 50 Minutes Servings: 4

✓ Cook chopped onion and carrots 10 Minutes.
✓ Add peas, diced ham, collards, and Minced garlic. Cook 5 Minutes.
✓ Add broth, 3 cups water, and pepper. Bring to a boil; simmer 35 Minutes, adding water if needed.

Nutrition: Calories 86 Protein 15 g Fat 2 g Carbs 9 g

104)   *Spanish Stew*

Ingredients:

- 1.1/2 (12-oz) pkg smoked chicken sausage links
- 1 (5-oz) pkg baby spinach
- 1 (15-oz) can chickpeas
- 1 (14.5-oz) can tomatoes with basil, garlic, and oregano
- 1/2 tsp. smoked paprika
- 1/2 tsp. cumin
- 3/4 cup onions
- 1 tbsp. extra virgin olive oil

Direction: Preparation Time: 10 Minutes Cooking

Time: 25 Minutes Servings: 4

✓ Cook sliced the sausage in hot oil until browned. Remove from pot.
✓ Add chopped onions; cook until tender.
✓ Add sausage, drained and rinsed chickpeas, diced tomatoes, paprika, and ground cumin. Cook 15 Minutes.
✓ Add in spinach; cook 1 to 2 Minutes.

Nutrition: Calories 200 / Protein 10 g / Fat 20 g / Carbs 1 g

105) *Creamy Taco Soup*

Ingredients:

- 3/4 lb. ground sirloin
- 1/2 (8-oz) cream cheese
- 1/2 onion
- 1 clove garlic
- 1 (10-oz) can tomatoes and green chiles
- 1 (14.5-oz) can beef broth
- 1/4 cup heavy cream
- 1,5 tsp. cumin
- 1/2 tsp. chili powder

Direction: Preparation Time: 10 Minutes

Cooking Time: 20 Minutes Servings: 4

✓ Cook beef, chopped onion, and Minced garlic until meat is browned and crumbly; drain and return to pot.
✓ Add ground cumin, chili powder, and cream cheese cut into small pieces and softened, stirring until cheese is melted.
✓ Add diced tomatoes, broth, and cream; bring to a boil, and simmer 10 Minutes. Season with pepper and salt to taste.

Nutrition: Calories 60 / Protein 3 g / Fat 1 g / Carbs 8 g

106) *Chicken with Caprese Salsa*

Ingredients:

- 3/4 lb. boneless, skinless chicken breasts
- 2 big tomatoes
- 1/2 (8-oz) ball fresh mozzarella cheese
- 1/4 cup red onion
- 2 tbsp. fresh basil
- 1 tbsp. balsamic vinegar
- 2 tbsp. extra virgin olive oil (divided)
- 1/2 tsp. salt (divided)

- 1/4 tsp. pepper (divided)

Direction: Preparation Time: 15 Minutes

Cooking Time: 5 Minutes Servings: 4

✓ Sprinkle cut in half lengthwise chicken with 1/4 tsp. salt and 1/8 tsp. pepper.
✓ Heat 1 tbsp. olive oil, cook chicken 5 Minutes.
✓ Meanwhile, mix chopped tomatoes, diced cheese, finely chopped onion, chopped basil, vinegar, 1 tbsp. oil, and 1/4 tsp. salt and 1/8 tsp. pepper.
✓ Spoon salsa over chicken.

Nutrition: Calories 210 / Protein 28 g / Fat 17 g / Carbs 0, 1 g

107) *Balsamic-Roasted Broccoli*

Ingredients:

- 1 lb. broccoli
- 1 tbsp. extra virgin olive oil
- 1 tbsp. balsamic vinegar
- 1 clove garlic
- 1/8 tsp. salt
- Pepper to taste

Direction: Preparation Time: 10 Minutes

Cooking Time: 15 Minutes Servings: 4

✓ Preheat oven to 450F.
✓ Combine broccoli, olive oil, vinegar, Minced garlic, salt, and pepper; toss.
✓ Spread broccoli on a baking sheet.
✓ Bake 12 to 15 Minutes.

Nutrition: Calories 27 / Protein 3 g / Fat 0, 3 g / Carbs 4 g

108) *Hearty Beef and Vegetable Soup*

Ingredients:

- 1/2 lb. lean ground beef
- 2 cups beef broth
- 1,5 tbsp. vegetable oil (divided)
- 1 cup green bell pepper
- 1/2 cup red onion
- 1 cup green cabbage
- 1 cup frozen mixed vegetables
- 1/2 can tomatoes
- 1,5 tsp. Worcestershire sauce
- 1 small bay leaf

- 1,8 tsp. pepper
- 2 tbsp. ketchup

Direction: Preparation Time: 10 Minutes

Cooking Time: 30 Minutes Servings: 4

✓ Cook beef in 1/2 tbsp. hot oil 2 Minutes.
✓ Stir in chopped bell pepper and chopped onion; cook 4 Minutes.
✓ Add chopped cabbage, mixed vegetables, stewed tomatoes, broth, Worcestershire sauce, bay leaf, and pepper; bring to a boil.
✓ Reduce heat to medium; cover, and cook 15 Minutes.
✓ Stir in ketchup and 1 tbsp. oil, and remove from heat. Let stand 10 Minutes.

Nutrition: Calories 170 / Protein 17 g / Fat 8 g / Carbs 3 g

109) *Cauliflower Muffin*

Ingredients:

- 2,5 cup cauliflower
- 2/3 cup ham
- 2,5 cups of cheese
- 2/3 cup champignon
- 1,5 tbsp. flaxseed
- 3 eggs
- 1/4 tsp. salt
- 1/8 tsp. pepper

Direction: Preparation Time: 15 Minutes

Cooking Time: 30 Minutes Servings: 4

✓ Preheat oven to 375 F.
✓ Put muffin liners in a 12-muffin tin.
✓ Combine diced cauliflower, ground flaxseed, beaten eggs, cup diced ham, grated cheese, and diced mushrooms, salt, pepper.
✓ Divide mixture rightly between muffin liners.
✓ Bake 30 Minutes.

Nutrition: Calories 116 / Protein 10 g / Fat 7 g / Carbs 3 g

110) *Ham and Egg Cups*

Ingredients:

- 5 slices ham
- 4 tbsp. cheese
- 1,5 tbsp. cream
- 3 egg whites
- 1,5 tbsp. pepper (green)

- 1 tsp. salt
- pepper to taste

Direction: Preparation Time: 10 Minutes

Cooking Time: 15 Minutes Servings: 4

✓ Preheat oven to 350 F.
✓ Arrange each slice of thinly sliced ham into 4 muffin tin.
✓ Put 1/4 of grated cheese into ham cup.
✓ Mix eggs, cream, salt and pepper and divide it into 2 tins.
✓ Bake in oven 15 Minutes; after baking, sprinkle with green onions.

Nutrition: Calories 180 / Protein 13 g / Fat 13 g / Carbs 2 g

111) *Cauliflower Rice with Chicken*

Ingredients:

- 1/2 large cauliflower
- 3/4 cup cooked meat
- 1/2 bell pepper
- 1 carrot
- 2 ribs celery
- 1 tbsp. stir fry sauce (low carb)
- 1 tbsp. extra virgin olive oil
- Salt and pepper to taste

Direction: Preparation Time: 15 Minutes Cooking Time: 15 Minutes Servings: 4

✓ Chop cauliflower in a processor to "rice." Place in a bowl.
✓ Properly chop all vegetables in a food processor into thin slices.
✓ Chop cauliflower in a processor to "rice." Place in a bowl.
✓ Properly chop all vegetables in a food processor into thin slices.
✓ Add cauliflower and other plants to WOK with heated oil. Fry until all veggies are tender.
✓ Add chopped meat and sauce to the wok and fry 10 Minutes and Serve. This dish is very mouth-watering!

Nutrition: Calories 200 / Protein 10 g / Fat 12 g /Carbs 10 g

112) *Turkey with Fried Eggs*

Ingredients:

- 4 large potatoes

- 1 cooked turkey thigh
- 1 large onion (about 2 cups diced)
- butter
- Chile flakes
- 4 eggs
- salt to taste
- pepper to taste

Direction: Preparation Time: 10 Minutes

Cooking Time: 20 Minutes Servings: 4

- ✓ Rub the cold boiled potatoes on the coarsest holes of a box grater. Dice the turkey.
- ✓ Cook the onion in as much unsalted butter as you feel comfortable with until it's just fragrant and translucent.
- ✓ Add the rubbed potatoes and a cup of diced cooked turkey, salt and pepper to taste, and cook 20 Minutes.

Nutrition: Calories 170 / Protein 19 g / Fat 7 g / Carbs 6 g

DINNER

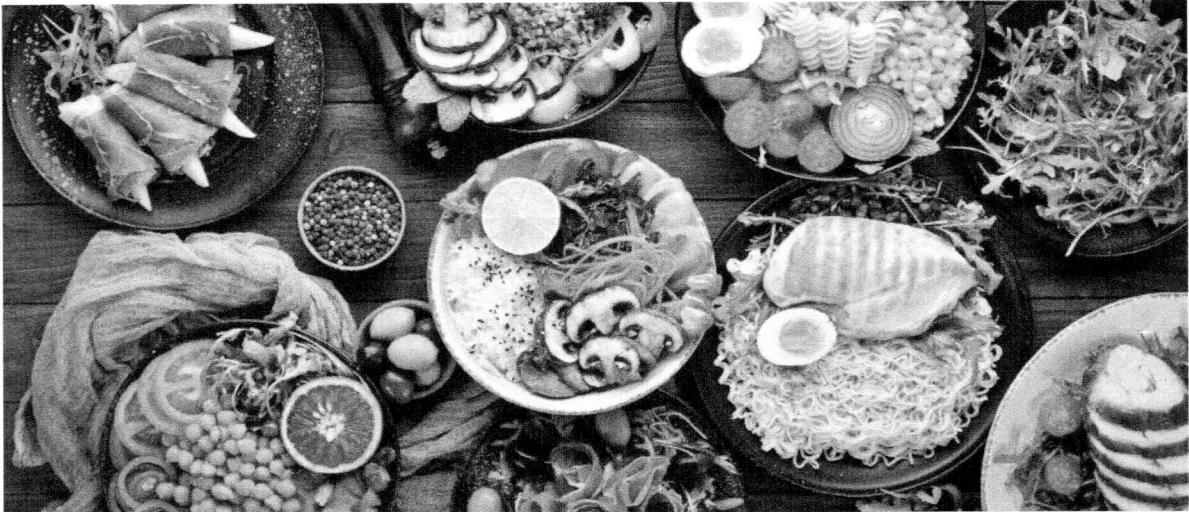

113)   *Salmon with Asparagus*

Ingredients:

- 1 lb. Salmon, sliced into fillets
- 1 tbsp. Olive Oil
- Salt & Pepper, as needed
- 1 bunch of Asparagus, trimmed
- 2 cloves of Garlic, minced
- Zest & Juice of 1/2 Lemon
- 1 tbsp. Butter, salted

Direction: Preparation Time: 5 Minutes

Cooking Time: 10 Minutes Servings: 3

- ✓ Spoon in the butter and olive oil into a large pan and heat it over medium-high heat.
- ✓ Once it becomes hot, place the salmon and season it with salt and pepper.
- ✓ Cook for 4 minutes per side and then cook the other side.
- ✓ Stir in the garlic and lemon zest to it.
- ✓ Cook for further 2 minutes or until lightly browned.
- ✓ Off the heat and squeeze the lemon juice over it.
- ✓ Serve it hot.

Nutrition: Calories: 409Kcal; Carbohydrates: 2.7g; Proteins: 32.8g; Fat: 28.8g; Sodium: 497mg

114)   *Shrimp in Garlic Butter*

Ingredients:

- 1 lb. Shrimp, peeled & deveined
- ¼ tsp. Red Pepper Flakes
- 6 tbsp. Butter, divided
- 1/2 cup Chicken Stock
- Salt & Pepper, as needed
- 2 tbsp. Parsley, minced
- 5 cloves of Garlic, minced
- 2 tbsp. Lemon Juice

Direction: Preparation Time: 5 Minutes

Cooking Time: 20 Minutes Servings: 4

- ✓ Heat a large bottomed skillet over medium-high heat.
- ✓ Spoon in two tablespoons of the butter and melt it. Add the shrimp.
- ✓ Season it with salt and pepper. Sear for 4 minutes or until shrimp gets cooked.
- ✓ Transfer the shrimp to a plate and stir in the garlic.
- ✓ Sauté for 30 seconds or until aromatic.
- ✓ Pour the chicken stock and whisk it well. Allow it to simmer for 5 to 10 minutes or until it has reduced to half.
- ✓ Spoon the remaining butter, red pepper, and lemon juice to the sauce. Mix.
- ✓ Continue cooking for another 2 minutes.
- ✓ Take off the pan from the heat and add the cooked shrimp to it.
- ✓ Garnish with parsley and transfer to the serving bowl.

Nutrition: Calories: 307Kcal; Carbs: 3g; Proteins: 27g; Fat: 20g; Sodium: 522mg

115)   *Cobb Salad*

Ingredients:

- 4 Cherry Tomatoes, chopped
- ¼ cup Bacon, cooked & crumbled
- 1/2 of 1 Avocado, chopped
- 2 oz. Chicken Breast, shredded
- 1 Egg, hardboiled
- 2 cups Mixed Green salad
- 1 oz. Feta Cheese, crumbled

Direction: Preparation Time: 5 Minutes

Cooking Time: 5 Minutes Servings: 1

- ✓ Toss all the ingredients for the Cobb salad in a large mixing bowl and toss well.
- ✓ Serve and enjoy it.

Nutrition: Calories: 307Kcal; Carbs: 3g; Proteins: 27g; Fat: 20g; Sodium: 522mg

116)   *Seared Tuna Steak*

Ingredients:

- 1 tsp. Sesame Seeds
- 1 tbsp. Sesame Oil
- 2 tbsp. Soya Sauce
- Salt & Pepper, to taste
- 2 × 6 oz. Ahi Tuna Steaks

Direction: Preparation Time: 10 Minutes

Cooking Time: 10 Minutes Serving Size: 2

- ✓ Seasoning the tuna steaks with salt and pepper. Keep it aside on a shallow bowl.
- ✓ In another bowl, mix soya sauce and sesame oil.
- ✓ pour the sauce over the salmon and coat them generously with the sauce.
- ✓ Keep it aside for 10 to 15 minutes and then heat a large skillet over medium heat.

✓ Once hot, keep the tuna steaks and cook them for 3 minutes or until seared underneath.

✓ Flip the fillets and cook them for a further 3 minutes.

✓ Transfer the seared tuna steaks to the serving plate and slice them into 1/2 inch slices. Top with sesame seeds.

Nutrition: Calories: 255Kcal; Fat: 9g; Carbs: 1g; Proteins: 40.5g; Sodium: 293mg

117) *Beef Chili*

Ingredients:

- 1/2 tsp. Garlic Powder
- 1 tsp. Coriander, grounded
- 1 lb. Beef, grounded
- 1/2 tsp. Sea Salt
- 1/2 tsp. Cayenne Pepper
- 1 tsp. Cumin, grounded
- 1/2 tsp. Pepper, grounded
- 1/2 cup Salsa, low-carb & no-sugar

Direction: Preparation Time: 10 Minutes Cooking Time: 20 Minutes Serving Size: 4

✓ Heat a large-sized pan over medium-high heat and cook the beef in it until browned.

✓ Stir in all the spices and cook them for 7 minutes or until everything is combined.

✓ When the beef gets cooked, spoon in the salsa.

✓ Bring the mixture to a simmer and cook for another 8 minutes or until everything comes together.

✓ Take it from heat and transfer to a serving bowl

Nutrition: Calories: 229Kcal; Fat: 10g; Carbs: 2g; Proteins: 33g; Sodium: 675mg

118) *Greek Broccoli Salad*

Ingredients:

- 1 ¼ lb. Broccoli, sliced into small bites
- ¼ cup Almonds, sliced
- 1/3 cup Sun-dried Tomatoes
- ¼ cup Feta Cheese, crumbled
- ¼ cup Red Onion, sliced

For the dressing:
- 1/4 cup Olive Oil
- Dash of Red Pepper Flakes
- 1 Garlic clove, minced
- ¼ tsp. Salt

- 2 tbsp. Lemon Juice
- 1/2 tsp. Dijon Mustard
- 1 tsp. Low Carb Sweetener Syrup
- 1/2 tsp. Oregano, dried

Direction: Preparation Time: 10 Minutes Cooking Time: 15 Minutes Servings: 4

✓ Mix broccoli, onion, almonds and sun-dried tomatoes in a large mixing bowl.

✓ In another small-sized bowl, combine all the dressing ingredients until emulsified. ✓ Spoon the dressing over the broccoli salad.

✓ Allow the salad to rest for half an hour before serving.

Nutrition: Calories: 272Kcal; Carbohydrates: 11.9g; Proteins: 8g

119) *Cheesy Cauliflower Gratin*

Ingredients:

- 6 deli slices Pepper Jack Cheese
- 4 cups Cauliflower florets
- Salt and Pepper, as needed
- 4 tbsp. Butter
- 1/3 cup Heavy Whipping Cream

Direction: Preparation Time: 5 Minutes Cooking Time: 25 Minutes Servings: 6

✓ Mix the cauliflower, cream, butter, salt, and pepper in a safe microwave bowl and combine well.

✓ Microwave the cauliflower mixture for 25 minutes on high until it becomes soft and tender.

✓ Remove the ingredients from the bowl and mash with the help of a fork.

✓ Taste for seasonings and spoon in salt and pepper as required.

✓ Arrange the slices of pepper jack cheese on top of the cauliflower mixture and microwave for 3 minutes until the cheese starts melting.

✓ Serve warm.

Nutrition: Calories: 421Kcal; Carbs: 3g; Proteins: 19g; Fat: 37g; Sodium: 111mg

120) *Strawberry Spinach Salad*

Ingredients:

- 4 oz. Feta Cheese, crumbled
- 8 Strawberries, sliced
- 2 oz. Almonds
- 6 Slices Bacon, thick-cut, crispy and crumbled
- 10 oz. Spinach leaves, fresh
- 2 Roma Tomatoes, diced
- 2 oz. Red Onion, sliced thinly

Direction: Preparation Time: 5 Minutes

Cooking Time: 10 Minutes Servings: 4

✓ For making this healthy salad, mix all the ingredients needed to make the salad in a large-sized bowl and toss them well.
✓ Enjoy

Nutrition: Calories – 255kcal; Fat – 16g; Carbs – 8g; Proteins – 14g; Sodium: 27mg

121) *Cauliflower Mac & Cheese*

Ingredients:

- 1 Cauliflower Head, torn into florets
- Salt & Black Pepper, as needed
- ¼ cup Almond Milk, unsweetened
- ¼ cup Heavy Cream
- 3 tbsp. Butter, preferably grass-fed
- 1 cup Cheddar Cheese, shredded

Direction: Preparation Time: 5 Minutes Cooking Time: 25 Minutes Serving Size: 4

✓ Preheat the oven to 450 F.
✓ Melt the butter in a small microwave-safe bowl and heat it for 30 seconds.
✓ Pour the melted butter over the cauliflower florets along with salt and pepper. Toss them well.
✓ Place the cauliflower florets in a parchment paper-covered large baking sheet.
✓ Bake them for 15 minutes or until the cauliflower is crisp-tender.
✓ Once baked, mix the heavy cream, cheddar cheese, almond milk, and the remaining butter in a large microwave-safe bowl and heat it on high heat for 2 minutes or until the cheese mixture is smooth. Repeat the procedure until the cheese has melted.
✓ Finally, stir in the cauliflower to the sauce mixture and coat well.

Nutrition: Calories: 294Kcal; Fat: 23g; Carbohydrates: 7g; Proteins: 11g

122) *Easy Egg Salad*

Ingredients:

- 6 Eggs, preferably free-range
- ¼ tsp. Salt
- 2 tbsp. Mayonnaise
- 1 tsp. Lemon juice
- 1 tsp. Dijon mustard
- Pepper, to taste
- Lettuce leaves, to serve

Direction: Preparation Time: 5 Minutes Cooking Time: 15 to 20 Minutes Servings: 4

✓ Keep the eggs in a saucepan of water and pour cold water until it covers the egg by another 1 inch.
✓ Bring to a boil and then remove the eggs from heat.
✓ Peel the eggs under cold running water.
✓ Transfer the cooked eggs into a food processor and pulse them until chopped.
✓ Stir in the mayonnaise, lemon juice, salt, Dijon mustard, and pepper and mix them well.
✓ Taste for seasoning and add more if required.
✓ Serve in the lettuce leaves.

Nutrition: Calories – 166kcal; Fat – 14g; Carbs - 0.85g; Proteins – 10g; Sodium 132mg

123) *Baked Chicken Legs*

Ingredients:

- 6 Chicken Legs
- ¼ tsp. Black Pepper
- ¼ cup Butter
- 1/2 tsp. Sea Salt
- 1/2 tsp. Smoked Paprika
- 1/2 tsp. Garlic Powder

Direction: Preparation Time: 10 Minutes

Cooking Time: 40 Minutes Servings: 6

✓ Preheat the oven to 425 F.
✓ Pat the chicken legs with a paper towel to absorb any excess moisture.
✓ Marinate the chicken pieces by first applying the butter over them and then with the seasoning. Set it aside for a few minutes.
✓ Bake them for 25 minutes. Turnover and bake for further 10 minutes or until the internal temperature reaches 165 F.
✓ Serve them hot.

Nutrition: Calories – 236kL; Fat – 16g; Carbs – 0g; Protein – 22g; Sodium – 314mg

124) *Creamed Spinach*

Ingredients:

- 3 tbsp. Butter
- ¼ tsp. Black Pepper
- 4 cloves of Garlic, minced
- ¼ tsp. Sea Salt
- 10 oz. Baby Spinach, chopped
- 1 tsp. Italian Seasoning

- 1/2 cup Heavy Cream
- 3 oz. Cream Cheese

Direction: Preparation Time: 5 Minutes

Cooking Time: 10 Minutes Servings: 4

✓ Melt butter in a large sauté pan over medium heat.
✓ Once the butter has melted, spoon in the garlic and sauté for 30 seconds or until aromatic.
✓ Spoon in the spinach and cook for 3 to 4 minutes or until wilted.
✓ Add all the remaining ingredients to it and continuously stir until the cream cheese melts and the mixture gets thickened.
✓ Serve hot

Nutrition: Calories – 274kL; Fat – 27g; Carbs – 4g; Protein – 4g; Sodium – 114mg

125) *Stuffed Mushrooms*

Ingredients:

- 4 Portobello Mushrooms, large
- 1/2 cup Mozzarella Cheese, shredded
- 1/2 cup Marinara, low-sugar
- Olive Oil Spray

Direction: Preparation Time: 10 Minutes

Cooking Time: 20 Minutes Servings: 4

✓ Preheat the oven to 375 F.
✓ Take out the dark gills from the mushrooms with the help of a spoon.
✓ Keep the mushroom stem upside down and spoon it with two tablespoons of marinara sauce and mozzarella cheese.
✓ Bake for 18 minutes or until the cheese is bubbly.

Nutrition: Calories – 113kL; Fat – 6g; Carbs – 4g; Protein – 7g; Sodium – 14mg

126) *Vegetable Soup*

Ingredients:

- 8 cups Vegetable Broth
- 2 tbsp. Olive Oil
- 1 tbsp. Italian Seasoning
- 1 Onion, large & diced
- 2 Bay Leaves, dried
- 2 Bell Pepper, large & diced
- Sea Salt & Black Pepper, as needed
- 4 cloves of Garlic, minced

- 28 oz. Tomatoes, diced
- 1 Cauliflower head, medium & torn into florets
- 2 cups Green Beans, trimmed & chopped

Direction: Preparation Time: 10 Minutes Cooking Time: 30 Minutes Servings: 5

✓ Heat oil in a Dutch oven over medium heat.
✓ Once the oil becomes hot, stir in the onions and pepper.
✓ Cook for 10 minutes or until the onion is softened and browned.
✓ Spoon in the garlic and sauté for a minute or until fragrant.
✓ Add all the remaining ingredients to it. Mix until everything comes together.
✓ Bring the mixture to a boil. Lower the heat and cook for further 20 minutes or until the vegetables have softened.
✓ Serve hot.

Nutrition: Calories – 79kL; Fat – 2g; Carbs – 8g; Protein – 2g; Sodium – 187mg

127) *Misto Quente*

Ingredients:

- 4 slices of bread without shell
- 4 slices of turkey breast
- 4 slices of cheese
- 2 tbsp. cream cheese
- 2 spoons of butter

Direction: Preparation time: 5 minutes

Cooking time: 10 minutes Servings: 4

✓ Preheat the air fryer. Set the timer of 5 minutes and the temperature to 200C.
✓ Pass the butter on one side of the slice of bread, and on the other side of the slice, the cream cheese.
✓ Mount the sandwiches placing two slices of turkey breast and two slices cheese between the breads, with the cream cheese inside and the side with butter.
✓ Place the sandwiches in the basket of the air fryer. Set the timer of the air fryer for 5 minutes and press the power button.

Nutrition: Calories: 340 Fat: 15g Carbs: 32g Protein: 15g Sugar: 0g Cholesterol: 0mg

128) *Garlic Bread*

Ingredients: Garlic Bread

- 2 stale French rolls
- 4 tbsp. crushed or crumpled garlic

- 1 cup of mayonnaise
- Powdered grated Parmesan
- 1 tbsp. olive oil

Direction: Preparation time: 10 minutes Cooking time: 15 minutes Servings: 4-5

✓ Preheat the air fryer. Set the time of 5 minutes and the temperature to 2000C.
✓ Mix mayonnaise with garlic and set aside.
✓ Cut the baguettes into slices, but without separating them completely.
✓ Fill the cavities of equals. Brush with olive oil and sprinkle with grated cheese.
✓ Place in the basket of the air fryer. Set the timer to 10 minutes, adjust the temperature to 1800C and press the power button.

Nutrition: Calories: 340 Fat: 15g Carbs: 32g Protein: 15g Sugar: 0g Cholesterol: 0mg

129) *Bruschetta*

Ingredients:

- 4 slices of Italian bread
- 1 cup chopped tomato tea
- 1 cup grated mozzarella tea
- Olive oil
- Oregano, salt, and pepper
- 4 fresh basil leaves

Direction: Preparation time: 5 minutes| Cooking time: 10 minutes Servings: 2

✓ Preheat the air fryer. Set the timer of 5 minutes and the temperature to 2000C.
✓ Sprinkle the slices of Italian bread with olive oil. Divide the chopped tomatoes and mozzarella between the slices. Season with salt, pepper, and oregano.
✓ Put oil in the filling. Place a basil leaf on top of each slice.
✓ Put the bruschetta in the basket of the air fryer being careful not to spill the filling. Set the timer of 5 minutes, set the temperature to 180C, and press the power button.
✓ Transfer the bruschetta to a plate and serve.

Nutrition: Calories: 434 Fat: 14g Carbohydrates: 63g Protein: 11g Sugar: 8g Cholesterol: 0mg

130) *Cauliflower Potato Mash*

Ingredients:

- 2 cups potatoes, peeled and cubed
- 2 tbsp. butter
- ¼ cup milk

- 10 oz. cauliflower florets
- ¾ tsp. salt

Direction: Preparation Time: 30 minutes Servings:4 Cooking Time: 5 minutes

✓ Add water to the saucepan and bring to boil.
✓ Reduce heat and simmer for 10 minutes.
✓ Drain vegetables well. Transfer vegetables, butter, milk, and salt in a blender and blend until smooth.

Nutrition: Calories 128 Fat 6.2 g, Sugar 3.3 g, Protein 3.2 g, Cholesterol 17 mg

131) *Cream Buns with Strawberries*

Ingredients:

- 240g all-purpose flour
- 50g granulated sugar
- 8g baking powder
- 1g of salt
- 85g chopped cold butter
- 84g chopped fresh strawberries
- 120 ml whipping cream
- 2 large eggs
- 10 ml vanilla extract
- 5 ml of water

Direction: Preparation time: 10 minutes Cooking time: 12 minutes Servings: 6

✓ Sift flour, sugar, baking powder and salt in a large bowl. Put the butter with the flour with the use of a blender or your hands until the mixture resembles thick crumbs.
✓ Mix the strawberries in the flour mixture. Set aside for the mixture to stand. Beat the whipping cream, 1 egg and the vanilla extract in a separate bowl.
✓ Put the cream mixture in the flour mixture until they are homogeneous, and then spread the mixture to a thickness of 38 mm.
✓ Use a round cookie cutter to cut the buns. Spread the buns with a combination of egg and water. Set aside
✓ Preheat the air fryer, set it to 180C.
✓ Place baking paper in the preheated inner basket.
✓ Place the buns on top of the baking paper and cook for 12 minutes at 180C, until golden brown.

Nutrition: Calories: 150 Fat: 14g Carbs: 3g Protein: 11g Sugar: 8g Cholesterol: 0mg

132) *Blueberry Buns*

Ingredients:

240g all-purpose flour
- 50g granulated sugar
- 8g baking powder
- 2g of salt
- 85g chopped cold butter
- 85g of fresh blueberries
- 3g grated fresh ginger
- 113 ml whipping cream
- 2 large eggs
- 4 ml vanilla extract
- 5 ml of water

Direction: Preparation time: 10 minutes
Cooking time: 12 minutes Servings: 6

✓ Put sugar, flour, baking powder and salt in a large bowl.
✓ Put the butter with the flour using a blender or your hands until the mixture resembles thick crumbs.
✓ Mix the blueberries and ginger in the flour mixture and set aside
✓ Mix the whipping cream, 1 egg and the vanilla extract in a different container.
✓ Put the cream mixture with the flour mixture until combined.
✓ Shape the dough until it reaches a thickness of approximately 38 mm and cut it into eighths.
✓ Spread the buns with a combination of egg and water. Set aside Preheat the air fryer set it to 180C.
✓ Place baking paper in the preheated inner basket and place the buns on top of the paper. Cook for 12 minutes at 180C, until golden brown

Nutrition: Calories: 105 Fat: 1.64g Carbs: 20.09g Protein: 2.43g Sugar: 2.1g Cholesterol: 0mg

133) *French toast in Sticks*

Ingredients:

- 4 slices of white bread, 38 mm thick, preferably hard
- 2 eggs
- 60 ml of milk
- 15 ml maple sauce
- 2 ml vanilla extract
- Nonstick Spray Oil
- 38g of sugar
- 3 ground cinnamon
- Maple syrup, to serve
- Sugar to sprinkle

Direction: Preparation time: 5 minutes
Cooking time: 10 minutes Servings: 4

✓ Cut each slice of bread into thirds making 12 pieces. Place sideways
✓ Beat the eggs, milk, maple syrup and vanilla.
✓ Preheat the air fryer, set it to 175C.
✓ Dip the sliced bread in the egg mixture and place it in the preheated air fryer. Sprinkle French toast generously with oil spray.
✓ Cook French toast for 10 minutes at 175C. Turn the toast halfway through cooking.
✓ Mix the sugar and cinnamon in a bowl.
✓ Cover the French toast with the sugar and cinnamon mixture when you have finished cooking.
✓ Serve with Maple syrup and sprinkle with powdered sugar

Nutrition: : Calories 128, Fat 6.2 g, Carbs 16.3 g, Sugar 3.3 g, Protein 3.2 g

134) *Muffins Sandwich*

Ingredients:

- Nonstick Spray Oil
- 1 slice of white cheddar cheese
- 1 slice of Canadian bacon
- 1 English muffin, divided
- 15 ml hot water
- 1 large egg
- Salt and pepper to taste

Direction: Preparation time: 2 minutes

Cooking time: 10 minutes Servings: 1

✓ Spray the inside of an 85g mold with oil spray and place it in the air fryer.
✓ Preheat the air fryer, set it to 160C.
✓ Add the Canadian cheese and bacon in the preheated air fryer.
✓ Pour the hot water and the egg into the hot pan and season with salt and pepper.
✓ Select Bread, set to 10 minutes.
✓ Take out the English muffins after 7 minutes, leaving the egg for the full time.
✓ Build your sandwich by placing the cooked egg on top of the English muffins and serve

Nutrition: Calories 400 Fat 26g, Carbs 26g, Sugar 15 g, Protein 3 g, Cholesterol 155 mg

135) *Bacon BBQ*

Ingredients:

- 13g dark brown sugar
- 5g chili powder

- 1g ground cumin
- 1g cayenne pepper
- 4 slices of bacon, cut in half

Direction: Preparation time: 2 minutes Cooking time: 8 minutes Servings: 2

- ✓ Mix seasonings until well combined.
- ✓ Dip the bacon in the dressing until it is completely covered. Leave aside.
- ✓ Preheat the air fryer, set it to 160C.
- ✓ Place the bacon in the preheated air fryer
- ✓ Select Bacon and press Start/Pause.

Nutrition: Calories: 1124 Fat: 72g Carbs: 59g Protein: 49g Sugar: 11g Cholesterol 77mg

136) *Stuffed French toast*

Ingredients:

- 1 slice of brioche bread,
- 64 mm thick, preferably rancid
- 113g cream cheese
- 2 eggs
- 15 ml of milk
- 30 ml whipping cream
- 38g of sugar
- 3g cinnamon
- 2 ml vanilla extract
- Nonstick Spray Oil
- Pistachios chopped to cover
- Maple syrup, to serve

Direction: Preparation time: 4 minutes Cooking time: 10 minutes Servings: 1

- ✓ Preheat the air fryer, set it to 175C.
- ✓ Cut a slit in the middle of the muffin.
- ✓ Fill the inside of the slit with cream cheese. Leave aside.
- ✓ Mix the eggs, milk, whipping cream, sugar, cinnamon, and vanilla extract.
- ✓ Moisten the stuffed French toast in the egg mixture for 10 seconds on each side.
- ✓ Sprinkle each side of French toast with oil spray.
- ✓ Place the French toast in the preheated air fryer and cook for 10 minutes at 175C
- ✓ Stir the French toast carefully with a spatula when you finish cooking.
- ✓ Serve topped with chopped pistachios and acrid syrup.

Nutrition: Calories: 159 Fat: 7.5g Carbs: 25.2g Protein: 14g Sugar: 0g Cholesterol 90mg

137) *Scallion Sandwich*

Ingredients:

- 2 slices wheat bread
- 2 teaspoons butter, low fat
- 2 scallions, sliced thinly
- 1 tablespoon of parmesan cheese, grated
- 3/4 cup of cheddar cheese, reduced fat, grated

Direction: Preparation Time: 10 minutes Cooking Time: 10 minutes Servings: 1

- ✓ Preheat the Air fryer to 356 degrees.
- ✓ Spread butter on a slice of bread. Place inside the cooking basket with the butter side facing down.
- ✓ Place cheese and scallions on top. Spread the rest of the butter on the other slice of bread Put it on top of the sandwich and sprinkle with parmesan cheese.
- ✓ Cook for 10 minutes.

Nutrition: Calorie: 154 Carbohydrate: 9g Fat: 2.5g Protein: 8.6g

138) *Lean Lamb and Turkey Meatballs with Yogurt*

Ingredients:

- 1 egg white
- 4 ounces ground lean turkey
- 1 pound of ground lean lamb
- 1 teaspoon each of cayenne pepper, ground coriander, red chili paste, salt, and ground cumin
- 2 garlic cloves, minced
- 1 1/2 tablespoons parsley, chopped
- 1/4 cup of olive oil
- 1 tablespoon mint, chopped,

For the yogurt

- 2 tablespoons of buttermilk
- 1 garlic clove, minced
- 1/4 cup mint, chopped
- 1/2 cup of Greek yogurt, non-fat
- Salt to taste

Direction: Preparation Time: 10 minutes Servings: 4 Cooking Time: 8 minutes

- ✓ Set the Air Fryer to 390 degrees.
- ✓ Mix all the ingredients for the meatballs in a bowl. Roll and mold them into golf-size round pieces. Arrange in the cooking basket. Cook for 8 minutes.
- ✓ While waiting, combine all the ingredients for the

mint yogurt in a bowl. Mix well.

✓ Serve the meatballs with the mint yogurt. Top with olives and fresh mint.

Nutrition: Calorie: 154 Carbohydrate: 9g Fat: 2.5g Protein: 8.6g Fiber: 2.4g

139) *Air Fried Section and Tomato*

Ingredients:

- 1 aubergine, sliced thickly into 4 disks
- 1 tomato, sliced into 2 thick disks
- 2 tsp. feta cheese, reduced fat
- 2 fresh basil leaves, minced
- 2 balls, small buffalo mozzarella, reduced fat, roughly torn
- Pinch of salt
- Pinch of black pepper

Direction: Preparation Time: 10 minutes Cooking Time: 5 minutes Servings: 2

✓ Preheat Air Fryer to 330 degrees F.

✓ Spray small amount of oil into the Air fryer basket. Fry aubergine slices for 5 minutes or until golden brown on both sides. Transfer to a plate.

✓ Fry tomato slices in batches for 5 minutes or until seared on both sides.

✓ To serve, stack salad starting with an aubergine base, buffalo mozzarella, basil leaves, tomato slice, and 1/2-teaspoon feta cheese.

✓ Top of with another slice of aborigine and 1/2 tsp. feta cheese. Serve.

Nutrition: Calorie: 140.3 Carbohydrate: 26.6 Fat: 3.4g Protein: 4.2g Fiber: 7.3g

140) *Cheesy Salmon Fillets*

Ingredients:

Ingredients: For the salmon fillets

- 2 pieces, 4 oz. each salmon fillets, choose even cuts
- 1/2 cup sour cream, reduced fat
- ¼ cup cottage cheese, reduced fat
- ¼ cup Parmigiano-Reggiano cheese, freshly grated

Garnish:

- Spanish paprika
- 1/2 piece lemon, cut into wedges

Direction: Preparation Time: 15 minutes Cooking Time: 20 minutes Servings: 2-3

✓ Preheat Air Fryer to 330 degrees F.

✓ To make the salmon fillets, mix sour cream, cottage cheese, and Parmigiano-Reggiano cheese in a bowl.

✓ Layer salmon fillets in the Air fryer basket. Fry for 20 minutes or until cheese turns golden brown.

✓ To assemble, place a salmon fillet and sprinkle paprika. Garnish with lemon wedges and squeeze lemon juice on top. Serve.

Nutrition: Calorie: 274 Carbohydrate: 1g Fat: 19g Protein: 24g

APPETIZERS AND SALADS

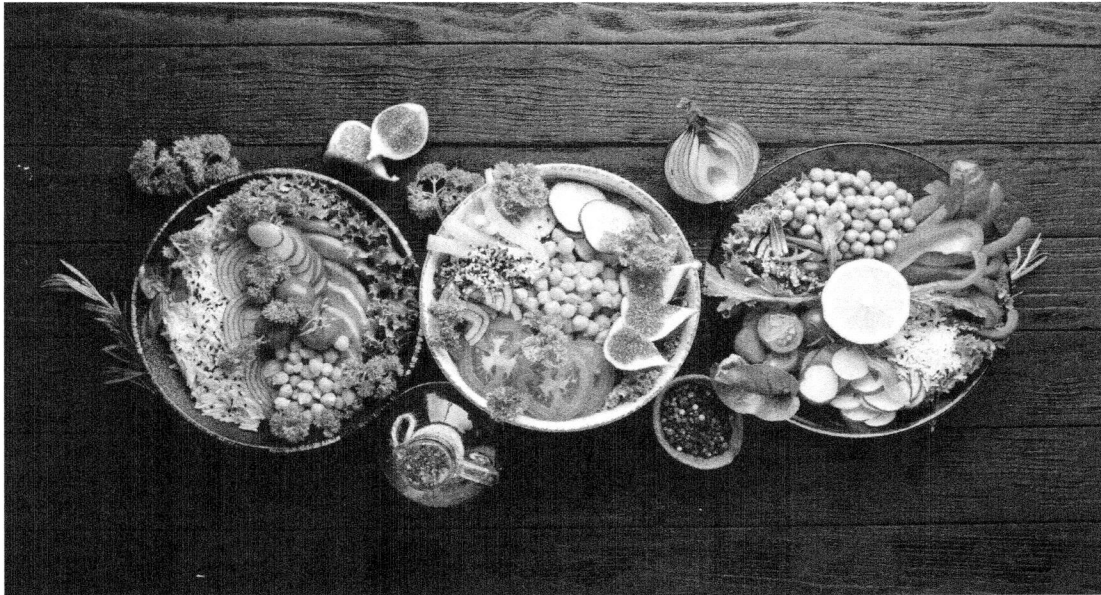

141) *Tuna Salad Recipe 1*

Ingredients:

- 1 can tuna (6 oz.)
- 1/3 cup fresh cucumber, chopped
- 1/3 cup fresh tomato, chopped
- 1/3 cup avocado, chopped
- 1/3 cup celery, chopped
- 2 garlic cloves, minced
- 4 tsp. olive oil
- 2 tbsp. lime juice
- Pinch of black pepper

Direction: Preparation Time: 10 minutes

Cooking time: none Servings: 3

✓ Prepare the dressing by combining olive oil, lime juice, minced garlic and black pepper.
✓ Mix the salad ingredients in a salad bowl and drizzle with the dressing.

Nutrition: Carbohydrates: 4.8 g Protein: 14.3 g Total sugars: 1.1 g Calories: 212 g

142) *Roasted Portobello Salad*

Ingredients:

- 1 1/2 lb. Portobello mushrooms, stems trimmed
- 3 heads Belgian endive, sliced
- 1 small red onion, sliced
- 4 oz. blue cheese
- 8 oz. mixed salad greens
Dressing:
- 3 tbsp. red wine vinegar
- 1 tbsp. Dijon mustard
- 2/3 cup olive oil
- Salt and pepper to taste

Direction: Preparation Time: 10 minutes Cooking time: none Servings: 4

✓ Preheat the oven to 450F.
✓ Prepare the dressing by whisking together vinegar, mustard, salt and pepper. Slowly add olive oil while whisking.
✓ Cut the mushrooms and arrange them on a baking sheet, stem-side up. Coat the mushrooms with some dressing and bake for 15 minutes.
✓ In a salad bowl toss the salad greens with onion, endive and cheese. Sprinkle with the dressing.
✓ Add mushrooms to the salad bowl.

Nutrition: Carbohydrates: 22.3 g Protein: 14.9 g Total sugars: 2.1 g Calories: 501

143) *Shredded Chicken Salad*

Ingredients:

- 2 chicken breasts, boneless, skinless
- 1 head iceberg lettuce, cut into strips
- 2 bell peppers, cut into strips
- 1 fresh cucumber, quartered, sliced
- 3 scallions, sliced
- 2 tbsp. chopped peanuts
- 1 tbsp. peanut vinaigrette
- Salt to taste
- 1 cup water

Direction: Preparation Time: 5 minutes

Cooking time: 10 minutes Servings: 6

✓ In a skillet simmer one cup of salted water.
✓ Add the chicken breasts, cover and cook on low for 5 minutes. Remove the cover. Then remove the chicken from the skillet and shred with a fork.
✓ In a salad bowl mix the vegetables with the cooled chicken, season with salt and sprinkle with peanut vinaigrette and chopped peanuts.

Nutrition: Carbohydrates: 9 g Protein: 11.6 g Total Calories: 117

144) *Broccoli Salad 1*

Ingredients:

- 1 medium head broccoli, raw, florets only
- 1/2 cup red onion, chopped
- 12 oz. turkey bacon, chopped, fried until crisp
- 1/2 cup cherry tomatoes, halved
- ¼ cup sunflower kernels
- ¾ cup raisins
- ¾ cup mayonnaise
- 2 tbsp. white vinegar

Direction: Preparation Time: 10 minutes Cooking time: none Servings: 6

✓ In a salad bowl combine the broccoli, tomatoes and onion.
✓ Mix mayo with vinegar and sprinkle over the broccoli.
✓ Add the sunflower kernels, raisins and bacon and toss well.

Nutrition: Carbohydrates: 17.3 g Protein: 11 g Total sugars: 10 g Calories: 220

145) *Cherry Tomato Salad*

Ingredients:

- 40 cherry tomatoes, halved
- 1 cup mozzarella balls, halved
- 1 cup green olives, sliced
- 1 can (6 oz.) black olives, sliced
- 2 green onions, chopped
- 3 oz. roasted pine nuts

Dressing:

- 1/2 cup olive oil
- 2 tbsp. red wine vinegar
- 1 tsp. dried oregano
- Salt and pepper to taste

Direction: Preparation Time: 10 minutes Cooking time: none Servings: 6

- ✓ In a salad bowl, combine the tomatoes, olives and onions.
- ✓ Prepare the dressing by combining olive oil with red wine vinegar, dried oregano, salt and pepper.
- ✓ Sprinkle with the dressing and add the nuts.
- ✓ Let marinate in the fridge for 1 hour.

Nutrition: Carbohydrates: 10.7 g Protein: 2.4 g Total sugars: 3.6 g

146) *Ground Turkey Salad*

Ingredients:

- 1 lb. lean ground turkey
- 1/2 inch ginger, minced
- 2 garlic cloves, minced
- 1 onion, chopped
- 1 tbsp. olive oil
- 1 bag lettuce leaves (for serving)
- ¼ cup fresh cilantro, chopped
- 2 tsp. coriander powder
- 1 tsp. red chili powder
- 1 tsp. turmeric powder
- Salt to taste
- 4 cups water
- Dressing:
- 2 tbsp. fat free yogurt
- 1 tbsp. sour cream, non-fat
- 1 tbsp. low fat mayonnaise
- 1 lemon, juiced
- 1 tsp. red chili flakes
- Salt and pepper to taste

Direction: Preparation Time: 10 minutes Cooking time: 35 minutes Servings: 6

- ✓ In a skillet sauté the garlic and ginger in olive oil for 1 minute. Add onion and season with salt. Cook for 10 minutes over medium heat.
- ✓ Add the ground turkey and sauté for 3 more minutes. Add the spices (turmeric, red chili powder and coriander powder).
- ✓ Add 4 cups water and cook for 30 minutes, covered.
- ✓ Prepare the dressing by combining yogurt, sour cream, mayo, lemon juice, chili flakes, salt and pepper.
- ✓ To serve arrange the salad leaves on serving plates and place the cooked ground turkey on them. Top with dressing.

Nutrition: Carbohydrates: 9.1 g Protein: 17.8 g Total sugars: 2.5 g Calories: 176

147) *Asian Cucumber Salad*

Ingredients:

- 1 lb. cucumbers, sliced
- 2 scallions, sliced
- 2 tbsp. sliced pickled ginger, chopped
- ¼ cup cilantro
- 1/2 red jalapeño, chopped
- 3 tbsp. rice wine vinegar
- 1 tbsp. sesame oil
- 1 tbsp. sesame seeds

Direction: Preparation Time: 10 minutes Cooking time: none Servings: 6

- ✓ In a salad bowl combine all ingredients and toss together.
- ✓ Enjoy!

Nutrition: Carbohydrates: 5.7 g Protein: 1 g Total sugars: 3.1 g Calories: 52

148) *Cauliflower Tofu Salad*

Ingredients:

- 2 cups cauliflower florets, blended
- 1 fresh cucumber, diced
- 1/2 cup green olives, diced
- 1/3 cup red onion, diced
- 2 tbsp. toasted pine nuts
- 2 tbsp. raisins
- 1/3 cup feta, crumbled
- 1/2 cup pomegranate seeds
- 2 lemons (juiced, zest grated)

- 8 oz. tofu
- 2 tsp. oregano
- 2 garlic cloves, minced
- 1/2tsp. red chili flakes
- 3 tbsp. olive oil
- Salt and pepper to taste

Direction: Preparation time: 10 minutes Cooking time: 15 minutes Servings: 4

✓ Season the processed cauliflower with salt and transfer to a strainer to drain.
✓ Prepare the marinade for tofu by combining 2 tbsp. lemon juice, 1.5 tbsp. olive oil, minced garlic, chili flakes, oregano, salt and pepper. Coat tofu in the marinade and set aside.
✓ Preheat the oven to 450F.
✓ Bake tofu on a baking sheet for 12 minutes.
✓ In a salad bowl mix the remaining marinade with onions, cucumber, cauliflower, olives and raisins. Add in the remaining olive oil and grated lemon zest.
✓ Top with tofu, pine nuts, and feta and pomegranate seeds.

Nutrition: Carbohydrates: 34.1 g Protein: 11.1 g Total sugars: 11.5 g Calories: 328

149)   *Scallop Caesar Salad*

Ingredients:

- 8 sea scallops
- 4 cups romaine lettuce
- 2 tsp. olive oil
- 3 tbsp. Caesar Salad Dressing
- 1 tsp. lemon juice
- Salt and pepper to taste

Direction: Preparation Time: 5 minutes Cooking Time: 2 minutes Servings: 2

✓ In a frying pan heat olive oil and cook the scallops in one layer no longer than 2 minutes per both sides. Season with salt and pepper to taste.
✓ Arrange lettuce on plates and place scallops on top.
✓ Pour over the Caesar dressing and lemon juice.

Nutrition: Carbohydrates: 14 g Protein: 30.7 g Total sugars: 2.2 g Calories: 340 g

150)   *Chicken Avocado Salad*

Ingredients:

- 1 lb. chicken breast, cooked, shredded
- 1 avocado, pitted, peeled, sliced
- 2 tomatoes, diced

- 1 cucumber, peeled, sliced
- 1 head lettuce, chopped
- 3 tbsp. olive oil
- 2 tbsp. lime juice
- 1 tbsp. cilantro, chopped
- Salt and pepper to taste

Direction: Preparation Time: 30 minutes

Cooking time: 15 minutes Servings: 4

✓ In a bowl whisk together oil, lime juice, cilantro, salt, and a pinch of pepper.
✓ Combine lettuce, tomatoes, cucumber in a salad bowl and toss with half of the dressing.
✓ Toss chicken with the remaining dressing and combine with vegetable mixture.
✓ Top with avocado.

Nutrition: Carbohydrates: 10 g Protein: 38 g Total sugars: 11.5 g Calories: 380

151)   *California Wraps*

Ingredients:

- 4 slices turkey breast, cooked
- 4 slices ham, cooked
- 4 lettuce leaves
- 4 slices tomato
- 4 slices avocado
- 1 tsp. lime juice
- A handful watercress leaves
- 4 tbsp. Ranch dressing, sugar free

Direction: Preparation Time: 5 minutes Cooking Time: 15 minutes Servings: 4

✓ Top a lettuce leaf with turkey slice, ham slice and tomato.
✓ In a bowl combine avocado and lime juice and place on top of tomatoes. Top with water cress and dressing.
✓ Repeat with the remaining ingredients for 4. Topping each lettuce leaf with a turkey slice, ham slice, tomato and dressing.

Nutrition: Carbohydrates: 4 g Protein: 9 g Total sugars: 0.5 g Calories: 140

152)   *Chicken Breast Salad*

Ingredients:

- 1/2 chicken breast, skinless, boiled and shredded
- 2 long cucumbers, cut into 8 thick rounds each, scooped out (won't use in a).
- 1 tsp. ginger, minced

- 1 tsp. lime zest, grated
- 4 tsp. olive oil
- 1 tsp. sesame oil
- 1 tsp. lime juice
- Salt and pepper to taste

Direction: Preparation Time: 5 minutes Cooking Time: 15 minutes Servings: 4

✓ In a bowl combine lime zest, juice, olive and sesame oils, ginger, and season with salt.
✓ Toss the chicken with the dressing and fill the cucumber cups with the salad.

Nutrition: Carbohydrates: 4 g Protein: 12 g Total sugars: 0.5 g Calories: 116 g

153) *Sunflower Seeds and Arugula Garden Salad*

Ingredients:

- ¼ tsp. black pepper
- ¼ tsp. salt
- 1 tsp. fresh thyme, chopped
- 2 tbsp. sunflower seeds, toasted
- 2 cups red grapes, halved
- 7 cups baby arugula, loosely packed
- 1 tbsp. coconut oil
- 2 tsp. honey
- 3 tbsp. red wine vinegar
- 1/2tsp. stone-ground mustard

Direction: Preparation time: 5 minutes

Cooking time: 10 minutes Servings: 6

✓ In a small bowl, whisk together mustard, honey and vinegar. Slowly pour oil as you whisk.
✓ In a large salad bowl, mix thyme, seeds, grapes and arugula.
✓ Drizzle with dressing and serve.

Nutrition: Calories: 86.7g Protein: 1.6g Carbs: 13.1g Fat: 3.1g.

154) *Supreme Caesar Salad*

Ingredients:

- ¼ cup olive oil
- ¾ cup mayonnaise
- 1 head romaine lettuce, torn into bite sized pieces
- 1 tbsp. lemon juice
- 1 tsp. Dijon mustard
- 1 tsp. Worcestershire sauce

- 3 cloves garlic, peeled and minced
- 3 cloves garlic, peeled and quartered
- 4 cups day old bread, cubed
- 5 anchovy filets, minced
- 6 tbsp. grated parmesan cheese, divided
- Ground black pepper to taste
- Salt to taste

Direction: Preparation time: 5 minutes Cooking time: 10 minutes Servings: 4

✓ In a small bowl, whisk well lemon juice, mustard, Worcestershire sauce, 2 tbsp. parmesan cheese, anchovies, mayonnaise, and minced garlic. Season with pepper and salt to taste. Set aside in the ref.
✓ On medium fire, place a large nonstick saucepan and heat oil.
✓ Sauté quartered garlic until browned around a minute or two. Remove and discard.
✓ Add bread cubes in same pan, sauté until lightly browned. Season with pepper and salt. Transfer to a plate.
✓ In large bowl, place lettuce and pour in dressing. Toss well to coat. Top with remaining parmesan cheese.
✓ Garnish with bread cubes, serve, and enjoy.

Nutrition: Calories: 443.3g Fat: 32.1g Protein: 11.6g Carbs: 27g

155) *Tabbouleh- Arabian Salad*

Ingredients:

- ¼ cup chopped fresh mint
- 1 2/3 cups boiling water
- 1 cucumber, peeled, seeded and chopped
- 1 cup bulgur
- 1 cup chopped fresh parsley
- 1 cup chopped green onions
- 1 tsp. salt
- 1/3 cup lemon juice
- 1/3 cup olive oil
- 3 tomatoes, chopped
- Ground black pepper to taste

Direction: Preparation time: 5 minutes

Cooking time: 10 minutes Servings: 6

✓ In a large bowl, mix together boiling water and bulgur. Let soak and set aside for an hour while covered.
✓ After one hour, toss in cucumber, tomatoes, mint, parsley, onions, lemon juice and oil. Then season with black pepper and salt to taste. Toss well and

refrigerate for another hour while covered before serving.

Nutrition: Calories: 185.5g fat: 13.1g Protein: 4.1g Carbs: 12.8g

156)   *Broccoli Salad 2*

Ingredients:

- 8 cups broccoli florets
- 3 strips of bacon, cooked and crumbled
- ¼ cup sunflower kernels
- 1 bunch of green onion, sliced

What you will need from the store cupboard:

- 3 tablespoons seasoned rice vinegar
- 3 tablespoons canola oil
- 1/2 cup dried cranberries

Direction: Preparation Time: 10 minutes, Cooking Time: 10 minutes; Servings: 10

- ✓ Combine the green onion, cranberries, and broccoli in a bowl.
- ✓ Whisk the vinegar, and oil in another bowl. Blend well.
- ✓ Now drizzle over the broccoli mix.
- ✓ Coat well by tossing.
- ✓ Sprinkle bacon and sunflower kernels before serving.

Nutrition: Calories 121, Carbs 14g, Cholesterol 2mg, Fiber 3g, Sugar 1g, Fat 7g, Protein 3g, Sodium 233mg

157)   *Tenderloin Grilled Salad*

Ingredients:

- 1 lb. pork tenderloin
- 10 cups mixed salad greens
- 2 oranges, seedless, cut into bite-sized pieces
- 1 tablespoon orange zest, grated

What you will need from the store cupboard:

- 2 tablespoons of cider vinegar
- 2 tablespoons olive oil
- 2 teaspoons Dijon mustard
- 1/2 cup juice of an orange
- 2 teaspoons honey
- 1/2 teaspoon ground pepper

Direction:

- ✓ Bring together all the dressing ingredients in a bowl.
- ✓ Grill each side of the pork covered over medium heat for 9 minutes.

- ✓ Slice after 5 minutes.
- ✓ Slice the tenderloin thinly.
- ✓ Keep the greens on your serving plate.
- ✓ Top with the pork and oranges.
- ✓ Sprinkle nuts (optional).

Nutrition: Calories 211, Carbs 13g, Cholesterol 51mg, Fiber 3g, Sugar 0.8g, Fat 9g, Protein 20g, Sodium 113mg

158)   *Barley Veggie Salad*

Ingredients:

- 1 tomato, seeded and chopped
- 2 tablespoons parsley, minced
- 1 yellow pepper, chopped
- 1 tablespoon basil, minced
- ¼ cup almonds, toasted

What you will need from the store cupboard:

- 1-1/4 cups vegetable broth
- 1 cup barley
- 1 tablespoon lemon juice
- 2 tablespoons of white wine vinegar
- 3 tablespoons olive oil
- ¼ teaspoon pepper
- 1/2 teaspoon salt
- 1 cup of water

Direction: Preparation Time: 10 minutes, Cooking Time: 20 minutes; Servings: 6

- ✓ Boil the broth, barley, and water in a saucepan.
- ✓ Reduce heat. Cover and let it simmer for 10 minutes.
- ✓ Take out from the heat.
- ✓ In the meantime, bring together the parsley, yellow pepper, and tomato in a bowl.
- ✓ Stir the barley in.
- ✓ Whisk the vinegar, oil, basil, lemon juice, water, pepper and salt in a bowl.
- ✓ Pour this over your barley mix. Toss to coat well.
- ✓ Stir the almonds in before serving.

Nutrition: Calories 211, Carbs 27g, Cholesterol 0mg, Fiber 7g, Sugar 0g, Fat 10g, Protein 6g, Sodium 334mg

159)   *Spinach Shrimp Salad*

Ingredients:

- 1 lb. uncooked shrimp, peeled and deveined
- 2 tablespoons parsley, minced
- ¾ cup halved cherry tomatoes
- 1 medium lemon

• 4 cups baby spinach

What you will need from the store cupboard:

- 2 tablespoons butter
- 3 minced garlic cloves
- ¼ teaspoon pepper
- ¼ teaspoon salt

Direction:

✓ Melt the butter over medium temperature in a nonstick skillet.
✓ Add the shrimp.
✓ Now cook the shrimp for 3 minutes until your shrimp becomes pink.
✓ Add the parsley and garlic.
✓ Cook for another minute. Take out from the heat.
✓ Keep the spinach in your salad bowl.
✓ Top with the shrimp mix and tomatoes.
✓ Drizzle lemon juice on the salad.
✓ Sprinkle pepper and salt.

Nutrition: Calories 201, Carbs 6g, Cholesterol 153mg, Fiber 2g, Sugar 0g, Fat 10g, Protein 21g, Sodium 350mg

160) *Sweet Potato and Roasted Beet Salad*

Ingredients:

- 2 beets
- 1 sweet potato, peeled and cubed
- 1 garlic clove, minced
- 2 tablespoons walnuts, chopped and toasted
- 1 cup fennel bulb, sliced

What you will need from the store cupboard:

- 3 tablespoons balsamic vinegar
- 1 teaspoon Dijon mustard
- 1 tablespoon honey
- 3 tablespoons olive oil
- ¼ teaspoon pepper
- ¼ teaspoon salt
- 3 tablespoons water

Direction: Preparation Time: 20 minutes, Cooking Time: 20-30 minutes; Servings: 6

✓ Scrub the beets. Trim the tops to 1 inch.
✓ Wrap in foil and keep on a baking sheet.
✓ Bake until tender. Take off the foil.
✓ Combine water and sweet potato in a bowl.
✓ Cover. Microwave for 5 minutes. Drain off.
✓ Now peel the beets. Cut into small wedges.
✓ Arrange the fennel, sweet potato and beets on 4 salad plates.
✓ Sprinkle nuts.
✓ Whisk the honey, mustard, vinegar, water, garlic, pepper and salt.
✓ Whisk in oil gradually.
✓ Drizzle over the salad.

Nutrition: Calories 270, Carbs 37g, Cholesterol 0mg, Fiber 6g, Sugar 0.3g, Fat 13g, Protein 5g, Sodium 309mg

161) *Potato Calico Salad*

Ingredients:

- 4 red potatoes, peeled and cooked
- 1-1/2 cups kernel corn, cooked
- 1/2 cup green pepper, diced
- 1/2 cup red onion, chopped
- 1 cup carrot, shredded

What you will need from the store cupboard:

- 1/2 cup olive oil
- ¼ cup vinegar
- 1-1/2 teaspoons chili powder
- 1 teaspoon salt
- Dash of hot pepper sauce

Direction: Preparation Time: 15 minutes, Cooking Time: 5 minutes; Servings: 14

✓ Keep all the ingredients together in a jar.
✓ Close it and shake well.
✓ Cube the potatoes. Combine with the carrot, onion, and corn in your salad bowl.
✓ Pour the dressing over.
✓ Now toss lightly.

Nutrition: Calories 146, Carbs 17g, Cholesterol 0mg, Fiber 0g, Sugar 0g, Fat 9g, Protein 2g, Sodium 212mg

162) *Mango and Jicama Salad*

Ingredients:

- 1 jicama, peeled
- 1 mango, peeled
- 1 teaspoon ginger root, minced
- 1/3 cup chives, minced
- 1/2 cup cilantro, chopped

What you will need from the store cupboard:

- ¼ cup canola oil
- 1/2 cup white wine vinegar

- 2 tablespoons of lime juice
- ¼ cup honey
- 1/8 teaspoon pepper
- ¼ teaspoon salt

Direction: Preparation Time: 15 minutes, Cooking Time: 5 minutes; Servings: 8

✓ Whisk together the vinegar, honey, canola oil, gingerroot, paper, and salt.
✓ Cut the mango and jicama into matchsticks.
✓ Keep in a bowl.
✓ Now toss with the lime juice.
✓ Add the dressing and herbs. Combine well by tossing.

Nutrition: Calories 143, Carbs 20g, Cholesterol 0mg, Fiber 3g, Sugar 1.6g, Fat 7g, Protein 1g, Sodium 78mg

163) *Asian Crispy Chicken Salad*

Ingredients:

- 2 chicken breast halved, skinless
- 1/2 cup panko bread crumbs
- 4 cups spring mix salad greens
- 4 teaspoons of sesame seeds
- 1/2 cup mushrooms, sliced

What you will need from the store cupboard:

- 1 teaspoon sesame oil
- 2 teaspoons of canola oil
- 2 teaspoons hoisin sauce
- ¼ cup sesame ginger salad dressing

Direction: Preparation Time: 15 minutes, Cooking Time: 5 minutes; Servings: 2

✓ Flatten the chicken breasts to half-inch thickness.
✓ Mix the sesame oil and hoisin sauce. Brush over the chicken.
✓ Combine the sesame seeds and panko in a bowl.
✓ Now dip the chicken mix in it.
✓ Cook each side of the chicken for 5 minutes.
✓ In the meantime, divide the salad greens between two plates.
✓ Top with mushroom.
✓ Slice the chicken and keep on top. Drizzle the dressing.

Nutrition: Calories 386, Carbs 29g, Cholesterol 63mg, Fiber 6g, Sugar 1g, Fat 17g, Protein 30g, Sodium 620mg

164) *Kale, Grape and Bulgur Salad*

Ingredients:

- 1 cup bulgur
- 1 cup pecan, toasted and chopped
- ¼ cup scallions, sliced
- 1/2 cup parsley, chopped
- 2 cups California grapes, seedless and halved

What you will need from the store cupboard:

- 2 tablespoons of extra virgin olive oil
- ¼ cup of juice from a lemon
- Pinch of kosher salt
- Pinch of black pepper
- 2 cups of water

Direction: Preparation Time: 18 minutes, Cooking Time: 10 minutes; Servings: 8

✓ Boil 2 cups of water in a saucepan.
✓ Stir the bulgur in and 1/2 teaspoon of salt.
✓ Take out from the heat.
✓ Keep covered. Drain.
✓ Stir in the other ingredients.
✓ Season with pepper and salt.

Nutrition: Calories 289, Carbohydrates 33g, Fat 17g, Protein 6g,

165) *Strawberry Salsa*

Ingredients:

- 4 tomatoes, seeded and chopped
- 1-pint strawberry, chopped
- 1 red onion, chopped
- 2 tablespoons of juice from a lime

What you will need from the store cupboard:

- 1 tablespoon olive oil
- 2 garlic cloves, minced
- 1 jalapeno pepper, minced

Direction: Preparation Time: 12 minutes, Cooking Time: 10 minutes; Servings: 4

✓ Bring together the strawberries, tomatoes, jalapeno, and onion in the bowl.
✓ Stir in the garlic, oil, and lime juice.
✓ Refrigerate. Serve with separately cooked pork or poultry.

Nutrition: Calories 19, Carbs 3g, Fiber 1g, Sugar 0.2g, Cholesterol 0mg, Total Fat 1g, Protein 0g

166)   *Garden Wraps*

Ingredients:

- 1 cucumber, chopped
- 1 sweet corn
- 1 cabbage, shredded
- 1 tablespoon lettuce, minced
- 1 tomato, chopped

What you will need from the store cupboard:

- 3 tablespoons of rice vinegar
- 2 teaspoons peanut butter
- 1/3 cup onion paste
- 1/3 cup chili sauce
- 2 teaspoons of low-sodium soy sauce

Direction: Preparation Time: 20 minutes, Cooking Time: 10 minutes; Servings: 8

- ✓ Cut corn from the cob. Keep in a bowl.
- ✓ Add the tomato, cabbage, cucumber, and onion paste.
- ✓ Now whisk the vinegar, peanut butter, and chili sauce together.
- ✓ Pour this over the vegetable mix. Toss for coating.
- ✓ Let this stand for 10 minutes.
- ✓ Take your slotted spoon and place 1/2 cup salad in every lettuce leaf.
- ✓ Fold the lettuce over your filling.

Nutrition: Calories 64, Carbs 13g, Fiber 2g, Sugar 1g, Cholesterol 0mg, Total Fat 1g, Protein 2g

167)   *Party Shrimp*

Ingredients:

- 16 oz. uncooked shrimp, peeled and deveined
- 1-1/2 teaspoons of juice from a lemon
- 1/2 teaspoon basil, chopped
- 1 teaspoon coriander, chopped
- 1/2 cup tomato

What you will need from the store cupboard:

- 1 tablespoon of olive oil
- 1/2 teaspoon Italian seasoning
- 1/2 teaspoon paprika
- 1 sliced garlic clove
- ¼ teaspoon pepper

Direction: Preparation Time: 15 minutes, Cooking Time: 10 minutes; Servings: 30

- ✓ Bring together everything except the shrimp in a dish or bowl.

- ✓ Add the shrimp. Coat well by tossing. Set aside.
- ✓ Drain the shrimp. Discard the marinade.
- ✓ Keep them on a baking sheet. It should not be greased.
- ✓ Broil each side for 4 minutes. The shrimp should become pink.

Nutrition: Calories 14, Carbs 0g, Fiber 0g, Sugar 0g, Cholesterol 18mg

168)   *Zucchini Mini Pizzas*

Ingredients:

- 1 zucchini, cut into ¼ inch slices diagonally
- 1/2 cup pepperoni, small slices
- 1 teaspoon basil, minced
- 1/2 cup onion, chopped
- 1 cup tomatoes

What you will need from the store cupboard:

- 1/8 teaspoon pepper
- 1/8 teaspoon salt
- 3/4 cup mozzarella cheese, shredded
- 1/3 cup pizza sauce

Direction: Preparation Time: 20 minutes, Cooking Time: 5-10 minutes; Servings: 2

- ✓ Preheat your broiler. Keep the zucchini in 1 layer on your greased baking sheet.
- ✓ Add the onion and tomatoes. Broil each side for 1 to 2 minutes till they become tender and crisp.
- ✓ Now sprinkle pepper and salt.
- ✓ Top with cheese, pepperoni, and sauce.
- ✓ Broil for a minute. The cheese should melt.
- ✓ Sprinkle basil on top.

Nutrition: Calories 29, Carbs 1g, Fiber 0g, Sugar 1g, Cholesterol 5mg, Total Fat 2g, Protein 2g

169)   *Garlic-Sesame Pumpkin Seeds*

Ingredients:

- 1 egg white
- 1 teaspoon onion, minced
- 1/2 teaspoon caraway seeds
- 2 cups pumpkin seeds
- 1 teaspoon sesame seeds

What you will need from the store cupboard:

- 1 garlic clove, minced
- 1 tablespoon of canola oil

- ¾ teaspoon of kosher salt

Direction: Preparation Time: 10 minutes

Cooking Time: 20 minutes Servings: 2

✓ Preheat your oven to 350 °F .
✓ Whisk together the oil and egg white in a bowl.
✓ Include pumpkin seeds. Coat well by tossing.
✓ Now stir in the onion, garlic, sesame seeds, caraway seeds, and salt ✓   Spread in 1 layer in your parchment-lined baking pan.
✓ Bake for 15 minutes until it turns golden brown.

Nutrition: Calories 95, Carbs 9g, Fiber 3g, Sugar 0g, Cholesterol 0mg, Total Fat 5g, Protein 4g

170)   *Tuna Salad Recipe2*

Ingredients:

- 2 (5-ounce) cans water packed tuna, drained
- 2 tablespoons fat-free plain Greek yogurt
- Salt and ground black pepper, as required •   2 medium carrots, peeled and shredded
- 2 apples, cored and chopped
- 2 cups fresh spinach, torn

Direction: Preparation Time: 15 minutes

Servings: 2

✓ In a large bowl, add the tuna, yogurt, salt and black pepper and gently, stir to combine.   ✓   Add the carrots and apples and stir to combine.
✓ Serve immediately.

Nutrition: Calories 306; Total Fat 1.8g ; Saturated Fat 0 g ; Cholesterol 63 mg ; Total Carbs 38 g Sugar 26 g ; Fiber 7.6 g ; Sodium 324 mg ; Potassium 602 mg ; Protein 35.8 g

POULTRY

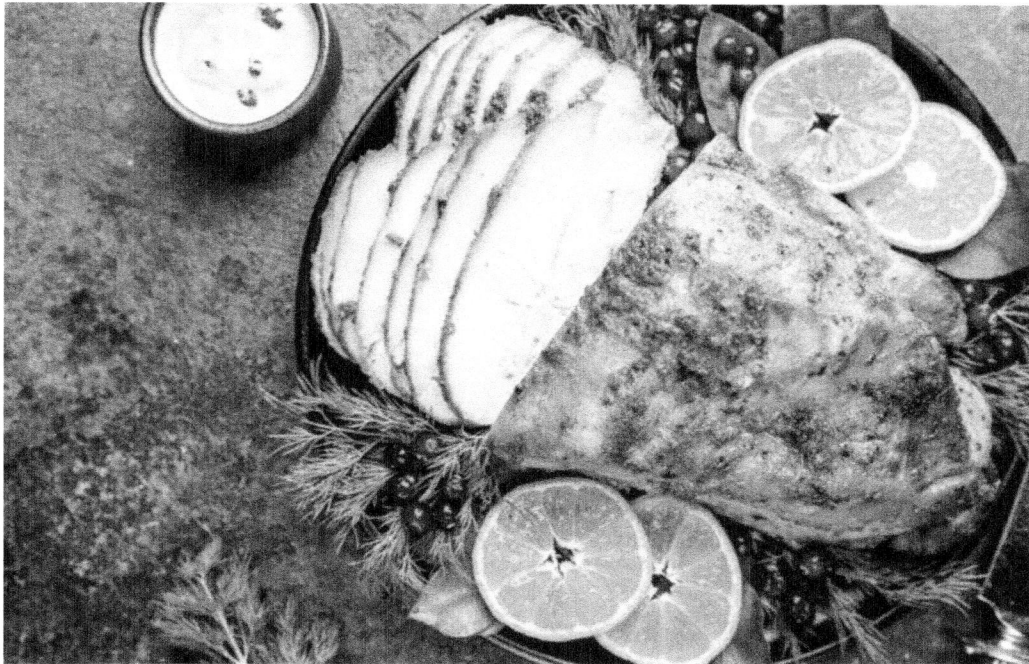

171)   Chicken Soup

Ingredients:

- 1 tablespoon olive oil
- 1 small carrot, peeled and chopped ½ cup onion, chopped
- 1 celery stalk, chopped 2 garlic cloves, minced
- 1 tablespoon fresh thyme, chopped 1 tablespoon fresh rosemary, chopped
- ½ teaspoon ground cumin
- ¼ teaspoon red pepper flakes, crushed lime zest, grated finely
- 5 cups low-sodium chicken broth
- 1¼ cups cooked chicken, chopped
- 2 cups fresh spinach, torn
- 1¼ cups zucchini, chopped
- Ground black pepper, as required
- 2 tablespoons fresh lime juice

Direction: Preparation Time: 15 minutes Cooking Time: 23 minutes Servings: 4

- ✓ In a large soup pan, heat the oil over medium heat and sauté the carrot, onion and celery for about 8-9 minutes.
- ✓ Add the garlic, rosemary and spices and sauté for about 1 minute.
- ✓ Add the broth and bring to a boil over high heat.
- ✓ Now, reduce the heat to medium-low and simmer for about 5 minutes.
- ✓ Add the cooked chicken, spinach and zucchini and simmer for about 6-8 minutes.
- ✓ Stir in the black pepper and lime juice and remove from heat.
- ✓ Serve hot with the garnishing of lime zest. Meal Prep Tip: Transfer the soup into a large bowl and set aside to cool.
- ✓ Divide the soup into 4 containers evenly. Cover the containers and refrigerate for 1-2 days. Reheat in the microwave before serving.

Nutrition: Calories 224 Total Fat 6.8g Total Carbs 7.5 g Sugar 2 g Fiber 2.2 g Protein 31.8 g

172)   Chicken Chili

Ingredients:

- 4 cups low-sodium chicken broth, divided
- 3 cups boiled black beans, divided 1 tablespoon extra-virgin olive oil
- 1 large onion, chopped 1 jalapeño pepper, seeded and chopped
- 4 garlic cloves, minced 1 teaspoon dried thyme, crushed

- 1½ tablespoons ground coriander
- 1 tablespoon ground cumin
- ½ tablespoon red chili powder
- 4 cups cooked chicken, shredded
- 1 tablespoon fresh lime juice
- ¼ cup fresh cilantro, chopped

Direction: Preparation Time: 15 minutes Cooking Time: 40 minutes Servings: 6

- ✓ In a food processor, add 1 cup of broth and 1 can of black beans and pulse until smooth. Transfer the beans puree into a bowl and set aside.
- ✓ In a large pan, heat the oil over medium heat and sauté the onion and jalapeño for about 4-5 minutes.
- ✓ Add the garlic, spices and sea salt and sauté for about 1 minute.
- ✓ Add the beans puree and remaining broth and bring to a boil. Now, reduce the heat to low and simmer for about 20 minutes.
- ✓ Stir in the remaining can of beans, chicken and lime juice and bring to a boil.
- ✓ Now, reduce the heat to low and simmer for about 5-10 minutes.
- ✓ Serve hot with the garnishing of cilantro.
- ✓ Meal Prep Tip: Transfer the chili into a large bowl and set aside to cool.
- ✓ Divide the chili into 6 containers evenly. Cover the containers and refrigerate for 1-2 days.
- ✓ Reheat in the microwave before serving.

Nutrition: Calories 356 Total Fat 7.1 g Carbs 33 g S Protein 39.6 g

173)   Chicken with Chickpeas

Ingredients:

- 2 tablespoons olive oil
- 1 pound skinless, boneless chicken breast, cubed
- 2 carrots, peeled and sliced 1 onion, chopped
- 2 celery stalks, chopped 2 garlic cloves, chopped
- 1 tablespoon fresh ginger root, minced
- ½ teaspoon dried oregano, crushed
- ¾ teaspoon ground cumin
- ½ teaspoon paprika
- ¼-13 teaspoon cayenne pepper
- ¼ teaspoon ground turmeric
- 1 cup tomatoes, crushed
- 1½ cups low-sodium chicken broth
- 1 zucchini, sliced
- 1 cup boiled chickpeas, drained
- 1 tablespoon fresh lemon juice

Direction: Preparation Time: 15 minutes Cooking Time: 36 minutes Servings: 4

- ✓ In a large nonstick pan, heat the oil over medium heat and cook the chicken cubes for about 4-5 minutes.
- ✓ With a slotted spoon, transfer the chicken cubes onto a plate.
- ✓ In the same pan, add the carrot, onion, celery and garlic and sauté for about 4-5 minutes.
- ✓ Add the ginger, oregano and spices and sauté for about 1 minute.
- ✓ Add the chicken, tomato and broth and bring to a boil. Now, reduce the heat to low and simmer for about 10 minutes.
- ✓ Add the zucchini and chickpeas and simmer, covered for about 15 minutes. Stir in the lemon juice and serve hot.

Meal Prep Tip:

- ✓ Transfer the chicken mixture into a large bowl and set aside to cool. Divide the mixture into 4 containers evenly. Cover the containers and refrigerate for 1-2 days. Reheat in the microwave before serving.

Nutrition: Calories 308 Total Fat 12.3 g Saturated Fat 2.7 g Cholesterol 66 mg Total Carbs 19 g Sugar 5.3g Fiber 4.7 g Sodium 202 mg Protein 30.7 g

174)   *Chicken & Broccoli Bake*

Ingredients:

- 6 (6-ounce) boneless, skinless chicken breasts
- 3 broccoli heads, cut into florets
- 4 garlic cloves, minced
- ¼ cup olive oil
- 1 teaspoon dried oregano, crushed
- 1 teaspoon dried rosemary, crushed
- Sea Salt and ground black pepper, as required

Direction: Preparation Time: 15 minutes Cooking Time: 45 minutes Servings: 6

- ✓ Preheat the oven to 375 degrees F. Grease a large baking dish. In a large bowl, add all the ingredients and toss to coat well.
- ✓ In the bottom of prepared baking dish, arrange the broccoli florets and top with chicken breasts in a single layer.
- ✓ Bake for about 45 minutes
- ✓ Remove from the oven and set aside for about 5 minutes before serving.

Meal Prep Tip:

- ✓ Remove the baking dish from the oven and set aside to cool completely. In 6 containers, divide the chicken breasts and broccoli evenly and refrigerate

for about 2 days.
- ✓ Reheat in microwave before serving.

Nutrition: Calories 443 Total Fat 21.5 g Saturated Fat 4.7 g Cholesterol 151 mg Total Carbs 9.4 g Sugar 2.2g Fiber 3.6 g Sodium 189 mg Potassium 831 mg Protein 53 g

175)   *Meatballs Curry*

Ingredients:

For Meatballs:

- 1 pound lean ground chicken
- 1 tablespoon onion paste
- 1 teaspoons fresh ginger paste
- 1 teaspoons garlic paste 1 green chili, chopped finely
- 1 tablespoon fresh cilantro leaves, chopped
- 1 teaspoon ground coriander
- ½ teaspoon cumin seeds
- ½ teaspoon red chili powder
- ½ teaspoon ground turmeric
- 1/8 teaspoon salt

For Curry:

- 3 tablespoons olive oil
- ½ teaspoon cumin seeds
- 1 (1-inch) cinnamon stick
- 2 onions, chopped 1 teaspoons fresh ginger, minced
- 1 teaspoons garlic, minced
- 4 tomatoes, chopped finely
- 2 teaspoons ground coriander
- 1 teaspoon garam masala powder
- ½ teaspoon ground nutmeg
- ½ teaspoon red chili powder
- ½ teaspoon ground turmeric
- Salt, as required 1 cup filtered water 3 tablespoons fresh cilantro, chopped

Direction: Preparation Time: 20 minutes Cooking Time: 25 minutes Servings: 6

For meatballs:

- ✓ In a large bowl, add all ingredients and mix until well combined.
- ✓ Make small equal-sized meatballs from mixture. In a large deep skillet, heat the oil over medium heat and cook the meatballs for about 3-5 minutes or until browned from all sides.
- ✓ Transfer the meatballs into a bowl. In the same skillet, add the cumin seeds and cinnamon stick and sauté for about 1 minute.
- ✓ Add the onions and sauté for about 4-5 minutes.
- ✓ Add the ginger and garlic paste and sauté for about 1

minute.

- ✓ Add the tomato and spices and cook, crushing with the back of spoon for about 2-3 minutes.
- ✓ Add the water and meatballs and bring to a boil.
- ✓ Now, reduce the heat to low and simmer for about 10 minutes.
- ✓ Serve hot with the garnishing of cilantro.

Meal Prep Tip:

- ✓ Transfer the curry into a large bowl and set aside to cool. Divide the curry into 5 containers evenly.
- ✓ Cover the containers and refrigerate for 1-2 days. Reheat in the microwave before serving.

Nutrition: Calories 196 Total Fat 11.4 g Saturated Fat 2.4 g Cholesterol 53 mg Total Carbs 7.9 g Sugar 3.9 g Fiber 2.1 g Sodium 143 mg Potassium 279 mg Protein 16.7 g

176) *Chicken, Oats & Chickpeas Meatloaf*

Ingredients:

- ½ cup cooked chickpeas
- 2 egg whites
- 2½ teaspoons poultry seasoning
- Ground black pepper, as required
- 10 ounce lean ground chicken 1 cup red bell pepper, seeded and minced
- 1 cup celery stalk, minced
- 1/3 cup steel-cut oats 1 cup tomato puree, divided
- 2 tablespoons dried onion flakes, crushed
- 1 tablespoon prepared mustard

Direction: Preparation Time: 20 minutes Cooking Time: 1¼ hours Servings: 4

- ✓ Preheat the oven to 350 degrees F. Grease a 9x5-inch loaf pan. In a food processor, add chickpeas, egg whites, poultry seasoning and black pepper and pulse until smooth.
- ✓ Transfer the mixture into a large bowl. Add the chicken, veggies oats, ½ cup of tomato puree and onion flakes and mix until well combined.
- ✓ Transfer the mixture into prepared loaf pan evenly.
- ✓ With your hands, press, down the mixture slightly. In another bowl mix together mustard and remaining tomato puree. Place the mustard mixture over loaf pan evenly.
- ✓ Bake for about 1-1¼ hours or until desired doneness. Remove from the oven and set aside for about 5 minutes before slicing..
- ✓ Cut into desired sized slices and serve.

Meal Prep Tip:

- ✓ In a resealable plastic bag, place the cooled meatloaf slices and seal the bag. Refrigerate for about 2-4 days. Reheat in the microwave on High for about 1 minute before serving.

Nutrition: Calories 229 Total Fat 5.6 g Saturated Fat 1.4 g Cholesterol 50 mg Total Carbs 23.7 g Sugar 5.2 g Fiber 4.7 g Sodium 227 mg Potassium 509 mg Protein 21.4 g

177) *Herbed Turkey Breast*

Ingredients:

- ½ cup olive oil
- 2 tablespoons fresh lemon juice
- 1 tablespoon scallion, chopped
- ½ teaspoon dried marjoram, crushed
- ½ teaspoon dried sage, crushed
- ½ teaspoon dried thyme, crushed
- Salt and ground black pepper, as required
- 1 (2-pound) boneless, skinless turkey breast half

Direction: Preparation Time: 15 minutes Cooking Time: 1 hour 50 minutes Servings: 6

- ✓ Preheat the oven to 325 degrees F. Arrange a rack into a greased shallow roasting pan. In a small pan, all the ingredients except turkey breast over medium heat and bring to a boil, stirring frequently.
- ✓ Remove from the heat and set aside to cool. Place turkey breast into the prepared roasting pan. Place some of the herb mixture over the top of turkey breast.
- ✓ Cover the roasting pan and bake for about 1¼-1¾ hours, basting with the remaining herb mixture occasionally.
- ✓ Remove from the oven and set aside for about 10-15 minutes before slicing.
- ✓ With a sharp knife, cut into desired slices and serve.

Meal Prep Tip:

- ✓ Transfer the turkey breast slices onto a wire rack to cool completely.
- ✓ With foil pieces, wrap the turkey breast slices and refrigerate for about 1-2 days. Reheat in the microwave before serving.

Nutrition: Calories 319 Total Fat 17.5 g Saturated Fat 2.4 g Cholesterol 93 mg Total Carbs 0.3 g Sugar 0.1 g Fiber 0.1 g Sodium 75 mg

178) *Turkey with Lentils*

Ingredients:

- 3 tablespoons olive oil, divided 1 onion, chopped
- 1 tablespoon fresh ginger, minced
- 4 garlic cloves, minced

- 3 plum tomatoes, chopped finely
- 2 cups dried red lentils, soaked for 30 minutes and drained
- 2 cups filtered water
- 2 teaspoons cumin seeds
- ½ teaspoon cayenne pepper
- 1 pound lean ground turkey
- 1 jalapeño pepper, seeded and chopped
- 2 scallions, chopped
- ¼ cup fresh cilantro, chopped

Direction: Preparation Time: 15 minutes Cooking Time: 51 minutes Servings: 7

✓ In a Dutch oven, heat 1 tablespoon of oil over medium heat and sauté the onion, ginger and garlic for about 5 minutes.

✓ Stir in tomatoes, lentils and water and bring to a boil Now, reduce the heat to medium-low and simmer, covered for about 30 minutes.

✓ Meanwhile, in a skillet, heat remaining oil over medium heat and sauté the cumin seeds and cayenne pepper for about 1 minute.

✓ Transfer the mixture into a small bowl and set aside. In the same skillet, add turkey and cook for about 4-5 minutes

✓ Add the jalapeño and scallion and cook for about 4-5 minutes. Add the spiced oil mixture and stir to combine well.

✓ Transfer the turkey mixture in simmering lentils and simmer for about 10-15 minutes or until desired doneness.

✓ Serve hot.

Meal Prep Tip:

✓ Transfer the turkey mixture into a large bowl and set aside to cool. Divide the mixture into 4 containers evenly. Cover the containers and refrigerate for 1-2 days. Reheat in the microwave before serving.

Nutrition: Calories 361 Total Fat 11.5.4 g Saturated Fat 2.4 g Cholesterol 46 mg Total Carbs 37 g Sugar 3.4 g Fiber 18 g Sodium 937mg Potassium 331 mg Protein 27.9 g

179) *Stuffed Chicken Breasts Greek-style*

Ingredients:

- 4 oz. chicken breasts, skinless and boneless
- ¼ cup onion, minced
- 4 artichoke hearts, minced
- 1 teaspoon oregano, crushed
- 4 lemon slices

What you will need from the store cupboard:

- 1 cup canned chicken broth, fat-free
- 1-1/2 lemon juice
- 1 tablespoon olive oil
- 2 teaspoons of cornstarch
- Ground pepper Salt, optional

Direction: Servings: 4 Cooking Time: 20 Minutes

✓ Take out all the fat from the chicken. Wash and pat dry. Season your chicken with pepper and salt.

✓ Pound the chicken to make it flat and thin. Bring together the oregano, onion, and artichoke hearts.

✓ Now spoon equal amounts of the mix at the center of your chicken.

✓ Roll up the log and secure using a skewer or toothpick. Heat oil in your skillet over medium temperature.

✓ Add the chicken. Brown all sides evenly.

✓ Pour the lemon juice and broth.

✓ Add lemon slices on top of the chicken.

✓ Simmer covered for 10 minutes. Transfer to a platter.

✓ Remove the skewers or toothpick.

✓ Mix cornstarch with a fork. Transfer to skillet and stir over high temperature. Put lemon sauce on the chicken.

Nutrition: Calories 224, Carbohydrates 8g, Fiber 1g, Cholesterol 82mg, Total Fat 5g, Protein 21g, Sodium 339mg

180) *Chicken & Tofu*

Ingredients:

- 2 tablespoons olive oil, divided 2 tablespoons orange juice
- 1 tablespoon Worcestershire sauce 1 tablespoon low-sodium soy sauce
- 1 teaspoon ground turmeric 1 teaspoon dry mustard
- 8 oz. chicken breast, cooked and sliced into cubes
- 8 oz. extra-firm tofu, drained and sliced into cubed
- 2 carrots, sliced into thin strips 1 cup mushroom, sliced
- 2 cups fresh bean sprouts
- 3 green onions, sliced
- 1 red sweet pepper, sliced into strips

Direction: Preparation Time: 1 hour and 15 minutes Cooking Time: 25 minutes Servings: 6

✓ In a bowl, mix half of the oil with the orange juice, Worcestershire sauce, soy sauce, turmeric and mustard.

✓ Coat all sides of chicken and tofu with the sauce.

✓ Marinate for 1 hour. In a pan over medium heat, add 1 tablespoon oil.

✓ Add carrot and cook for 2 minutes.

✓ Add mushroom and cook for another 2 minutes.

✓ Add bean sprouts, green onion and sweet pepper.

✓ Cook for two to three minutes. Stir in the chicken and heat through.

Nutrition: Calories 285 Total Fat 9 g Saturated Fat 1 g Cholesterol 32 mg Sodium 331 mg Total Carbohydrate 30 g Dietary Fiber 4 g Total Sugars 4 g Protein 20 g Potassium 559 mg

181)　　　*Chicken & Peanut Stir-Fry*

Ingredients:

- 3 tablespoons lime juice
- ½ teaspoon lime zest
- 4 cloves garlic, minced
- 2 teaspoons chili bean sauce
- 1 tablespoon fish sauce
- 1 tablespoon water
- 2 tablespoons peanut butter
- 3 teaspoons oil, divided
- 1 lb. chicken breast, sliced into strips
- 1 red sweet pepper, sliced into strips
- 3 green onions, sliced thinly
- 2 cups broccoli, shredded
- 2 tablespoons peanuts, chopped

Direction: Preparation Time: 15 minutes Cooking Time: 15 minutes Servings: 4

✓ In a bowl, mix the lime juice, lime zest, garlic, chili bean sauce, fish sauce, water and peanut butter.

✓ Mix well. In a pan over medium high heat, add 2 teaspoons of oil.

✓ Cook the chicken until golden on both sides.

✓ Pour in the remaining oil. Add the pepper and green onions.

✓ Add the chicken, broccoli and sauce. Cook for 2 minutes. Top with peanuts before serving.

Nutrition: Calories 368 Total Fat 11 g Saturated Fat 2 g Cholesterol 66 mg Sodium 556 mg Total Carbohydrate 34 g Dietary Fiber 3 g Total Sugars 4 g Protein 32 g Potassium 482 mg

182)　　　*Honey Mustard Chicken*

Ingredients:

- 2 tablespoons honey mustard
- 2 teaspoons olive oil
- Salt to taste
- 1 lb. chicken tenders
- 1 lb. baby carrots, steamed

- Chopped parsley

Direction: Preparation Time: 15 minutes Cooking Time: 12 minutes Servings: 4

✓ Preheat your oven to 450 degrees F.

✓ Mix honey mustard, olive oil and salt.

✓ Coat the chicken tenders with the mixture. Place the chicken on a single layer on the baking pan.

✓ Bake for 10 to 12 minutes. Serve with steamed carrots and garnish with parsley.

Nutrition: Calories 366 Total Fat 8 g Saturated Fat 2 g Cholesterol 63 mg Sodium 543 mg Total Carbohydrate 46 g Dietary Fiber 8 g Total Sugars 13 g Protein 33 g Potassium 377 mg

183)　　　*Lemon Garlic Turkey*

Ingredients:

- 4 turkey breasts fillet
- 2 cloves garlic, minced
- 1 tablespoon olive oil
- 3 tablespoons lemon juice
- 1 oz. Parmesan cheese, shredded Pepper to taste
- 1 tablespoon fresh sage, snipped 1 teaspoon lemon zest

Direction: Preparation Time: 1 hour and 10 minutes Cooking Time: 5 minutes Servings: 4

✓ Pound the turkey breast until flat. In a bowl, mix the olive oil, garlic and lemon juice.

✓ Add the turkey to the bowl. Marinate for 1 hour.

✓ Broil for 5 minutes until turkey is fully cooked.

✓ Sprinkle cheese on top on the last minute of cooking. In a bowl, mix the pepper, sage and lemon zest.

✓ Sprinkle this mixture on top of the turkey before serving.

Nutrition: Calories 188 Total Fat 7 g Saturated Fat 2 g Cholesterol 71 mg Sodium 173 mg Total Carbohydrate 2 g Dietary Fiber 0 g Total Sugars 0 g Protein 29 g Potassium 264 mg

184)　　　*Chicken & Spinach*

Ingredients:

- 2 tablespoons olive oil
- 1 lb. chicken breast fillet, sliced into small pieces
- Salt and pepper to taste
- 4 cloves garlic, minced
- 1 tablespoon lemon juice
- ½ cup dry white wine
- 1 teaspoon lemon zest

- 10 cups fresh spinach, chopped
- 4 tablespoons Parmesan cheese, grated

Direction: Preparation Time: 15 minutes Cooking Time: 13 minutes Servings: 4

✓ Pour oil in a pan over medium heat. Season chicken with salt and pepper.
✓ Cook in the pan for 7 minutes until golden on both sides.
✓ Add the garlic and cook for 1 minute. Stir in the lemon juice and wine.
✓ Sprinkle lemon zest on top. Simmer for 5 minutes.
✓ Add the spinach and cook until wilted.
✓ Serve with Parmesan cheese

Nutrition: Calories 334 Total Fat 12 g Saturated Fat 3 g Cholesterol 67 mg Total Carbohydrate 25 g Dietary Fiber 2 g Total Sugars 1 g Protein 29 g

185)   *Balsamic Chicken 2*

Ingredients:
- 6 chicken breast halves, skin removed
- 1 onion, sliced into wedges 1 tablespoon tapioca (quick cooking), crushed
- Salt and pepper to taste
- 1 teaspoon dried thyme, crushed
- 1 teaspoon dried rosemary, crushed
- ¼ cup balsamic vinegar
- 2 tablespoons chicken broth 9 oz. frozen Italian green beans
- 1 red sweet pepper, sliced into strips

Direction: Preparation Time: 15 minutes Cooking Time: 5 hours Servings: 6
✓ Put the chicken, onion and tapioca inside a slow cooker. Season with the salt, pepper, thyme and rosemary.
✓ Seal the pot and cook on low setting for 4 hours and 30 minutes.
✓ Add the sweet pepper and green beans.
✓ Cook for 30 more minutes.
✓ Pour sauce over the chicken and vegetables before serving.

Nutrition: Calories 234 Total Fat 2 g Saturated Fat 1 g Cholesterol 100 mg Sodium 308 mg Total Carbohydrate 10 g Dietary Fiber 2 g Total Sugars 5 g Protein 41 g Potassium 501 mg

186)   *Greek Chicken Lettuce Wraps*

Ingredients:

- 2 tablespoons freshly squeezed lemon juice
- 1 teaspoon lemon zest
- 5 teaspoons olive oil, divided

- 3 teaspoons garlic, minced and divided
- 1 teaspoon dried oregano
- ¼ teaspoon red pepper, crushed
- 1 lb. chicken tenders
- 1 cucumber, sliced in half and grated
- Salt and pepper to taste
- ¾ cup non-fat Greek yogurt
- 2 teaspoons fresh mint, chopped
- 2 teaspoons fresh dill, chopped
- 4 lettuce leaves
- ½ cup red onion, sliced 1 cup tomatoes, chopped

Direction: Preparation Time: 1 hour and 15 minutes Cooking Time: 8 minutes Servings: 4
✓ In a bowl, mix the lemon juice, lemon zest, half of oil, half of garlic, and red pepper. Coat the chicken with the marinade.
✓ Marinate it for 1 hour. Toss grated cucumber in salt. Squeeze to release liquid.
✓ Add the yogurt, dill, salt, pepper, remaining garlic and remaining oil.
✓ Grill the chicken for 4 minutes per side.
✓ Shred the chicken and put on top of the lettuce leaves.
✓ Top with the yogurt mixture, onion and tomatoes.
✓ Wrap the lettuce leaves and secure with a toothpick.

Nutrition: Calories 353 Total Fat 9 g Total Carbohydrate 33 g Dietary Fiber 6 g Total Sugars 6 g Protein 37 g

187)   *Lemon Chicken with Kale*

Ingredients:
- 1 tablespoon olive oil
- 1 lb. chicken thighs, trimmed
- Salt and pepper to taste
- ½ cup low-sodium chicken stock
- 1 lemon, sliced
- 1 tablespoon fresh tarragon, chopped
- 4 cloves garlic, minced
- 6 cups baby kale

Direction: Preparation Time: 10 minutes Cooking Time: 19 minutes Servings: 4
✓ Pour olive oil in a pan over medium heat. Season chicken with salt and pepper.
✓ Cook until golden brown on both sides.
✓ Pour in the stock. Add the lemon, tarragon and garlic. Simmer for 15 minutes.
✓ Add the kale and cook for 4 minutes.

Nutrition: Calories 374 Total Fat 19 g Saturated Fat Cholesterol 76 mg Sodium 378 mg Total Carbohydrate 26 g Dietary Fiber 3 g Total Sugars 2 g Protein 25 g Potassium 677 m

Meat Recipes

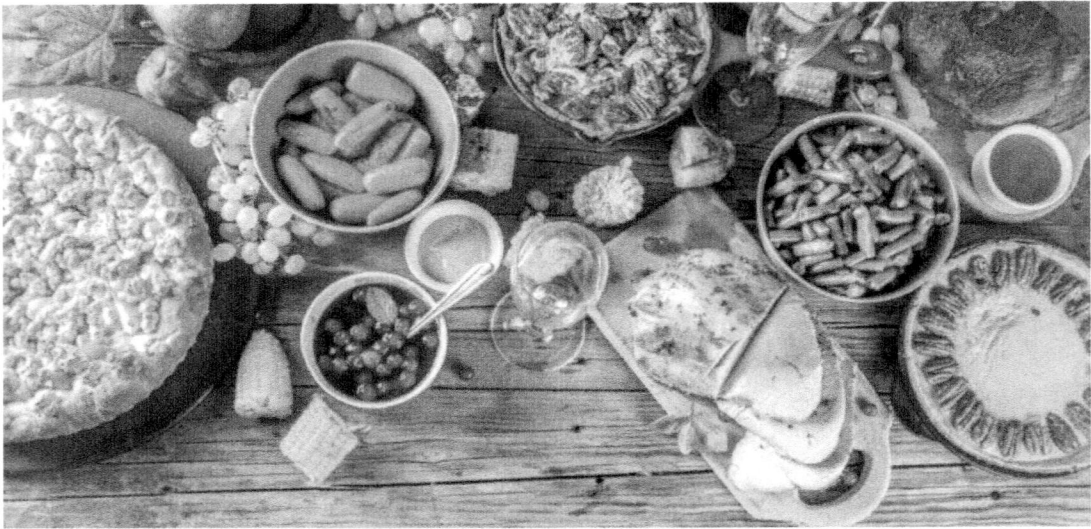

188)   *Pork Chops with Grape Sauce*

Ingredients:

- Cooking spray
- 4 pork chops
- ¼ cup onion, sliced
- 1 clove garlic, minced
- 1/2 cup low-sodium chicken broth
- ¾ cup apple juice
- 1 tablespoon cornstarch
- 1 tablespoon balsamic vinegar
- 1 teaspoon honey
- 1 cup seedless red grapes, sliced in half

Direction: Preparation Time: 15 minutes Cooking Time: 25 minutes Servings: 4

- ✓ Spray oil on your pan.
- ✓ Put it over medium heat.
- ✓ Add the pork chops to the pan.
- ✓ Cook for 5 minutes per side.
- ✓ Remove and set aside.
- ✓ Add onion and garlic.
- ✓ Cook for 2 minutes.
- ✓ Pour in the broth and apple juice.
- ✓ Bring to a boil.
- ✓ Reduce heat to simmer.
- ✓ Put the pork chops back to the skillet.
- ✓ Simmer for 4 minutes.
- ✓ In a bowl, mix the cornstarch, vinegar and honey.
- ✓ Add to the pan.
- ✓ Cook until the sauce has thickened.
- ✓ Add the grapes.
- ✓ Pour sauce over the pork chops before serving.

Nutrition: Calories 188; Total Fat 4 g; Saturated Fat 1 g; Cholesterol 47 mg; Sodium 117 mg; Total Carbohydrate 18 g; Dietary Fiber 1 g; Total Sugars 13 g; Protein 19 g; Potassium 759 mg

189)   *Roasted Pork & Apples*

Ingredients:

- Salt and pepper to taste
- 1/2 teaspoon dried, crushed
- 1 lb. pork tenderloin
- 1 tablespoon canola oil
- 1 onion, sliced into wedges
- 3 cooking apples, sliced into wedges
- 2/3 cup apple cider
- Sprigs fresh sage

Direction: Preparation Time: 15 minutes Cooking Time: 30 minutes Servings: 4

- ✓ In a bowl, mix salt, pepper and sage.
- ✓ Season both sides of pork with this mixture.
- ✓ Place a pan over medium heat.
- ✓ Brown both sides.
- ✓ Transfer to a roasting pan.
- ✓ Add the onion on top and around the pork.
- ✓ Drizzle oil on top of the pork and apples.
- ✓ Roast in the oven at 425 degrees F for 10 minutes.
- ✓ Add the apples, roast for another 15 minutes.
- ✓ In a pan, boil the apple cider and then simmer for 10 minutes.
- ✓ Pour the apple cider sauce over the pork before serving.

Nutrition: Calories 239; Total Fat 6 g; Saturated Fat 1 g; Cholesterol 74 mg; Sodium 209 mg; Total Carbohydrate 22 g; Dietary Fiber 3 g; Total Sugars 16 g; Protein 24 g; Potassium 655 mg

190)   *Pork with Cranberry Relish*

Ingredients:

- 12 oz. pork tenderloin, fat trimmed and sliced crosswise
- Salt and pepper to taste
- ¼ cup all-purpose flour
- 2 tablespoons olive oil
- 1 onion, sliced thinly
- ¼ cup dried cranberries
- ¼ cup low-sodium chicken broth
- 1 tablespoon balsamic vinegar

Direction: Preparation Time: 30 minutes Cooking Time: 30 minutes Servings: 4

- ✓ Flatten each slice of pork using a mallet.
- ✓ In a dish, mix the salt, pepper and flour.
- ✓ Dip each pork slice into the flour mixture.
- ✓ Add oil to a pan over medium high heat.
- ✓ Cook pork for 3 minutes per side or until golden crispy.
- ✓ Transfer to a serving plate and cover with foil.
- ✓ Cook the onion in the pan for 4 minutes.
- ✓ Stir in the rest of the ingredients.
- ✓ Simmer until the sauce has thickened.

Nutrition: Calories 211; Total Fat 9 g; Saturated Fat 2 g; Sodium 116 mg; Total Carbohydrate 15 g; Dietary Fiber 1 g; Total Sugars 6 g; Protein 18 g; Potassium 378 mg

191) Sesame Pork with Mustard Sauce

Ingredients:

- 2 tablespoons low-sodium teriyaki sauce
- ¼ cup chili sauce
- 2 cloves garlic, minced
- 2 teaspoons ginger, grated
- 2 pork tenderloins
- 2 teaspoons sesame seeds
- ¼ cup low fat sour cream
- 1 teaspoon Dijon mustard
- Salt to taste
- 1 scallion, chopped

Direction: Preparation Time: 25 minutes

Cooking Time: 25 minutes Servings: 4

- ✓ Preheat your oven to 425 degrees F.
- ✓ Mix the teriyaki sauce, chili sauce, garlic and ginger.
- ✓ Put the pork on a roasting pan.
- ✓ Brush the sauce on both sides of the pork.
- ✓ Bake in the oven for 15 minutes.
- ✓ Brush with more sauce.
- ✓ Top with sesame seeds.
- ✓ Roast for 10 more minutes.
- ✓ Mix the rest of the ingredients.
- ✓ Serve the pork with mustard sauce.

Nutrition: Calories 135 ; Total Fat 3 g; Saturated Fat 1 g; Cholesterol 56X mg; Sodium 302 mg; Total Carbohydrate 7 g; Dietary Fiber 1 g; Total Sugars 15 g; Protein 20 g; Potassium 755 mg

192) Steak with Mushroom Sauce

Ingredients:

- 12 oz. sirloin steak, sliced and trimmed
- 2 teaspoons grilling seasoning
- 2 teaspoons oil
- 6 oz. broccoli, trimmed
- 2 cups frozen peas
- 3 cups fresh mushrooms, sliced
- 1 cup beef broth (unsalted)
- 1 tablespoon mustard
- 2 teaspoons cornstarch
- Salt to taste

Direction: Preparation Time: 20 minutes Cooking

Time: 5 minutes Servings: 4

- ✓ Preheat your oven to 350 degrees F.
- ✓ Season meat with grilling seasoning.
- ✓ In a pan over medium high heat, cook the meat and broccoli for 4 minutes.
- ✓ Sprinkle the peas around the steak.
- ✓ Put the pan inside the oven and bake for 8 minutes.
- ✓ Remove both meat and vegetables from the pan.
- ✓ Add the mushrooms to the pan.
- ✓ Cook for 3 minutes.
- ✓ Mix the broth, mustard, salt and cornstarch.
- ✓ Add to the mushrooms.
- ✓ Cook for 1 minute.
- ✓ Pour sauce over meat and vegetables before serving.

Nutrition: Calories 226; Total Fat 6 ; Saturated Fat 2 g; Cholesterol 51 mg ; Sodium 356 mg; Total Carbohydrate 16 g; Dietary Fiber 5 g; Total Sugars 6 g; Protein 26 g; Potassium 780 mg

193) Steak with Tomato & Herbs

Ingredients:

- 8 oz. beef loin steak, sliced in half
- Salt and pepper to taste
- Cooking spray
- 1 teaspoon fresh basil, snipped
- ¼ cup green onion, sliced
- 1/2 cup tomato, chopped

Direction: Preparation Time: 30 minutes

Cooking Time: 30 minutes Servings: 2

- ✓ Season the steak with salt and pepper.
- ✓ Spray oil on your pan.
- ✓ Put the pan over medium high heat.
- ✓ Once hot, add the steaks.
- ✓ Reduce heat to medium.
- ✓ Cook for 10 to 13 minutes for medium, turning once.
- ✓ Add the basil and green onion.
- ✓ Cook for 2 minutes.
- ✓ Add the tomato.
- ✓ Cook for 1 minute.
- ✓ Let cool a little before slicing.

Nutrition: Calories 170; Total Fat 6 g; Saturated Fat 2 g; Cholesterol 66 mg; Sodium 207 mg; Total Carbohydrate 3 g; Dietary Fiber 1 g; Total Sugars 5 g; Protein 25 g; Potassium 477 mg

194) Barbecue Beef Brisket

Ingredients:

- 4 lb. beef brisket (boneless), trimmed and sliced
- 1 bay leaf
- 2 onions, sliced into rings
- 1/2 teaspoon dried thyme, crushed
- ¼ cup chili sauce
- 1 clove garlic, minced
- Salt and pepper to taste
- 2 tablespoons light brown sugar
- 2 tablespoons cornstarch
- 2 tablespoons cold water

Direction: Preparation Time: 25 minutes

Cooking Time: 10 hours Servings: 10

- ✓ Put the meat in a slow cooker.
- ✓ Add the bay leaf and onion.
- ✓ In a bowl, mix the thyme, chili sauce, salt, pepper and sugar.
- ✓ Pour the sauce over the meat.
- ✓ Mix well.
- ✓ Seal the pot and cook on low heat for 10 hours.
- ✓ Discard the bay leaf.
- ✓ Pour cooking liquid in a pan.
- ✓ Add the mixed water and cornstarch.
- ✓ Simmer until the sauce has thickened.
- ✓ Pour the sauce over the meat.

Nutrition: Calories 182; Total Fat 6 g; Saturated Fat 2 g; Cholesterol 57 mg; Sodium 217 mg; Total Sugars 4 g; Protein 20 g; Potassium 383 mg

195)   *Beef & Asparagus*

Ingredients:

- 2 teaspoons olive oil
- 1 lb. lean beef sirloin, trimmed and sliced
- 1 carrot, shredded
- Salt and pepper to taste
- 12 oz. asparagus, trimmed and sliced
- 1 teaspoon dried herbs de Provence, crushed
- 1/2 cup Marsala
- ¼ teaspoon lemon zest

Direction: Preparation Time: 15 minutes Cooking Time: 10 minutes Servings: 4

- ✓ Pour oil in a pan over medium heat.
- ✓ Add the beef and carrot.
- ✓ Season with salt and pepper.
- ✓ Cook for 3 minutes.
- ✓ Add the asparagus and herbs.

- ✓ Cook for 2 minutes.
- ✓ Add the Marsala and lemon zest.
- ✓ Cook for 5 minutes, stirring frequently.

Nutrition: Calories 327; Total Fat 7 g; Saturated Fat 2 g; Cholesterol 69 mg ; Sodium 209 mg; Total Carbohydrate 29 g; Dietary Fiber 2 g; Total Sugars 3 g; Protein 28 g; Potassium 576 mg

196)   *Italian Beef*

Ingredients:

- Cooking spray
- 1 lb. beef round steak, trimmed and sliced
- 1 cup onion, chopped
- 2 cloves garlic, minced
- 1 cup green bell pepper, chopped
- 1/2 cup celery, chopped
- 2 cups mushrooms, sliced
- 14 1/2 oz. canned diced tomatoes
- 1/2 teaspoon dried basil
- ¼ teaspoon dried oregano
- 1/8 teaspoon crushed red pepper
- 2 tablespoons Parmesan cheese, grated

Direction: Preparation Time: 20 minutes Cooking Time: 1 hour and 20 minutes Servings: 4

- ✓ Spray oil on the pan over medium heat.
- ✓ Cook the meat until brown on both sides.
- ✓ Transfer meat to a plate.
- ✓ Add the onion, garlic, bell pepper, celery and mushroom to the pan.
- ✓ Cook until tender.
- ✓ Add the tomatoes, herbs, and pepper.
- ✓ Put the meat back to the pan.
- ✓ Simmer while covered for 1 hour and 15 minutes.
- ✓ Stir occasionally.
- ✓ Sprinkle Parmesan cheese on top of the dish before serving.

Nutrition: Calories 212; Total Fat 4 g; Saturated Fat 1 g; Cholesterol 51 mg; Total Sugars 6 g; Protein 30 g;

197)   *Lamb with Broccoli & Carrots*

Ingredients:

- 2 cloves garlic, minced
- 1 tablespoon fresh ginger, grated
- ¼ teaspoon red pepper, crushed
- 2 tablespoons low-sodium soy sauce

- 1 tablespoon white vinegar
- 1 tablespoon cornstarch
- 12 oz. lamb meat, trimmed and sliced
- 2 teaspoons cooking oil
- 1 lb. broccoli, sliced into florets
- 2 carrots, sliced into strips
- ¾ cup low-sodium beef broth
- 4 green onions, chopped
- 2 cups cooked spaghetti squash pasta

Direction: Preparation Time: 20 minutes Cooking Time: 10 minutes Servings: 4

✓ Combine the garlic, ginger, red pepper, soy sauce, vinegar and cornstarch in a bowl.
✓ Add lamb to the marinade.
✓ Marinate for 10 minutes.
✓ Discard marinade.
✓ In a pan over medium heat, add the oil.
✓ Add the lamb and cook for 3 minutes.
✓ Transfer lamb to a plate.
✓ Add the broccoli and carrots.
✓ Cook for 1 minute.
✓ Pour in the beef broth.
✓ Cook for 5 minutes.
✓ Put the meat back to the pan.
✓ Sprinkle with green onion and serve on top of spaghetti squash.

Nutrition: Calories 205; Total Fat 6 g; Saturated Fat 1 g; Cholesterol 40 mg; Sodium 659 mg; Total Carb. 17 g

198) *Rosemary Lamb*

Ingredients:

- Salt and pepper to taste
- 2 teaspoons fresh rosemary, snipped
- 5 lb. whole leg of lamb, trimmed and cut with slits on all sides
- 3 cloves garlic, slivered
- 1 cup water

Direction: Preparation Time: 15 minutes Cooking Time: 2 hours Servings: 14

✓ Preheat your oven to 375 degrees F.
✓ Mix salt, pepper and rosemary in a bowl.
✓ Sprinkle mixture all over the lamb.
✓ Insert slivers of garlic into the slits.
✓ Put the lamb on a roasting pan.
✓ Add water to the pan.
✓ Roast for 2 hours.

Nutrition: Calories 136; Total Fat 4 g; Saturated Fat 1g cholesterol 71 mg; Sodium 218 mg; Protein 23 g;

199) *Mediterranean Lamb Meatballs*

Ingredients:

- 12 oz. roasted red peppers
- 1 1/2 cups whole wheat breadcrumbs
- 2 eggs, beaten
- 1/3 cup tomato sauce
- 1/2 cup fresh basil
- ¼ cup parsley, snipped
- Salt and pepper to taste
- 2 lb. lean ground lamb

Direction: Preparation Time: 10 minutes

Cooking Time: 20 minutes Servings: 8

✓ Preheat your oven to 350 degrees F.
✓ In a bowl, mix all the ingredients and then form into meatballs.
✓ Put the meatballs on a baking pan.
✓ Bake in the oven for 20 minutes.

Nutrition: Calories 94; Total Fat 3 g; Saturated Fat 1 g; Cholesterol 35 mg Sodium 170 mg; Total Carbohydrate 2 g; Dietary Fiber 1 g; Total Sugars 0 g

200) *Shredded Beef*

Ingredients:

- 1.5lb lean steak 1 cup low sodium gravy
- 2tbsp mixed spices

Direction: Servings: 2 Cooking Time: 35 Minutes

✓ Mix all the ingredients in your Instant Pot. Cook on Stew for 35 minutes.
✓ Release the pressure naturally. Shred the beef.

Nutrition: Calories: 200 Carbs: 2 Sugar: 0 Fat: 5 Protein: 48 GL: 1

201) *Classic Mini Meatloaf*

Ingredients:

- 1 pound 80/20 ground beef
- ¼ medium yellow onion, peeled and diced
- ½ medium green bell pepper, seeded and diced 1 large egg
- 3 tablespoons blanched finely ground almond flour
- 1 tablespoon Worcestershire sauce

- ½ teaspoon garlic powder
- 1 teaspoon dried parsley
- 2 tablespoons tomato paste
- ¼ cup water
- 1 tablespoon powdered erythritol

Direction: Servings: 6 Cooking Time: 25 Minutes

✓ In a large bowl, combine ground beef, onion, pepper, egg, and almond flour. Pour in the

✓ Worcestershire sauce and add the garlic powder and parsley to the bowl.

✓ Mix until fully combined. Divide the mixture into two and place into two (4") loaf baking pans.

✓ In a small bowl, mix the tomato paste, water, and erythritol. Spoon half the mixture over each loaf.

✓ Working in batches if necessary, place loaf pans into the air fryer basket.

✓ Adjust the temperature to 350°F and set the timer for 25 minutes or until internal temperature is 180°F. Serve warm.

Nutrition: Calories: 170 Protein: 14.9 G Fiber: 0.9 G Net Carbohydrates: 2.6 G Sugar Alcohol: 1.5 G Fat: 9.4 G Sodium: 85 Mg Carbohydrates: 5.0 G Sugar: 1.5 G

202) *Skirt Steak With Asian Peanut Sauce*

Ingredients:

- ⅓ cup light coconut milk
- 1 teaspoon curry powder
- 1 teaspoon coriander powder
- 1 teaspoon reduced-sodium soy sauce
- 1¼ pound skirt steak Cooking spray
- ½ cup Asian Peanut Sauce

Direction: Servings: 4 Cooking Time: 15 Minutes

✓ In a large bowl, whisk together the coconut milk, curry powder, coriander powder, and soy sauce.

✓ Add the steak and turn to coat.

✓ Cover the bowl and refrigerate for at least 30 minutes and no longer than 24 hours.

✓ Preheat the barbecue or coat a grill pan with cooking spray and place the steak over medium-high heat.

✓ Grill the meat until it reaches an internal temperature of 145°F, about 3 minutes per side.

✓ Remove the steak from the grill and let it rest for 5 minutes. Slice the steak into 5-ounce pieces and serve each with 2 tablespoons of the Asian Peanut Sauce.

✓ REFRIGERATE: Store the cooled steak in a reseal able container for up to 1 week. Reheat each piece in the microwave for 1 minute.

Nutrition: Calories: 361 Fat: 22g Saturated Fat: 7g Protein: 36g Total Carbs: 8g Fiber: 2g Sodium: 349mg

203) *Roasted Pork Loin With Grainy Mustard Sauce*

Ingredients:

- (2-pound) boneless pork loin roast Sea salt
- Freshly ground black pepper
- 3 tablespoons olive oil
- 1½ cups heavy (whipping) cream
- 3 tablespoons grainy mustard, such as Pommery

Direction: Servings: 8 Cooking Time: 70 Minutes

✓ Preheat the oven to 375°F. Season the pork roast all over with sea salt and pepper.

✓ Place a large skillet over medium-high heat and add the olive oil.

✓ Brown the roast on all sides in the skillet, about 6 minutes in total, and place the roast in a baking dish.

✓ Roast until a meat thermometer inserted in the thickest part of the roast reads 155°F, about 1 hour.

✓ When there is approximately 15 minutes of roasting time left, place a small saucepan over medium heat and add the heavy cream and mustard. Stir the sauce until it simmers, then reduce the heat to low.

✓ Simmer the sauce until it is very rich and thick, about 5 minutes.

✓ Remove the pan from the heat and set aside. Let the pork rest for 10 minutes before slicing and serve with the sauce.

Nutrition: Calories 368 Fat: 29g Protein: 25g Carbs: 2g Fiber: 0g Net Carbs: 2g Fat 70%/Protein 25%/Carbs 5%

204) *Meatballs In Tomato Gravy*

Ingredients:

For Meatballs:

- 1 pound lean ground lamb
- 1 tablespoon homemade tomato paste
- ¼ cup fresh cilantro leaves, chopped 1 small onion, chopped finely
- 2 garlic cloves, minced
- ½ teaspoon ground cumin
- 1/8 teaspoon salt Ground black pepper, as required

For Tomato Gravy:

- 3 tablespoons olive oil, divided 2 medium onions, chopped finely
- 2 garlic cloves, minced

- ½ tablespoon fresh ginger, minced
- 1 teaspoon dried thyme, crushed
- 1 teaspoon dried oregano, crushed
- 3 large tomatoes, chopped finely Ground black pepper, as required
- 1½ cups warm low-sodium chicken broth

Direction: Servings: 6 Cooking Time: 30 Minutes

✓ For meatballs: in a large bowl, add all the ingredients and mix until well combined. Make small equal-sized balls from mixture and set aside.

✓ For gravy: in a large pan, heat 1 tablespoon of oil over medium heat.

✓ Add the meatballs and cook for about 4-5 minutes or until lightly browned from all sides. With a slotted spoon, transfer the meatballs onto a plate.

✓ In the same pan, heat the remaining oil over medium heat and sauté the onion for about 8-10 minutes. Add the garlic, ginger and herbs and sauté for about 1 minute.

✓ Add the tomatoes and cook for about 3-4 minutes, crushing with the back of spoon. Add the warm broth and bring to a boil.

✓ Carefully, place the meatballs and cook for 5 minutes, without stirring.

✓ Now, reduce the heat to low and cook partially covered for about 15-20 minutes, stirring gently 2-3 times. Serve hot.

Meal Prep Tip:

✓ Transfer the meatballs mixture into a large bowl and set aside to cool. Divide the mixture into 6 containers evenly. Cover the containers and refrigerate for 1-2 days.

✓ Reheat in the microwave before serving.

Nutrition: Calories 248 Total Fat 12.9 g Saturated Fat 3 g Cholesterol 68 mg Total Carbs 10 g Sugar 4.8 g Fiber 2.5 g Sodium 138 mg

205)   *Garlic-braised Short Rib*

Ingredients:

- 4 (4-ounce) beef short ribs
- Sea salt
- Freshly ground black pepper
- 1 tablespoon olive oil
- 2 teaspoons minced garlic
- ½ cup dry red wine
- 3 cups Rich Beef Stock (here)

Direction: Servings: 4 Cooking Time: 2 Hours, 20 Minutes

✓ Preheat the oven to 325°F. Season the beef ribs on all sides with salt and pepper.

✓ Place a deep ovenproof skillet over medium-high heat and add the olive oil.

✓ Sear the ribs on all sides until browned, about 6 minutes in total.

✓ Transfer the ribs to a plate. Add the garlic to the skillet and sauté until translucent, about 3 minutes.

✓ Whisk in the red wine to deglaze the pan.

✓ Be sure to scrape all the browned bits from the meat from the bottom of the pan.

✓ Simmer the wine until it is slightly reduced, about 2 minutes.

✓ Add the beef stock, ribs, and any accumulated juices on the plate back to the skillet and bring the liquid to a boil.

✓ Cover the skillet and place it in the oven to braise the ribs until the meat is fall-off-the-bone tender, about 2 hours.

✓ Serve the ribs with a spoonful of the cooking liquid drizzled over each serving.

Nutrition: Calories: 481 Fat: 38g Protein: 29g Carbs: 5g Fiber: 3g Net Carbs: 2g Fat 70%/Protein 25%/Carbs 5%

206)   *Pulled Pork*

Ingredients:

- 2 tablespoons chili powder
- 1 teaspoon garlic powder
- ½ teaspoon onion powder
- ½ teaspoon ground black pepper
- ½ teaspoon cumin

Direction: Servings: 8 Cooking Time: 2½ Hours

✓ (4-pound) pork shoulder In a small bowl, mix chili powder, garlic powder, onion powder, pepper, and cumin.

✓ Rub the spice mixture over the pork shoulder, patting it into the skin.

✓ Place pork shoulder into the air fryer basket.

✓ Adjust the temperature to 350°F and set the timer for 150 minutes.

✓ Pork skin will be crispy and meat easily shredded with two forks when done.

✓ The internal temperature should be at least 145°F.

Nutrition: Calories: 537 Protein: 42.6 G Fiber: 0.8 G Net Carbohydrates: 0.7 G Fat: 35.5 G Sodium: 180 Mg Carbohydrates: 1.5 G Sugar: 0.2 G

207)   *Rosemary-garlic Lamb Racks*

Ingredients:

- 4 tablespoons extra-virgin olive oil
- 2 tablespoons finely chopped fresh rosemary
- 2 teaspoons minced garlic Pinch sea salt
- 2 (1-pound) racks
- French-cut lamb chops (8 bones each)

Direction: Servings: 4 Cooking Time: 25 Minutes

✓ In a small bowl, whisk together the olive oil, rosemary, garlic, and salt. Place the racks in a sealable freezer bag and pour the olive oil mixture into the bag.

✓ Massage the meat through the bag so it is coated with the marinade. Press the air out of the bag and seal it.

✓ Marinate the lamb racks in the refrigerator for 1 to 2 hours. Preheat the oven to 450°F. Place a large ovenproof skillet over medium-high heat

✓ Take the lamb racks out of the bag and sear them in the skillet on all sides, about 5 minutes in total.

✓ Arrange the racks upright in the skillet, with the bones interlaced, and roast them in the oven until they reach your desired doneness, about 20 minutes for medium-rare or until the internal temperature reaches 125°F.

✓ Let the lamb rest for 10 minutes and then cut the racks into chops. Serve 4 chops per person.

Nutrition: Calories: 354 Fat: 30g Protein: 21g Carbs: 0g Fiber: 0g Net Carbs: 0g

208) *Irish Pork Roast*

Ingredients:

- 1 ½ lb. parsnips, peeled and sliced into small pieces
- 1 ½ lb. carrots, sliced into small pieces
- 3 tablespoons olive oil,
- divided 2 teaspoons fresh thyme leaves, divided
- Salt and pepper to taste
- 2 lb. pork loin roast
- 1 teaspoon honey
- 1 cup dry hard cider Applesauce

Direction: Preparation Time: 40 minutes Cooking Time: 1 hour Servings: 8

✓ Preheat your oven to 400 degrees F.

✓ Drizzle half of the oil over the parsnips and carrots. Season with half of thyme, salt and pepper.

✓ Arrange on a roasting pan. Rub the pork with the remaining oil.

✓ Season with the remaining thyme.

✓ Season with salt and pepper. Put it on the roasting pan on top of the vegetables.

✓ Roast for 65 minutes.

✓ Let cool before slicing.

✓ Transfer the carrots and parsnips in a bowl and mix with honey.

✓ Add the cider. Place in a pan and simmer over low heat until the sauce has thickened.

✓ Serve the pork with the vegetables and applesauce.

Nutrition: Calories 272 Total Fat 8 g Saturated Fat 2 g Cholesterol 61 mg Sodium 327 mg Total Carbohydrate 23 g Dietary Fiber 6 g Total Sugars 10 g Protein 24 g

209) *Lamb & Chickpeas*

Ingredients:

- 1 lb. lamb leg (boneless), trimmed and sliced into small pieces
- 2 tablespoons olive oil
- 1 teaspoon ground coriander
- Salt and pepper to taste
- ½ teaspoon ground cumin
- ¼ teaspoon red pepper, crushed
- ¼ cup fresh mint, chopped
- 2 teaspoons lemon zest
- 2 cloves garlic, minced
- 30 oz. unsalted chickpeas, rinsed and drained
- 1 cup tomatoes, chopped
- 1 cup English cucumber, chopped
- ¼ cup fresh parsley, snipped 1 tablespoon red wine vinegar

Direction: Preparation Time: 30 minutes Cooking Time: 30 minutes Servings: 4

✓ Preheat your oven to 375 degrees F.

✓ Place the lamb on a baking dish.

✓ Toss in half of the following: oil, cumin and coriander.

✓ Season with red pepper, salt and pepper.

✓ Mix well. Roast for 20 minutes. In a bowl, combine the rest of the ingredients with the remaining seasonings.

✓ Add salt and pepper. Serve lamb with chickpea mixture.

Nutrition: Calories 366 Total Fat 15 g Saturated Fat 3 g Cholesterol 74 mg Sodium 369 mg Total Carbohydrate 27 g Dietary Fiber 7 g Protein 32 g

210) *Braised Lamb with Vegetables*

Ingredients:

- Salt and pepper to taste
- 2 ½ lb. boneless lamb leg, trimmed and sliced into

cubes
- 1 tablespoon olive oil
- 1 onion, chopped
- 1 carrot, chopped
- 14 oz. canned diced tomatoes
1 cup low-sodium beef broth
- 1 tablespoon fresh rosemary
- chopped 4 cloves garlic, minced
- 1 cup pearl onions
- 1 cup baby turnips, peeled and sliced into wedges
- 1 ½ cups baby carrots
- 1 ½ cups peas
- 2 tablespoons fresh parsley, chopped

Direction: Preparation Time: 30 minutes Cooking Time: 2 hours and 15 minutes Servings: 6

- ✓ Sprinkle salt and pepper on both sides of the lamb. Pour oil in a deep skillet.
- ✓ Cook the lamb for 6 minutes. Transfer lamb to a plate.
- ✓ Add onion and carrot. Cook for 3 minutes. Stir in the tomatoes, broth, rosemary and garlic. Simmer for 5 minutes.
- ✓ Add the lamb back to the skillet.
- ✓ Reduce heat to low. Simmer for 1 hour and 15 minutes. Add the pearl onion, baby carrot and baby turnips.
- ✓ Simmer for 30 minutes. Add the peas.
- ✓ Cook for 1 minute. Garnish with parsley before serving.

Nutrition: Calories 420 Total Fat 14 g Saturated Fat 4 g Cholesterol 126 mg Sodium 529 mg Total Carbohydrate 16 g Dietary Fiber 4 g Total Sugars 7 g Protein 43 g Potassium 988 mg

211)   *Beef Salad*

Ingredients:

For Steak:
- 1½ pounds skirt steak, trimmed and cut into 4 pieces
Salt and ground black pepper, as required
For Salad:
- 2 medium green bell pepper, seeded and sliced thinly
- 2 large tomatoes, sliced
- 1 cup onion, sliced thinly
- 8 cups mixed fresh baby greens
For Dressing:
- 2 teaspoons Dijon mustard
- 4 tablespoons balsamic vinegar

- ½ cup olive oil
- Salt and ground black pepper, as required

Direction: Preparation Time: 20 minutes Cooking Time: 8 minutes Servings: 6

- ✓ Preheat the grill to medium-high heat. Grease the grill grate. Sprinkle the beef steak with a little salt and black pepper. Place the steak onto the grill and cook, covered for about 3-4 minutes per side. Transfer the steak onto a cutting board for about 10 minutes before slicing. With a sharp knife, cut the beef steaks into thin slices.
- ✓ Meanwhile, in a large bowl, mix together all salad ingredients. For dressing: in another bowl, add all the ingredients and beat until well combined.
- ✓ Pour the dressing over salad and gently toss to coat well. Divide the salad onto serving plates evenly. Top each plate with the steak slices and serve.
- ✓ Meanwhile, in a large bowl, mix together all salad ingredients. For dressing: in another bowl, add all the ingredients and beat until well combined. Pour the dressing over salad and gently toss to coat well. Divide the salad onto serving plates evenly. Top each plate with the steak slices and serve.

Nutrition: Calories 313 Total Fat 21.4 g Saturated Fat 5.1 g Cholesterol 50 mg Total Carbs 6.4 g Sugar 3.4 g Fiber 1.7 g Protein 24 g

212)   *Beef Curry*

Ingredients:

- 1 cup fat-free plain Greek yogurt
- ½ teaspoon garlic paste
- ½ teaspoon ginger paste
- ½ teaspoon ground cloves
- ½ teaspoon ground cumin
- 2 teaspoons red pepper flakes, crushed
- ¼ teaspoon ground turmeric
- Salt, as required
- 2 pounds round steak, cut into pieces
- ¼ cup olive oil
- 1 medium yellow onion, thinly sliced
- 1½ tablespoons fresh lemon juice
- ¼ cup fresh cilantro, chopped

Direction: Preparation Time: 20 minutes Cooking Time: 40 minutes Servings: 6

- ✓ In a large bowl, add the yogurt, garlic paste, ginger paste and spices and mix well.
- ✓ Add the steak pieces and generously coat with the yogurt mixture. Set aside for at least 15 minutes.
- ✓ In a large skillet, heat the oil over medium-high heat and sauté the onion for about 4-5 minutes.

✓ Add the steak pieces with marinade and stir to combine. Immediately, adjust the heat to low and simmer, covered and cook for about 25 minutes, stirring occasionally.

✓ Stir in the lemon juice and simmer for about 10 more minutes.

✓ Garnish with fresh cilantro and serve hot.

Meal Prep Tip:

✓ Transfer the curry into a large bowl and set aside to cool.

✓ Divide the curry into 6 containers evenly.

✓ Cover the containers and refrigerate for 1-2 days.

✓ Reheat in the microwave before serving.

Nutrition: Calories 389 Total Fat 18.2 g Saturated Fat 4.8 g Cholesterol 136 mg Total Carbs 4.3 g Sugar 2.4 g Fiber 0.7 g 149 mg

213)   *Beef with Barley & Veggies*

Ingredients:

- ¾ cup filtered water
- ¼ cup pearl barley
- 2 teaspoons olive oil
- 7 ounces lean ground beef
- 1 cup fresh mushrooms, sliced
- ¾ cup onion, chopped
- 2 cups frozen green beans
- ¼ cup low-sodium beef broth
- 2 tablespoon fresh parsley, chopped

Direction: Preparation Time: 15 minutes Cooking Time: 1 hour 5 minutes Servings: 2

✓ In a pan, add water, barley and pinch of salt and bring to a boil over medium heat.

✓ Now, reduce the heat to low and simmer, covered for about 30-40 minutes or until all the liquid is absorbed.

✓ Remove from heat and set aside.

✓ In a skillet, heat oil over medium-high heat and cook beef for about 8-10 minutes.

✓ Add the mushroom and onion and cook f or about 6-7 minutes.

✓ Add the green beans and cook for about 2-3 minutes. Stir in cooked barley and broth and cook for about 3-5 minutes more.

✓ Stir in the parsley and serve hot.

Meal Prep Tip:

✓ Transfer the beef mixture into a large bowl and set aside to cool.

✓ Divide the mixture into 2 containers evenly. Cover the containers and refrigerate for 1-2 days. Reheat in the microwave before serving.

Nutrition: Calories 374 Total Fat 11.4 g Saturated Fat 3.1 g Cholesterol 89 mg Total Carbs 32.7g Sugar 1.1 g Fiber 4.2 g Sodium 136 mg Potassium 895 mg Protein 36.6 g

214)   *Beef with Broccoli*

Ingredients:

- 2 tablespoons olive oil, divided
- 2 garlic cloves, minced
- 1 pound beef sirloin steak, trimmed and sliced into thin strips
- ¼ cup low-sodium chicken broth
- 2 teaspoons fresh ginger, grated
- 1 tablespoon ground flax seeds
- ½ teaspoon red pepper flakes, crushed
- Salt and ground black pepper, as required
- 1 large carrot, peeled and sliced thinly
- 2 cups broccoli florets
- 1 medium scallion, sliced thinly

Direction: Preparation Time: 10 minutes Cooking Time: 14 minutes Servings: 4

✓ In a large skillet, heat 1 tablespoon of oil over medium-high heat and sauté the garlic for about 1 minute.

✓ Add the beef and cook for about 4-5 minutes or until browned. With a slotted spoon, transfer the beef into a bowl.

✓ Remove the excess liquid from skillet. In a bowl, add the broth, ginger, flax seeds, red pepper flakes, salt and black pepper.

✓ In the same skillet, heat remaining oil over medium heat.

✓ Add the carrot, broccoli and ginger mixture and cook for about 3-4 minutes or until desired doneness. Stir in beef and scallion and cook for about 3-4 minutes.

Meal Prep Tip:

✓ Transfer the beef mixture into a large bowl and set aside to cool.

✓ Divide the mixture into 4 containers evenly. Cover the containers and refrigerate for 1-2 days. Reheat in the microwave before serving.

Nutrition: Calories 211 Total Fat 14.9 g Saturated Fat 3.9 g Cholesterol 101 mg Total Carbs 6.9 g Sugar 1.9 g Fiber 2.4 g Sodium 108 mg Potassium 706 mg Protein 36.5 g

215)   *Pan Grilled Steak*

Ingredients:

- 8 medium garlic cloves, crushed

- 1 (2-inch) piece fresh ginger, sliced thinly
- ¼ cup olive oil
- Salt and ground black pepper, as required
- ½ pounds flank steak, trimmed

Direction: Preparation Time: 10 minutes Cooking Time: 16 minutes Servings: 4

✓ In a large sealable bag, mix together all ingredients except steak.

✓ Add the steak and coat with marinade generously. Seal the bag and refrigerate to marinate for about 24 hours.

✓ Remove from refrigerator and keep in room temperature for about 15 minutes.

✓ Discard the excess marinade from steak. Heat a lightly greased grill pan over medium-high heat and cook the steak for about 6-8 minutes per side.

✓ Remove from grill pan and set aside for about 10 minutes before slicing.

✓ With a sharp knife cut into desired slices and serve.

Meal Prep Tip:

✓ Transfer the teak slices onto a wire rack to cool completely. With foil pieces, wrap the steak slices and refrigerate for about 1-2 days. Reheat in the microwave before serving.

Nutrition: Calories 447 Total Fat 26.8 g Saturated Fat 7.7 g Cholesterol 94 mg Total Carbs 2.1g Sugar 0.1 g Fiber 0.2 g Sodium 96 mg Potassium 601 mg Protein 47.7 g

216)   *Lamb Stew Recipe1*

Ingredients:

- 1 teaspoon ground cumin
- 1 teaspoon ground coriander
- ½ teaspoon cayenne pepper
- ½ teaspoon ground cinnamon
- 2 tablespoons olive oil
- 3 pounds lamb stew meat, trimmed and cubed
- Sea Salt and ground black pepper, as required
- 1 onion, chopped
- 2 garlic cloves, minced
- 2¼ cups low-sodium chicken broth
- 2 cups tomatoes, chopped finely
- 1 medium head cauliflower, cut into 1-inch florets

Direction: Preparation Time: 15 minutes Cooking Time: 2¼ hours Servings: 8

✓ Preheat the oven to 300 degrees F.

✓ In a small bowl, mix together spices and set aside.

✓ In a large ovenproof pan, heat oil over medium heat and cook the lamb with a little salt and black pepper for about 10 minutes or until browned from all sides.

✓ With a slotted spoon, transfer the lamb into a bowl.

✓ In the same pan, add onion and sauté for about 3-4 minutes. Add the garlic and spice mixture and sauté for about 1 minute.

✓ Add the cooked lamb, broth and tomatoes and bring to a gentle boil.

✓ Immediately, cover the pan and transfer into oven. Bake for about 1½ hours.

✓ Remove from oven and stir in cauliflower. Bake for about 30 minutes more or until cauliflower is done completely. Serve hot.

Meal Prep Tip:

✓ Transfer the stew into a large bowl and set aside to cool. Divide the stew into 8 containers evenly.

✓ Cover the containers and refrigerate for 1-2 days. Reheat in the microwave before serving.

Nutrition: Calories 375 Total Fat 16.2 g Saturated Fat 5 g Cholesterol 153 mg Total Carbs 5.6 g Sugar 2.6 g Fiber 1.8 g Sodium 162 mg Potassium 808 mg Protein 49.7 g

217)   *Lamb Curry*

Ingredients:

For Spice Mixture:

- 2 teaspoons ground coriander
- 2 teaspoons ground cumin
- 1 teaspoon ground cinnamon
- ½ teaspoon ground ginger
- 1 tablespoons sweet paprika
- ½ tablespoon cayenne pepper
- 1 teaspoon red chili powder

For Curry:

- 1 tablespoon olive oil
- 2 pounds boneless lamb, trimmed and cubed into
- 1-inch size
- 2 cups onions, chopped
- ½ cup fat-free plain
- Greek yogurt, whipped
- 1½ cups water
- Salt and ground black pepper, as required

Direction: Preparation Time: 15 minutes Cooking Time: 2¼ hours Servings: 8

✓ For spice mixture: in a bowl, add all spices and mix well. Set aside. In a large

✓ Dutch oven, heat the oil over medium-high heat and stir fry the lamb cubes for about 5 minutes.

✓ Add the onion and cook for about 4-5 minutes. Stir

in the spice mixture and cook for about 1 minute.

✓ Add the yogurt and water and bring to a boil over high heat.

✓ Now, reduce the heat to low and simmer, covered for about 1-2 hours or until desired doneness of lamb. Uncover and simmer for about 3-4 minutes. Serve hot.

Meal Prep Tip:

✓ Transfer the curry into a large bowl and set aside to cool.

✓ Divide the curry into 8 containers evenly.

✓ Cover the containers and refrigerate for 1-2 days. Reheat in the microwave before serving.

Nutrition: Calories 254 Total Fat 10.5 g Saturated Fat 3.3 g Cholesterol 102 mg Total Carbs 4.7 g Sugar 1.9 g Fiber 1.4 g Sodium 99 mg Protein 34 g

218) *Yummy Meatballs in Tomato Gravy*

Ingredients:

For Meatballs:

- 1 pound lean ground lamb
- 1 tablespoon homemade tomato paste
- ¼ cup fresh cilantro leaves, chopped
- 1 small onion, chopped finely
- 2 garlic cloves, minced
- ½ teaspoon ground cumin
- 1/8 teaspoon salt
- Ground black pepper, as required

For Tomato Gravy:

- 3 tablespoons olive oil, divided
- 2 medium onions, chopped finely
- 2 garlic cloves, minced
- ½ tablespoon fresh ginger, minced
- 1 teaspoon dried thyme, crushed
- 1 teaspoon dried oregano, crushed
- 3 large tomatoes, chopped finely
- Ground black pepper, as required
- 1½ cups warm low-sodium chicken broth

Direction: Preparation Time: 20 minutes Cooking Time: 30 minutes Servings: 6

✓ For meatballs: in a large bowl, add all the ingredients and mix until well combined.

✓ Make small equal-sized balls from mixture and set aside.

✓ For gravy: in a large pan, heat 1 tablespoon of oil over medium heat.

✓ Add the meatballs and cook for about 4-5 minutes

or until lightly browned from all sides.

✓ With a slotted spoon, transfer the meatballs onto a plate. In the same pan, heat the remaining oil over medium heat and sauté the onion for about 8-10 minutes.

✓ Add the garlic, ginger and herbs and sauté for about 1 minute.

✓ Add the tomatoes and cook for about 3-4 minutes, crushing with the back of spoon.

✓ Add the warm broth and bring to a boil. Carefully, place the meatballs and cook for 5 minutes, without stirring.

✓ Now, reduce the heat to low and cook partially covered for about 15-20 minutes, stirring gently 2-3 times. Serve hot.

Meal Prep Tip:

✓ Transfer the meatballs mixture into a large bowl and set aside to cool. Divide the mixture into 6 containers evenly. Cover the containers and refrigerate for 1-2 days. Reheat in the microwave before serving.

Nutrition: Calories 248 Total Fat 12.9 g Total Carbs 10 g Fiber 2.5 g Protein 23.4 g

219) *Spiced Leg of Lamb*

Ingredients:

For Marinade:

- 2/3 cup fat-free plain Greek yogurt
- 1 tablespoon homemade tomato puree
- 1 tablespoon fresh lemon juice
- 3-4 garlic cloves, minced
- 2 tablespoons fresh rosemary, chopped
- 2 teaspoons ground coriander
- 1 teaspoon ground cumin
- 1 teaspoon ground cinnamon 1 teaspoon red pepper flakes, crushed
- ¼ teaspoon sweet paprika
- Sea salt and freshly ground black pepper, as required
- 1 (4½-pound) bone-in leg of lamb

Direction: Preparation Time: 15 minutes Cooking Time: 1 hour 40 minutes Servings: 6

✓ In a large bowl, add yogurt, tomato puree, lemon juice, garlic, rosemary, and spices and mix until well combined.

✓ Add leg of lamb and coat with marinade generously. Cover and refrigerate to marinate for about 8-10 hours, flipping occasionally.

✓ Remove the marinated leg of lamb from refrigerator and keep in room temperature for about 25-30 minutes before roasting.

✓ Preheat the oven to 425 degree F. Line a large roasting pan with a greased foil piece.

✓ Arrange the leg of lamb into prepared roasting pan. Roast for 20 minutes.

✓ Remove the roasting pan from oven and change the side of leg of lamb.

✓ Now, Now, reduce the temperature of oven to 325 degree F.

✓ Roast for 40 minutes. Now loosely cover the roasting pan with a large piece of foil. Roast for 40 minutes more. Remove from oven and place onto a cutting board for about 10-15 minutes before slicing.

✓ With a sharp knife cut the leg of lamb in desired sized slices and serve.

Meal Prep Tip:

✓ Transfer the leg slices onto a wire rack to cool completely. With foil pieces, wrap the leg slices and refrigerate for about 1-2 days. Reheat in the microwave before serving.

Nutrition: Calories 478 Total Fat 15.5 g Saturated Fat 6.1 g Cholesterol 226 mg Total Carbs 3.3 g Sugar 1.3 g Fiber 0.9 g Sodium 226 mg Potassium 48 mg Protein 72.3 g

220)   *Baked Lamb & Spinach*

Ingredients:

- 2 tablespoons olive oil
- 2 pounds lamb necks, trimmed and cut into
- 2-inch pieces crosswise
- Salt, as required
- 2 medium onions, chopped
- 3 tablespoons fresh ginger, minced
- 4 garlic cloves, minced
- 2 tablespoons ground coriander
- 1 tablespoon ground cumin
- 1 teaspoon ground turmeric
- ¼ cup fat-free plain Greek yogurt
- ½ cup tomatoes, chopped 2 cups boiling water
- 30 ounces frozen spinach, thawed and squeezed
- 1½ tablespoons garam masala
- 1 tablespoon fresh lemon juice Ground black pepper, as required

Direction: Preparation Time: 15 minutes Cooking Time: 2 hours 55 minutes Servings: 6

✓ Preheat the oven to 300 degrees F. In a large

✓ Dutch oven, heat the oil over medium-high heat and stir fry the lamb necks with a little salt for about 4-5 minutes or until browned completely.

✓ With a slotted spoon, transfer the lamb onto a plate and Now, reduce the heat to medium.

✓ In the same pan, add the onion and sauté for about 10 minutes.

✓ Add the ginger, garlic and spices and sauté for about 1 minute.

✓ Add the yogurt and tomatoes and cook for about 3-4 minutes.

✓ With an immersion blender, blend the mixture until smooth. Add the lamb, boiling water and salt and bring to a boil. Cover the pan and transfer into the oven.

✓ Bake for about 2½ hours. Now, remove the pan from oven and place over medium heat. Stir in spinach and garam masala and cook for about 3-5 minutes. Stir in lemon juice, salt and black pepper and remove from heat.

✓ Serve hot.

Meal Prep Tip:

✓ Transfer the lamb mixture into a large bowl and set aside to cool. Divide the mixture into 6 containers evenly. Cover the containers and refrigerate for 1-2 days. Reheat in the microwave before serving.

Nutrition: Calories 469 Total Fat 32.4 g Saturated Fat 13.4 g Cholesterol 0 mg Total Carbs 12.9 g Sugar 3.1 g Fiber 4.7 g Sodium 304 mg Potassium 957 mg Protein 34.1 g

221)   *Pork Salad*

Ingredients:

- 1½ pounds pork tenderloin, trimmed and sliced thinly
- Salt and ground black pepper, as required
- 3 tablespoon olive oil
- 2 carrots, peeled and grated
- 3 cups Napa cabbage, shredded
- 2 scallions, chopped
- 2 tablespoon fresh lime juice
- ¼ cup fresh mint leaves, chopped

Direction: Preparation Time: 15 minutes Cooking Time: 6 minutes Servings: 5

✓ Season the pork with salt and black pepper lightly.

✓ In a large skillet, heat the oil over medium heat and cook the pork slices for about 2-3 minutes per sides or until cooked through.

✓ Remove from the heat and set aside to cool slightly.

✓ In a large bowl, add the pork and remaining ingredients except mint leaves and toss to coat well. Serve with the garnishing of mint leaves.

Meal Prep Tip:

✓ In 5 containers, divide salad. Refrigerate the containers for about 1 day. Just before serving, stir the salad well

Nutrition: Calories 292 Total Fat 13.3 g Saturated Fat 2.9 g Cholesterol 99 mg Total Carbs 5.7 g Sugar 2.7 g Fiber 2.1 g Sodium 104 mg Protein 36.6 g

222) *Pork with Bell Peppers*

Ingredients:

- 1 tablespoon fresh ginger, chopped finely
- 4 garlic cloves, chopped finely
- 1 cup fresh cilantro, chopped and divided
- ¼ cup plus
- 1 tablespoon olive oil, divided
- 1 pound tender pork, trimmed, sliced thinly
- 2 onions, sliced thinly
- 1 green bell pepper, seeded and sliced thinly
- 1 red bell pepper, seeded and sliced thinly
- 1 tablespoon fresh lime juice

Direction: Preparation Time: 15 minutes Cooking Time: 13 minutes Servings: 4

- ✓ In a large bowl, mix together ginger, garlic, ½ cup of cilantro and ¼ cup of oil.
- ✓ Add the pork and coat with mixture generously.
- ✓ Refrigerate to marinate for about 2 hours.
- ✓ Heat a large skillet over medium-high heat and stir fry the pork mixture for about 4-5 minutes.
- ✓ Transfer the pork into a bowl. In the same skillet, heat remaining oil over medium heat and sauté the onion for about 3 minutes. Stir in the bell pepper and stir fry for about 3 minutes.
- ✓ Stir in the pork, lime juice and remaining cilantro and cook for about 2 minutes.
- ✓ Serve hot.

Meal Prep Tip:
- ✓ Transfer the pork mixture into a large bowl and set aside to cool.
- ✓ Divide the mixture into 4 containers evenly.
- ✓ Cover the containers and refrigerate for 1-2 days. Reheat in the microwave before serving

Nutrition: Calories 360 Total Fat 21.8 g Cholesterol 83 mg Total Carbs 11 g Protein 31.2 g

223) *Roasted Pork Shoulder*

Ingredients:

- 1 head garlic, peeled and crushed
- ¼ cup fresh rosemary, minced
- 2 tablespoons fresh lemon juice
- 2 tablespoons balsamic vinegar
- 1 (4-pound) pork shoulder, trimmed

Direction: Preparation Time: 10 minutes Cooking Time: 6 hours Servings: 12

- ✓ In a bowl, add all the ingredients except pork shoulder and mix well.
- ✓ In a large roasting pan place pork shoulder and coat with marinade generously. With a large plastic wrap, cover the roasting pan and refrigerate to marinate for at least 1-2 hours.
- ✓ Remove the roasting pan from refrigerator.
- ✓ Remove the plastic wrap from roasting pan and keep in room temperature for 1 hour. Preheat the oven to 275 degrees F.
- ✓ Arrange the roasting pan in oven and roast for about 6 hours.
- ✓ Remove from the oven and set aside for about 15-20 minutes. With a sharp knife, cut the pork shoulder into desired slices and serve.

Meal Prep Tip:
- ✓ Transfer the pork slices onto a wire rack to cool completely. With foil pieces, wrap the pork slices and refrigerate for about 1-2 days. Reheat in the microwave before serving.

Nutrition: Calories 450 Total Fat 32.6g Saturated Fat 12 g Cholesterol 136 mg Total Carbs 1.5 g Sugar 0.1 g Fiber 0.6 g Sodium 104 mg Potassium 522 mg Protein 35.4 g

224) *Pork Chops in Peach Glaze*

Ingredients:

- 2 (6-ounce) boneless pork chops, trimmed
- Sea Salt and ground black pepper, as required
- ½ of ripe yellow peach, peeled, pitted and chopped
- 1 tablespoon olive oil
- 2 tablespoons shallot, minced
- 2 tablespoons garlic, minced
- 2 tablespoons fresh ginger, minced
- 4-6 drops liquid stevia
- 1 tablespoon balsamic vinegar
- ¼ teaspoon red pepper flakes, crushed
- ¼ cup filtered water

Direction: Preparation Time: 15 minutes Cooking Time: 16 minutes Servings: 2

- ✓ Season the pork chops with sea salt and black pepper generously. In a blender, add the peach pieces and pulse until a puree forms.
- ✓ Reserve the remaining peach pieces. In a skillet, heat the oil over medium heat and sauté the shallots for about 1-2 minutes.
- ✓ Add the garlic and ginger and sauté for about 1

minute. Stir in the remaining ingredients and bring to a boil.

✓ Now, reduce the heat to medium-low and simmer for about 4-5 minutes or until a sticky glaze forms.

✓ Remove from the heat and reserve 1/3 of the glaze and set aside. Coat the chops with remaining glaze.

✓ Heat a nonstick skillet over medium-high heat and sear the chops for about 4 minutes per side.

✓ Transfer the chops onto a plate and coat with the remaining glaze evenly. Serve immediately.

Meal Prep Tip:

✓ Transfer the pork chops into a large bowl and set aside to cool.

✓ Divide the chops into 2 containers evenly.

✓ Cover the containers and refrigerate for 1-2 days. Reheat in the microwave before serving.

Nutrition: Calories 359 Total Fat 13.5 g Saturated Fat 3.2 g Cholesterol 124 mg Total Carbs 12 g Sugar 3.8 g Protein 46.2 g

225)   *Ground Pork with Spinach*

Ingredients:

• 1 tablespoon olive oil

• ½ of white onion, chopped

• 2 garlic cloves, chopped finely

• 1 jalapeño pepper, chopped finely

• 1 pound lean ground pork

• 1 teaspoon ground coriander

• 1 teaspoon ground cumin

• 1 teaspoon fresh lemon juice

• ½ teaspoon ground turmeric

• ½ teaspoon ground cinnamon

• ½ teaspoon ground fennel seeds

• Salt and ground black pepper, as required

• ½ cup fresh cherry tomatoes, quartered

• 1¼ pounds collard greens leaves, stemmed and chopped

Direction: Preparation Time: 15 minutes Cooking Time: 15 minutes Servings: 4

✓ In a large skillet, heat the oil over medium heat and sauté the onion for about 4 minutes.

✓ Add the garlic and jalapeño pepper and sauté for about 1 minute.

✓ Add the pork and spices and cook for about 6 minutes breaking into pieces with the spoon.

✓ Stir in the tomatoes and greens and cook, stirring gently for about 4 minutes. Stir in the lemon juice and remove from heat. Serve hot.

Meal Prep Tip:

✓ Transfer the pork mixture into a large bowl and set aside to cool. Divide the mixture into 4 containers evenly. Cover the containers and refrigerate for 1-2 days. Reheat in the microwave before serving.

Nutrition: Calories 316 Total Fat 21.8 g Saturated Fat 0.5 g Cholesterol 0 mg Total Carbs 11.4 g Sugar 1.4 g Fiber 5.7 g Protein 23 g

FISH AND SEAFOOD

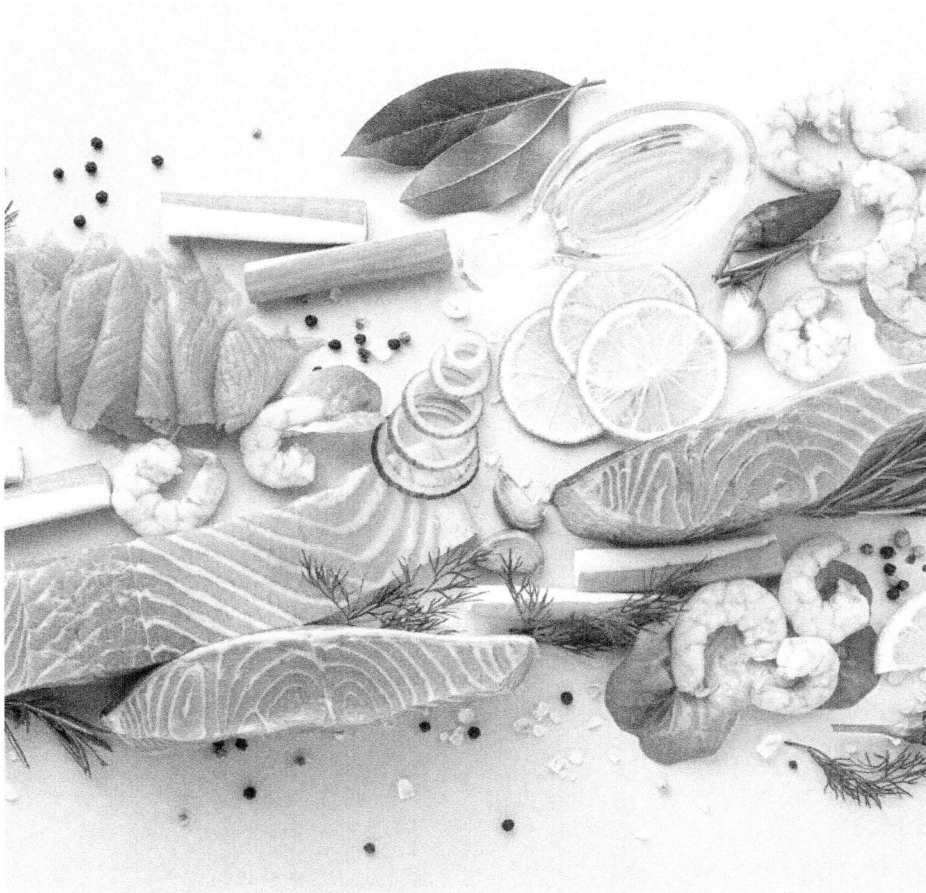

226) Baked Salmon with Garlic Parmesan Topping

Ingredients:

- 1 lb. wild caught salmon filets
- 2 tbsp. margarine
- What you'll need from store cupboard:
- ¼ cup reduced fat parmesan cheese, grated
- ¼ cup light mayonnaise
- 2-3 cloves garlic, diced
- 2 tbsp. parsley
- Salt and pepper

Direction: Preparation time: 5 minutes,

Cooking time: 20 minutes, Servings: 4

- ✓ Heat oven to 350 and line a baking pan with parchment paper.
- ✓ Place salmon on pan and season with salt and pepper.
- ✓ In a medium skillet, over medium heat, melt butter. Add garlic and cook, stirring 1 minute.
- ✓ Reduce heat to low and add remaining Ingredients. Stir until everything is melted and combined.
- ✓ Spread evenly over salmon and bake 15 minutes for thawed fish or 20 for frozen. Salmon is done when it flakes easily with a fork. Serve.

Nutrition: Calories 408; Total Carbs 4g; Protein 41g; Fat 24g; Sugar 1g; Fiber 0g

227) Blackened Shrimp

Ingredients:

- 1 1/2 lbs. shrimp, peel & devein
- 4 lime wedges
- 4 tbsp. cilantro, chopped
- What you'll need from store cupboard:
- 4 cloves garlic, diced
- 1 tbsp. chili powder
- 1 tbsp. paprika
- 1 tbsp. olive oil
- 2 tsp. Splenda brown sugar
- 1 tsp. cumin
- 1 tsp. oregano
- 1 tsp. garlic powder
- 1 tsp. salt
- 1/2tsp. pepper

Direction: Preparation time: 5 minutes Cooking time: 5 minutes Servings: 4

- ✓ In a small bowl combine seasonings and Splenda

brown sugar.

- ✓ Heat oil in a skillet over med-high heat. Add shrimp, in a single layer, and cook 1-2 minutes per side.
- ✓ Add seasonings, and cook, stirring, 30 seconds.
- ✓ Serve garnished with cilantro and a lime wedge.

Nutrition: Calories 252; Total Carbs 7g; Net Carbs 6g; Protein 39g; Fat 7g; Sugar 2g; Fiber 1g

228) Cajun Catfish

Ingredients:

- 4 (8 oz.) catfish fillets
- What you'll need from store cupboard:
- 2 tbsp. olive oil
- 2 tsp. garlic salt
- 2 tsp. thyme
- 2 tsp. paprika
- 1/2tsp. cayenne pepper
- 1/2tsp. red hot sauce
- ¼ tsp. black pepper
- Nonstick cooking spray

Direction: Preparation time: 5 minutes

Cooking time: 15 minutes Servings: 4

- ✓ Heat oven to 450 degrees. Spray a 9x13-inch baking dish with cooking spray.
- ✓ In a small bowl whisk together everything but catfish. Brush both sides of fillets, using all the spice mix.
- ✓ Bake 10-13 minutes or until fish flakes easily with a fork. Serve.

Nutrition: Calories 366; Total Carbs 0g; Protein 35g; Fat 24g; Sugar 0g; Fiber 0g

229) Cajun Flounder & Tomatoes

Ingredients:

- 4 flounder fillets
- 2 1/2 cups tomatoes, diced
- ¾ cup onion, diced
- ¾ cup green bell pepper, diced
- What you'll need from store cupboard:
- 2 cloves garlic, diced fine
- 1 tbsp. Cajun seasoning
- 1 tsp. olive oil

Direction: Preparation time: 10 minutes Cooking time: 15 minutes Servings: 4

- ✓ Heat oil in a large skillet over med-high heat. Add

onion and garlic and cook 2 minutes, or until soft. Add tomatoes, peppers and spices, and cook 2-3 minutes until tomatoes soften.

✓ Lay fish over top. Cover, reduce heat to medium and cook, 5-8 minutes, or until fish flakes easily with a fork. Transfer fish to serving plates and top with sauce.

Nutrition: Calories 194; Total Carbs 8g; Net Carbs 6g; Protein 32g; Fat 3g; Sugar 5g; Fiber 2g

230)   *Cajun Shrimp & Roasted Vegetables*

Ingredients:

- 1 lb. large shrimp, peeled and deveined
- 2 zucchinis, sliced
- 2 yellow squash, sliced
- 1/2 bunch asparagus, cut into thirds
- 2 red bell pepper, cut into chunks
- What you'll need from store cupboard:
- 2 tbsp. olive oil
- 2 tbsp. Cajun Seasoning
- Salt & pepper, to taste

Direction: Preparation time: 5 minutes Cooking time: 15 minutes Servings: 4

✓ Heat oven to 400 degrees.
✓ Combine shrimp and vegetables in a large bowl. Add oil and seasoning and toss to coat.
✓ Spread evenly in a large baking sheet and bake 15-20 minutes, or until vegetables are tender. Serve.

Nutrition: Calories 251; Total Carbs 13g; Net Carbs 9g; Protein 30g; Fat 9g; Sugar 6g; Fiber 4g

231)   *Cilantro Lime Grilled Shrimp*

Ingredients:

- 1 1/2 lbs. large shrimp raw, peeled, deveined with tails on
- Juice and zest of 1 lime
- 2 tbsp. fresh cilantro chopped
- What you'll need from store cupboard:
- ¼ cup olive oil
- 2 cloves garlic, diced fine
- 1 tsp. smoked paprika
- ¼ tsp. cumin
- 1/2 teaspoon salt
- ¼ tsp. cayenne pepper

Direction: Preparation time: 5 minutes, Cooking time: 5 minutes, Servings: 6

✓ Place the shrimp in a large Ziploc bag.
✓ Mix remaining Ingredients in a small bowl and pour over shrimp. Let marinate 20-30 minutes.
✓ Heat up the grill. Skewer the shrimp and cook 2-3 minutes, per side, just until they turn pick. Be careful not to overcook them. Serve garnished with cilantro.

Nutrition: Calories 317; Total Carbs 4g; Protein 39g; Fat 15g; Sugar 0g; Fiber 0g

232)   *Crab Frittata*

Ingredients:

- 4 eggs
- 2 cups lump crabmeat
- 1 cup half-n-half
- 1 cup green onions, diced
- What you'll need from store cupboard:
- 1 cup reduced fat parmesan cheese, grated
- 1 tsp. salt
- 1 tsp. pepper
- 1 tsp. smoked paprika
- 1 tsp. Italian seasoning
- Nonstick cooking spray

Direction: Preparation time: 10 minutes

Cooking time: 50 minutes Servings: 4

✓ Heat oven to 350 degrees. Spray an 8-inch springform pan, or pie plate with cooking spray.
✓ In a large bowl, whisk together the eggs and half-n-half. Add seasonings and parmesan cheese, stir to mix.
✓ Stir in the onions and crab meat. Pour into prepared pan and bake 35-40 minutes, or eggs are set and top is lightly browned.
✓ Let cool 10 minutes, then slice and serve warm or at room temperature.

Nutrition: Calories 276; Total Carbs 5g; Net Carbs 4g; Protein 25g; Fat 17g Sugar 1g, Fiber 1g

233)   *Crunchy Lemon Shrimp*

Ingredients:

- 1 lb. raw shrimp, peeled and deveined
- 2 tbsp. Italian parsley, roughly chopped
- 2 tbsp. lemon juice, divided

What you'll need from store cupboard:

- 2/3 cup panko bread crumbs

- 21/2 tbsp. olive oil, divided
- Salt and pepper, to taste

Direction: Preparation time: 5 minutes Cooking time: 10 minutes, Servings: 4

✓ Heat oven to 400 degrees.
✓ Place the shrimp evenly in a baking dish and sprinkle with salt and pepper.
✓ Drizzle on 1 tablespoon lemon juice and 1 tablespoon of olive oil. Set aside.
✓ In a medium bowl, combine parsley, remaining lemon juice, bread crumbs, remaining olive oil, and ¼ tsp. each of salt and pepper. Layer the panko mixture evenly on top of the shrimp.
✓ Bake 8-10 minutes or until shrimp are cooked through and the panko is golden brown.

Nutrition: Calories 283; Total Carbs 15g; Net Carbs 14g; Protein 28g; Fat 12g; Sugar 1g; Fiber 1g

234) *Grilled Tuna Steaks*

Ingredients:

- 6 6 oz. tuna steaks
- 3 tbsp. fresh basil, diced
- What you'll need from store cupboard:
- 4 1/2tsp. olive oil
- ¾ tsp. salt
- ¼ tsp. pepper
- Nonstick cooking spray

Direction: Preparation time: 5 minutes

Cooking time: 10 minutes, Servings: 6

✓ Heat grill to medium heat. Spray rack with cooking spray.
✓ Drizzle both sides of the tuna with oil. Sprinkle with basil, salt and pepper.
✓ Place on grill and cook 5 minutes per side, tuna should be slightly pink in the center. Serve.

Nutrition: Calories 343; Total Carbs 0g; Protein 51g; Fat 14g; Sugar 0g; Fiber 0g

235) *Red Clam Sauce & Pasta*

Ingredients:

- 1 onion, diced
- ¼ cup fresh parsley, diced
- What you'll need from store cupboard:
- 2 6 1/2 oz. cans clams, chopped, undrained
- 14 1/2 oz. tomatoes, diced, undrained
- 6 oz. tomato paste

- 2 cloves garlic, diced
- 1 bay leaf
- 1 tbsp. sunflower oil
- 1 tsp. Splenda
- 1 tsp. basil
- 1/2tsp. thyme
- 1/2 Homemade Pasta, cook & drain

Direction: Preparation time: 10 minutes,

Cooking time: 3 hours, Servings: 4

✓ Heat oil in a small skillet over med-high heat. Add onion and cook until tender,
✓ Add garlic and cook 1 minute more. Transfer to crock pot.
✓ Add remaining Ingredients, except pasta, cover and cook on low 3-4 hours.
✓ Discard bay leaf and serve over cooked pasta.

Nutrition: Calories 223; Total Carbs 32g; Net Carbs 27g; Protein 12g; Fat 6g; Sugar 15g Fiber 5g

236) *Salmon Milano*

Ingredients:

- 2 1/2 lb. salmon filet
- 2 tomatoes, sliced
- 1/2 cup margarine
- What you'll need from store cupboard:
- 1/2 cup basil pesto

Direction: Preparation time: 10 minutes,

Cooking time: 20 minutes, Servings: 6

✓ Heat the oven to 400 degrees. Line a 9x15-inch baking sheet with foil, making sure it covers the sides. Place another large piece of foil onto the baking sheet and place the salmon filet on top of it.
✓ Place the pesto and margarine in blender or food processor and pulse until smooth. Spread evenly over salmon.
✓ Place tomato slices on top.
✓ Wrap the foil around the salmon, tenting around the top to prevent foil from touching the salmon as much as possible.
✓ Bake 15-25 minutes, or salmon flakes easily with a fork. Serve.

Nutrition: Calories 444; Total Carbs 2g; Protein 55g; Fat 24g; Sugar 1g; Fiber 0g

237) *Shrimp & Artichoke Skillet*

Ingredients:

- 1 1/2 cups shrimp, peel & devein

- 2 shallots, diced
- 1 tbsp. margarine
- What you'll need from store cupboard
- 2 12 oz. jars artichoke hearts, drain & rinse
- 2 cups white wine
- 2 cloves garlic, diced fine

Direction: Preparation time: 5 minutes Cooking time: 10 minutes Servings: 4

✓ Melt margarine in a large skillet over med-high heat. Add shallot and garlic and cook until they start to brown, stirring frequently.

✓ Add artichokes and cook 5 minutes. Reduce heat and add wine. Cook 3 minutes, stirring occasionally.

✓ Add the shrimp and cook just until they turn pink. Serve.

Nutrition: Calories 487; Total Carbs 26g; Protein 64g; Fat 5;

238)   *Tuna Carbonara*

Ingredients:

- 1/2 lb. tuna fillet, cut in pieces
- 2 eggs
- 4 tbsp. fresh parsley, diced
- What you'll need from store cupboard:
- 1/2 Homemade Pasta, cook & drain,
- 1/2 cup reduced fat parmesan cheese
- 2 cloves garlic, peeled
- 2 tbsp. extra virgin olive oil
- Salt & pepper, to taste

Direction: Preparation time: 5 minutes Cooking time: 25 minutes Servings: 4

✓ In a small bowl, beat the eggs, parmesan and a dash of pepper.

✓ Heat the oil in a large skillet over med-high heat.

✓ Add garlic and cook until browned. Add the tuna and cook 2-3 minutes, or until tuna is almost cooked through. Discard the garlic.

✓ Add the pasta and reduce heat. Stir in egg mixture and cook, stirring constantly, 2 minutes. If the sauce is too thick, thin with water, a little bit at a time, until it has a creamy texture.

✓ Salt and pepper to taste and serve garnished with parsley.

Nutrition: Calories 409; Total Carbs 7g; Net Carbs 6g; Protein 25g

239)   *Mediterranean Fish Fillets*

Ingredients:

- 4 cod fillets

- 1 lb. grape tomatoes, halved
- 1 cup olives, pitted and sliced
- 2 tbsp. capers
- 1 tsp. dried thyme
- 2 tbsp. olive oil
- 1 tsp. garlic, minced
- Pepper
- Salt

Direction: Preparation Time: 10 minutes Cooking Time: 3 minutes Servings: 4

✓ Pour 1 cup water into the instant pot then place steamer rack in the pot.

✓ Spray heat-safe baking dish with cooking spray.

✓ Add half grape tomatoes into the dish and season with pepper and salt.

✓ Arrange fish fillets on top of cherry tomatoes. Drizzle with oil and season with garlic, thyme, capers, pepper, and salt.

✓ Spread olives and remaining grape tomatoes on top of fish fillets.

✓ Place dish on top of steamer rack in the pot.

✓ Seal pot with a lid and select manual and cook on high for 3 minutes.

✓ Once done, release pressure using quick release. Remove lid.

✓ Serve and enjoy.

Nutrition: Calories 212; Fat 11.9 g; Carbs 7.1 g; Sugar 3 g; Protein 21.4

240)   *Lemony Salmon*

Ingredients:

- 1 pound salmon fillet, cut into 3 pieces
- 3 teaspoons fresh dill, chopped
- 5 tablespoons fresh lemon juice, divided
- Salt and ground black pepper, as required

Direction: Preparation Time: 10 minutes Cooking Time: 3 Minutes Servings: 3

✓ Arrange a steamer trivet in Instant Pot and pour ¼ cup of lemon juice.

✓ Season the salmon with salt and black pepper evenly.

✓ Place the salmon pieces on top of trivet, skin side down and drizzle with remaining lemon juice.

✓ Now, sprinkle the salmon pieces with dill evenly.

✓ Close the lid and place the pressure valve to "Seal" position.

✓ Press "Steam" and use the default time of 3 minutes.

✓ Press "Cancel" and allow a "Natural" release.

✓ Open the lid and serve hot.

Nutrition: Calories 20 Fats 9.6g, Carbs 1.1g, Sugar

0.5g, Proteins 29.7g, Sodium 74mg

241) *Shrimp with Green Beans*

Ingredients:

- ¾ pound fresh green beans, trimmed
- 1 pound medium frozen shrimp, peeled and deveined
- 2 tablespoons fresh lemon juice
- 2 tablespoons olive oil
- Salt and ground black pepper, as required

Direction: Preparation Time: 10 minutes Cooking Time: 2 Minutes Servings: 4

- ✓ Arrange a steamer trivet in the Instant Pot and pour cup of water.
- ✓ Arrange the green beans on top of trivet in a single layer and top with shrimp.
- ✓ Drizzle with oil and lemon juice.
- ✓ Sprinkle with salt and black pepper.
- ✓ Close the lid and place the pressure valve to "Seal" position.
- ✓ Press "Steam" and just use the default time of 2 minutes.
- ✓ Press "Cancel" and allow a "Natural" release.
- ✓ Open the lid and serve.

Nutrition: Calories 223, Fats 1g, Carbs 7.9g, Sugar 1.4g, Proteins 27.4g, Sodium 322mg

242) *Crab Curry*

Ingredients:

- 0.5lb chopped crab
- 1 thinly sliced red onion
- 0.5 cup chopped tomato
- 3tbsp curry paste
- 1tbsp oil or ghee

Direction: Preparation Time: 10 minutes

Cooking Time: 20 Minutes Servings: 2

- ✓ Set the Instant Pot to sauté and add the onion, oil, and curry paste.
- ✓ When the onion is soft, add the remaining ingredients and seal.
- ✓ Cook on Stew for 20 minutes.
- ✓ Release the pressure naturally.

Nutrition: Calories 2; Carbs 11; Sugar 4; Fat 10; Protein 24; GL 9

243) *Mixed Chowder*

Ingredients:

- 1lb fish stew mix
- 2 cups white sauce   •   3tbsp old bay seasoning

Direction: Preparation Time: 10 minutes

Cooking Time: 35 Minutes Servings: 2

- ✓ Mix all the ingredients in your Instant Pot.
- ✓ Cook on Stew for 35 minutes.
- ✓ Release the pressure naturally.

Nutrition: : Calories 320; Carbs 9; Sugar 2; Fat 16; Protein GL 4

244) *Mussels in Tomato Sauce*

Ingredients:

- 2 tomatoes, seeded and chopped finely
- 2 pounds mussels, scrubbed and de-bearded
- 1 cup low-sodium chicken broth
- 1 tablespoon fresh lemon juice
- 2 garlic cloves, minced

Direction: Preparation Time: 10 minutes

Cooking Time: 3 Minutes Servings: 4

- ✓ In the pot of Instant Pot, place tomatoes, garlic, wine and bay leaf and stir to combine.
- ✓ Arrange the mussels on top.
- ✓ Close the lid and place the pressure valve to "Seal" position.
- ✓ Press "Manual" and cook under "High Pressure" for about 3 minutes.
- ✓ Press "Cancel" and carefully allow a "Quick" release.
- ✓ Open the lid and serve hot.

Nutrition: Calories 213, Fats 25.2g, Carbs 11g, Sugar 1. Proteins 28.2g, Sodium 670mg

245) *Citrus Salmon*

Ingredients:

- 4 (4-ounce) salmon fillets
- 1 cup low-sodium chicken broth
- 1 teaspoon fresh ginger, minced
- 2 teaspoons fresh orange zest, grated finely
- 3 tablespoons fresh orange juice
- 1 tablespoon olive oil
- Ground black pepper, as required

Direction: Preparation Time: 10 minutes Cooking Time: 7 Minutes Servings: 4

- ✓ In Instant Pot, add all ingredients and mix.
- ✓ Close the lid and place the pressure valve to "Seal"

position.
- ✓ Press "Manual" and cook under "High Pressure" for about 7 minutes. ✓ Press "Cancel" and allow a "Natural" release.
- ✓ Open the lid and serve the salmon fillets with the topping of cooking sauce.

Nutrition: Calories 190, Fats 10.5g, Carbs 1.8g, Sugar 1g, Proteins 22. Sodium 68mg

246)   *Herbed Salmon*

Ingredients:

- 4 (4-ounce) salmon fillets
- ¼ cup olive oil
- 2 tablespoons fresh lemon juice
- 1 garlic clove, minced
- ¼ teaspoon dried oregano
- Salt and ground black pepper, as required
- 4 fresh rosemary sprigs
- 4 lemon slices

Direction: Preparation Time: 10 minutes Cooking Time: 3 Minutes Servings: 4

- ✓ For dressing: in a large bowl, add oil, lemon juice, garlic, oregano, salt and black pepper and beat until well co combined.
- ✓ Arrange a steamer trivet in the Instant Pot and pour 11/2 cups of water in Instant Pot.
- ✓ Place the salmon fillets on top of trivet in a single layer and top with dressing.
- ✓ Arrange 1 rosemary sprig and 1 lemon slice over each fillet.
- ✓ Close the lid and place the pressure valve to "Seal" position.
- ✓ Press "Steam" and just use the default time of 3 minutes.
- ✓ Press "Cancel" and carefully allow a "Quick" release.
- ✓ Open the lid and serve hot.

Nutrition: Calories 262, Fats 17g, Carbs 0.7g, Sugar 0.2g, Proteins 22.1g, Sodium 91mg

247)   *Salmon in Green Sauce*

Ingredients:

- 4 (6-ounce) salmon fillets
- 1 avocado, peeled, pitted and chopped
- 1/2 cup fresh basil, chopped
- 3 garlic cloves, chopped
- 1 tablespoon fresh lemon zest, grated finely

Direction: Preparation Time: 10 minutes Cooking Time: 12 Minutes Servings: 4

- ✓ Grease a large piece of foil.
- ✓ In a large bowl, add all ingredients except salmon and water and with a fork, mash completely.
- ✓ Place fillets in the center of foil and top with avocado mixture evenly.
- ✓ Fold the foil around fillets to seal them.
- ✓ Arrange a steamer trivet in the Instant Pot and pour 1/2 cup of water.
- ✓ Place the foil packet on top of trivet.
- ✓ Close the lid and place the pressure valve to "Seal" position.
- ✓ Press "Manual" and cook under "High Pressure" for about minutes.
- ✓ Meanwhile, preheat the oven to broiler.
- ✓ Press "Cancel" and allow a "Natural" release.
- ✓ Open the lid and transfer the salmon fillets onto a broiler pan.
- ✓ Broil for about 3-4 minutes.
- ✓ Serve warm.

Nutrition: Calories 333, Fats 20.3g, Carbs 5.5g, Sugar 0.4g, Proteins 34.2g, Sodium 79mg

248)   *Braised Shrimp*

Ingredients:

- 1 pound frozen large shrimp, peeled and deveined
- 2 shallots, chopped
- ¾ cup low-sodium chicken broth
- 2 tablespoons fresh lemon juice
- 2 tablespoons olive oil
- 1 tablespoon garlic, crushed
- Ground black pepper, as required

Direction: Preparation Time: 10 minutes Cooking Time: 4 Minutes Servings: 4

- ✓ In the Instant Pot, place oil and press "Sauté". Now add the shallots and cook for about 2 minutes.
- ✓ Add the garlic and cook for about 1 minute.
- ✓ Press "Cancel" and stir in the shrimp, broth, lemon juice and black pepper.
- ✓ Close the lid and place the pressure valve to "Seal" position.
- ✓ Press "Manual" and cook under "High Pressure" for about 1 minute.
- ✓ Press "Cancel" and carefully allow a "Quick" release.
- ✓ Open the lid and serve hot.

Nutrition: Calories 209, Fats 9g, Carbs 4.3g, Sugar 0.2g, Proteins 26.6g, Sodium 293mg

249)   *Shrimp Coconut Curry*

Ingredients:

- 0.5lb cooked shrimp
- 1 thinly sliced onion
- 1 cup coconut yogurt
- 3tbsp curry paste
- 1tbsp oil or ghee

Direction: Preparation Time: 10 minutes

Cooking Time: 20 Minutes Servings: 2

- ✓ Set the Instant Pot to sauté and add the onion, oil, and curry paste.
- ✓ When the onion is soft, add the remaining ingredients and seal.
- ✓ Cook on Stew for 20 minutes.
- ✓ Release the pressure naturally.

Nutrition: Calories: 380 Carbs 13; Sugar 4; Fat 22; Protein 40; GL 14

250)   *Trout Bake*

Ingredients:

- 1lb trout fillets, boneless
- 1lb chopped winter vegetables
- 1 cup low sodium fish broth
- 1tbsp mixed herbs
- sea salt as desired

Direction: Preparation Time: 10 minutes

Cooking Time: 35 Minutes Servings: 2

- ✓ Mix all the ingredients except the broth in a foil pouch.
- ✓ Place the pouch in the steamer basket your Instant Pot.
- ✓ Pour the broth into the Instant Pot.
- ✓ Cook on Steam for 35 minutes.
- ✓ Release the pressure naturally.

Nutrition: : Calories 310; Carbs 14; Sugar 2; Fat 12; Protein 40; GL 5

251)   *Sardine Curry*

Ingredients:

- 5 tins of sardines in tomato
- 1lb chopped vegetables
- 1 cup low sodium fish broth
- 3tbsp curry paste

Direction: Preparation Time: 10 minutes Cooking

Time: 35 Minutes Servings: 2

- ✓ Mix all the ingredients in your Instant Pot.
- ✓ Cook on Stew for 35 minutes.
- ✓ Release the pressure naturally.

Nutrition: Calories 320; Carbs 8; Sugar 2; Fat 16; Protein GL 3

252)   *Swordfish Steak*

Ingredients:

- 1lb swordfish steak, whole
- 1lb chopped Mediterranean vegetables
- 1 cup low sodium fish broth
- 2tbsp soy sauce

Direction: Preparation Time: 10 minutes Cooking Time: 35 Minutes Servings: 2

- ✓ Mix all the ingredients except the broth in a foil pouch.
- ✓ Place the pouch in the steamer basket for your Instant Pot.
- ✓ Pour the broth into the Instant Pot. Lower the steamer basket into the Instant Pot.
- ✓ Cook on Steam for 35 minutes.
- ✓ Release the pressure naturally.

Nutrition: Calories 270; Carbs 5; Sugar 1; Fat 10; Protein 48; GL 1

253)   *Lemon Sole*

Ingredients:

- 1lb sole fillets, boned and skinned
- 1 cup low sodium fish broth
- 2 shredded sweet onions
- juice of half a lemon
- 2tbsp dried cilantro

Direction: Preparation Time: 10 minutes

Cooking Time: 5 Minutes Servings: 2

- ✓ Mix all the ingredients in your Instant Pot.
- ✓ Cook on Stew for 5 minutes.
- ✓ Release the pressure naturally.

Nutrition: Calories 230; Carbs Sugar 1; Fat 6; Protein 46; GL 1

254)   *Tuna Sweet corn Casserole*

Ingredients:

- 3 small tins of tuna

- 0.5lb sweet corn kernels
- 1lb chopped vegetables
- 1 cup low sodium vegetable broth
- 2tbsp spicy seasoning

Direction: Preparation Time: 10 minutes

Cooking Time: 35 Minutes Servings: 2

✓ Mix all the ingredients in your Instant Pot.
✓ Cook on Stew for 35 minutes.
✓ Release the pressure naturally.

Nutrition: Calories: 300;Carbs: 6 ;Sugar: 1 ;Fat: 9 ;Protein: ;GL: 2

255)   *Lemon Pepper Salmon*

Ingredients:

- 3 tbsps. ghee or avocado oil
- 1 lb. skin-on salmon filet
- 1 julienned red bell pepper
- 1 julienned green zucchini
- 1 julienned carrot
- ¾ cup water
- A few sprigs of parsley, tarragon, dill, basil or a combination
- 1/2 sliced lemon
- 1/2 tsp. black pepper
- ¼ tsp. sea salt

Direction: Preparation Time: 10 minutes Cooking Time: 10 Minutes Servings: 4

✓ Add the water and the herbs into the bottom of the Instant Pot and put in a wire steamer rack making sure the handles extend upwards.
✓ Place the salmon filet onto the wire rack, with the skin side facing down.
✓ Drizzle the salmon with ghee, season with black pepper and salt, and top with the lemon slices.
✓ Close and seal the Instant Pot, making sure the vent is turned to "Sealing".
✓ Select the "Steam" setting and cook for 3 minutes.
✓ While the salmon cooks, julienne the vegetables, and set aside.
✓ Once done, quick release the pressure, and then press the "Keep Warm/Cancel" button.
✓ Uncover and wearing oven mitts, carefully remove the steamer rack with the salmon.
✓ Remove the herbs and discard them.
✓ Add the vegetables to the pot and put the lid back on.
✓ Select the "Sauté" function and cook for 1-2 minutes.

✓ Serve the vegetables with salmon and add the remaining fat to the pot.
✓ Pour a little of the sauce over the fish and vegetables if desired.

Nutrition: Calories 296, Carbs 8g, Fat 15 g, Protein 31 g, Potassium (K) 1084 mg, Sodium (Na) 284 mg

256)   *Almond Crusted Baked Chili Mahi Mahi*

Ingredients:

- 4 mahi mahi fillets 1 lime
- 2 teaspoons olive oil Salt and pepper to taste
- ½ cup almonds
- ¼ teaspoon paprika
- ¼ teaspoon onion powder
- ¾ teaspoon chili powder
- ½ cup red bell pepper, chopped
- ¼ cup onion, chopped
- ¼ cup fresh cilantro, chopped

Direction: Preparation Time: 20 minutes Cooking Time: 15 minutes Servings: 4

✓ Preheat your oven to 325 degrees F. Line your baking pan with parchment paper. Squeeze juice from the lime.
✓ Grate zest from the peel. Put juice and zest in a bowl. Add the oil, salt and pepper. In another bowl, add the almonds, paprika, onion powder and chili powder.
✓ Put the almond mixture in a food processor. Pulse until powdery.
✓ Dip each fillet in the oil mixture.
✓ Dredge with the almond and chili mixture.
✓ Arrange on a single layer in the oven. Bake for 12 to 15 minutes or until fully cooked.
✓ Serve with red bell pepper, onion and cilantro.

Nutrition: Calories 322 Total Fat 12 g Saturated Fat 2 g Cholesterol 83 mg Sodium 328 mg Total Carbohydrate 28 g Dietary Fiber 4 g Total Sugars 10 g Protein 28 g Potassium 829 mg

257)   *Salmon & Asparagus*

Ingredients:

- 2 salmon fillets
- 8 spears asparagus, trimmed
- 2 tablespoons balsamic vinegar
- 1 teaspoon olive oil
- 1 teaspoon dried dill
- Salt and pepper to taste

Direction: Preparation Time: 15 minutes Cooking Time: 10 minutes Servings: 2

- ✓ Preheat your oven to 325 degrees F.
- ✓ Dry salmon with paper towels.
- ✓ Arrange the asparagus around the salmon fillets on a baking pan. In a bowl, mix the rest of the ingredients.
- ✓ Pour mixture over the salmon and vegetables.
- ✓ Bake in the oven for 10 minutes or until the fish is fully cooked.

Nutrition: Calories 328 Total Fat 15 g Saturated Fat 3 g Cholesterol 67 mg Sodium 365 mg Total Carbohydrate 6 g Dietary Fiber 4 g Total Sugars 5 g Protein 28 g Potassium 258 mg

258)   *Halibut with Spicy Apricot Sauce*

Ingredients:

- 4 fresh apricots, pitted
- ⅓ cup apricot preserves
- ½ cup apricot nectar
- ½ teaspoon dried oregano
- 3 tablespoons scallion, sliced
- 1 teaspoon hot pepper sauce Salt to taste
- 4 halibut steaks
- 1 tablespoon olive oil

Direction: Preparation Time: 15 minutes Cooking Time: 17 minutes Servings: 4

- ✓ Put the apricots, preserves, nectar, oregano, scallion, hot pepper sauce and salt in a saucepan.
- ✓ Bring to a boil and then simmer for 8 minutes. Set aside.
- ✓ Brush the halibut steaks with olive oil.
- ✓ Grill for 7 to 9 minutes or until fish is flaky.
- ✓ Brush one tablespoon of the sauce on both sides of the fish. Serve with the reserved sauce.

Nutrition:: Calories 304 Total Fat 8 g Saturated Fat 1 g Cholesterol 73 mg Sodium 260 mg Total Carbohydrate 27 g Dietary Fiber 2 g Total Sugars 16 g Protein 29 g Potassium 637 mg

259)   *Popcorn Shrimp*

Ingredients:

- Cooking spray
- ½ cup all-purpose flour
- 2 eggs, beaten
- 2 tablespoons water
- 1 ½ cups panko breadcrumbs

- 1 tablespoon garlic powder
- 1 tablespoon ground cumin
- 1 lb. shrimp, peeled and deveined
- ½ cup ketchup
- 2 tablespoons fresh cilantro, chopped
- 2 tablespoons lime juice Salt to taste

Direction: Preparation Time: 15 minutes Cooking Time: 8 minutes Servings: 4

- ✓ Coat the air fryer basket with cooking spray
- ✓ Put the flour in a dish. In the second dish, beat the eggs and water.
- ✓ In the third dish, mix the breadcrumbs, garlic powder and cumin.
- ✓ Dip each shrimp in each of the three dishes, first in the dish with flour, then the egg and then breadcrumb mixture.
- ✓ Place the shrimp in the air fryer basket.
- ✓ Cook at 360 degrees F for 8 minutes, flipping once halfway through.
- ✓ Combine the rest of the ingredients as dipping sauce for the shrimp.

Nutrition: Calories 297 Total Fat 4 g Saturated Fat 1 g Cholesterol 276 mg Sodium 291 mg Total Carbohydrate 35 g Dietary Fiber 1 g Total Sugars 9 g Protein 29 g Potassium 390 mg

260)   *Shrimp Lemon Kebab*

Ingredients:

- 1 ½ lb. shrimp, peeled and deveined but with tails intact
- ⅓ cup olive oil
- ¼ cup lemon juice
- 2 teaspoons lemon zest
- 1 tablespoon fresh parsley, chopped
- 8 cherry tomatoes, quartered
- 2 scallions, sliced

Direction: Preparation Time: 10 minutes Cooking Time: 5 minutes Servings: 4

- ✓ Mix the olive oil, lemon juice, lemon zest and parsley in a bowl.
- ✓ Marinate the shrimp in this mixture for 15 minutes.
- ✓ Thread each shrimp into the skewers.
- ✓ Grill for 4 to 5 minutes, turning once halfway through.
- ✓ Serve with tomatoes and scallions.

Nutrition: Calories 271 Total Fat 12 g Saturated Fat 2 g Cholesterol 259 mg Sodium 255 mg Total Carbohydrate 4 g Dietary Fiber 1 g Total Sugars 1 g Protein 25 g Potassium 429 mg

261) *Grilled Herbed Salmon with Raspberry Sauce & Cucumber Dill Dip*

Ingredients:

- 3 salmon fillets
- 1 tablespoon olive oil
- Salt and pepper to taste
- 1 teaspoon fresh sage, chopped
- 1 tablespoon fresh parsley, chopped
- 2 tablespoons Apple juice
- 1 cup raspberries
- 1 teaspoon Worcestershire sauce
- 1 cup cucumber, chopped
- 2 tablespoons light mayonnaise
- ½ teaspoon dried dill

Direction: Preparation Time: 15 minutes Cooking Time: 30 minutes Servings: 4

✓ Coat the salmon fillets with oil. Season with salt, pepper, sage and parsley.
✓ Cover the salmon with foil.
✓ Grill for 20 minutes or until fish is flaky.
✓ While waiting, mix the apple juice, raspberries and Worcestershire sauce.
✓ Pour the mixture into a saucepan over medium heat. Bring to a boil and then simmer for 8 minutes.
✓ In another bowl, mix the rest of the ingredients.
✓ Serve salmon with raspberry sauce and cucumber dip.

Nutrition: Calories 256 Total Fat 15 g Saturated Fat 3 g Cholesterol 68 mg Sodium 176 mg Total Carbohydrate 6 g Dietary Fiber 1 g Total Sugars 5 g Protein 23 g Potassium 359 mg

262) *Tarragon Scallops*

Ingredients:

- 1 cup water
- 1 lb. asparagus spears, trimmed
- 2 lemons 1
- ¼ lb. scallops
- Salt and pepper to taste
- 1 tablespoon olive oil
- 1 tablespoon fresh tarragon, chopped

Direction: Preparation Time: 10 minutes Cooking Time: 15 minutes Servings: 4

✓ Pour water into a pot. Bring to a boil. Add asparagus spears. Cover and cook for 5 minutes.
✓ Drain and transfer to a plate. Slice one lemon into wedges.
✓ Squeeze juice and shred zest from the remaining lemon.
✓ Season the scallops with salt and pepper.
✓ Put a pan over medium heat.
✓ Add oil to the pan.
✓ Cook the scallops until golden brown.
✓ Transfer to the same plate, putting scallops beside the asparagus.
✓ Add lemon zest, juice and tarragon to the pan. Cook for 1 minute.
✓ Drizzle tarragon sauce over the scallops and asparagus.

Nutrition: Calories 253 Total Fat 12 g Saturated Fat 2 g Cholesterol 47 mg Sodium 436 mg Total Carbohydrate 14 g Dietary Fiber 5 g Total Sugars 3 g Protein 27 g Potassium 773 mg

263) *Garlic Shrimp & Spinach*

Ingredients:

- 3 tablespoons olive oil, divided
- 6 clove garlic, sliced and divided
- 1 lb. spinach Salt to taste
- 1 tablespoons lemon juice
- 1 lb. shrimp, peeled and deveined
- ¼ teaspoon red pepper, crushed
- 1 tablespoon parsley, chopped
- 1 teaspoon lemon zest

Direction: Preparation Time: 10 minutes Cooking Time: 10 minutes Servings: 4

✓ Pour 1 tablespoon olive oil in a pot over medium heat.
✓ Cook the garlic for 1 minute.
✓ Add the spinach and season with salt.
✓ Cook for 3 minutes. Stir in lemon juice.
✓ Transfer to a bowl. Pour the remaining oil.
✓ Add the shrimp. Season with salt and add red pepper.
✓ Cook for 5 minutes.
✓ Sprinkle parsley and lemon zest over the shrimp before serving

Nutrition: Calories 226 Total Fat 12 g Saturated Fat 2 g Cholesterol 183 mg Sodium 444 mg Total Carbohydrate 6 g Dietary Fiber 3 g Total Sugars 1 g Protein 26 g Potassium 963 mg

264) *Herring & Veggies Soup*

Ingredients:

- 2 tablespoons olive oil
- 1 shallot, chopped
- 2 small garlic cloves, minced
- 1 jalapeño pepper, chopped
- 1 head cabbage, chopped 1 small red bell pepper, seeded and chopped finely
- 1 small yellow bell pepper, seeded and chopped finely
- 5 cups low-sodium chicken broth 2 (4-ounce) boneless herring fillets, cubed
- ¼ cup fresh cilantro, minced
- 2 tablespoons fresh lemon juice
- Ground black pepper, as required
- 2 scallions, chopped

Direction: Preparation Time: 15 minutes Cooking Time: 25 minutes Servings: 5

- ✓ In a large soup pan, heat the oil over medium heat and sauté shallot and garlic for 2-3 minutes.
- ✓ Add the cabbage and bell peppers and sauté for about 3-4 minutes.
- ✓ Add the broth and bring to a boil over high heat.
- ✓ Now, reduce the heat to medium-low and simmer for about 10 minutes.
- ✓ Add the herring cubes and cook for about 5-6 minutes.
- ✓ Stir in the cilantro, lemon juice, salt and black pepper and cook for about 1-2 minutes.
- ✓ Serve hot with the topping of scallion.

Meal Prep Tip:

- ✓ Transfer the soup into a large bowl and set aside to cool. Divide the soup into 5 containers evenly. Cover the containers and refrigerate for 1-2 days. Reheat in the microwave before serving.

Nutrition: Calories 215 Total Fat 11.2g Saturated Fat 2.1 g Cholesterol 35 mg Total Carbs 14.7 g Sugar 7 g Fiber 4.5 g Sodium 152 mg Potassium 574 mg Protein 15.1 g

265) Salmon Soup

Ingredients:

- 1 tablespoon olive oil
- 1 yellow onion, chopped
- 1 garlic clove, minced
- 4 cups low-sodium chicken broth
- 1 pound boneless salmon, cubed
- 2 tablespoon fresh cilantro, chopped
- Ground black pepper, as required
- 1 tablespoon fresh lime juice

Direction: Preparation Time: 15 minutes Cooking Time: 20 minutes Servings: 4

- ✓ In a large pan heat the oil over medium heat and sauté the onion for about 5 minutes.
- ✓ Add the garlic and sauté for about 1 minute.
- ✓ Stir in the broth and bring to a boil over high heat. Now, reduce the heat to low and simmer for about 10 minutes.
- ✓ Add the salmon, and soy sauce and cook for about 3-4 minutes. Stir in black pepper, lime juice, and cilantro and serve hot.

Meal Prep Tip:

- ✓ Transfer the soup into a large bowl and set aside to cool.
- ✓ Divide the soup into 4 containers evenly.
- ✓ Cover the containers and refrigerate for 1-2 days. Reheat in the microwave before serving.

Nutrition: Calories 208 Total Fat 10.5 g Saturated Fat 1.5 g Cholesterol 50 mg Total Carbs 3.9 g Sugar 1.2 g Fiber 0.6 g Sodium 121 mg Potassium 331 mg Protein 24.4 g

266) Salmon Curry

Ingredients:

- 6 (4-ounce) salmon fillets
- 1 teaspoon ground turmeric, divided Salt, as required
- 3 tablespoon olive oil, divided
- 1 yellow onion, chopped finely
- 1 teaspoon garlic paste
- 1 teaspoon fresh ginger paste
- 3-4 green chilies, halved
- 1 teaspoon red chili powder
- ½ teaspoon ground cumin
- ½ teaspoon ground cinnamon
- ¾ cup fat-free plain Greek yogurt, whipped
- ¾ cup filtered water 3 tablespoon fresh cilantro, chopped

Direction: Preparation Time: 15 minutes Cooking Time: 30 minutes Servings: 6

- ✓ Season each salmon fillet with ½ teaspoon of the turmeric and salt.
- ✓ In a large skillet, melt 1 tablespoon of the butter over medium heat and cook the salmon fillets for about 2 minutes per side.
- ✓ Transfer the salmon onto a plate. In the same skillet, melt the remaining butter over medium heat and sauté the onion for about 4-5 minutes.
- ✓ Add the garlic paste, ginger paste, green chilies, remaining turmeric and spices and sauté for about 1 minute.

✓ Now, reduce the heat to medium-low. Slowly, add the yogurt and water, stirring continuously until smooth.

✓ Cover the skillet and simmer for about 10-15 minutes or until desired doneness of the sauce.

✓ Carefully, add the salmon fillets and simmer for about 5 minutes. Serve hot with the garnishing of cilantro.

Meal Prep Tip:

✓ Transfer the curry into a large bowl and set aside to cool. Divide the curry into 6 containers evenly.

✓ Cover the containers and refrigerate for 1-2 days. Reheat in the microwave before serving.

Nutrition: Calories 242 Total Fat 14.3 g Saturated Fat 2 g Sugar 2 g Fiber 0.8 g mg Protein 25.4 g

267)   *Salmon with Bell Peppers*

Ingredients:

- 6 (3-ounce) salmon fillets Pinch of salt
- Ground black pepper, as required
- 1 yellow bell pepper, seeded and cubed
- 1 red bell pepper, seeded and cubed, 4 plum tomatoes, cubed
- 1 small onion, sliced thinly
- ½ cup fresh parsley, chopped
- ¼ cup olive oil
- 2 tablespoons fresh lemon juice

Direction: Preparation Time: 15 minutes Cooking Time: 20 minutes Servings: 6

✓ Preheat the oven to 400 degrees F. Season each salmon fillet with salt and black pepper lightly. In a bowl, mix together the bell peppers, tomato and onion.

✓ Arrange 6 foil pieces onto a smooth surface. Place 1 salmon fillet over each foil paper and sprinkle with salt and black pepper.

✓ Place veggie mixture over each fillet evenly and top with parsley and capers evenly.

✓ Drizzle with oil and lemon juice. Fold each foil around salmon mixture to seal it. Arrange the foil packets onto a large baking sheet in a single layer.

✓ Bake for about 20 minutes. Serve hot.

Meal Prep Tip:

✓ Transfer the salmon mixture into a large bowl and set aside to cool. Divide the salmon mixture into 6 containers evenly.

✓ Cover the containers and refrigerate for 1 day. Reheat in the microwave before serving.

Nutrition: Calories 220 Total Fat 14 g Saturated Fat 2 g Cholesterol 38 mg Total Carbs 7.7 g Sugar 4.8 g Fiber 2 g Sodium 74 mg Potassium 647 mg Protein 17.9 g

268)   *Shrimp Salad*

Ingredients:

- For Salad: 1 pound shrimp, peeled and deveined
- Salt and ground black pepper, as required
- 1 teaspoon olive oil
- 1½ cups carrots, peeled and julienned
- 1½ cups red cabbage, shredded1
- ½ cup cucumber, julienned
- 5 cups fresh baby arugula
- ¼ cup fresh basil, chopped
- ¼ cup fresh cilantro, chopped
- 4 cups lettuce, torn
- ¼ cup almonds, chopped

For Dressing:

- 2 tablespoons natural almond butter
- 1 garlic clove, crushed
- 1 tablespoon fresh cilantro, chopped
- 1 tablespoon fresh lime juice 1 tablespoon unsweetened applesauce
- 2 teaspoons balsamic vinegar
- ½ teaspoon cayenne pepper Salt, as required
- 1 tablespoon water 1/3 cup olive oil

Direction: Preparation Time: 20 minutes Cooking Time: 4 minutes Servings: 6

✓ Slowly, add the oil, beating continuously until smooth. For salad: in a bowl, add shrimp, salt, black pepper and oil and toss to coat well. Heat a skillet over medium-high heat and cook the shrimp for about 2 minutes per side.

✓ Remove from the heat and set aside to cool. In a large bowl, add the shrimp, vegetables and mix well. For dressing: in a bowl, add all ingredients except oil and beat until well combined.

✓ Place the dressing over shrimp mixture and gently, toss to coat well. Serve immediately.

Meal Prep Tip:

✓ Divide dressing in 6 large mason jars evenly. Place the remaining ingredients in the layers of carrots, followed by cabbage, cucumber, arugula, basil, cilantro, shrimp, lettuce and almonds.

✓ Cover each jar with the lid tightly and refrigerate for about 1 day. Shake the jars well just before serving.

Nutrition: Calories 274 Total Fat 17.7 g Saturated Fat 2.4 g Cholesterol 159 mg Total Carbs 10 g Sugar 3.8 g Fiber 2.9 g Sodium 242 mg Potassium 481 mg Protein 20.5 g

269) *Shrimp & Veggies Curry*

Ingredients:

- 2 teaspoons olive oil
- 1½ medium white onions, sliced
- 2 medium green bell peppers, seeded and sliced
- 3 medium carrots, peeled and sliced thinly
- 3 garlic cloves, chopped finely
- 1 tablespoon fresh ginger, chopped finely
- 2½ teaspoons curry powder
- 1½ pounds shrimp, peeled and deveined
- 1 cup filtered water
- 2 tablespoons fresh lime juice
- Salt and ground black pepper, as required
- 2 tablespoons fresh cilantro, chopped

Direction: Preparation Time: 20 minutes Cooking Time: 20 minutes Servings: 6

- ✓ In a large skillet, heat oil over medium-high heat and sauté the onion for about 4-5 minutes.
- ✓ Add the bell peppers and carrot and sauté for about 3-4 minutes. Add the garlic, ginger and curry powder and sauté for about 1 minute.
- ✓ Add the shrimp and sauté for about 1 minute. Stir in the water and cook for about 4-6 minutes, stirring occasionally.
- ✓ Stir in lime juice and remove from heat. Serve hot with the garnishing of cilantro.

Meal Prep Tip:
- ✓ Transfer the curry into a large bowl and set aside to cool. Divide the curry into 6 containers evenly.
- ✓ Cover the containers and refrigerate for 1-2 days. Reheat in the microwave before serving.

Nutrition: Calories 193 Total Fat 3.8 g Saturated Fat 0.9 g Cholesterol 239 mg Total Carbs 12 g Sugar 4.7 g Fiber 2.3 g Sodium 328 mg

270) *Shrimp with Zucchini*

Ingredients:

- 3 tablespoons olive oil
- 1 pound medium shrimp, peeled and deveined
- 1 shallot, minced 4 garlic cloves, minced
- ¼ teaspoon red pepper flakes, crushed
- Salt and ground black pepper, as required
- ¼ cup low-sodium chicken broth
- 2 tablespoons fresh lemon juice
- 1 teaspoon fresh lemon zest, grated finely
- ½ pound zucchini, spiralized with Blade C

Direction: Preparation Time: 20 minutes Cooking Time: 8 minutes Servings: 4

- ✓ In a large skillet, heat the oil and butter over medium-high heat and cook the shrimp, shallot, garlic, red pepper flakes, salt and black pepper for about 2 minutes, stirring occasionally.
- ✓ Stir in the broth, lemon juice and lemon zest and bring to a gentle boil.
- ✓ Stir in zucchini noodles and cook for about 1-2 minutes.
- ✓ Serve hot.

Meal Prep Tip:
- ✓ Transfer the shrimp mixture into a large bowl and set aside to cool.
- ✓ Divide the shrimp mixture into 4 containers. Cover the containers and refrigerate for about 1-2 days.
- ✓ Reheat in microwave before serving.

Nutrition: Calories 245 Total Fat 12.6 g Saturated Fat 2.2 g Cholesterol 239 mg Total Carbs 5.8 g Sugar 1.2 g Fiber 08 g Sodium 289 mg Potassium 381 mg Protein 27 g

271) *Shrimp with Broccoli*

Ingredients:

- 2 tablespoons olive oil, divided
- 4 cups broccoli, chopped
- 2-3 tablespoons filtered water
- 1½ pounds large shrimp, peeled and deveined
- 2 garlic cloves, minced
- 1 (1-inch) piece fresh ginger, minced
- Salt and ground black pepper, as required

Direction: Preparation Time: 15 minutes Cooking Time: 12 minutes Servings: 6

- ✓ : In a large skillet, heat 1 tablespoon of oil over medium-high heat and cook the broccoli for about 1-2 minutes stirring continuously.
- ✓ Stir in the water and cook, covered for about 3-4 minutes, stirring occasionally.
- ✓ With a spoon, push the broccoli to side of the pan. Add the remaining oil and let it heat.
- ✓ Add the shrimp and cook for about 1-2 minutes, tossing occasionally.
- ✓ Add the remaining ingredients and sauté for about 2-3 minutes. Serve hot.

Meal Prep Tip:
- ✓ Transfer the shrimp mixture into a large bowl and set aside to cool.
- ✓ Divide the shrimp mixture into 6 containers evenly.
- ✓ Cover the containers and refrigerate for 1 day. Reheat in the microwave before serving.

Nutrition: Calories 197 Total Fat 6.8 g Saturated Fat

1.3 g Cholesterol 239 mg Total Carbs 6.1 g Sugar 1.1g Fiber 1.6 g Sodium 324 mg Potassium 389 mg Protein 27.6 g

272) *Grilled Salmon with Ginger Sauce*

Ingredients:

- 1 tablespoon toasted sesame oil
- 1 tablespoon fresh cilantro, chopped
- 1 tablespoon lime juice
- 1 teaspoon fish sauce
- 1 clove garlic, mashed
- 1 teaspoon fresh ginger, grated
- 1 teaspoon jalapeño pepper, minced
- 4 salmon fillets
- 1 tablespoon olive oil
- Salt and pepper to taste

Direction: Preparation Time: 15 minutes Cooking Time: 8 minutes Servings: 4

- ✓ In a bowl, mix the sesame oil, cilantro, lime juice, fish sauce, garlic, ginger and jalapeño pepper.
- ✓ Preheat your grill.
- ✓ Brush oil on salmon. Season both sides with salt and pepper.
- ✓ Grill salmon for 6 to 8 minutes, turning once or twice.
- ✓ Take 1 tablespoon from the oil mixture.
- ✓ Brush this on the salmon while grilling.
- ✓ Serve grilled salmon with the remaining sauce.

Nutrition: Calories 204 Total Fat 11 g Saturated Fat 2 g Cholesterol 53 mg Sodium 320 mg Total Carbohydrate 2 g Dietary Fiber 0 g Total Sugars 2 g Protein 23 g Potassium 437 mg

273) *Swordfish with Tomato Salsa*

Ingredients:

- 1 cup tomato, chopped
- ¼ cup tomatillo, chopped
- 2 tablespoons fresh cilantro, chopped
- ¼ cup avocado, chopped
- 1 clove garlic, minced
- 1 jalapeño pepper, chopped
- 1 tablespoon lime juice
- Salt and pepper to taste
- 4 swordfish steaks
- 1 clove garlic, sliced in half
- 2 tablespoons lemon juice
- ½ teaspoon ground cumin

Direction: Preparation Time: 20 minutes Cooking Time: 12 minutes Servings: 4

- ✓ Preheat your grill. In a bowl, mix the tomato, tomatillo, cilantro, avocado, garlic, jalapeño, lime juice, salt and pepper.
- ✓ Cover the bowl with foil and put in the refrigerator.
- ✓ Rub each swordfish steak with sliced garlic. Drizzle lemon juice on both sides.
- ✓ Season with salt, pepper and cumin.
- ✓ Grill for 12 minutes or until the fish is fully cooked. Serve with salsa.

Nutrition: Calories 190 Total Fat 8 g Saturated Fat 2 g Cholesterol 43 mg Sodium 254 mg Total Carbohydrate 6 g Dietary Fiber 3 g Total Sugars 1 g Protein 24 g Potassium 453 mg

274) *Salmon & Shrimp Stew*

Ingredients:

- 2 tablespoons olive oil
- 1/2 cup onion, chopped finely
- 2 garlic cloves, minced
- 1 Serrano pepper, chopped
- 1 teaspoon smoked paprika
- 4 cups fresh tomatoes, chopped
- 4 cups low-sodium chicken broth
- 1 pound salmon fillets, cubed
- 1 pound shrimp, peeled and deveined
- 2 tablespoons fresh lime juice
- ¼ cup fresh basil, chopped
- ¼ cup fresh parsley, chopped
- Ground black pepper, as required
- 2 scallions, chopped

Direction: Preparation Time: 20 minutes

Cooking Time: 21 minutes Servings: 6

- ✓ In a large soup pan, melt coconut oil over medium-high heat and sauté the onion for about 5-6 minutes.
- ✓ Add the garlic, Serrano pepper and smoked paprika and sauté for about 1 minute.
- ✓ Add the tomatoes and broth and bring to a gentle simmer over medium heat.
- ✓ Simmer for about 5 minutes.
- ✓ Add the salmon and simmer for about 3-4 minutes.
- ✓ Stir in the remaining seafood and cook for about 4-5 minutes.
- ✓ Stir in the lemon juice, basil, parsley, sea salt and black pepper and remove from heat.
- ✓ Serve hot with the garnishing of scallion.

Nutrition: Calories 271; Total Fat 11 g; Saturated Fat

1.8 g; Cholesterol 193 mg; Total Carbs 8.6 g; Sugar
3.8 g; Fiber 2.1 g; Sodium 273 mg; Potassium 763
mg; Protein 34.7 g

275)   *Salmon Baked*

Ingredients:

- 6 (3-ounce) salmon fillets
- Pinch of salt
- Ground black pepper, as required
- 1 yellow bell pepper, seeded and cubed
- 1 red bell pepper, seeded and cubed
- 4 plum tomatoes, cubed
- •1 small onion, sliced thinly
- 1/2 cup fresh parsley, chopped
- ¼ cup olive oil
- 2 tablespoons fresh lemon juice

Direction: Preparation Time: 15 minutes

Cooking Time: 20 minutes Servings: 6

- ✓ Preheat the oven to 400 degrees F.
- ✓ Season each salmon fillet with salt and black pepper lightly.
- ✓ In a bowl, mix together the bell peppers, tomato and onion.
- ✓ Arrange 6 foil pieces onto a smooth surface.
- ✓ Place 1 salmon fillet over each foil paper and sprinkle with salt and black pepper.   ✓
      Place veggie mixture over each fillet evenly and top with parsley and capers evenly.
- ✓ Drizzle with oil and lemon juice.
- ✓ Fold each foil around salmon mixture to seal it.
- ✓ Arrange the foil packets onto a large baking sheet in a single layer.
- ✓ Bake for about 20 minutes.
- ✓ Serve hot.

**Nutrition: Calories 220; Total Fat 14 g; Saturated Fat
2 g ; Cholesterol 38 mg; Total Carbs 7.7 g; Sugar 4.8
g; Fiber 2 g; Sodium 74 mg; Potassium 647 mg;
Protein 17.9 g**

SIDE DISH

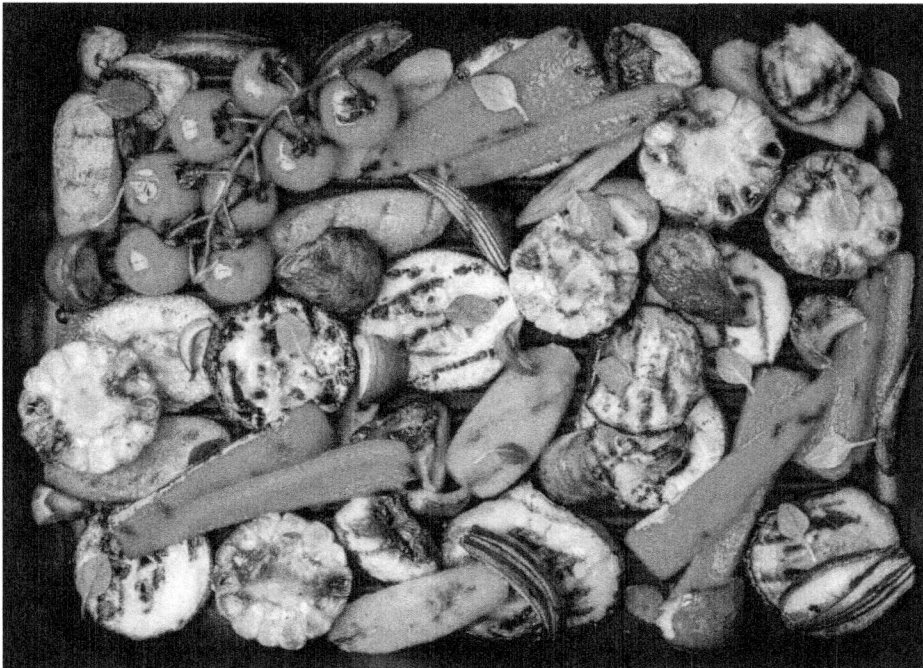

276)   *Lemon Garlic Green Beans*

Ingredients:

- 1 1/2 pounds green beans, trimmed
- 2 tablespoons olive oil
- 1 tablespoon fresh lemon juice
- 2 cloves minced garlic
- Salt and pepper

Direction: Preparation time: 5 minutes Cooking Time: 10 minutes Servings: 6

- ✓ Fill a large bowl with ice water and set aside.
- ✓ Bring a pot of salted water to boil then add the green beans.
- ✓ Cook for 3 minutes then drain and immediately place in the ice water.
- ✓ Cool the beans completely then drain them well.
- ✓ Heat the oil in a large skillet over medium-high heat.
- ✓ Add the green beans, tossing to coat, then add the lemon juice, garlic, salt, and pepper.
- ✓ Sauté for 3 minutes until the beans are tender-crisp then serve hot.

Nutrition: Calories 75, Total Fat 4.8g, Saturated Fat 0.7g, Total Carbs 8.5g, Net Carbs 4.6g, Protein 2.1g, Sugar 1.7g, Fiber 3.9g, Sodium 7mg

277)   *Brown Rice & Lentil Salad*

Ingredients:

- 1 cup water
- 1/2 cup instant brown rice
- 2 tablespoons olive oil
- 2 tablespoons red wine vinegar
- 1 tablespoon Dijon mustard
- 1 tablespoon minced onion
- 1/2 teaspoon paprika
- Salt and pepper
- 1 (15-ounce) can brown lentils, rinsed and drained
- 1 medium carrot, shredded
- 2 tablespoons fresh chopped parsley

Direction: Preparation time: 10 minutes

Cooking Time: 10 minutes Servings: 4

- ✓ Stir together the water and instant brown rice in a medium saucepan.
- ✓ Bring to a boil then simmer for 10 minutes, covered.
- ✓ Remove from heat and set aside while you prepare the salad.
- ✓ Whisk together the olive oil, vinegar, Dijon mustard,

onion, paprika, salt, and pepper in a medium bowl.
- ✓ Toss in the cooked rice, lentils, carrots, and parsley.
- ✓ Adjust seasoning to taste then stir well and serve warm.

Nutrition: Calories 145, Total Fat 7.7g, Saturated Fat 1g, Total Carbs 13.1g, Net Carbs 10.9g, Protein 6g, Sugar 1g, Fiber 2.2g, Sodium 57mg

278)   *Mashed Butternut Squash*

Ingredients:

- 3 pounds whole butternut squash (about 2 medium)
- 2 tablespoons olive oil
- Salt and pepper

Direction: Preparation time: 5 minutes Cooking Time: 25 minutes Servings: 6

- ✓ Preheat the oven to 400F and line a baking sheet with parchment.
- ✓ Cut the squash in half and remove the seeds.
- ✓ Cut the squash into cubes and toss with oil then spread on the baking sheet.
- ✓ Roast for 25 minutes until tender then place in a food processor.
- ✓ Blend smooth then season with salt and pepper to taste.

Nutrition: Calories 90, Total Fat 4.8g, Saturated Fat 0.7g, Total Carbs 12.3g, Net Carbs 10.2g, Protein 1.1g, Sugar 2.3g, Fiber 2.1g, Sodium 4mg

279)   *Cilantro Lime Quinoa*

Ingredients:

- 1 cup uncooked quinoa
- 1 tablespoon olive oil
- 1 medium yellow onion, diced
- 2 cloves minced garlic
- 1 (4-ounce) can diced green chiles, drained
- 1 1/2 cups fat-free chicken broth
- ¾ cup fresh chopped cilantro
- 1/2 cup sliced green onion
- 2 tablespoons lime juice
- Salt and pepper

Direction: Preparation time: 5 minutes

Cooking Time: 25 minutes Servings: 6

- ✓ Rinse the quinoa thoroughly in cool water using a fine mesh sieve.
- ✓ Heat the oil in a large saucepan over medium heat.
- ✓ Add the onion and sauté for 2 minutes then stir in the chile and garlic.

✓ Cook for 1 minute then stir in the quinoa and chicken broth.

✓ Bring to a boil then reduce heat and simmer, covered, until the quinoa absorbs the liquid – about 20 to 25 minutes.

✓ Remove from heat then stir in the cilantro, green onions, and lime juice.

✓ Season with salt and pepper to taste and serve hot.

Nutrition: Calories 150, Total Fat 4.1g, Saturated Fat 0.5g, Total Carbs 22.5g, Net Carbs 19.8g, Protein 6g, Sugar 1.7g, Fiber 2.7g, Sodium 179mg

280)   *Oven-Roasted Veggies*

Ingredients:

- 1 pound cauliflower florets
- 1/2 pound broccoli florets
- 1 large yellow onion, cut into chunks
- 1 large red pepper, cored and chopped
- 2 medium carrots, peeled and sliced
- 2 tablespoons olive oil
- 2 tablespoons apple cider vinegar
- Salt and pepper

Direction: Preparation time: 5 minutes Cooking Time: 25 minutes Servings: 6

✓ Preheat the oven to 425F and line a large rimmed baking sheet with parchment.

✓ Spread the veggies on the baking sheet and drizzle with oil and vinegar.

✓ Toss well and season with salt and pepper.

✓ Spread the veggies in a single layer then roast for 20 to 25 minutes, stirring every 10 minutes, until tender.

✓ Adjust seasoning to taste and serve hot.

Nutrition: Calories 100, Total Fat 5g, Saturated Fat 0.7g, Total Carbs 12.4g, Net Carbs 8.2g, Protein 3.2g, Sugar 5.5g, Fiber 4.2g, Sodium 51mg

281)   *Vegetable Rice Pilaf*

Ingredients:

- 1 tablespoon olive oil
- 1/2 medium yellow onion, diced
- 1 cup uncooked long-grain brown rice
- 2 cloves minced garlic
- 1/2 teaspoon dried basil
- Salt and pepper
- 2 cups fat-free chicken broth
- 1 cup frozen mixed veggies

Direction: Preparation time: 5 minutes

Cooking Time: 25 minutes Servings: 6

✓ Heat the oil in a large skillet over medium heat.

✓ Add the onion and sauté for 3 minutes until translucent.

✓ Stir in the rice and cook until lightly toasted.

✓ Add the garlic, basil, salt, and pepper then stir to combined.

✓ Stir in the chicken broth then bring to a boil.

✓ Reduce heat and simmer, covered, for 10 minutes.

✓ Stir in the frozen veggies then cover and cook for another 10 minutes until heated through. Serve hot.

Nutrition: Calories 90, Total Fat 2.7g, Saturated Fat 0.4g, Total Carbs 12.6g, Net Carbs 10.4g, Protein 3.9g, Sugar 1.5g, Fiber 2.2g, Sodium 143mg

282)   *Curry Roasted Cauliflower Florets*

Ingredients:

- 8 cups cauliflower florets
- 2 tablespoons olive oil
- 1 teaspoon curry powder
- 1/2 teaspoon garlic powder
- Salt and pepper

Direction: Preparation time: 5 minutes Cooking Time: 25 minutes Servings: 6

✓ Preheat the oven to 425F and line a baking sheet with foil.

✓ Toss the cauliflower with the olive oil and spread on the baking sheet.

✓ Sprinkle with curry powder, garlic powder, salt, and pepper.

✓ Roast for 25 minutes or until just tender. Serve hot.

Nutrition: Calories 75, Total Fat 4.9g, Saturated Fat 0.7g, Total Carbs 7.4g, Net Carbs 3.9g, Protein 2.7g, Sugar 3.3g, Fiber 3.5g, Sodium 40mg

283)   *Mushroom Barley Risotto*

Ingredients:

- 4 cups fat-free beef broth
- 2 tablespoons olive oil
- 1 small onion, diced well
- 2 cloves minced garlic
- 8 ounces thinly sliced mushrooms
- ¼ tsp. dried thyme
- Salt and pepper
- 1 cup pearled barley
- 1/2 cup dry white wine

Direction: Preparation time: 5 minutes

Cooking Time: 25 minutes Servings: 8

- ✓ Heat the beef broth in a medium saucepan and keep it warm.
- ✓ Heat the oil in a large, deep skillet over medium heat.
- ✓ Add the onions and garlic and sauté for 2 minutes then stir in the mushrooms and thyme.
- ✓ Season with salt and pepper and sauté for 2 minutes more.
- ✓ Add the barley and sauté for 1 minute then pour in the wine.
- ✓ Ladle about 1/2 cup of beef broth into the skillet and stir well to combine.
- ✓ Cook until most of the broth has been absorbed then add another ladle.
- ✓ Repeat until you have used all of the broth and the barley is cooked to al dente.
- ✓ Adjust seasoning to taste with salt and pepper and serve hot.

Nutrition: Calories 155, Total Fat 4.4g, Saturated Fat 0.6g, Total Carbs 21.9g, Net Carbs 17.5g, Protein 5.5g, Sugar 1.2g, Fiber 4.4g, Sodium 455mg

284)   *Braised Summer Squash*

Ingredients:

- 3 tablespoons olive oil
- 3 cloves minced garlic
- ¼ teaspoon crushed red pepper flakes
- 1 pound summer squash, sliced
- 1 pound zucchini, sliced
- 1 teaspoon dried oregano
- Salt and pepper

Direction: Preparation time: 10 minutes Cooking Time: 20 minutes Servings: 6

- ✓ Heat the oil in a large skillet over medium heat.
- ✓ Add the garlic and crushed red pepper and cook for 2 minutes.
- ✓ Add the summer squash and zucchini and cook for 15 minutes, stirring often, until just tender.
- ✓ Stir in the oregano then season with salt and pepper to taste. serve hot.

Nutrition: Calories 90, Total Fat 7.4g, Saturated Fat 1.1g, Total Carbs 6.2g, Net Carbs 4.4g, Protein 1.8g, Sugar 4g, Fiber 1.8g, Sodium 10mg

285)   *Parsley Tabbouleh*

Ingredients:

- 1 cup water
- 1/2 cup bulgur
- ¼ cup fresh lemon juice
- 2 tablespoons olive oil
- 2 cloves minced garlic
- Salt and pepper
- 2 cups fresh chopped parsley
- 2 medium tomatoes, died
- 1 small cucumber, diced
- ¼ cup fresh chopped mint

Direction: Preparation time: 5 minutes

Cooking Time: 25 minutes Servings: 6

- ✓ Bring the water and bulgur to a boil in a small saucepan then remove from heat.
- ✓ Cover and let stand until the water is fully absorbed, about 25 minutes.
- ✓ Meanwhile, whisk together the lemon juice, olive oil, garlic, salt, and pepper in a medium bowl.
- ✓ Toss in the cooked bulgur along with the parsley, tomatoes, cucumber, and mint.
- ✓ Season with salt and pepper to taste and serve.

Nutrition: Calories 110, Total Fat 5.3g, Saturated Fat 0.9g, Total Carbs 14.4g, Net Carbs 10.5g, Protein 3g, Sugar 2.4g, Fiber 3.9g, Sodium 21mg

286)   *Garlic Sautéed Spinach*

Ingredients:

- 1 1/2 tablespoons olive oil
- 4 cloves minced garlic
- 6 cups fresh baby spinach
- Salt and pepper

Direction: Preparation time: 5 minutes Cooking Time: 10 minutes Servings: 4

- ✓ Heat the oil in a large skillet over medium-high heat.
- ✓ Add the garlic and cook for 1 minute.
- ✓ Stir in the spinach and season with salt and pepper.
- ✓ Sauté for 1 to 2 minutes until just wilted. Serve hot.

Nutrition: Calories 60, Total Fat 5.5g, Saturated Fat 0.8g, Total Carbs 2.6g, Net Carbs 1.5g, Protein 1.5g, Sugar 0.2g, Fiber 1.1g, Sodium 36mg

287)   *French Lentils*

Ingredients:

- 2 tablespoons olive oil
- 1 medium onion, diced

- 1 medium carrot, peeled and diced
- 2 cloves minced garlic
- 5 1/2 cups water
- 2 ¼ cups French lentils, rinsed and drained
- 1 teaspoon dried thyme
- 2 small bay leaves
- Salt and pepper

Direction: Preparation time: 5 minutes

Cooking Time: 25 minutes Servings: 10

✓ Heat the oil in a large saucepan over medium heat.
✓ Add the onions, carrot, and garlic and sauté for 3 minutes.
✓ Stir in the water, lentils, thyme, and bay leaves – season with salt.
✓ Bring to a boil then reduce to a simmer and cook until tender, about 20 minutes.
✓ Drain any excess water and adjust seasoning to taste. Serve hot.

Nutrition: Calories 185, Total Fat 3.3g, Saturated Fat 0.5g, Total Carbs 27.9g, Net Carbs 14.2g, Protein 11.4g, Sugar 1.7g, Fiber 13.7g, Sodium 11mg

288) *Grain-Free Berry Cobbler*

Ingredients:

- 4 cups fresh mixed berries
- 1/2 cup ground flaxseed
- ¼ cup almond meal
- ¼ cup unsweetened shredded coconut
- 1/2 tablespoon baking powder
- 1 teaspoon ground cinnamon
- ¼ teaspoon salt
- Powdered stevia, to taste
- 6 tablespoons coconut oil

Direction: Preparation time: 5 minutes

Cooking Time: 25 minutes Servings: 10

✓ Preheat the oven to 375F and lightly grease a 10-inch cast-iron skillet.
✓ Spread the berries on the bottom of the skillet.
✓ Whisk together the dry ingredients in a mixing bowl.
✓ Cut in the coconut oil using a fork to create a crumbled mixture.
✓ Spread the crumble over the berries and bake for 25 minutes until hot and bubbling.
✓ Cool the cobbler for 5 to 10 minutes before serving.

Nutrition: Calories 215 Total Fat 16.8g, Saturated Fat 10.4g, Total Carbs 13.1g, Net Carbs 6.7g, Protein 3.7g, Sugar 5.3g, Fiber 6.4g, Sodium 61mg

289) *Spicy Spinach*

Ingredients:

- 1 tablespoon olive oil
- 1 red onion, chopped finely
- 6 garlic cloves, minced
- 1 (1-inch) piece fresh ginger, minced
- 1 teaspoon garam masala
- 1 teaspoon ground coriander
- ½ teaspoon ground cumin
- ¼ teaspoon ground turmeric
- 6 cups fresh spinach, chopped
- Salt and ground black pepper, as required
- 1-2 tablespoons water

Direction: Preparation Time: 10 minutes Cooking Time: 20 minutes Servings: 3

✓ Heat the olive oil in a large nonstick skillet over medium heat and sauté the onion for about 6-7 minutes.
✓ Add the garlic, ginger and spices and sauté for about 1 minute.
✓ Add the spinach, salt and black pepper and water and cook, covered for about 10 minutes.
✓ Uncover and stir fry for about 2 minutes. Serve hot.

Meal Prep Tip:
✓ Transfer the spinach mixture into a large bowl and set aside to cool completely. Divide the mixture into 3 containers evenly.
✓ Cover the containers and refrigerate for about 1-2 days. Reheat in the microwave before serving.

Nutrition: Calories 80 Total Fat 5.1 g Saturated Fat 0.7 g Cholesterol 0 mg Total Carbs 8 g Sugar 1.9 g Fiber 2.3 g Sodium 52 mg Potassium 331 mg Protein 2.6 g

290) *Herbed Asparagus*

Ingredients:

- 2 tablespoons olive oil
- 2 tablespoons fresh lemon juice
- 1 tablespoon balsamic vinegar
- 1 teaspoon garlic, minced
- 1 tablespoon fresh parsley, chopped
- 1 teaspoon dried oregano
- Salt and ground black pepper, as required
- 1 pound fresh asparagus, ends removed

Direction: Preparation Time: 10 minutes Cooking Time: 10 minutes Servings: 4

✓ Preheat oven to 400 degrees F and lightly grease a

rimmed baking sheet.

✓ Place the oil, lemon juice, vinegar, garlic, herbs, salt and black pepper in a bowl and beat until well combined.

✓ Arrange the asparagus onto the prepared baking sheet in a single layer. Top with half of the herb mixture and toss to coat.

✓ Roast for about 8-10 minutes. Remove from the oven and transfer the asparagus onto a platter. Drizzle with the remaining herb mixture and serve.

Meal Prep Tip:

✓ Transfer the asparagus into a large bowl and set aside to cool completely.

✓ Divide the asparagus into 4 containers evenly. Cover the containers and refrigerate for about 1-2 days. Reheat in the microwave before serving.

Nutrition: Calories 88 Total Fat 7.3 g Saturated Fat 1.1 g Cholesterol 0 mg Total Carbs 5.1 g Sugar 2.4 g Fiber 2.6 g Sodium 5 mg Potassium 256 mg Protein 2.7 g

291)   *Lemony Brussels Sprout*

Ingredients:

- ½ pound Brussels sprouts, halved
- 1 tablespoon olive oil
- 1 garlic clove, minced
- ½ teaspoon red pepper flakes, crushed
- Salt and ground black pepper, as required
- 1 tablespoon fresh lemon juice

Direction: Preparation Time: 10 minutes Cooking Time: 7 minutes Servings: 2

✓ : Heat the olive oil in a large skillet over medium heat and cook the garlic and red pepper flakes for about 1 minute, stirring continuously.

✓ Stir in the Brussels sprouts, salt and black pepper and sauté for about 4-5 minutes.

✓ Stir in lemon juice and sauté for about 1 minute more. Serve hot.

Meal Prep Tip:

✓ Transfer the Brussels sprouts into a large bowl and set aside to cool completely.

✓ Divide the Brussels sprouts into 2 containers evenly. Cover the containers and refrigerate for about 1-2 days.

✓ Reheat in the microwave before serving.

Nutrition: Calories 114 Total Fat 7.5 g Saturated Fat 1.2 g Cholesterol 0 mg Total Carbs 11.2 g Sugar 2.7 g Fiber 4.4 g Sodium 108 mg Potassium 465 mg Protein 4.1 g

292)   *Gingered Cauliflower*

Ingredients:

- 2 cups cauliflower, cut into
- 1-inch florets Salt, as required
- 2 tablespoons olive oil
- 1 teaspoon fresh ginger root, sliced thinly
- 2 fresh thyme sprigs

Direction: Preparation Time: 0 minutes Cooking Time: 0 minutes Servings: 2

✓ In a pan of the water, add the cauliflower and salt over medium heat and bring to a boil.

✓ Cover and cook for about 10-12 minutes.

✓ Drain the cauliflower well and transfer onto a serving platter.

✓ Meanwhile, in a small skillet, melt the coconut oil over medium-low heat.

✓ Add the ginger and thyme sprigs and swirl the pan occasionally for about 2-3 minutes.   ✓ Discard the ginger and thyme sprigs.

✓ Pour the oil over cauliflower and serve immediately.

Meal Prep Tip:

✓ Transfer the cauliflower into a large bowl and set aside to cool completely.

✓ Divide the cauliflower into 2 containers evenly.

✓ Cover the containers and refrigerate for about 1-2 days. Reheat in the microwave before serving.

Nutrition: Calories 147 Total Fat 14.2 g Saturated Fat 2 g Cholesterol 0 mg Total Carbs 5.7 g Sugar 2.4 g Fiber 2.7 g Sodium 108 mg Potassium 310 mg Protein 2 g

293)   *Roasted Broccoli*

Ingredients:

- 2 cups fresh broccoli florets
- 1 small yellow onion, cut into wedges
- ¼ teaspoon garlic powder
- 1/8 teaspoon paprika
- 1/8 teaspoon freshly ground black pepper
- 2 tablespoons olive oil

Direction: Preparation Time: 10 minutes Cooking Time: 15 minutes Servings: 2

✓ Preheat the grill to medium heat. In a large bowl, add all the ingredients and toss to coat well.

✓ Transfer the broccoli mixture over a double thickness of a foil paper.

✓ Fold the foil paper around broccoli mixture to seal it.

✓ Grill for about 10-15 minutes. Serve hot.

Meal Prep Tip:
- ✓ Transfer the broccoli mixture into a large bowl and set aside to cool completely.
- ✓ Divide the broccoli mixture into 2 containers evenly.
- ✓ Cover the containers and refrigerate for about 1-2 days. Reheat in the microwave before serving.

Nutrition: Calories 167 Total Fat 14.4 g Saturated Fat 2 g Cholesterol 0 mg Total Carbs 9.7 g Sugar 3.1 g Fiber 3.2 g Sodium 32 mg Potassium 348 mg Protein 3 g

294) *Garlicky Cabbage*

Ingredients:

- 1 tablespoon olive oil
- 2 garlic cloves, minced
- 1 pound cabbage, shredded
- 2-3 tablespoons filtered water
- 1½ tablespoons fresh lemon juice
- Salt and ground black pepper, as required

Direction: Preparation Time: 10 minutes Cooking Time: 10 minutes Servings: 4

- ✓ In a large skillet, heat the oil over medium heat and sauté the garlic for about 1 minute.
- ✓ Stir in the cabbage and cook, covered for about 2-3 minute.
- ✓ Stir in the water and cook for about 2-3 minutes, stirring continuously.
- ✓ Increase the heat to high and stir in the lemon juice, salt and black pepper.
- ✓ Cook for about 2-3 minutes, stirring continuously. Serve hot.

Meal Prep Tip:
- ✓ Transfer the cabbage mixture into a large bowl and set aside to cool completely. Divide the cabbage mixture into 2 containers evenly. Cover the containers and refrigerate for about 1-2 days. Reheat in the microwave before serving.

Nutrition: Calories 62 Total Fat 3.7 g Saturated Fat 0.6 g Cholesterol 0 mg Total Carbs 7.2 g Sugar 3.8 g Fiber 2.9 g Sodium 168 mg Potassium 206 mg Protein 1.6 g

295) *Stir Fried Zucchini*

Ingredients:

- 1 tablespoon olive oil
- ½ cup yellow onion, sliced
- 4 cups zucchini, sliced
- 1½ teaspoons garlic, minced
- ¼ cup water

- Salt and ground black pepper, as required

Direction: Preparation Time: 10 minutes Cooking Time: 10 minutes Servings: 4

- ✓ In a large skillet, heat the oil over medium-high heat and sauté the onion and zucchini for about 4-5 minutes.
- ✓ Add the garlic and sauté for about 1 minute.
- ✓ Add the remaining ingredients and stir to combine.
- ✓ Now, reduce the heat to medium and cook for about 3-4 minutes, stirring occasionally.
- ✓ Serve hot. Meal Prep Tip: Transfer the zucchini mixture into a large bowl and set aside to cool completely.
- ✓ Divide the zucchini mixture into 4 containers evenly.
- ✓ Cover the containers and refrigerate for about 1-2 days. Reheat in the microwave before serving.

Nutrition: Calories 55 Total Fat 3.7 g Saturated Fat 0.5 g Cholesterol 0 mg Total Carbs 5.5 g Sugar 2.6 g Fiber 1.6 g Sodium 51 mg Protein 1.6 g

296) *Green Beans with Tomatoes*

Ingredients:

- ¼ teaspoon fresh lemon peel, grated finely
- 2 teaspoons olive oil
- Salt and freshly ground white pepper, as required
- 4 cups grape tomatoes
- 1½ pounds fresh green beans, trimmed

Direction: Preparation Time: 15 minutes Cooking Time: 40 minutes Servings: 8

- ✓ Preheat the oven to 350 degrees F. In a large bowl, mix together lemon peel, oil, salt and white pepper.
- ✓ Add the cherry tomatoes and toss to coat well.
- ✓ Transfer the tomato mixture into a roasting pan.
- ✓ Roast for about 35-40 minutes, stirring once in the middle way.
- ✓ Meanwhile, in a pan of boiling water, arrange a steamer basket.
- ✓ Place the green beans in steamer basket and steam, covered for about 7-8 minutes.
- ✓ Drain the green beans well.
- ✓ Divide the green beans and tomatoes onto serving plates and serve. Meal Prep Tip:
- ✓ Transfer the green beans and tomatoes into a large bowl and set aside to cool completely.
- ✓ Divide the green beans and tomatoes into 8 containers evenly.
- ✓ Cover the containers and refrigerate for about 1-2 days. Reheat in the microwave before serving.

Nutrition: Calories 53 Total Fat 1.5 g Saturated Fat 0.2 g cholesterol 0 mg Total Carbs 9.6 g Sugar 3.6 g Fiber 4 g Sodium 29 mg Protein 2.3 g

SOUPS AND STEWS

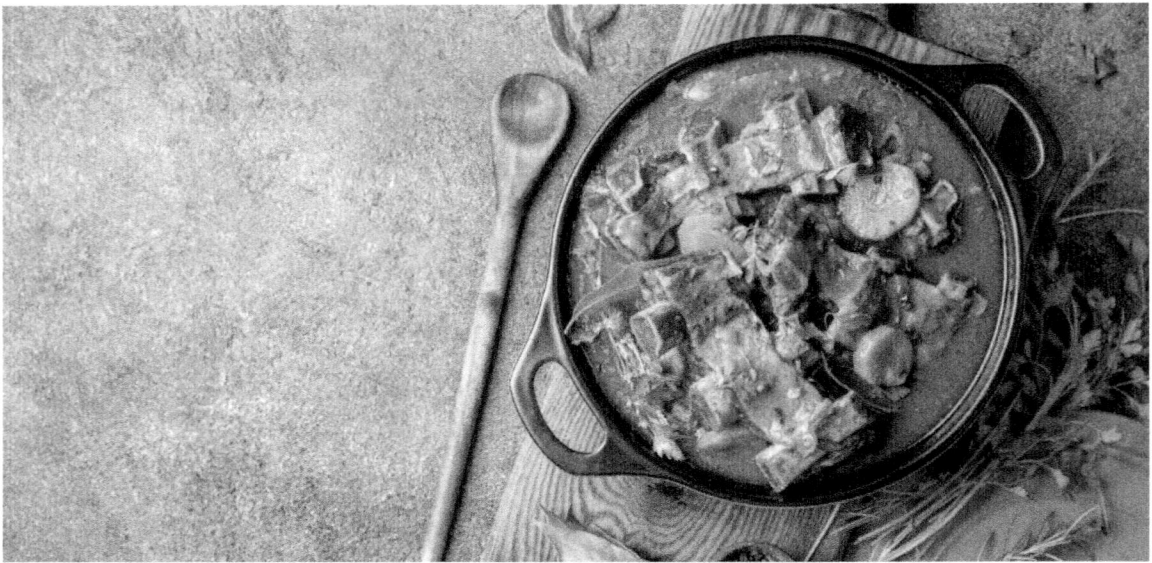

297)   *Kidney Bean Stew*

Ingredients:

- 1lb cooked kidney beans
- 1 cup tomato passata
- 1 cup low sodium beef broth
- 3tbsp Italian herbs

Direction: Preparation time: 15 minutes

Cooking time: 15 minutes Servings: 2

✓ Mix all the ingredients in your Instant Pot.
✓ Cook on Stew for 15 minutes.
✓ Release the pressure naturally.

Nutrition: Calories: 270; Carbs: 16; Sugar: 3; Fat: 10; Protein: 23; GL: 8

298)   *Cabbage Soup*

Ingredients:

- 1lb shredded cabbage
- 1 cup low sodium vegetable broth
- 1 shredded onion
- 2tbsp mixed herbs
- 1tbsp black pepper

Direction: Preparation time: 15 minutes

Cooking time: 35 minutes Servings: 2

✓ Mix all the ingredients in your Instant Pot.
✓ Cook on Stew for 35 minutes.
✓ Release the pressure naturally.

Nutrition: Calories: 60; Carbs: 2; Sugar: 0; Fat: 2; Protein: 4; GL: 1

299)   *Pumpkin Spice Soup*

Ingredients:

- 1lb cubed pumpkin
- 1 cup low sodium vegetable broth
- 2tbsp mixed spice

Direction: Preparation time: 10 minutes

Cooking time: 35 minutes Servings: 2

✓ Mix all the ingredients in your Instant Pot.
✓ Cook on Stew for 35 minutes.
✓ Release the pressure naturally.
✓ Blend the soup.

Nutrition: Calories: 100; Carbs: 7; Sugar: 1; Fat: 2; Protein: 3; GL: 1

300)   *Cream of Tomato Soup*

Ingredients:

- 1lb fresh tomatoes, chopped
- 1.5 cups low sodium tomato puree
- 1tbsp black pepper

Direction: Preparation time: 15 minutes

Cooking time: 15 minutes Servings: 2

✓ Mix all the ingredients in your Instant Pot.
✓ Cook on Stew for 15 minutes.
✓ Release the pressure naturally.
✓ Blend.

Nutrition: Calories: 20; Carbs: 2; Sugar: 1; Fat: 0; Protein: 3; GL: 1

301)   *Shiitake Soup*

Ingredients:

- 1 cup shiitake mushrooms
- 1 cup diced vegetables
- 1 cup low sodium vegetable broth
- 2tbsp 5 spice seasoning

Direction: Preparation time: 15 minutes

Cooking time: 35 minutes Servings: 2

✓ Mix all the ingredients in your Instant Pot.
✓ Cook on Stew for 35 minutes.
✓ Release the pressure naturally.

Nutrition: Calories: 70; Carbs: 5; Sugar: 1; Fat: 2; Protein: 2; GL: 1

302)   *Spicy Pepper Soup*

Ingredients:

- 1lb chopped mixed sweet peppers
- 1 cup low sodium vegetable broth
- 3tbsp chopped chili peppers
- 1tbsp black pepper

Direction: Preparation time: 15 minutes

Cooking time: 15 minutes Servings: 2

✓ Mix all the ingredients in your Instant Pot.
✓ Cook on Stew for 15 minutes.
✓ Release the pressure naturally. Blend.

Nutrition: Calories: 100; Carbs: 11; Sugar: 4; Fat: 2; Protein: 3; GL: 6

303) Zoodle Won-Ton Soup

Ingredients:

- 1lb spiralized zucchini
- 1 pack unfried won-tons
- 1 cup low sodium beef broth
- 2tbsp soy sauce

Direction: Preparation time: 15 minutes

Cooking time: 5 minutes Servings: 2

✓ Mix all the ingredients in your Instant Pot.
✓ Cook on Stew for 5 minutes.
✓ Release the pressure naturally.

Nutrition: Calories: 300; Carbs: 6; Sugar: 1; Fat: 9; Protein: 43; GL: 2

304) Broccoli Stilton Soup

Ingredients:

- 1lb chopped broccoli
- 0.5lb chopped vegetables
- 1 cup low sodium vegetable broth
- 1 cup Stilton

Direction: Preparation time: 15 minutes

Cooking time: 35 minutes Servings: 2

✓ Mix all the ingredients in your Instant Pot.
✓ Cook on Stew for 35 minutes.
✓ Release the pressure naturally.
✓ Blend the soup.
Nutrition: Calories: 280; Carbs: 9; Sugar: 2; Fat: 22; Protein: 13; GL: 4

305) Lamb Stew Recipe 2

Ingredients:

- 1lb diced lamb shoulder
- 1lb chopped winter vegetables
- 1 cup low sodium vegetable broth
- 1tbsp yeast extract
- 1tbsp star anise spice mix

Direction: Preparation time: 15 minutes

Cooking time: 35 minutes Servings: 2

✓ Mix all the ingredients in your Instant Pot.
✓ Cook on Stew for 35 minutes.
✓ Release the pressure naturally.

Nutrition: Calories: 320; Carbs: 10; Sugar: 2; Fat: 8; Protein: 42; GL: 3

306) Irish Stew

Ingredients:

- 1.5lb diced lamb shoulder
- 1lb chopped vegetables
- 1 cup low sodium beef broth
- 3 minced onions
- 1tbsp ghee

Direction: Preparation time: 15 minutes

Cooking time: 35 minutes Servings: 2

✓ Mix all the ingredients in your Instant Pot.
✓ Cook on Stew for 35 minutes.
✓ Release the pressure naturally.
Nutrition: Calories: 330; Carbs: 9; Sugar: 2; Fat: 12; Protein: 49; GL: 3

307) Sweet And Sour Soup

Ingredients:

- 1lb cubed chicken breast
- 1lb chopped vegetables
- 1 cup low carb sweet and sour sauce
- 0.5 cup diabetic marmalade

Direction: Preparation time: 15 minutes

Cooking time: 35 minutes Servings: 2

✓ Mix all the ingredients in your Instant Pot.
✓ Cook on Stew for 35 minutes.
✓ Release the pressure naturally.

308) Meatball Stew

Ingredients:

- 1lb sausage meat
- 2 cups chopped tomato
- 1 cup chopped vegetables
- 2tbsp Italian seasonings
- 1tbsp vegetable oil

Direction: Preparation time: 15 minutes

Cooking time: 25 minutes Servings: 2

✓ Roll the sausage into meatballs.
✓ Put the Instant Pot on Sauté and fry the meatballs in the oil until brown.
✓ Mix all the ingredients in your Instant Pot.
✓ Cook on Stew for 25 minutes.
✓ Release the pressure naturally.

Nutrition: Calories: 300; Carbs: 4; Sugar: 1; Fat: 12; Protein: 40; GL: 2

309)   *Kebab Stew*

Ingredients:

- 1lb cubed, seasoned kebab meat
- 1lb cooked chickpeas
- 1 cup low sodium vegetable broth
- 1tbsp black pepper

Direction: Preparation time: 15 minutes

Cooking time: 35 minutes Servings: 2

✓ Mix all the ingredients in your Instant Pot.
✓ Cook on Stew for 35 minutes.
✓ Release the pressure naturally.

Nutrition: Calories: 290; Carbs: 22; Sugar: 4; Fat: 10; Protein: 34; GL: 6

310)   *French Onion Soup*

Ingredients:

- 6 onions, chopped finely
- 2 cups vegetable broth
- 2tbsp oil
- 2tbsp Gruyere

Direction: Preparation time: 35 minutes Cooking time: 35 minutes Servings: 2

✓ Place the oil in your Instant Pot and cook the onions on Sauté until soft and brown.
✓ Mix all the ingredients in your Instant Pot.
✓ Cook on Stew for 35 minutes.
✓ Release the pressure naturally.

Nutrition: Calories: 110; Carbs: 8; Sugar: 3; Fat: 10; Protein: 3; GL: 4

311)   *Meatless Ball Soup*

Ingredients:

- 1lb minced tofu
- 0.5lb chopped vegetables
- 2 cups low sodium vegetable broth
- 1tbsp almond flour
- salt and pepper

Direction: Preparation time: 15 minutes

Cooking time: 15 minutes Servings: 2

✓ Mix the tofu, flour, salt and pepper.
✓ Form the meatballs.
✓ Place all the ingredients in your Instant Pot.
✓ Cook on Stew for 15 minutes.
✓ Release the pressure naturally.

Nutrition: Calories: 240; Carbs: 9; Sugar: 3; Fat: 10; Protein: 35; GL: 5

312)   *Fake-On Stew*

Ingredients:

- 0.5lb soy bacon
- 1lb chopped vegetables
- 1 cup low sodium vegetable broth
- 1tbsp nutritional yeast

Direction: Preparation time: 15 minutes Cooking time: 25 minutes Servings: 2

✓ Mix all the ingredients in your Instant Pot.
✓ Cook on Stew for 25 minutes.
✓ Release the pressure naturally.

Nutrition: Calories: 200; Carbs: 12; Sugar: 3; Fat: 7; Protein: 41; GL: 5

313)   *Chickpea Soup*

Ingredients:

- 1lb cooked chickpeas
- 1lb chopped vegetables
- 1 cup low sodium vegetable broth
- 2tbsp mixed herbs

Direction: Preparation time: 15 minutes

Cooking time: 35 minutes Servings: 2

✓ Mix all the ingredients in your Instant Pot.
✓ Cook on Stew for 35 minutes.
✓ Release the pressure naturally.

Nutrition: Calories: 310; Carbs: 20; Sugar: 3; Fat: 5; Protein: 27; GL: 5

314)   *Chicken Zoodle Soup*

Ingredients:

- 1lb chopped cooked chicken
- 1lb spiralized zucchini
- 1 cup low sodium chicken soup
- 1 cup diced vegetables

Direction: Preparation time: 15 minutes

Cooking time: 35 minutes Servings: 2

- ✓ Mix all the ingredients except the zucchini in your Instant Pot.
- ✓ Cook on Stew for 35 minutes.
- ✓ Release the pressure naturally.
- ✓ Stir in the zucchini and allow to heat thoroughly.

Nutrition: Calories: 250; Carbs: 5; Sugar: 0; Fat: 10; Protein: 40; GL: 1

SMOOTHIES & JUICES

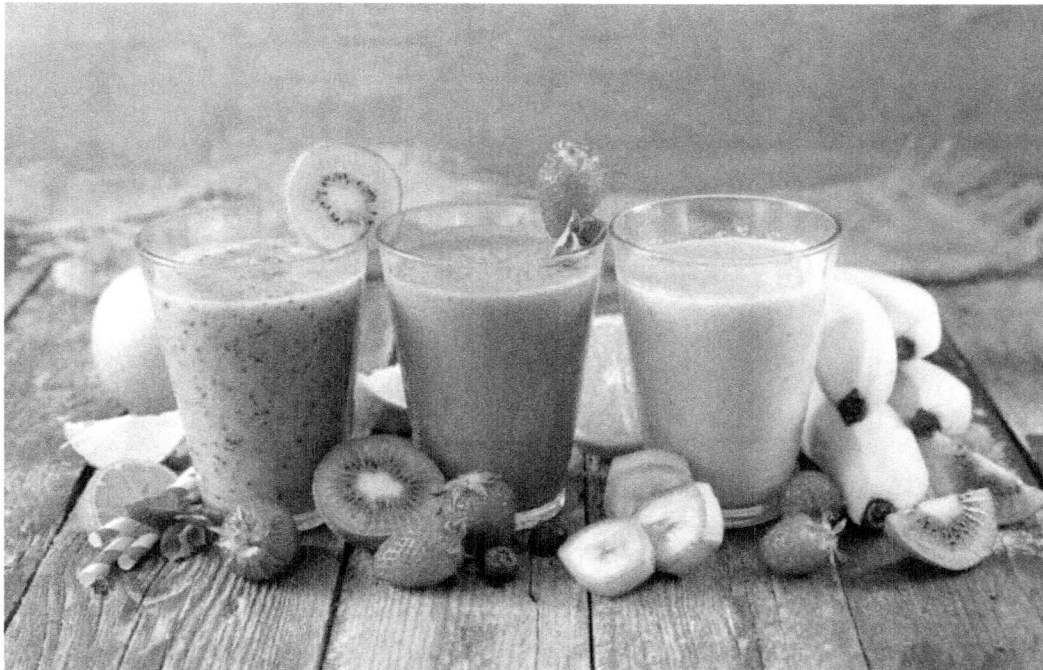

315) *Strawberry Smoothie*

Ingredients:

- 5 Strawberries, medium
- 6 Ice Cubes
- 1 cup Soy Milk, unsweetened
- 1/2 cup Greek Yoghurt, low-fat

Direction: Preparation Time: 5 Minutes

Cooking Time: 5 Minutes Servings: 1

- ✓ Place strawberries, yogurt, milk, and ice cubes in a high-speed blender.
- ✓ Blend them for 2 to 3 minutes or until you get a smooth and luscious smoothie.
- ✓ Transfer to a serving glass and enjoy it.

Nutrition: Calories 167Kcal; Carbohydrates 11g; Proteins 16g; Fat 6g; Sodium 161mg

316) *Berry Mint Smoothie*

Ingredients:

- 1 tbsp. Low-carb Sweetener of your choice
- 1 cup Kefir or Low Fat-Yoghurt
- 2 tbsp. Mint
- ¼ cup Orange
- 1 cup Mixed Berries

Direction: Preparation Time: 5 Minutes Cooking Time: 5 Minutes Servings: 2

- ✓ Place all of the ingredients in a high-speed blender and then blend it until smooth.
- ✓ Transfer the smoothie to a serving glass and enjoy it.

Nutrition: Calories: 137Kcal; Carbohydrates: 11g; Proteins: 6g; Fat: 1g; Sodium: 64mg

317) *Greenie Smoothie*

Ingredients:

- 1 1/2 cup Water
- 1 tsp. Stevia
- 1 Green Apple, ripe
- 1 tsp. Stevia
- 1 Green Pear, chopped into chunks
- 1 Lime
- 2 cups Kale, fresh
- ¾ tsp. Cinnamon
- 12 Ice Cubes
- 20 Green Grapes
- 1/2 cup Mint, fresh

Direction: Preparation Time: 5 Minutes

Cooking Time: 5 Minutes Servings: 2

- ✓ Pour water, kale, and pear in a high-speed blender and blend them for 2 to 3 minutes until mixed.
- ✓ Stir in all the remaining ingredients into it and blend until it becomes smooth.
- ✓ Transfer the smoothie to serving glass.

Nutrition: Calories: 123Kcal; Carbohydrates: 27g; Proteins: 2g; Fat: 2g; Sodium: 30mg

318) *Coconut Spinach Smoothie*

Ingredients:

- 1 ¼ cup Coconut Milk
- 2 Ice Cubes
- 2 tbsp. Chia Seeds
- 1 scoop of Protein Powder, preferably vanilla
- 1 cup Spin

Direction: Preparation Time: 5 Minutes Cooking Time: 5 Minutes Servings: 2

- ✓ Pour coconut milk along with spinach, chia seeds, protein powder, and ice cubes in a high-speed blender.
- ✓ Blend for 2 minutes to get a smooth and luscious smoothie.
- ✓ Serve in a glass and enjoy it.

Nutrition: Calories 251Kcal; Carbs 10.9g; Proteins 20.3g; Fat 15.1g; Sodium: 102mg

319) *Oats Coffee Smoothie*

Ingredients:

- 1 cup Oats, uncooked & grounded
- 2 tbsp. Instant Coffee
- 3 cup Milk, skimmed
- 2 Banana, frozen & sliced into chunks
- 2 tbsp. Flax Seeds, grounded

Direction: Preparation Time: 5 Minutes

Cooking Time: 5 Minutes Servings: 2

- ✓ Place all of the ingredients in a high-speed blender and blend for 2 minutes or until smooth and luscious.
- ✓ Serve and enjoy.

Nutrition: Calories: 251Kcal; Carbs 10.9g; Proteins: 20.3g; Fat: 15.1g; Sodium: 102mg

320) *Veggie Smoothie*

Ingredients:

- ¼ of 1 Red Bell Pepper, sliced
- 1/2 tbsp. Coconut Oil
- 1 cup Almond Milk, unsweetened
- ¼ tsp. Turmeric
- 4 Strawberries, chopped
- Pinch of Cinnamon
- 1/2 of 1 Banana, preferably frozen

Direction: Preparation Time: 5 Minutes Cooking Time: 5 Minutes Servings: 1

- ✓ Combine all the ingredients required to make the smoothie in a high-speed blender.
- ✓ Blend for 3 minutes to get a smooth and silky mixture.
- ✓ Serve and enjoy.

Nutrition: Calories: 169cal; Carbs: 17g; Proteins: 2.3g; Fat: 9.8g; Sodium: 162mg

321) *Avocado Smoothie*

Ingredients:

- 1 Avocado, ripe & pit removed
- 2 cups Baby Spinach
- 2 cups Water
- 1 cup Baby Kale
- 1 tbsp. Lemon Juice
- 2 sprigs of Mint
- 1/2 cup Ice Cubes

Direction: Preparation Time: 10 Minutes

Cooking Time: 0 Minutes Servings: 2

- ✓ Place all the ingredients needed to make the smoothie in a high-speed blender then blend until smooth.
- ✓ Transfer to a serving glass and enjoy it.

Nutrition: Calories: 214cal; Carbohydrates: 15g; Proteins: 2g; Fat: 17g; Sodium: 25mg

322) *Orange Carrot Smoothie*

Ingredients:

- 1 1/2 cups Almond Milk
- ¼ cup Cauliflower, blanched & frozen
- 1 Orange
- 1 tbsp. Flax Seed
- 1/3 cup Carrot, grated
- 1 tsp. Vanilla Extract

Direction: Preparation Time: 5 Minutes

Cooking Time: 0 Minutes Servings: 1

- ✓ Mix all the ingredients in a high-speed blender and blend for 2 minutes or until you get the desired consistency.
- ✓ Transfer to a serving glass and enjoy it.

Nutrition: Calories: 216cal; Carbohydrates: 10g; Proteins: 15g; Fat: 7g; Sodium: 25mg

323) *Blackberry Smoothie*

Ingredients:

- 1 1/2 cups Almond Milk
- 1/2 tsp. Vanilla Extract
- 3 oz. Black berries, frozen
- 1 tbsp. Lemon Juice
- 1 tsp. Vanilla Extract

Direction: Preparation Time: 5 Minutes Cooking Time: 0 Minutes Servings: 1

- ✓ Place all the ingredients needed to make the blackberry smoothie in a high-speed blender and blend for 2 minutes until you get a smooth mixture.
- ✓ Transfer to a serving glass and enjoy it.

Nutrition: Calories: 275cal; Carbohydrates: 9g; Proteins: 11g; Fat: 17g; Sodium: 73mg

324) *Key Lime Pie Smoothie*

Ingredients:

- 1/2 cup Cottage Cheese
- 1 tbsp. Sweetener of your choice
- 1/2 cup Water
- 1/2 cup Spinach
- 1 tbsp. Lime Juice
- 1 cup Ice Cubes

Direction: Preparation Time: 5 Minutes Cooking Time: 2 Minutes Servings: 2

- ✓ Spoon in the ingredients to a high-speed blender and blend until silky smooth.
- ✓ Transfer to a serving glass and enjoy it.

Nutrition: Calories: 180 cal; Carbohydrates: 7g; Proteins: 36g; Fat: 1 g; Sodium: 35mg

325) *Cinnamon Roll Smoothie*

Ingredients:

- 1 tsp. Flax Meal or oats, if preferred

- 1 cup Almond Milk
- 1/2 tsp. Cinnamon
- 2 tbsp. Protein Powder
- 1 cup Ice
- ¼ tsp. Vanilla Extract
- 4 tsp. Sweetener of your choice

Direction: Preparation Time: 5 Minutes
Cooking Time: 0 Minutes Servings: 1

✓ Pour the milk into the blender, followed by the protein powder, sweetener, flax meal, cinnamon, vanilla extract, and ice.
✓ Blend for 40 seconds or until smooth.
✓ Serve and enjoy.

Nutrition: : Calories: 145cal; Carbs: 1.6g; Proteins: 26.5g; Fat: 3.25g; Sodium: 30mg

326) *Strawberry Cheesecake Smoothie*

Ingredients:

- ¼ cup Soy Milk, unsweetened
- 1/2 cup Cottage Cheese, low-fat
- 1/2 tsp. Vanilla Extract
- 2 oz. Cream Cheese
- 1 cup Ice Cubes
- 1/2 cup Strawberries
- 4 tbsp. Low-carb Sweetener of your choice

Direction: Preparation Time: 5 Minutes
Cooking Time: 0 Minutes Servings: 1

✓ Add all the ingredients for making the strawberry cheesecake smoothie to a high-speed blender until you get the desired smooth consistency.
✓ Serve and enjoy.

Nutrition: Calories: 347cal; Carbs: 10.05g; Proteins: 17.5g; Fat: 24g; Sodium: 45mg

327) *Peanut Butter Banana Smoothie*

Ingredients:

- ¼ cup Greek Yoghurt, plain
- 1/2 tbsp. Chia Seeds
- 1/2 cup Ice Cubes
- 1/2 of 1 Banana
- 1/2 cup Water
- 1 tbsp. Peanut Butter

Direction: Preparation Time: 5 Minutes

Cooking Time: 2 Minutes Servings: 1

✓ Place all the ingredients needed to make the smoothie in a high-speed blender and blend to get a smooth and luscious mixture.
✓ Transfer the smoothie to a serving glass and enjoy it.

Nutrition: Calories: 202cal; Carbohydrates: 14g; Proteins: 10g; Fat: 9g; Sodium: 30mg

328) *Avocado Turmeric Smoothie*

Ingredients:

- 1/2 of 1 Avocado
- 1 cup Ice, crushed
- ¾ cup Coconut Milk, full-fat
- 1 tsp. Lemon Juice
- ¼ cup Almond Milk
- 1/2 tsp. Turmeric
- 1 tsp. Ginger, freshly grated

Direction: Preparation Time: 5 Minutes

Cooking Time: 2 Minutes Servings: 1

✓ Place all the ingredients excluding the crushed ice in a high-speed blender and blend for 2 to 3 minutes or until smooth.
✓ Transfer to a serving glass and enjoy it.

Nutrition: Calories: 232cal; Carbs: 4.1g; Proteins: 1.7g; Fat: 22.4g; Sodium: 25mg

329) *Blueberry Smoothie*

Ingredients:

- 1 tbsp. Lemon Juice
- 1 ¾ cup Coconut Milk, full-fat
- 1/2 tsp. Vanilla Extract
- 3 oz. Blueberries, frozen

Direction: Preparation Time: 5 Minutes

Cooking Time: 2 Minutes Servings: 2

✓ Combine coconut milk, blueberries, lemon juice, and vanilla extract in a high-speed blender.
✓ Blend for 2 minutes for a smooth and luscious smoothie.
✓ Serve and enjoy.

Nutrition: Calories: 275cal; Carbohydrates: 9g; Proteins: 11g; Fat: 17g; Sodium: 73mg

330)   *Matcha Green Smoothie*

Ingredients:

- ¼ cup Heavy Whipping Cream
- 1/2 tsp. Vanilla Extract
- 1 tsp. Matcha Green Tea Powder
- 2 tbsp. Protein Powder
- 1 tbsp. Hot Water
- 1 ¼ cup Almond Milk, unsweetened
- 1/2 of 1 Avocado, medium

Direction: Preparation Time: 5 Minutes

Cooking Time: 2 Minutes Servings: 2

- ✓ Place all the ingredients in the high-blender for one to two minutes.
- ✓ Serve and enjoy.

Nutrition: Calories: 229cal; Carbs: 1.5g; Proteins: 14.1g; Fat: 43g; Sodium: 35mg

DESSERTS

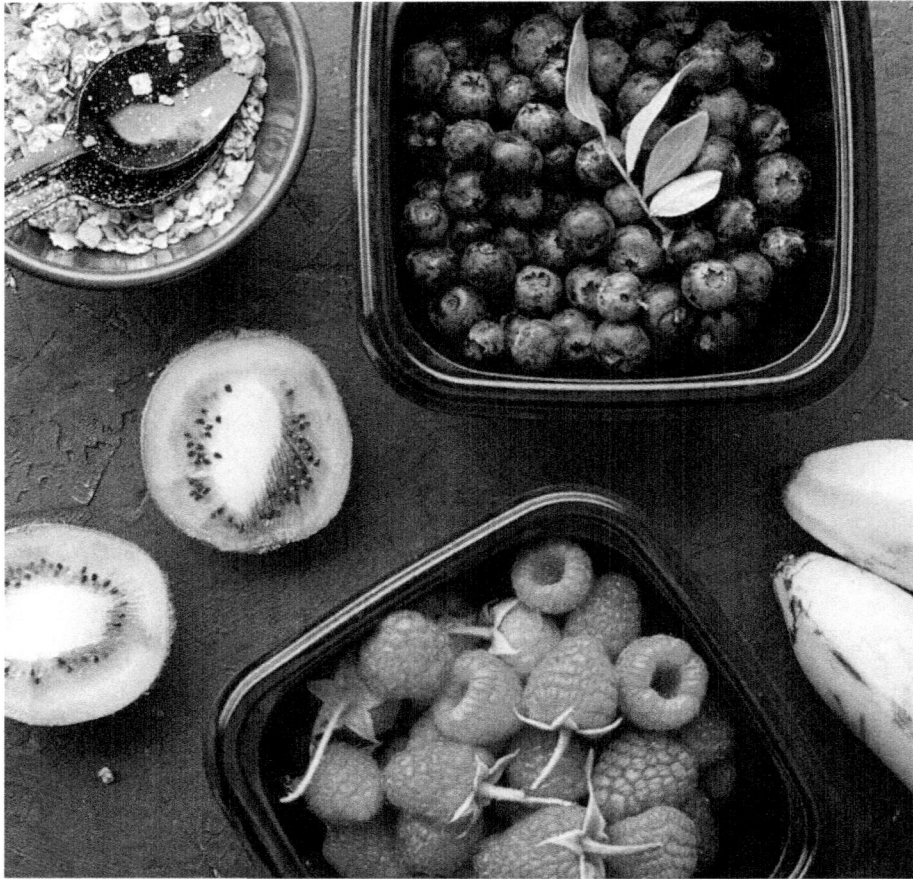

331)   *Slow Cooker Peaches*

Ingredients:

- 4 cups peaches, sliced
- 2/3 cup rolled oats
- 1/3 cup Bisques
- 1/4 teaspoon cinnamon
- 1/2 cup brown sugar
- 1/2 cup granulated sugar

Direction: Preparation Time: 10 minutes

Cooking time: 4 hours 20 minutes Servings: 4-6

✓ Spray the slow cooker pot with a cooking spray.
✓ Mix oats, Bisques, cinnamon and all the sugars in the pot.
✓ Add peaches and stir well to combine. Cook on low for 4-6 hours.

Nutrition: 617 calories; 3.6 g fat; 13 g total carbs; 9 g protein

332)   *Pumpkin Custard 1*

Ingredients:

- 1/2 cup almond flour
- 4 eggs
- 1 cup pumpkin puree
- 1/2 cup stevia/erythritol blend, granulated
- 1/8 teaspoon sea salt
- 1 teaspoon vanilla extract or maple flavoring
- 4 tablespoons butter, ghee, or coconut oil melted
- 1 teaspoon pumpkin pie spice

Direction: Preparation Time: 10 minutes Cooking time: 2 hours 30 minutes Servings: 6

✓ Grease or spray a slow cooker with butter or coconut oil spray.
✓ In a medium mixing bowl, beat the eggs until smooth. Then add in the sweetener.
✓ To the egg mixture, add in the pumpkin puree along with vanilla or maple extract.
✓ Then add almond flour to the mixture along with the pumpkin pie spice and salt. Add melted butter, coconut oil or ghee.
✓ Transfer the mixture into a slow cooker. Close the lid. Cook for 2-2 ¾ hours on low.
✓ When through, serve with whipped cream, and then sprinkle with little nutmeg if need be. Enjoy!
✓ Set slow-cooker to the low setting. Cook for 2-2.45 hours, and begin checking at the two hour mark. Serve warm with stevia sweetened whipped cream and a sprinkle of nutmeg.

Nutrition: 147 calories; 12 g fat; 4 g total carbs; 5 g

protein

333)   *Blueberry Lemon Custard Cake*

Ingredients:

- 6 eggs, separated
- 2 cups light cream
- 1/2 cup coconut flour
- 1/2 teaspoon salt
- 2 teaspoon lemon zest
- 1/2 cup granulated sugar substitute
- 1/3 cup lemon juice
- 1/2 cup blueberries fresh
- 1 teaspoon lemon liquid stevia

Direction: Preparation Time: 10 minutes Cooking time: 3 hours Servings: 12

✓ Into a stand mixer, add the egg whites and whip them well until stiff peaks have formed; set aside.
✓ Whisk the yolks together with the remaining ingredients except blueberries, to form batter.
✓ When done, fold egg whites into the formed batter a little at a time until slightly combined.
✓ Grease the crock pot and then pour in the mixture. Then sprinkle batter with the blueberries.
✓ Close the lid then cook for 3 hours on low. When the cooking time is over, open the lid and let cool for an hour, and then let chill in the refrigerator for at least 2 hours or overnight.
✓ Serve cold with little sugar free whipped cream and enjoy!

Nutrition: 165 calories; 10 g fat; 14 g total carbs; 4 g protein

334)   *Sugar Free Carrot Cake*

Ingredients:

- 2 eggs
- 1 1/2 almond flour
- 1/2 cup butter, melted
- ¼ cup heavy cream
- 1 teaspoon baking powder
- 1 teaspoon vanilla extract or almond extract, optional
- 1 cup sugar substitute
- 1 cup carrots, finely shredded
- 1 teaspoon cinnamon
- ¼ teaspoon nutmeg

- 1/8 teaspoon allspice
- 1 teaspoon ginger
- 1/2 teaspoon baking soda
- For cream cheese frosting:
- 1 cup confectioner's sugar substitute
- ¼ cup butter, softened
- 1 teaspoon almond extract
- 4 oz. cream cheese, softened

Direction: Cooking time: 4 hours Servings: 8 Ingredients

✓ Grease a loaf pan well and then set it aside.

✓ Using a mixer, combine butter together with eggs, vanilla, sugar substitute and heavy cream in a mixing bowl, until well blended.

✓ Combine almond flour together with baking powder, spices and the baking soda in a another bowl until well blended.

✓ When done, combine the wet ingredients together with the dry ingredients until well blended, and then stir in carrots.

✓ Pour the mixer into the prepared loaf pan, and then place the pan into a slow cooker on a trivet. Add 1 cup water inside.

✓ Cook for about 4-5 hours on low. Be aware that the cake will be very moist.

✓ When the cooking time is over, let the cake cool completely.

✓ To prepare the cream cheese frosting: blend the cream cheese together with extract, butter and powdered sugar substitute until frosting is formed.

✓ Top the cake with the frosting.

Nutrition: 299 calories; 25.4 g fat; 15 g total carbs; 4 g protein

335) *Sugar Free Chocolate Molten Lava Cake*

Ingredients:

- 3 egg yolks
- 1 1/2 cups Swerve sweetener, divided
- 1 teaspoon baking powder
- 1/2 cup flour, gluten free
- 3 whole eggs
- 5 tablespoons cocoa powder, unsweetened, divided
- 4 oz. chocolate chips, sugar free
- 1/2 teaspoon salt
- 1/2 teaspoon vanilla liquid stevia
- 1/2 cup butter, melted, cooled

- 2 cups hot water
- 1 teaspoon vanilla extract

Direction: Preparation Time: 10 minutes

Cooking time: 3 hours Servings: 12

✓ Grease the crockpot well with cooking spray.

✓ Whisk 1 ¼ cups of swerve together with flour, salt, baking powder and 3 tablespoons cocoa powder in a bowl.

✓ Stir the cooled melted butter together with eggs, yolks, liquid stevia and the vanilla extract in a separate bowl.

✓ When done, add the wet ingredients to the dry ingredient until nicely combined, and then pour the mixture into the prepared crock pot.

✓ Then top the mixture in the crockpot with chocolate chips.

✓ Whisk the rest of the swerve sweetener and the remaining cocoa powder with the hot water, and then pour this mixture over the chocolate chips top.

✓ Close the lid and cook for 3 hours on low. When the cooking time is over, let cool a bit and then serve. Enjoy!

Nutrition: 157 calories; 13 g fat; 10.5 g total carbs; 3.9 g protein

336) *Chocolate Quinoa Brownies*

Ingredients:

- 2 eggs
- 3 cups quinoa, cooked
- 1 teaspoon vanilla liquid stevia
- 1 ¼ chocolate chips, sugar free
- 1 teaspoon vanilla extract
- 1/3 cup flaxseed ground
- ¼ teaspoon salt
- 1/3 cup cocoa powder, unsweetened
- 1/2 teaspoon baking powder
- 1 teaspoon pure stevia extract
- 1/2 cup applesauce, unsweetened
- Sugar- frees frosting:
- ¼ cup heavy cream
- 1 teaspoon chocolate liquid stevia
- ¼ cup cocoa powder, unsweetened
- 1/2 teaspoon vanilla extract

Direction: Preparation Time: 10 minutes

Cooking time: 2 hours Servings: 16

✓ Add all the ingredients to a food processor. Then process until well incorporated.

✓ Line a crock pot with a parchment paper, and then spread the batter into the lined pot.

✓ Close the lid and cook for 4 hours on LOW or 2 hours on HIGH. Let cool.

✓ Prepare the frosting. Whisk all the ingredients together and then microwave for 20 seconds. Taste and adjust on sweetener if desired.

✓ When the frosting is ready, stir it well again and then pour it over the sliced brownies.

✓ Serve and enjoy!

Nutrition: 133 calories; 7.9 g fat; 18.4 g total carbs; 4.3 g protein

337)   *Blueberry Crisp*

Ingredients:

- 1/4 cup butter, melted
- 24 oz. blueberries, frozen
- 3/4 teaspoon salt
- 1 1/2 cups rolled oats, coarsely ground
- 3/4 cup almond flour, blanched
- 1/4 cup coconut oil, melted
- 6 tablespoons sweetener
- 1 cup pecans or walnuts, coarsely chopped

Direction: Preparation Time: 10 minutes

Cooking time: 3-4 hours Servings: 10

✓ Using a non-stick cooking spray, spray the slow cooker pot well.

✓ Into a bowl, add ground oats and chopped nuts along with salt, blanched almond flour, brown sugar, stevia granulated sweetener, and then stir in the coconut/butter mixture. Stir well to combine.

✓ When done, spread crisp topping over blueberries. Cook for 3-4 hours, until the mixture has become bubbling hot and you can smell the blueberries.

✓ Serve while still hot with the whipped cream or the ice cream if desired. Enjoy!

Nutrition: 261 calories; 16.6 g fat; 32 g total carbs; 4 g protein

338)   *Maple Custard*

Ingredients:

- 1 teaspoon maple extract
- 2 egg yolks
- 1 cup heavy cream
- 2 eggs
- 1/2 cup whole milk
- 1/4 teaspoon salt
- 1/4 cup Sukrin Gold or any sugar-free brown sugar

substitute
- 1/2 teaspoon cinnamon

Direction: Preparation Time: 10 minutes Cooking time: 2 hours Servings: 6

✓ Combine all ingredients together in a blender, process well.

✓ Grease 6 ramekins and then pour the batter evenly into each ramekin.

✓ To the bottom of the slow cooker, add 4 ramekins and then arrange the remaining 2 against the side of a slow cooker, and not at the top of bottom ramekins.

✓ Close the lid and cook on high for 2 hours, until the center is cooked through but the middle is still jiggly.

✓ Let cool at a room temperature for an hour after removing from the slow cooker, and then chill in the fridge for at least 2 hours.

✓ Serve and enjoy with a sprinkle of cinnamon and little sugar free whipped cream.

Nutrition: 190 calories; 18 g fat; 2 g total carbs; 4 g protein

339)   *Raspberry Cream Cheese Coffee Cake*

Ingredients:

- 1 1/4 almond flour
- 2/3 cup water
- 1/2 cup Swerve
- 3 eggs
- 1/4 cup coconut flour
- 1/4 cup protein powder
- 1/4 teaspoon salt
- 1/2 teaspoon vanilla extract
- 1 1/2 teaspoon baking powder
- 6 tablespoons butter, melted

For the Filling:
- 1 1/2 cup fresh raspberries
- 8 oz. cream cheese
- 1 large egg
- 1/3 cup powdered Swerve
- 2 tablespoon whipping cream

Direction: Preparation Time: 10 minutes Cooking time: 4 hours Servings: 12

✓ Grease the slow cooker pot. Prepare the cake batter. In a bowl, combine almond flour together with coconut flour, sweetener, baking powder, protein powder and salt, and then stir in the melted butter along with eggs and water until well combined. Set aside.

✓ Prepare the filling.

✓ Beat cream cheese thoroughly with the sweetener until have smoothened, and then beat in whipping cream along with the egg and vanilla extract until well combined.

✓ Assemble the cake. Spread around 2/3 of batter in the slow cooker as you smoothen the top using a spatula or knife.

✓ Pour cream cheese mixture over the batter in the pan, evenly spread it, and then sprinkle with raspberries. Add the rest of batter over filling.

✓ Cook for 3-4 hours on low. Let cool completely.

✓ Serve and enjoy!

Nutrition: 239 calories; 19.18 g fat; 6.9 g total carbs; 7.5 g protein

340) *Pumpkin Pie Bars*

Ingredients:

- For the Crust:
- 3/4 cup coconut, shredded
- 4 tablespoons butter, unsalted, softened
- 1/4 cup cocoa powder, unsweetened
- 1/4 teaspoon salt
- 1/2 cup raw sunflower seeds or sunflower seed flour
- 1/4 cup confectioners Swerve
- Filling:
- 2 teaspoons cinnamon liquid stevia
- 1 cup heavy cream
- 1 can pumpkin puree
- 6 eggs
- 1 tablespoon pumpkin pie spice
- 1/2 teaspoon salt
- 1 tablespoon vanilla extract
- 1/2 cup sugar-free chocolate chips, optional

Direction: Preparation Time: 10 minutes

Cooking time: 3 hours Servings: 16

✓ Add all the crust ingredients to a food processor. Then process until fine crumbs are formed.

✓ Grease the slow cooker pan well. When done, press crust mixture onto the greased bottom.

✓ In a stand mixer, combine all the ingredients for the filling, and then blend well until combined.

✓ Top the filling with chocolate chips if using, and then pour the mixture onto the prepared crust.

✓ Close the lid and cook for 3 hours on low. Open the lid and let cool for at least 30 minutes, and then place the slow cooker into the refrigerator for at least 3 hours.

✓ Slice the pumpkin pie bar and serve it with sugar free whipped cream. Enjoy!

Nutrition: 169 calories; 15 g fat; 6 g total carbs; 4 g protein

341) *Dark Chocolate Cake*

Ingredients:

- 1 cup almond flour
- 3 eggs
- 2 tablespoons almond flour
- 1/4 teaspoon salt
- 1/2 cup Swerve Granular
- 3/4 teaspoon vanilla extract
- 2/3 cup almond milk, unsweetened
- 1/2 cup cocoa powder
- 6 tablespoons butter, melted
- 1 1/2 teaspoon baking powder
- 3 tablespoon unflavored whey protein powder or egg white protein powder
- 1/3 cup sugar-free chocolate chips, optional

Direction: Preparation Time: 10 minutes

Cooking time: 3 hours Servings: 10

✓ Grease the slow cooker well.

✓ Whisk the almond flour together with cocoa powder, sweetener, whey protein powder, salt and baking powder in a bowl. Then stir in butter along with almond milk, eggs and the vanilla extract until well combined, and then stir in the chocolate chips if desired.

✓ When done, pour into the slow cooker. Allow to cook for 2-2 1/2 hours on low.

✓ When through, turn off the slow cooker and let the cake cool for about 20-30 minutes.

✓ When cooled, cut the cake into pieces and serve warm with lightly sweetened whipped cream. Enjoy!

Nutrition: 205 calories; 17 g fat; 8.4 g total carbs; 12 g protein

342) *Lemon Custard*

Ingredients:

- 2 cups whipping cream or coconut cream
- 5 egg yolks
- 1 tablespoon lemon zest
- 1 teaspoon vanilla extract
- 1/4 cup fresh lemon juice, squeezed
- 1/2 teaspoon liquid stevia
- Lightly sweetened whipped cream

Direction: Preparation Time: 10 minutes Cooking time: 3 hours Servings: 4

- ✓ Whisk egg yolks together with lemon zest, liquid stevia, lemon zest and vanilla in a bowl, and then whisk in heavy cream.
- ✓ Divide the mixture among 4 small jars or ramekins.
- ✓ To the bottom of a slow cooker add a rack, and then add ramekins on top of the rack and add enough water to cover half of ramekins.
- ✓ Close the lid and cook for 3 hours on low. Remove ramekins.
- ✓ Let cool to room temperature, and then place into the refrigerator to cool completely for about 3 hours.
- ✓ When through, top with the whipped cream and serve. Enjoy!

Nutrition: 319 calories; 30 g fat; 3 g total carbs; 7 g protein

343) *Coffee & Chocolate Ice Cream*

Ingredients:

- 3 cups brewed coffee
- ½ cup low calorie chocolate flavored syrup
- ¾ cup low fat half and half

Direction: Preparation Time: 4 minutes Cooking Time: 0 minutes Servings: 15

- ✓ Mix the ingredients in a bowl.
- ✓ Pour into popsicle molds. Freeze for 4 hours.

Nutrition: Calories 21 Total Fat 0 g Saturated Fat 0 g Cholesterol 1 mg Sodium 28 mg Total Carbohydrate 4 g Dietary Fiber 0 g Total Sugars 3 g Protein 0 g Potassium 450 mg

344) *Choco Banana Bites*

Ingredients:

- 2 bananas, sliced into rounds
- ¼ cup dark chocolate cubes

Direction: Preparation Time: 2 hours and 5 minutes Cooking Time: 5 minutes Servings: 4

- ✓ Melt chocolate in the microwave or in a saucepan over medium heat.
- ✓ Coat each banana slice with melted chocolate.
- ✓ Place on a metal pan. Freeze for 2 hours.

Nutrition: Calories 102 Total Fat 3 g Saturated Fat 2 g Cholesterol 0 mg Sodium 4 mg Total Carbohydrate 20 g Dietary Fiber 2 g Total Sugars 13 g Protein 1 g Potassium 211 mg

345) *Blueberries with Yogurt*

Ingredients:

- 1 cup nonfat Greek yogurt
- ¼ cup blueberries
- ¼ cup almonds

Direction: Preparation Time: 5 minutes Cooking Time: 0 minute Serving: 1

- ✓ Add yogurt and blueberries in a food processor.
- ✓ Pulse until smooth. Top with almonds before serving.

Nutrition: Calories 154 Total Fat 1 g Saturated Fat 0 g Cholesterol 11 mg Sodium 81 mg Total Carbohydrate 13 g Dietary Fiber 1 g Total Sugars 11 g Protein 23 g Potassium 346 mg

346) *Roasted Mangoes*

Ingredients:

- 2 mangoes, peeled and sliced into cubes
- 2 tablespoons coconut flakes
- 2 teaspoons crystallized ginger, chopped
- 2 teaspoons orange zest

Direction: Preparation Time: 5 minutes Cooking Time: 10 minutes Servings: 4

- ✓ Preheat your oven to 350 degrees F. Put the mango cubes in custard cups.
- ✓ Top with the ginger and orange zest. Bake in the oven for 10 minutes.

Nutrition: Calories 89 Total Fat 2 g Saturated Fat 1 g Cholesterol 0 mg Sodium 14 mg Total Carbohydrate 20 g Dietary Fiber 2 g Total Sugars 17 g Protein 1 g Potassium 177 mg

347) *Figs with Yogurt*

Ingredients:

- 8 oz. low fat yogurt
- ½ teaspoon vanilla
- 2 figs, sliced
- 1 tablespoon walnuts, toasted and chopped
- Lemon zest

Direction: Preparation Time: 8 hours and 5 minutes Cooking Time: 0 minutes Servings: 2

- ✓ Refrigerate yogurt in a bowl for 8 hours.
- ✓ After 8 hours, take it out of the refrigerator and stir in yogurt and vanilla.
- ✓ Stir in the figs. Sprinkle walnuts and lemon zest on top before serving.

Nutrition: Calories 157 Total Fat 4 g Saturated Fat 1 g

Cholesterol 7 mg Sodium 80 mg Total Carbohydrate 24 g Dietary Fiber 2 g Total Sugars 1 g Protein 7 g Potassium 557mg

348) *Grilled Peaches*

Ingredients:

- 1 cup balsamic vinegar
- ⅛ teaspoon ground cinnamon
- 1 tablespoon honey
- 3 peaches, pitted and sliced in half
- 2 teaspoons olive oil
- 6 gingersnaps, crushed

Direction: Preparation Time: 5 minutes Cooking Time: 3 minutes Servings: 6

- ✓ Pour the vinegar into a saucepan. Bring it to a boil. Lower heat and simmer for 10 minutes.
- ✓ Remove from the stove. Stir in cinnamon and honey.
- ✓ Coat the peaches with oil. Grill peaches for 2 to 3 minutes.
- ✓ Drizzle each one with syrup. Top with the gingersnaps.

Nutrition: : Calories 135 Total Fat 3 g Saturated Fat 1 g Cholesterol 0 mg Sodium 42 mg Total Carbohydrate 25 g Dietary Fiber 2 g Total Sugars 18 g Protein 1 g Potassium 251 mg

349) *Fruit Salad*

Ingredients:

- 8 oz. light cream cheese
- 6 oz. Greek yogurt
- 1 tablespoon honey
- 1 teaspoon orange zest
- 1 teaspoon lemon zest
- 1 orange, sliced into sections
- 3 kiwi fruit, peeled and sliced 1 mango, cubed
- 1 cup blueberries

Direction: Preparation Time: 5 minutes Cooking Time: 0 minute Servings: 6

- ✓ Beat cream cheese using an electric mixer.
- ✓ Add yogurt and honey. Beat until smooth.
- ✓ Stir in the orange and lemon zest.
- ✓ Toss the fruits to mix.
- ✓ Divide in glass jars. Top with the cream cheese mixture.

Nutrition: Calories 131 Total Fat 3 g Saturated Fat 2 g Cholesterol 9 mg Sodium 102 mg Total Carbohydrate 23 g Dietary Fiber 3 g Total Sugars 18 g Protein 5 g Potassium 234 mg

350) *Strawberry & Watermelon Pops*

Ingredients:

- ¾ cup strawberries, sliced
- 2 cups watermelon, cubed
- ¼ cup lime juice
- 2 tablespoons brown sugar
- ⅛ teaspoon salt

Direction: Preparation Time: 6 hours and 10 minutes Cooking Time: 0 minutes Servings: 6

- ✓ Put the strawberries inside popsicle molds. In a blender, pulse the rest of the ingredients until well mixed
- ✓ Pour the puree into a sieve before pouring into the molds. Freeze for 6 hours.

Nutrition: Calories 57 Total Fat 0 g Saturated Fat 0 g Cholesterol 0 mg Sodium 180 mg Total Carbohydrate 14 g Dietary Fiber 2 g Total Sugars 11 g Protein 1 g Potassium 180 mg

351) *Frozen Vanilla Yogurt*

Ingredients:

- 3 cups fat-free plain Greek yogurt
- 4-6 drops liquid stevia
- 1 teaspoon organic vanilla extract
- ¼ cup fresh strawberries, hulled and sliced

Direction: Preparation Time: 10 minutes Servings: 6

- ✓ In a bowl, add all the ingredients except strawberries and mix until well combined.
- ✓ Transfer the mixture into an ice cream maker and process according to manufacturer's directions.
- ✓ Transfer the mixture into a bowl and freeze, covered for about 30-40 minutes or until desired consistency.
- ✓ Garnish with strawberry slices and serve. Meal Prep Tip: Line a cookie sheet with parchment paper. With a cookie scooper, place the yogurt portion onto the prepared cookie sheet.
- ✓ Freeze overnight. Remove from the freezer and transfer the frozen yogurt balls into an airtight container. Store in freezer up to 1 week. Remove from the freezer and set aside for 15-20 minutes before serving.

Nutrition: Calories 74 Total Fat 0.3 g Saturated Fat 0 g Cholesterol 4mg Total Carbs 5.6 g Sugar 4.9 g Fiber 0.1 g Sodium 58 mg Potassium 10 mg Protein 12 g

352)   *Spinach Sorbet*

Ingredients:

- 3 cups fresh spinach, chopped
- 1 tablespoon fresh basil leaves
- ½ of avocado, peeled, pitted and chopped
- ¾ cup unsweetened almond milk 20 drops liquid stevia
- 1 teaspoon almonds, chopped very finely
- 1 teaspoon organic vanilla extract 1 cup ice cubes

Direction: Preparation Time: 15 minutes Servings: 4

- ✓ : In a blender, add all ingredients and pulse until creamy and smooth.
- ✓ Transfer into an ice cream maker and process according to manufacturer's directions. Transfer into an airtight container and freeze for at least 4-5 hours before serving.

Meal Prep Tip:

Transfer the sorbet into a shallow, flat container.

- ✓ With a plastic wrap, cover the ice cream and store in the back of the freezer.

Nutrition: Calories 70 Total Fat 5.9 g Saturated Fat 1.1 g Cholesterol 0 mg Total Carbs 3.6 g Sugar 0.4 g Fiber 2.4 g Sodium 53 mg Potassium 290 mg Protein 1.4 g

353)   *Avocado Mousse*

Ingredients:

- 2 ripe Haas avocados, peeled, pitted and chopped roughly
- 1 teaspoon liquid stevia
- 1 teaspoon organic vanilla extract Pinch of salt

Direction: Preparation Time: 15 minutes Servings: 3

- ✓ In a high-speed blender, add all the ingredients and pulse until smooth.
- ✓ Transfer the pudding into a serving bowl. Cover the bowl and refrigerate to chill for at least 2 hours before serving. Meal Prep Tip:
- ✓ Transfer the mousse into an airtight container.
- ✓ Cover the containers and refrigerate for about 1 day.

Nutrition: Calories 277 Total Fat 26.1 g Saturated Fat 5.5 g Cholesterol 0 mg Total Carbs 11.7 g Sugar 0.9 g Fiber 8 g Sodium 59 mg Potassium 652 mg Protein 2.6g

354)   *Strawberry Mousse*

Ingredients:

- 1½ cups fresh strawberries, hulled

- 1 2/3 cups chilled unsweetened almond milk
- 2-3 drops liquid stevia
- 1 teaspoon organic vanilla extract

Direction: Preparation Time: 15 minutes Servings: 6

- ✓ In a food processor, add all the ingredients and pulse until smooth.
- ✓ Transfer into serving bowls and serve.

Meal Prep Tip:

- ✓ Transfer the mousse into an airtight container.
- ✓ Cover the containers and refrigerate for up to 3 days.

Nutrition: Calories 25 Total Fat 1.1g Saturated Fat 0.1 g Cholesterol 0 mg Total Carbs 3.4 g Sugar 1.9 g Fiber 1 g Sodium 50 mg Potassium 109 mg Protein 0.5 g

355)   *Blueberries Pudding*

Ingredients:

- 1 small avocado, peeled, pitted and chopped
- 1 cup frozen blueberries
- ¼ teaspoon fresh ginger, grated freshly
- 1 teaspoon lime zest, grated finely
- 2 tablespoons fresh lime juice
- 10 drops liquid stevia
- 5 tablespoons filtered water

Direction: Preparation Time: 10 minutes Servings: 3

- ✓ In a blender, add all the ingredients and pulse till creamy and smooth.
- ✓ Transfer into serving bowls and serve.

Meal Prep Tip:

- ✓ Transfer the pudding into an airtight container.
- ✓ Cover the containers and refrigerate for up to 2 days.

Nutrition: Calories 166 Total Fat 13.3 g Saturated Fat 4.2.8 g Cholesterol 0 mg Total Carbs 13.1 g Sugar 5.2 g Fiber 5.8 g Potassium 331 mg Protein 1.7 g

356)   *Raspberry Chia Pudding*

Ingredients:

- 1½ cups unsweetened almond milk
- 1¼ cups fresh raspberries
- ½ cup chia seeds
- 1 tablespoon flax meal
- 3-4 drops liquid stevia
- 2 teaspoons organic vanilla extract

Direction: Preparation Time: 10 minutes Servings:4

✓ In a blender, add the almond milk and raspberries and pulse until smooth.

✓ Transfer the milk mixture into a large bowl.

✓ Add the remaining ingredients except raspberries and stir until well combined.

✓ Refrigerate to chill for at least 1 hour before serving.

Meal Prep Tip:

✓ Transfer the pudding into an airtight container.

✓ Cover the containers and refrigerate for about 1 day.

Nutrition: Calories 107 Total Fat 7.2 g Saturated Fat 0.5 g Cholesterol 0 mg Total Carbs 12.1 g Sugar 2 g Fiber 8.4 g Sodium 68 mg Potassium 246 mg Protein 4.2 g

357) *Brown Rice Pudding*

Ingredients:

• 2 cups low-fat milk 1/3 cup Erythritol 1½ teaspoons organic vanilla extract

• ¼ teaspoon ground cinnamon 1 egg 2 cups cooked brown rice

Direction: Preparation Time: 15 minutes Cooking Time: 30 minutes Servings: 4

✓ In a medium pan, add the milk, Erythritol, vanilla extract and cinnamon over medium-high heat and bring to a boil, stirring continuously. Remove from the heat.

✓ In a large bowl, add the egg and beat well. Slowly, add the hot milk mixture, a little bit at a time and beat until well combined. In the same pan, add the milk mixture and rice and

✓ Place the 2 cups of cooked rice into the pan used to cook the milk mixture and stir to combine.

✓ Place the pan over medium-high heat and bring to a boil, stirring continuously.

✓ Reduce heat to low and simmer for about 15-20 minutes, stirring after every 5 minutes. Remove from the heat and transfer into a bowl. With a wax paper, cover the top of pudding and refrigerate to chill before serving.

Meal Prep Tip:

✓ Transfer the pudding into an airtight container. Cover the containers and refrigerate for up to 2 days.

Nutrition: Calories 416 Total Fat 4.8 g Saturated Fat 1.6 g Cholesterol 47 mg Total Carbs 78 g Sugar 6 g Fiber 3.3 g Sodium 73 mg Potassium 455 mg Protein 12.5 g

358) *Lemon Cookies*

Ingredients:

• ¼ cup unsweetened applesauce 1 cup cashew butter 1 teaspoon fresh lemon zest, grated finely

• 2 tablespoons fresh lemon juice Pinch of sea salt

Direction: Preparation Time: 10 minutes Cooking Time: 12 minutes Servings: 6

✓ Preheat the oven to 350 degrees F. Line a large cookie sheet with parchment paper. In a food processor, add all ingredients and pulse until smooth. With a tablespoon, place the mixture onto prepared cookie sheet in a single layer. Bake for about 12 minutes or until golden brown. Remove from oven and place the cookie sheet onto a wire rack to cool for about 5 minutes.

✓ Carefully invert the cookies onto wire rack to cool completely before serving. Meal Prep Tip: Store these cookies in an airtight container, by placing parchment papers between the cookies to avoid the sticking. These cookies can be stored in the refrigerator for up to 2 weeks.

Nutrition: : Calories 257 Total Fat 21.9 g Saturated Fat 4.2 g Cholesterol 0 mg Total Carbs 13.1 g Sugar 1.2 g Fiber 1 g Sodium 47 mg Potassium 248 mg Protein 7.6 g

359) *Yogurt Cheesecake*

Ingredients:

• 2½ cups fat-free plain Greek yogurt

• 6-8 drops liquid stevia 3 egg whites

• 1/3 cup cacao powder

• ¼ cup arrowroot starch

• 1 teaspoon organic vanilla extract

• Pinch of sea salt

Direction: Preparation Time: 15 minutes Cooking Time: 35 minutes Servings: 8

✓ Preheat the oven to 35 degrees F. Grease a 9-inch cake pan.

✓ In a large bowl, add all ingredients and mix until well combined.

✓ Place the mixture into the prepared pan evenly. Bake for about 30-35 minutes. Remove from oven and let it cool completely.

✓ Refrigerate to chill for about 3-4 hours or until set completely.

✓ Cut into 8 equal sized slices and serve.

Meal Prep Tip:

✓ With foil pieces, wrap the cheesecake slices and refrigerate for about 1-3 days. Reheat in the microwave before serving.

Nutrition: Calories 74 Total Fat 0.9g Saturated Fat 0.4 g Cholesterol 2 mg Total Carbs 8.5 g Sugar 3 g Fiber 1.1 g Sodium 89 mg Potassium 21 mg Protein 9.5 g

360) *Flourless Chocolate Cake*

Ingredients:

- 1/2 Cup of stevia
- 12 Ounces of unsweetened baking chocolate
- 2/3 Cup of ghee
- 1/3 Cup of warm water
- ¼ Teaspoon of salt
- 4 Large pastured eggs
- 2 Cups of boiling water

**Direction: Preparation time: 10 minutes
Cooking time: 45 minutes Yield: 6 Servings**

- ✓ Line the bottom of a 9-inch pan of a spring form with a parchment paper.
- ✓ Heat the water in a small pot; then add the salt and the stevia over the water until wait until the mixture becomes completely dissolved.
- ✓ Melt the baking chocolate into a double boiler or simply microwave it for about 30 seconds.
- ✓ Mix the melted chocolate and the butter in a large bowl with an electric mixer.
- ✓ Beat in your hot mixture; then crack in the egg and whisk after adding each of the eggs.
- ✓ Pour the obtained mixture into your prepared spring form tray.
- ✓ Wrap the spring form tray with a foil paper.
- ✓ Place the spring form tray in a large cake tray and add boiling water right to the outside; make sure the depth doesn't exceed 1 inch.
- ✓ Bake the cake into the water bath for about 45 minutes at a temperature of about 350 F.
- ✓ Remove the tray from the boiling water and transfer to a wire to cool.
- ✓ Let the cake chill for an overnight in the refrigerator.
- ✓ Serve and enjoy your delicious cake!

Nutrition: Calories: 295| Fat: 26g | Carbohydrates: 6g | Fiber: 4g |Protein: 8g

361) *Raspberry Cake With White Chocolate Sauce*

Ingredients:

- 5 Ounces of melted cacao butter
- 2 Ounces of grass-fed ghee
- 1/2 Cup of coconut cream
- 1 Cup of green banana flour
- 3 Teaspoons of pure vanilla
- 4 Large eggs
- 1/2 Cup of as Lakanto Monk Fruit
- 1 Teaspoon of baking powder
- 2 Teaspoons of apple cider vinegar
- 2 Cup of raspberries
- For the white chocolate sauce:
- 3 and 1/2 ounces of cacao butter
- 1/2 Cup of coconut cream
- 2 Teaspoons of pure vanilla extract
- 1 Pinch of salt

**Direction: Preparation time: 15 minutes
Cooking time: 60 minutes Yield: 5-6 Servings**

- ✓ Preheat your oven to a temperature of about 280 degrees Fahrenheit.
- ✓ Combine the green banana flour with the pure vanilla extract, the baking powder, the coconut cream, the eggs, the cider vinegar and the monk fruit and mix very well.
- ✓ Leave the raspberries aside and line a cake loaf tin with a baking paper .
- ✓ Pour in the batter into the baking tray and scatter the raspberries over the top of the cake.
- ✓ Place the tray in your oven and bake it for about 60 minutes; in the meantime, prepare the sauce by
- ✓ Directions for sauce:
- ✓ Combine the cacao cream, the vanilla extract, the cacao butter and the salt in a saucepan over a low heat.
- ✓ Mix all your ingredients with a fork to make sure the cacao butter mixes very well with the cream.
- ✓ Remove from the heat and set aside to cool a little bit; but don't let it harden.
- ✓ Drizzle with the chocolate sauce.
- ✓ Scatter the cake with more raspberries.
- ✓ Slice your cake; then serve and enjoy it!

Nutrition: Calories: 323| Fat: 31.5g | Carbohydrates: 9.9g | Fiber: 4g |Protein: 5g

362) *Ketogenic Lava Cake*

Ingredients:

- 2 Oz of dark chocolate; you should at least use chocolate of 85% cocoa solids
- 1 Tablespoon of super-fine almond flour
- 2 Oz of unsalted almond butter
- 2 Large eggs

Direction: Preparation time: 10 minutes Cooking time: 10 minutes Yield: 2 Servings

- ✓ Heat your oven to a temperature of about 350 Fahrenheit.
- ✓ Grease 2 heat proof ramekins with almond butter.
- ✓ Now, melt the chocolate and the almond butter and stir very well.

✓ Beat the eggs very well with a mixer.
✓ Add the eggs to the chocolate and the butter mixture and mix very well with almond flour and the swerve; then stir.
✓ Pour the dough into 2 ramekins.
✓ Bake for about 9 to 10 minutes.
✓ Turn the cakes over plates and serve with pomegranate seeds!

Nutrition: Calories: 459| Fat: 39g | Carbohydrates: 3.5g | Fiber: 0.8g |Protein: 11.7g

363) *Ketogenic Cheese Cake*

Ingredients:

- For the Almond Flour Cheesecake Crust:
- 2 Cups of Blanched almond flour
- 1/3 Cup of almond Butter
- 3 Tablespoons of Erythritol (powdered or granular)
- 1 Teaspoon of Vanilla extract
- For the Keto Cheesecake Filling:
- 32 Oz of softened Cream cheese
- 1 and ¼ cups of powdered erythritol
- 3 Large Eggs
- 1 Tablespoon of Lemon juice
- 1 Teaspoon of Vanilla extract

Direction: Preparation time: 15 minutes Cooking time: 50 minutes Yield: 6 Servings

✓ Preheat your oven to a temperature of about 350 degrees F.
✓ Grease a spring form pan of 9¨ with cooking spray or just line its bottom with a parchment paper.
✓ In order to make the cheesecake rust, stir in the melted butter, the almond flour, the vanilla extract and the erythritol in a large bowl.
✓ The dough will get will be a bit crumbly; so press it into the bottom of your prepared tray.
✓ Bake for about 12 minutes; then let cool for about 10 minutes.
✓ In the meantime, beat the softened cream cheese and the powdered sweetener at a low speed until it becomes smooth.
✓ Crack in the eggs and beat them in at a low to medium speed until it becomes fluffy. Make sure to add one a time.
✓ Add in the lemon juice and the vanilla extract and mix at a low to medium speed with a mixer.
✓ Pour your filling into your pan right on top of the crust. You can use a spatula to smooth the top of the cake.
✓ Bake for about 45 to 50 minutes.
✓ Remove the baked cheesecake from your oven and run a knife around its edge.

✓ Let the cake cool for about 4 hours in the refrigerator.

Nutrition: Calories: 325| Fat: 29g | Carbohydrates: 6g | Fiber: 1g |Protein: 7g

364) *Cake with Whipped Cream Icing*

Ingredients:

- ¾ Cup Coconut flour
- ¾ Cup of Swerve Sweetener
- 1/2 Cup of Cocoa powder
- 2 Teaspoons of Baking powder
- 6 Large Eggs
- 2/3 Cup of Heavy Whipping Cream
- 1/2 Cup of Melted almond Butter
- For the whipped Cream Icing:
- 1 Cup of Heavy Whipping Cream
- ¼ Cup of Swerve Sweetener
- 1 Teaspoon of Vanilla extract
- 1/3 Cup of Sifted Cocoa Powder

Direction: Preparation time: 20 minutes Cooking time: 25 minutes Yield: 7 Servings

✓ Pre-heat your oven to a temperature of about 350 F.
✓ Grease an 8x8 cake tray with cooking spray.
✓ Add the coconut flour, the Swerve sweetener; the cocoa powder, the baking powder, the eggs, the melted butter; and combine very well with an electric or a hand mixer.
✓ Pour your batter into the cake tray and bake for about 25 minutes.
✓ Remove the cake tray from the oven and let cool for about 5 minutes.
✓ For the Icing:
✓ Whip the cream until it becomes fluffy; then add in the Swerve, the vanilla and the cocoa powder.
✓ Add the Swerve, the vanilla and the cocoa powder; then continue mixing until your ingredients are very well combined.
✓ Frost your baked cake with the icing; then slice it; serve and enjoy your delicious cake!

Nutrition: Calories: 357| Fat: 33g | Carbohydrates: 11g | Fiber: 2g |Protein: 8g

365) *Walnut-Fruit Cake*

Ingredients:

- 1/2 Cup of almond butter (softened)
- ¼ Cup of so Nourished granulated erythritol

- 1 Tablespoon of ground cinnamon
- 1/2 Teaspoon of ground nutmeg
- ¼ Teaspoon of ground cloves
- 4 Large pastured eggs
- 1 Teaspoon of vanilla extract
- 1/2 Teaspoon of almond extract
- 2 Cups of almond flour
- 1/2 Cup of chopped walnuts
- ¼ Cup of dried of unsweetened cranberries
- ¼ Cup of seedless raisins

Direction:

✓ Preheat your oven to a temperature of about 350 F and grease an 8-inch baking tin of round shape with coconut oil.
✓ Beat the granulated erythritol on a high speed until it becomes fluffy.
✓ Add the cinnamon, the nutmeg, and the cloves; then blend your ingredients until they become smooth.
✓ Crack in the eggs and beat very well by adding one at a time, plus the almond extract and the vanilla.
✓ Whisk in the almond flour until it forms a smooth batter then fold in the nuts and the fruit.
✓ Spread your mixture into your prepared baking pan and bake it for about 20 minutes.
✓ Remove the cake from the oven and let cool for about 5 minutes.
✓ Dust the cake with the powdered erythritol.
✓ Serve and enjoy your cake!

Nutrition: Calories: 250| Fat: 11g | Carbohydrates: 12g | Fiber: 2g |Protein: 7g

366) *Ginger Cake*

Ingredients:

- 1/2 Tablespoon of unsalted almond butter to grease the pan
- 4 Large eggs
- ¼ Cup coconut milk
- 2 Tablespoons of unsalted almond butter
- 1 and 1/2 teaspoons of stevia
- 1 Tablespoon of ground cinnamon
- 1 Tablespoon of natural unweeded cocoa powder
- 1 Tablespoon of fresh ground ginger
- 1/2 Teaspoon of kosher salt
- 1 and 1/2 cups of blanched almond flour
- 1/2 Teaspoon of baking soda

Direction: Preparation time: 15 minutes Cooking time: 20 minutes Yield: 9 Servings

✓ Preheat your oven to a temperature of 325 F.

✓ Grease a glass baking tray of about 8X8 inches generously with almond butter.
✓ In a large bowl, whisk all together the coconut milk, the eggs, the melted almond butter, the stevia, the cinnamon, the cocoa powder, the ginger and the kosher salt.
✓ Whisk in the almond flour, then the baking soda and mix very well.
✓ Pour the batter into the prepared pan and bake for about 20 to 25 minutes.
✓ Let the cake cool for about 5 minutes; then slice; serve and enjoy your delicious cake.

Nutrition: Calories: 175| Fat: 15g | Carbohydrates: 5g | Fiber: 1.9g |Protein: 5g

367) *Ketogenic Orange Cake*

Ingredients:

- 2 and 1/2 cups of almond flour
- 2 Unwaxed washed oranges
- 5 Large separated eggs
- 1 Teaspoon of baking powder
- 2 Teaspoons of orange extract
- 1 Teaspoon of vanilla bean powder
- 6 Seeds of cardamom pods crushed
- 16 drops of liquid stevia; about 3 teaspoons
- 1 Handful of flaked almonds to decorate

Direction: Preparation time: 10 minutes Cooking time: 50 minutes Yield: 8 Servings

✓ Preheat your oven to a temperature of about 350 Fahrenheit.
✓ Line a rectangular bread baking tray with a parchment paper.
✓ Place the oranges into a pan filled with cold water and cover it with a lid.
✓ Bring the saucepan to a boil, then let simmer for about 1 hour and make sure the oranges are totally submerged.
✓ Make sure the oranges are always submerged to remove any taste of bitterness.
✓ Cut the oranges into halves; then remove any seeds; and drain the water and set the oranges aside to cool down.
✓ Cut the oranges in half and remove any seeds, then puree it with a blender or a food processor.
✓ Separate the eggs; then whisk the egg whites until you see stiff peaks forming.
✓ Add all your ingredients except for the egg whites to the orange mixture and add in the egg whites; then mix.
✓ Pour the batter into the cake tin and sprinkle with the flaked almonds right on top.
✓ Bake your cake for about 50 minutes.

✓ Remove the cake from the oven and set aside to cool for 5 minutes.

✓ Slice your cake; then serve and enjoy its incredible taste!

Nutrition: Calories: 164| Fat: 12g | Carbohydrates: 7.1 | Fiber: 2.7g |Protein: 10.9g

368)   *Lemon Cake*

Ingredients:

- 2 Medium lemons
- 4 Large eggs
- 2 Tablespoons of almond butter
- 2 Tablespoons of avocado oil
- 1/3 cup of coconut flour
- 4-5 tablespoons of honey (or another sweetener of your choice)
- 1/2 tablespoon of baking soda

Direction: Preparation time: 20 minutes Cooking time: 20 minutes Yield: 9 Servings

✓ Preheat your oven to a temperature of about 350 F.

✓ Crack the eggs in a large bowl and set two egg whites aside.

✓ Whisk the 2 whites of eggs with the egg yolks, the honey, the oil, the almond butter, the lemon zest and the juice and whisk very well together.

✓ Combine the baking soda with the coconut flour and gradually add this dry mixture to the wet ingredients and keep whisking for a couple of minutes.

✓ Beat the two eggs with a hand mixer and beat the egg into foam. Add the white egg foam gradually to the mixture with a silicone spatula.

✓ Transfer your obtained batter to tray covered with a baking paper.

✓ Bake your cake for about 20 to 22 minutes.

✓ Let the cake cool for 5 minutes; then slice your cake.

✓ Serve and enjoy your delicious cake!

Nutrition: Calories: 164| Fat: 12g | Carbohydrates: 7.1 | Fiber: 2.7g |Protein: 10.9g

369)   *Cinnamon Cake*

Ingredients:

- For the Cinnamon Filling:
- 3 Tablespoons of Swerve Sweetener
- 2 Teaspoons of ground cinnamon
- For the Cake:
- 3 Cups of almond flour
- ¾ Cup of Swerve Sweetener
- ¼ Cup of unflavoured whey protein powder

- 2 Teaspoon of baking powder
- 1/2 Teaspoon of salt
- 3 large pastured eggs
- 1/2 Cup of melted coconut oil
- 1/2 Teaspoon of vanilla extract
- 1/2 Cup of almond milk
- 1 Tablespoon of melted coconut oil

For the cream cheese Frosting:

- 3 Tablespoons of softened cream cheese
- 2 Tablespoons of powdered Swerve Sweetener
- 1 Tablespoon of coconut heavy whipping cream
- 1/2 Teaspoon of vanilla extract

Direction: Preparation time: 15 minutes

Cooking time: 35 minutes Yield: 8 Servings

✓ Preheat your oven to a temperature of about 325 F and grease a baking tray of 8x8 inch.

✓ For the filling, mix the Swerve and the cinnamon in a mixing bowl and mix very well; then set it aside.

✓ For the preparation of the cake; whisk all together the almond flour, the sweetener, the protein powder, the baking powder, and the salt in a mixing bowl.

✓ Add in the eggs, the melted coconut oil and the vanilla extract and mix very well.

✓ Add in the almond milk and keep stirring until your ingredients are very well combined.

✓ Spread about half of the batter in the prepared pan; then sprinkle with about two thirds of the filling mixture.

✓ Spread the remaining mixture of the batter over the filling and smooth it with a spatula.

✓ Bake for about 35 minutes in the oven.

✓ Brush with the melted coconut oil and sprinkle with the remaining cinnamon filling.

✓ Prepare the frosting by beating the cream cheese, the powdered erythritol, the cream and the vanilla extract in a mixing bowl until it becomes smooth.

✓ Drizzle frost over the cooled cake.

✓ Slice the cake; then serve and enjoy your cake!

Nutrition: Calories: 222| Fat: 19.2g | Carbohydrates: 5.4g | Fiber: 1.5g |Protein: 7.3g

370)   *Chocolate & Raspberry Ice Cream*

Ingredients:

- ¼ cup almond milk
- 2 egg yolks
- 2 tablespoons cornstarch
- ¼ cup honey

- ¼ teaspoon almond extract
- ⅛ teaspoon salt
- 1 cup fresh raspberries
- 2 oz. dark chocolate, chopped
- ¼ cup almonds, slivered and toasted

Direction: Preparation Time: 12 hours and 20 minutes Cooking Time: 0 minutes Servings: 8

- ✓ Mix almond milk, egg yolks, cornstarch and honey in a bowl.
- ✓ Pour into a saucepan over medium heat.
- ✓ Cook for 8 minutes.
- ✓ Strain through a sieve. Stir in salt and almond extract.
- ✓ Chill for 8 hours.
- ✓ Put into an ice cream maker.
- ✓ Follow manufacturer's directions.
- ✓ Stir in the rest of the ingredients.
- ✓ Freeze for 4 hours.

Nutrition: Calories 142 Total Fat 7 g Saturated Fat 2 g Cholesterol 70 mg Sodium 87 mg Total Carbohydrate 18 g Dietary Fiber 2 g Total Sugars 13 g Protein 3 g Potassium 150 mg

371) *Mocha Pops*

Ingredients:

- 3 cups brewed coffee
- ½ cup low calorie chocolate flavored syrup
- ¾ cup low fat half and half

Direction: Preparation Time: 4 minutes Cooking Time: 0 minutes Servings: 15

- ✓ Mix the ingredients in a bowl.
- ✓ Pour into popsicle molds. Freeze for 4 hours.

Nutrition: Calories 21 Total Fat 0 g Saturated Fat 0 g Cholesterol 1 mg Sodium 28 mg Total Carbohydrate 4 g Dietary Fiber 0 g Total Sugars 3 g Protein 0 g Potassiu

372) *Fruit Kebab*

Ingredients:

- 3 apples
- ¼ cup orange juice
- 1 ½ lb. watermelon is
- ¾ cup blueberries

Direction: Preparation Time: 30 minutes Cooking Time: 0 minutes Servings: 12

- ✓ Use a star-shaped cookie cutter to cut out stars from the apple and watermelon.
- ✓ Soak the apple stars in orange juice.
- ✓ Thread the apple stars, watermelon stars and blueberries into skewers.
- ✓ Refrigerate for 30 minutes before serving.

Nutrition: Calories 52 Total Fat 0 g Saturated Fat 0 g Cholesterol 0 mg Sodium 1 mg Total Carbohydrate 14 g Dietary Fiber 2 g Total Sugars 10 g Protein 1 g Potassium 134 mg

373) *Salad Preparation*

Ingredients:

- 8 oz. light cream cheese 6 oz. Greek yogurt 1 tablespoon honey
- 1 teaspoon orange zest
- 1 teaspoon lemon zest
- 1 orange, sliced into sections
- 3 kiwi fruit, peeled and sliced
- 1 mango, cubed 1 cup blueberries

Direction: Time: 5 minutes Cooking Time: 0 minute

Servings: 6

- ✓ Beat cream cheese using an electric mixer. Add yogurt and honey.
- ✓ Beat until smooth. Stir in the orange and lemon zest. Toss the fruits to mix.
- ✓ Divide in glass jars. Top with the cream cheese mixture.

Nutrition: Calories 131 Total Fat 3 g Saturated Fat 2 g Cholesterol 9 mg Sodium 102 mg Total Carbohydrate 23 g Dietary Fiber 3 g Total Sugars 18 g Protein 5 g Potassium 234 mg

MORE RECIPES

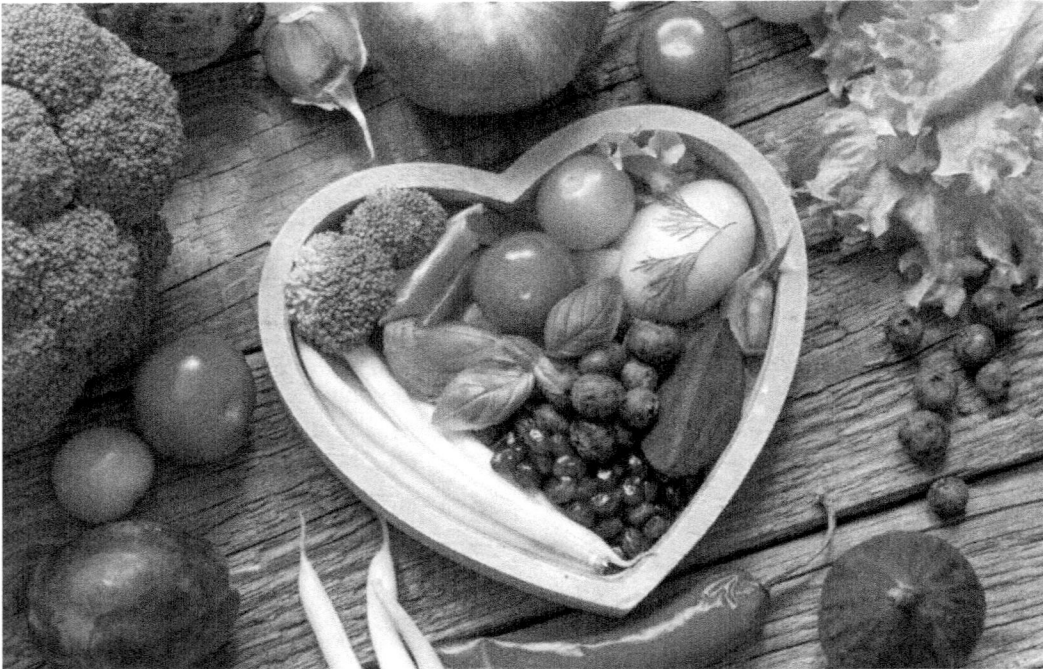

374) *Chili Chicken Wings*

Ingredients:

- 2 lbs chicken wings
- 1/8 tsp. paprika
- 1/2 cup coconut flour
- 1/4 tsp. garlic powder
- 1/4 tsp. chili powder

Direction: Preparation Time: 10 minutes Cooking Time: 1 hour 10 minutes Servings: 4

- ✓ Preheat the oven to 400 F/ 200 C.
- ✓ In a mixing bowl, add all ingredients except chicken wings and mix well.
- ✓ Add chicken wings to the bowl mixture and coat well and place on a baking tray.
- ✓ Bake in preheated oven for 55-60 minutes.
- ✓ Serve and enjoy.

Nutrition: Calories 440 Fat 17.1 g, Carbs 1.3 g, Sugar 0.2 g, Protein 65.9 g, Cholesterol 202 mg

375) *Garlic Chicken Wings*

Ingredients:

- 12 chicken wings
- 2 garlic clove, minced
- 3 tbsp. ghee
- 1/2 tsp. turmeric
- 2 tsp. cumin seeds

Direction: Preparation Time: 10 minutes Cooking Time: 55 minutes Servings: 6

- ✓ Preheat the oven to 425 F/ 215 C.
- ✓ In a large bowl, mix together 1 teaspoon cumin, 1 tbsp. ghee, turmeric, pepper, and salt.
- ✓ Add chicken wings to the bowl and toss well.
- ✓ Spread chicken wings on a baking tray and bake in preheated oven for 30 minutes.
- ✓ Turn chicken wings to another side and bake for 8 minutes more.
- ✓ Meanwhile, heat remaining ghee in a pan over medium heat.
- ✓ Add garlic and cumin to the pan and cook for a minute.
- ✓ Remove pan from heat and set aside.
- ✓ Remove chicken wings from oven and drizzle with ghee mixture/
- ✓ Bake chicken wings 5 minutes more.
- ✓ Serve and enjoy.

Nutrition: Calories 378 Fat 27.9 g, Carbs 11.4 g, Sugar 0 g, Protein 19.7 g, Cholesterol 94 mg

376) *Spinach Cheese Pie*

Ingredients:

- 6 eggs, lightly beaten
- 2 boxes frozen spinach, chopped
- 2 cup cheddar cheese, shredded
- 15 oz. cottage cheese
- 1 tsp. salt

Direction: Preparation Time: 10 minutes Cooking Time: 40 minutes Servings: 8

- ✓ Preheat the oven to 375 F/ 190 C.
- ✓ Spray an 8*8-inch baking dish with cooking spray and set aside.
- ✓ In a mixing bowl, combine together spinach, eggs, cheddar cheese, cottage cheese, pepper, and salt.
- ✓ Pour spinach mixture into the prepared baking dish and bake in preheated oven for 10 minutes.
- ✓ Serve and enjoy.

Nutrition: Calories 229 Fat 14 g, Carbs. 5.4 g, Sugar 0.9 g, Protein 21 g, Cholesterol 157 mg

377) *Tasty Harissa Chicken*

Ingredients:

- 1 lb. chicken breasts, skinless and boneless
- 1/2 tsp. ground cumin
- 1 cup harissa sauce
- 1/4 tsp. garlic powder
- 1/2 tsp. kosher salt

Direction: Preparation Time: 10 minutes

Cooking Time: 4 hours 10 minutes Servings: 4

- ✓ Season chicken with garlic powder, cumin, and salt.
- ✓ Place chicken to the slow cooker.
- ✓ Pour harissa sauce over the chicken.
- ✓ Cover slow cooker with lid and cook on low for 4 hours.
- ✓ Remove chicken from slow cooker and shred using a fork.
- ✓ Return shredded chicken to the slow cooker and stir well.
- ✓ Serve and enjoy.

Nutrition: Calories 232 Fat 9.7 g, Carbs 1.3 g, Sugar 0.1 g, Protein 32.9 g, Cholesterol 101 mg

378) Roasted Balsamic Mushrooms

Ingredients:

- 8 oz. mushrooms, sliced
- 1/2tsp. thyme
- 2 tbsp. balsamic vinegar
- 2 tbsp. extra virgin olive oil
- 2 onions, sliced

Direction: Preparation Time: 10 minutes

Cooking Time: 50 minutes Servings: 4

✓ Preheat the oven to 375 F/ 190 C.
✓ Line baking tray with aluminum foil and spray with cooking spray and set aside.
✓ In a mixing bowl, add all ingredients and mix well.
✓ Spread mushroom mixture onto a prepared baking tray.
✓ Roast in preheated oven for 45 minutes.
✓ Season with pepper and salt.
✓ Serve and enjoy.

Nutrition: Calories 96 Fat 7.2 g, Carbohydrates 7.2 g, Sugar 3.3 g, Protein 2.4 g, Cholesterol 0 mg

379) Roasted Cumin Carrots

Ingredients:

- 8 carrots, peeled and cut into 1/2 inch thick slices
- 1 tsp. cumin seeds
- 1 tbsp. olive oil
- 1/2tsp. kosher salt

Direction: Preparation Time: 10 minutes

Cooking Time: 45 minutes Servings: 4

✓ Preheat the oven to 400 F/ 200 C.
✓ Line baking tray with parchment paper.
✓ Add carrots, cumin seeds, olive oil, and salt in a large bowl and toss well to coat.
✓ Spread carrots on a prepared baking tray and roast in preheated oven for 20 minutes.
✓ Turn carrots to another side and roast for 20 minutes more.
✓ Serve and enjoy.

Nutrition: Calories 82 Fat 3.6 g, Carbohydrates 12.2 g, Sugar 6 g, Protein 1.1 g, Cholesterol 0 mg

380) Tasty & Tender Brussels Sprouts

Ingredients:

- 1 lb. Brussels sprouts, trimmed cut in half
- ¼ cup balsamic vinegar
- 1 onion, sliced
- 1 tbsp. olive oil

Direction: Preparation Time: 10 minutes

Cooking Time: 35 minutes Servings: 4

✓ Add water in a saucepan and bring to boil.
✓ Add Brussels sprouts and cook over medium heat for 20 minutes. Drain well.
✓ Heat oil in a pan over medium heat.
✓ Add onion and cook until softened. Add sprouts and vinegar and stir well and cook for 1-2 minutes.
✓ Serve and enjoy.

Nutrition: Calories 93 Fat 3.9 g, Carbohydrates 13 g, Sugar 3.7 g, Protein 4.2 g, Cholesterol 0 mg

381) Sautéed Veggies

Ingredients:

- 1/2 cup mushrooms, sliced
- 1 zucchini, diced
- 1 squash, diced
- 2 1/2 tsp. southwest seasoning
- 3 tbsp. olive oil

Direction: Preparation Time: 10 minutes

Cooking Time: 15 minutes Servings: 4

✓ In a medium bowl, whisk together southwest seasoning, pepper, olive oil, and salt.
✓ Add vegetables to a bowl and mix well to coat.
✓ Heat pan over medium-high heat.
✓ Add vegetables in the pan and sauté for 5-7 minutes.
✓ Serve and enjoy.

Nutrition: Calories 107, Fat 10.7 g, Carbs 3.6 g, Sugar 1.5 g, Protein 1.2 g, Cholesterol 0 mg

382) Mustard Green Beans

Ingredients:

- 1 lb. green beans, washed and trimmed
- 1 tsp. whole grain mustard
- 1 tbsp. olive oil
- 2 tbsp. apple cider vinegar
- 1/4 cup onion, chopped

Direction: Preparation Time: 10 minutes

Cooking Time: 20 minutes Servings: 4

✓ Steam green beans in the microwave until tender.
✓ Meanwhile, in a pan heat olive oil over medium heat.
✓ Add the onion in a pan sauté until softened.
✓ Add water, apple cider vinegar, and mustard in the pan and stir well.
✓ Add green beans and stir to coat and heat through.
✓ Season green beans with pepper and salt.
✓ Serve and enjoy.

Nutrition: Calories 71 Fat 3.7 g, Carbohydrates 8.9 g, Sugar 1.9 g, Protein 2.1 g, Cholesterol 0 mg

383)   *Zucchini Fries*

Ingredients:

- 1 egg
- 2 medium zucchini, cut into fries shape
- 1 tsp. Italian herbs
- 1 tsp. garlic powder
- 1 cup parmesan cheese, grated

Direction: Preparation Time: 10 minutes

Cooking Time: 40 minutes Servings: 4

✓ Preheat the oven to 425 F/ 218 C.
✓ Spray a baking tray with cooking spray and set aside.
✓ In a small bowl, add egg and lightly whisk it.
✓ In a separate bowl, mix together spices and parmesan cheese.
✓ Dip zucchini fries in egg then coat with parmesan cheese mixture and place on a baking tray.
✓ Bake in preheated oven for 25-30 minutes. Turn halfway through.
✓ Serve and enjoy.

Nutrition: Calories 184 Fat 10.3 g, Carbs 3.9 g, Sugar 2 g, Protein 14.7 g, Cholesterol 71 mg

384)   *Broccoli Nuggets*

Ingredients:

- 2 cups broccoli florets
- 1/4 cup almond flour
- 2 egg whites
- 1 cup cheddar cheese, shredded
- 1/8 tsp. salt

Direction: Preparation Time: 10 minutes

Cooking Time: 25 minutes Servings: 4

✓ Preheat the oven to 350 F/ 180 C.

✓ Spray a baking tray with cooking spray and set aside.
✓ Using potato masher breaks the broccoli florets into small pieces.
✓ Add remaining ingredients to the broccoli and mix well.
✓ Drop 20 scoops onto baking tray and press lightly into a nugget shape.
✓ Bake in preheated oven for 20 minutes.
✓ Serve and enjoy.

Nutrition: Calories 148 Fat 10.4 g, Carbs 3.9 g, Sugar 1.1 g, Protein 10.5 g, Cholesterol 30 mg

385)   *Zucchini Cauliflower Fritters*

Ingredients:

- 2 medium zucchini, grated and squeezed
- 3 cups cauliflower florets
- 1 tbsp. coconut oil
- 1/4 cup coconut flour
- 1/2 tsp. sea salt

Direction: Preparation Time: 10 minutes

Cooking Time: 15 minutes Servings: 4

✓ Steam cauliflower florets for 5 minutes.
✓ Add cauliflower into the food processor and process until it looks like rice.
✓ Add all ingredients except coconut oil to the large bowl and mix until well combined.
✓ Make small round patties from the mixture and set aside.
✓ Heat coconut oil in a pan over medium heat.
✓ Place patties in a pan and cook for 3-4 minutes on each side.
✓ Serve and enjoy.

Nutrition: Calories 68 Fat 3.8 g, Carbs 7.8 g, Sugar 3.6 g, Protein 2.8 g, Cholesterol 0 mg

386)   *Roasted Chickpeas*

Ingredients:

- 15 oz. can chickpeas, drained, rinsed and pat dry
- 1/2 tsp. paprika
- 1 tbsp. olive oil
- 1/2 tsp. pepper
- 1/2 tsp. salt

Direction: Preparation Time: 10 minutes

Cooking Time: 30 minutes Servings: 4

✓ Preheat the oven to 450 F/ 232 C.

✓ Spray a baking tray with cooking spray and set aside.

✓ In a large bowl, toss chickpeas with olive oil, paprika, pepper, and salt.

✓ Spread chickpeas on a prepared baking tray and roast in preheated oven for 25 minutes. Stir every 10 minutes.

✓ Serve and enjoy.

Nutrition: Calories 158 Fat 4.8 g, Carbs 24.4 g, Sugar 0 g, Protein 5.3 g, Cholesterol 0 mg

387) *Peanut Butter Mousse*

Ingredients:

- 1 tbsp. peanut butter
- 1 tsp. vanilla extract
- 1 tsp. stevia
- 1/2 cup heavy cream

Direction: Preparation Time: 10 minutes

Cooking Time: 10 minutes Servings: 2

✓ Add all ingredients into the bowl and whisk until soft peak forms.   ✓   Spoon into the serving bowls and enjoy.

Nutrition: Calories 157 Fat 15.1 g, Carbohydrates 5.2 g, Sugar 3.6 g, Protein 2.6 g, Cholesterol 41 mg

388) *Coffee Mousse*

Ingredients:

- 4 tbsp. brewed coffee
- 16 oz. cream cheese, softened
- 1/2 cup unsweetened almond milk
- 1 cup whipping cream
- 2 tsp. liquid stevia

Direction: Preparation Time: 10 minutes

Cooking Time: 20 minutes Servings: 8

✓ Add coffee and cream cheese in a blender and blend until smooth.

✓ Add stevia, and milk and blend again until smooth.

✓ Add cream and blend until thickened.   ✓
Pour into the serving glasses and place in the refrigerator.

✓ Serve chilled and enjoy.

Nutrition: Calories 244 Fat 24.6 g, Carbs 2.1 g, Sugar 0.1 g, Protein 4.7 g,

VEGETARIAN

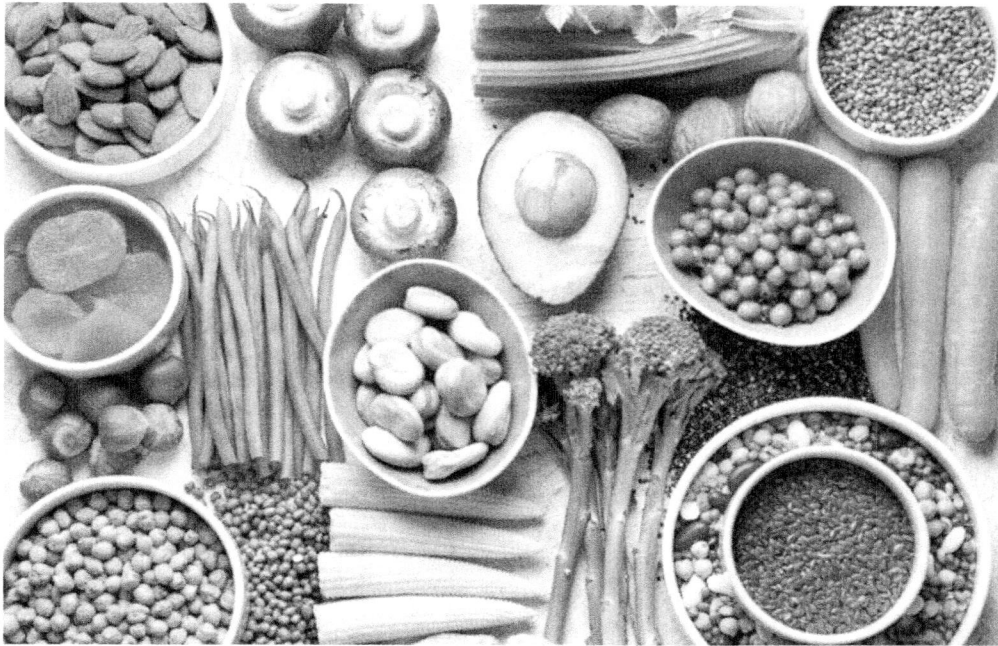

Ingredients:

- : ¾ cup amaranth 1 cup quinoa, rinsed
- ¼ cup wild rice
- 4¼ cups filtered water
- 2 teaspoons ground cumin
- ½ teaspoon paprika Salt, as required
- 1¼ cups boiled chickpeas
- 2 medium carrots, peeled and grated
- 1 garlic clove, minced
- Ground black pepper, as required

Direction: Preparation Time: 15 minutes Cooking Time: 35 minutes Servings: 6

- ✓ In a large pan, add the amaranth, quinoa, wild rice, water and spices over medium-high heat and bring to a boil.
- ✓ Now, reduce the heat to medium-low and simmer, covered for about 20-25 minutes.
- ✓ Stir in remaining ingredients and simmer for about 3-5 minutes. Serve hot.

Meal Prep Tip:

- ✓ Transfer the grains mixture into a large bowl and set aside to cool. Divide the mixture into 6 containers evenly.
- ✓ Cover the containers and refrigerate for 1 day. Reheat in the microwave before serving.

Nutrition: Calories 365 Total Fat 5.6 g Saturated Fat 0.6 g Cholesterol 0 mg Total Carbs 64 g Sugar 5.8 g Fiber 12 g Sodium 58 mg Potassium 686 mg Protein 16.4 g

389)   *Baked Beans*

Ingredients:

- ¼ pound dry lima beans, soaked overnight and drained
- ¼ pound dry red kidney beans, soaked overnight and drained
- 1¼ tablespoons oive oil 1 small onion, chopped
- 4 garlic cloves, minced 1 teaspoon dried thyme, crushed
- ½ teaspoon ground cumin
- ½ teaspoon red pepper flakes, crushed
- ¼ teaspoon paprika
- 1 tablespoon balsamic vinegar
- 1 cup homemade tomato puree
- 1 cup low-sodium vegetable broth
- Ground black pepper, as required
- 2 tablespoons fresh parsley, chopped

Direction: Preparation Time: 15 minutes Cooking Time: 2 hours 10 minutes Servings: 4

- ✓ In a large pan of the boiling water, add the beans over high heat and bring to a boil.
- ✓ Now, reduce the heat to low and simmer, covered for about 1 hour. Remove from the heat and drain the beans well.
- ✓ Preheat the oven to 325 degrees F. In a large ovenproof pan, heat the oil over medium heat and cook the onion for about 8-9 minutes, stirring frequently.
- ✓ Add the garlic, thyme and red spices and sauté for about 1 minute.
- ✓ Add the cooked beans and remaining ingredients and immediately remove from the heat.
- ✓ Cover the pan and transfer into the oven. Bake for about 1 hour. Serve with the garnishing of cilantro.

Meal Prep Tip:

- ✓ Transfer the beans mixture into a large bowl and set aside to cool. Divide the mixture into 4 containers evenly. Cover the containers and refrigerate for 1-2 days. Reheat in the microwave before serving.

Nutrition: Calories 136 Total Fat 4.3 g Saturated Fat 0.9 g Cholesterol 0 mg Total Carbs 19 g Sugar 4.7 g Fiber 4.6 g Sodium 112 mg Potassium 472 mg Protein 5.7 g Spicy

390)   *Grains Combo Black Beans*

Ingredients:

- 4 cups filtered water
- 1½ cups dried black beans, soaked for
- 8 hours and drained
- ½ teaspoon ground turmeric
- 3 tablespoons olive oil
- 1 small onion, chopped finely
- 1 green chili, chopped
- 1 (1-inch) piece fresh ginger, minced
- 2 garlic cloves, minced
- 1-1½ tablespoons ground coriander
- 1 teaspoon ground cumin
- ½ teaspoon cayenne pepper Sea salt, as required
- 2 medium tomatoes, chopped finely
- ½ cup fresh cilantro, chopped

Direction: Preparation Time: 15 minutes Cooking Time: 1½ hours Servings: 6

- ✓ In a large pan, add water, black beans and turmeric and bring to a boil on high heat.
- ✓ Now, reduce the heat to low and simmer, covered for about 1 hour or till desired doneness of beans. Meanwhile, in a skillet, heat the oil over medium

heat and sauté the onion for about 4-5 minutes.

✓ Add the green chili, ginger, garlic, spices and salt and sauté for about 1-2 minutes. Stir in the tomatoes and cook for about 10 minutes, stirring occasionally.

✓ Transfer the tomato mixture into the pan with black beans and stir to combine.

✓ Increase the heat to medium-low and simmer for about 15-20 minutes. Stir in the cilantro and simmer for about 5 minutes.

✓ Serve hot.

Meal Prep Tip:

✓ Transfer the beans mixture into a large bowl and set aside to cool. Divide the mixture into 6 containers evenly. Cover the containers and refrigerate for 1-2 days. Reheat in the microwave before serving.

Nutrition: Calories 160 Total Fat 8 g Saturated Fat 1 g Cholesterol 0 mg Total Carbs 17.9 g Sugar 2.4 g Fiber 6.2 g Sodium 50 mg Potassium 343 mg Protein 6 g

391)   *Lentils Chili*

Ingredients:

- 2 teaspoons olive oil
- 1 large onion, chopped 3 medium carrot, peeled and chopped
- 4 celery stalks, chopped 2 garlic cloves, minced
- 1 jalapeño pepper, seeded and chopped
- ½ tablespoon dried thyme, crushed 1 tablespoon chipotle chili powder
- ½ tablespoon cayenne pepper
- 1½ tablespoons ground coriander
- 1½ tablespoons ground cumin 1 teaspoon ground turmeric
- Ground black pepper, as required
- 1 tomato, chopped finely
- 1 pound lentils, rinsed
- 8 cups low-sodium vegetable broth
- 6 cups fresh spinach
- ½ cup fresh cilantro, chopped

Direction: Preparation Time: 15 minutes Cooking Time: 2 hours 20 minutes Servings: 8

✓ : In a large pan, heat the oil over medium heat and sauté the onion, carrot and celery for about 5 minutes.

✓ Add the garlic, jalapeño pepper, thyme and spices and sauté for about 1 minute.

✓ Add the tomato paste, lentils and broth and bring to a boil.

✓ Now, reduce the heat to low and simmer for about 2 hours.

✓ Stir in the spinach and simmer for about 3-5 minutes. Stir in cilantro and remove from the heat.

✓ Serve hot.

Meal Prep Tip:

✓ Transfer the chili into a large bowl and set aside to cool. Divide the chili into 8 containers evenly.

✓ Cover the containers and refrigerate for 1-2 days. Reheat in the microwave before serving.

Nutrition: Calories 259 Total Fat 2.3 g Saturated Fat 0.3 g Cholesterol 0 mg Total Carbs 41 g Sugar 3.6 g Fiber 19 g Sodium 118 mg Potassium 856 mg Protein 18.2 g

392)   *Quinoa in Tomato*

Ingredients:

- 2 tablespoons olive oil
- 1 cup quinoa, rinsed
- 1 green bell pepper, seeded and chopped
- 1 medium onion, chopped finely
- 3 garlic cloves, minced
- 2½ cups filtered water
- 2 cups tomatoes, crushed finely
- 1 teaspoon red chili powder
- ¼ teaspoon ground cumin
- ¼ teaspoon garlic powder
- Ground black pepper, as required

Direction: Sauce Preparation Time: 15 minutes Cooking Time: 40 minutes Servings: 4

✓ In a large pan, heat the oil over medium-high heat and cook the quinoa, onion, bell pepper and garlic for about 5 minutes, stirring frequently.

✓ Stir in the remaining ingredients and bring to a boil.

✓ Now, reduce the heat to medium-low. ✓ Cover the pan tightly and simmer for about 30 minutes, stirring occasionally. Serve hot.

Meal Prep Tip:

✓ Transfer the quinoa mixture into a large bowl and set aside to cool.

✓ Divide the chili into 4 containers evenly.

✓ Cover the containers and refrigerate for 1-2 days. Reheat in the microwave before serving.

Nutrition: Calories 260 Total Fat 10 g Saturated Fat 1.4 g Cholesterol 0 mg Total Carbs 36.9 g Sugar 5.2 g Fiber 5.4 g Sodium 16 mg Potassium 575 mg Protein 7.7 g

393)   *Barley Pilaf*

Ingredients:

- ½ cup pearl barley
- 1 cup low-sodium vegetable broth

- 2 tablespoons olive oil, divided
- 2 garlic cloves, minced finely
- ½ cup onion, chopped
- ½ cup eggplant, sliced thinly
- ½ cup green bell pepper, seeded and chopped
- ½ cup red bell pepper, seeded and chopped
- 2 tablespoons fresh cilantro, chopped
- 2 tablespoons fresh mint leaves, chopped

Direction: Preparation Time: 20 minutes Cooking Time: 1 hour 5 minutes Servings: 4

- ✓ In a pan, add the barley and broth over medium-high heat and bring to a boil. Immediately, reduce the heat to low and simmer, covered for about 45 minutes or until all the liquid is absorbed. In a large skillet, heat 1 tablespoon of oil over high heat and sauté the garlic for about 1 minute.
- ✓ Stir in the cooked barley and cook for about 3 minutes. Remove from heat and set aside. In another skillet, heat remaining oil over medium heat and sauté the onion for about 5-7 minutes.
- ✓ Add the eggplant and bell peppers and stir fry for about 3 minutes. Stir in the remaining ingredients except walnuts and cook for about 2-3 minutes. Stir in barley mixture and cook for about 2-3 minutes.
- ✓ Serve hot.

Meal Prep Tip:

- ✓ Transfer the pilaf into a large bowl and set aside to cool. Divide the pilaf into 4 containers evenly. Cover the containers and refrigerate for 1 day. Reheat in the microwave before serving.

Nutrition: Calories 168 Total Fat 7.4 g Saturated Fat 1.1 g Cholesterol 0 mg Total Carbs 23.5 g Sugar 1.9 g Fiber 5 g Sodium 22 mg Potassium 164 mg Protein 3.6 g

394) *Baked Veggies Combo*

Ingredients:

- 2 large zucchinis, sliced
- 1 large yellow squash, sliced
- 3 cups fresh broccoli florets
- 1-pound fresh asparagus, trimmed
- 2 garlic cloves, minced
- 1 tablespoon fresh rosemary, minced
- 1 tablespoon fresh thyme, minced
- ½ teaspoon ground cumin
- ½ teaspoon red pepper flakes, crushed
- ¼ teaspoon cayenne pepper
- 2 tablespoons olive oil
- Salt, as required

Direction: Preparation Time: 15 minutes Cooking

Time: 40 minutes Servings: 8

- ✓ Preheat the oven to 400 degrees F. Line 2 large baking sheets with aluminum foil. In a large bowl, add all ingredients and toss to coat well.
- ✓ Divide the vegetables mixture onto prepared baking sheets and spread in a single layer.
- ✓ Roast for about 35-40 minutes. Remove from oven and serve.

Meal Prep Tip:

- ✓ Remove from oven and set the veggies aside to cool completely.
- ✓ Transfer the veggie mixture into 8 containers and refrigerate for 2-3 days.
- ✓ Reheat in microwave before serving.

Nutrition: Calories 77 Total Fat 4 g Saturated Fat 0.6 g Cholesterol 0 mg Total Carbs 9.4 g Sugar 3.8 g Fiber 3.8 g Sodium 45 mg Potassium 554 mg Protein 3.8 g

395) *Mixed Veggie Salad*

Ingredients:

For Dressing:

- 1/3 cup olive oil ½ cup fresh lemon juice
- 1 tablespoon fresh ginger, grated
- 2 teaspoons mustard 4-6 drops liquid stevia
- ¼ teaspoon salt

For Salad:

- 2 avocados, peeled, pitted and chopped
- 2 tablespoons fresh lemon juice
- 2 cups fresh baby spinach, torn
- 2 cups small broccoli florets
- 1 cup red cabbage, shredded
- 1 cup purple cabbage, shredded
- 2 large carrots, peeled and grated
- 1 small orange bell pepper, seeded and sliced into matchsticks
- 1 small yellow bell pepper, seeded and sliced into matchsticks
- ½ cup fresh parsley leaves, chopped
- 1 cup walnuts, chopped

Direction: Preparation Time: 20 minutes Servings: 8

- ✓ For dressing: in a food processor, add all ingredients and pulse until well combined. In a large bowl, add the avocado slices and drizzle with lemon juice.
- ✓ Add the remaining vegetables and mix. Place the dressing and toss to coat well.
- ✓ Serve immediately.

Meal Prep Tip:

✓ Transfer dressing into a small jar and refrigerate for 1 day. In 8 containers, divide avocado and remaining vegetables.

✓ Refrigerate for 1 day. Before serving, drizzle each portion with dressing and serve.

Nutrition: Calories 314 Total Fat 28.1 g Saturated Fat 4 g Cholesterol 0 mg Total Carbs 14.1 g Sugar 4.3g Fiber 6.9 g Sodium 113 mg Potassium 642 mg Protein 6.8 g

396) *Tofu with Brussels Sprout*

Ingredients:

- 1 tablespoon olive oil, divided
- 8 ounces extra-firm tofu, drained, pressed and cut into slices
- 2 garlic cloves, chopped
- 1/3 cup pecans, toasted and chopped
- 1 tablespoon unsweetened applesauce
- ¼ cup fresh cilantro, chopped
- ¾ pound Brussels sprouts, trimmed and cut into wide ribbons

Direction: Preparation Time: 15 minutes Cooking Time: 15 minutes Servings: 4

✓ In a skillet, heat ½ tablespoon of the oil over medium heat and sauté the tofu and for about 6-7 minutes or until golden brown.

✓ Add the garlic and pecans and sauté for about 1 minute. Add the applesauce and cook for about 2 minutes.

✓ Stir in the cilantro and remove from heat. Transfer tofu into a plate and set aside In the same skillet, heat the remaining oil over medium-high heat and cook the Brussels sprouts for about 5 minutes.

✓ Stir in the tofu and remove from the heat. Serve immediately.

Meal Prep Tip:

✓ Remove the tofu mixture from heat and set aside to cool completely.

✓ In 4 containers, divide the tofu mixture evenly and refrigerate for about 2 days. Reheat in microwave before serving.

Nutrition: Calories 204 Total Fat 15.5 g Saturated Fat 1.8 g Cholesterol 0 mg Total Carbs 11.5 g Sugar 3 g Fiber 4.8 g Sodium 27 mg Potassium 468 mg Protein 9.9 g

397) *Beans, Walnuts & Veggie Burgers*

Ingredients:

- ½ cup walnuts
- 1 carrot, peeled and chopped
- 1 celery stalk, chopped
- 4 scallions, chopped
- 5 garlic cloves, chopped
- 2¼ cups cooked black beans
- 2½ cups sweet potato, peeled and grated
- ½ teaspoon red pepper flakes, crushed
- ¼ teaspoon cayenne pepper
- Salt and ground black pepper, as required

Direction: Preparation Time: 20 minutes Cooking Time: 25 minutes Servings: 8

✓ Preheat the oven to 400 degrees F. Line a baking sheet with parchment paper. In a food processor, add walnuts and pulse until finely ground. Add the carrot, celery, scallion and garlic and pulse until chopped finely.

✓ Transfer the vegetable mixture into a large bowl. In the same food processor, add beans and pulse until chopped. Add 1½ cups of sweet potato and pulse until a chunky mixture forms.

✓ Transfer the bean mixture into the bowl with vegetable mixture. Stir in the remaining sweet potato and spices and mix until well combined.

✓ Make 8 patties from mixture. Arrange the patties onto prepared baking sheet in a single layer. Bake for about 25 minutes. Serve hot.

Meal Prep Tip:

✓ Remove the burgers from oven and set aside to cool completely. Store these burgers in an airtight container, by placing parchment papers between the burgers to avoid the sticking.

✓ These burgers can be stored in the freezer for up to 3 weeks. Before serving, thaw the burgers and then reheat in microwave.

Nutrition: Calories 177 Total Fat 5 g Saturated Fat 0.3 g Cholesterol 0 mg Total Carbs 27.6 g Sugar 5.3 g Fiber 7.6 g Sodium 205 mg Potassium 398 mg Protein 8 g

DIABETIC AIR FRYER RECIPES

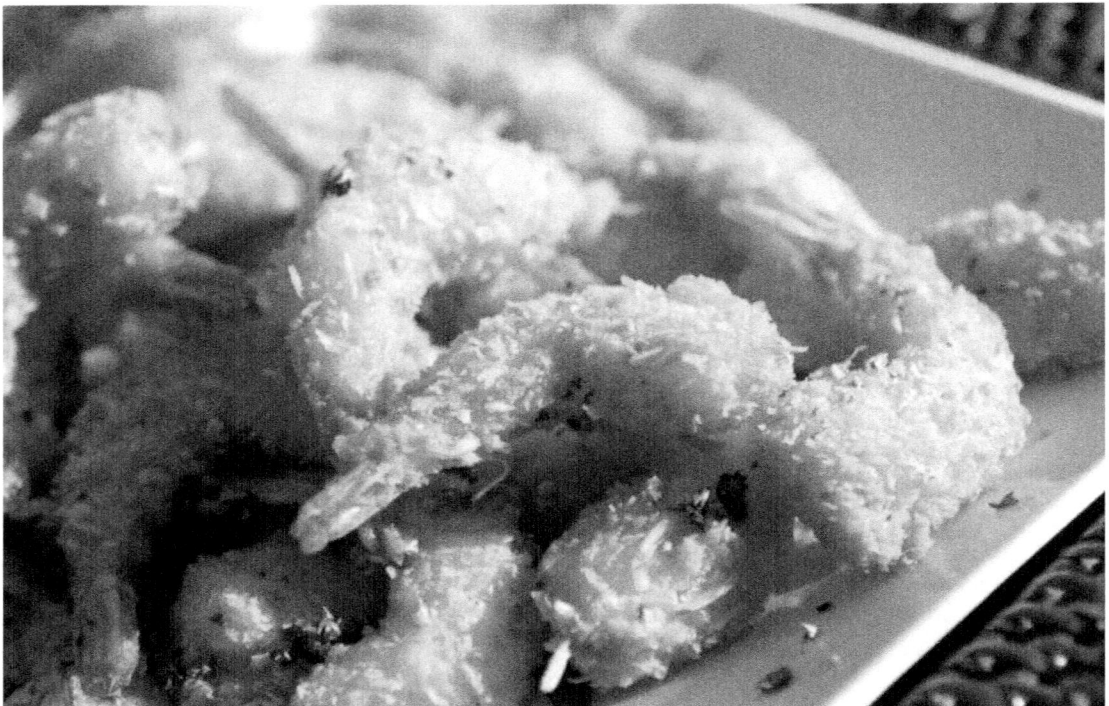

398) *Air-Fried Hot Wings*
Ingredients:
- (4 Servings)
- ¼ tsp celery salt
- ¼ tsp bay leaf powder
- Black pepper to taste
- ½ tsp cayenne pepper
- ¼ tsp allspice
- 1 tbsp thyme leaves
- 1 lb chicken wings

Direction:(Prep + Cook Time: 25 minutes)
- ✓ Preheat the air fryer to 360 F.
- ✓ In a bowl, mix celery salt, bay leaf powder, black pepper, paprika, thyme, cayenne pepper, and allspice.
- ✓ Coat the wings in the mixture.
- ✓ Arrange the wings on the greased frying basket and AirFry for 10 minutes.
- ✓ Flip and cook for 6-8 more minutes until crispy on the outside.

nutritional value: Calories 226.7 Total Fat 10.7 g Saturated Fat 3.7 g cholesterol 153.7 mg Total Carbs 14.2 g Dietary Fiber 0.6 g Sugar 4.6 g Protein 19.2 g % Copper 0.8 %

398) *Crispy Alfredo Chicken Wings*
Ingredients:
- (4 Servings)
- 1 ½ lb chicken wings, pat-dried
- Salt to taste
- ½ cup Alfredo sauce

Direction: (Prep + Cook Time: 25 minutes
- ✓ Preheat the air fryer to 370 F.
- ✓ Season the wings with salt.
- ✓ Arrange them in the greased frying basket, without overlapping, and AirFry for 12 minutes until no longer pink in the center Flip them, increase the heat to 390 F, and cook for 5 more minutes.
- ✓ Work in batches if needed.
- ✓ Plate the wings and drizzle with Alfredo sauce to serve.

nutritional value: Calories: 225 Net Carbs: 1g Carbs: 1g Fat : 17g Protein : 16g Fiber : 0g

399) *Crunchy Ranch Chicken Wings*
Ingredients:
- (4 Servings)
- 2 lb chicken wings
- 2 tbsp olive oil
- 1 tbsp ranch
- seasoning mix
- Salt to taste

Direction:(Prep + Cook Time: 25 minutes)
- ✓ Preheat the air fryer to 390 F.
- ✓ Put the ranch seasoning, olive oil, and salt in a large, resealable bag and mix well.

- ✓ Add the wings, seal the bag, and toss until the wings are thoroughly coated.
- ✓ Put the wings in the greased frying basket in one layer, spritz them with a nonstick cooking spray, and AirFry for 7 minutes.
- ✓ Turn them over and fry for 5-8 more minutes until the wings are light brown and crispy.
- ✓ Test for doneness with a meat thermometer.
- ✓ Serve with your favorite dipping sauce and enjoy!

nutritional value: Calories 774.37 Kcal Calories from Fat 513.56 Kcal Total Fat 57.06g cholesterol 245.06 mg Total Carbs 23.87g Sugar 5.7g Dietary Fiber 3.34g Protein 40.89g g 7 mg

400) *Korean Chili Chicken Wings*
Ingredients:
- (4 Servings)
- 8 chicken wings
- Salt to taste
- 1 tsp sesame oil
- Juice from half lemon
- ¼ cup sriracha chili sauce
- 1-inch piece ginger, grated
- 1 tsp garlic powder
- 1 tsp sesame seeds

Direction:(Prep + Cook Time: 20 minutes)
- ✓ Preheat the air fryer to 370 F.
- ✓ Grease the air frying basket with cooking spray. In a bowl, mix salt, ginger, garlic, lemon juice, sesame oil, and chili sauce.
- ✓ Coat the wings in thedTransfer the wings to the basket and AirFry for 15 minutes, flipping once.
- ✓ Sprinkle with sesame seeds and serve.

nutritional value: Calories 143 Total Fat 8.3g Saturated Fat 1.1g Trans Fat 0.1g cholesterol 38 mg g Total Carbs 8.8g Dietary Fiber 0.4g Sugar 4.6g Protein 7.7g

401) *Teriyaki Chicken Wings*
Ingredients:
- (4 Servings)
- 1 lb chicken wings
- 1 cup soy sauce.
- ½ cup brown Sugar
- ½ cup apple cider vinegar
- 2 tbsp fresh ginger,
- minced
- 1 garlic clove,
- minced
- Black pepper to taste
- 2 tbsp cornstarch
- 2 tbsp cold Water
- 1 tsp sesame seeds

Direction(Prep + Cook Time: 20 minutes)
- ✓ In a bowl, add the chicken wings and cover with half a cup of soy sauce.

- ✓ Refrigerate for 20 minutes.
- ✓ Drain and pat dry.
- ✓ Arrange them on the greased frying basket and AirFry for 14 minutes at 380 F, turning once halfway through cooking.
- ✓ In a skillet over medium heat, stir the Sugar , remaining soy sauce, vinegar, ginger, garlic, and black pepper, for 4 minutes.
- ✓ Dissolve 2 tbsp of cornstarch in cold Water and stir in the sauce until it thickens, about 2 minutes.
- ✓ Pour the sauce over the wings and sprinkle with sesame seeds.
- ✓ Serve hot.

nutritional value: Calories 699 Total Fat 53.4g Sat. Fat 10.5g Trans Fat 0g cholesterol 150.1 mg g Tot. Carb. 14.8g Dietary Fiber 0g Sugar 6.7g Protein 44.1g

402) *Chicken Wings with Gorgonzola Dip*

Ingredients:

- (4 Servings)
- 8 chicken wings
- 1 tsp cayenne pepper
- Salt to taste
- 2 tbsp olive oil
- 1 tsp red chili flakes
- 1 cup heavy cream
- 3 oz gorgonzola cheese, crumbled
- ½ lemon, juiced
- ½ tsp garlic powder

Direction:(Prep + Cook Time: 30 minutes)

- ✓ Preheat the air fryer to 380 F.
- ✓ Coat the wings with cayenne pepper, salt, and olive oil.
- ✓ Place in the fryer and AirFry for 16 minutes until crispy and golden brown, flipping once.
- ✓ In a bowl, mix heavy cream, gorgonzola cheese, chili flakes, lemon juice, and garlic powder.
- ✓ Serve the wings with the cheese dip.

nutritional value: Calories 78 Total Fat 6.7g Saturated Fat 1.4g Trans Fat 0g cholesterol 17 mg Total Carbs 0g Dietary Fiber 0g Total Sugar 0g Protein 4g

403) *Piri Piri Chicken Wings*

Ingredients:

- (2 Servings)
- 8 chicken wings
- Salt and black pepper to taste
- 1 tsp smoked paprika
- 1 tbsp lemon juice
- ½ tsp ground ginger
- ½ tsp red chili powder
- 1 tsp ground cumin
- 1 cup mayonnaise mixed with

Direction:(Prep + Cook Time: 25 minutes)

- ✓ Preheat the air fryer to 380 F.
- ✓ In a bowl, mix paprika, ginger, chili powder, cumin, salt, and pepper.
- ✓ Add the chicken wings and toss to coat.
- ✓ Place in the greased frying basket and AirFry for 16-18 minutes, flipping once halfway through.
- ✓ Let cool for a few minutes. Serve with lemon mayonnaise.

nutritional value: Calories 598 Total Fat 35.4g Saturated Fat 10.4g arbohydrates 0g Net carbs 0g Fiber 0g Protein 69.8g

404) *Air-Fried Chicken Thighs*

Ingredients:

- (4 Servings)
- 1 ½ lb chicken thighs
- 2 eggs, lightly beaten
- 1 cup seasoned breadcrumbs
- ½ tsp oregano
- Salt and black pepper to taste

Direction:(Prep + Cook Time: 20 minutes)

- ✓ Preheat the air fryer to 390 F.
- ✓ Season the thighs with oregano, salt, and black pepper.
- ✓ In a bowl, add the beaten eggs.
- ✓ In a separate bowl, add the breadcrumbs Dip the thighs in the egg wash. Then roll them in the breadcrumbs and press firmly, so the breadcrumbs stick well.
- ✓ Spray the thighs with cooking spray and arrange them in the frying basket in a single layer, skin-side up.
- ✓ AirFry for 12 minutes, turn the thighs over, and cook for 6-8 more minutes until crispy.
- ✓ Serve and enjoy!

nutritional value: Calories 243 Total Fat 16g Saturated Fat 5g cholesterol 145 mg Total Carbs 0.2g Dietary Fiber 0g Sugar s0.0g Protein 27g

405) *Mustard-Honey Chicken Thighs*

Ingredients:

- (4 Servings)
- 1 lb chicken thighs
- Salt and garlic powder to taste
- 2 tbsp olive oil
- 1 tsp yellow mustard
- 1 tsp honey
- ¼ cup mayo mixed with
- 2 tbsp hot sauce

Direction:(Prep + Cook Time: 30 minutes)

- ✓ Preheat the air fryer to 360 F.
- ✓ In a bowl, whisk the olive oil, honey, mustard, salt, and garlic powder.
- ✓ Add the thighs and stir to coat.
- ✓ Marinate for 10 minutes.
- ✓ Transfer the thighs to the greased frying basket, skin side down, and insert in the air fryer.

✓ AirFry for 18-20 minutes, flipping once until golden and crispy.

✓ Serve immediately with the hot mayo sauce. Enjoy!

nutritional value: Calories 163 Total Fat 2.6g Saturated Fat 0.6g *Trans Fat* 0g cholesterol 49 mg g Total Carbs 17g Dietary Fiber 0.7g Sugar 16g Protein 19g

406)   *Crispy Chicken Nuggets*
Ingredients:

- (4 Servings)
- 1 lb chicken breasts, cut into large cubes
- Salt and black pepper to taste
- 2 tbsp olive oil
- 5 tbsp plain breadcrumbs
- 2 tbsp panko breadcrumbs
- 2 tbsp grated Parmesan cheese

Direction:(Prep + Cook Time: 25 minutes)

✓ Preheat the air fryer to 380 F.

✓ Season the chicken with black pepper and salt.

✓ In a bowl, mix the breadcrumbs and Parmesan cheese.

✓ Coat the chicken pieces with the olive oil. Then dip into the breadcrumb mixture, shake off the excess, and place in the greased frying basket.

✓ Lightly spray the nuggets with cooking spray and AirFry for 13-15 minutes, flipping once.

✓ Serve warm

nutritional value: Calories 187.5 Total Fat 2.6 g Saturated Fat 0.6 g g cholesterol 66.0 Total Carbs 12.6 g Dietary Fiber 0.4 g Sugar 1.6 g Protein 27.3 g

407)   *Paprika Chicken Fingers*
Ingredients:

- (4 Servings)
- 2 chicken breasts, cut into chunks
- 1 tsp paprika
- 2 tbsp milk
- 2 eggs 1 tsp garlic powder
- Salt and black pepper to taste
- 1 cup flour
- 2 cups breadcrumbs

Direction:(Prep + Cook Time: 20 minutes + cooling time)

✓ Preheat the air fryer to 370 F.

✓ In a bowl, mix paprika, garlic powder, salt, pepper, flour, and breadcrumbs.

✓ In another bowl, beat eggs with milk.

✓ Dip the chicken in the egg mixture, then roll in the crumbs.

✓ Place in the frying basket and spray with cooking spray.

✓ AirFry for 14-16 minutes, flipping once. Yummy!

nutritional value: Calories 650 Total Fat 49g Saturated Fat 10g Trans Fat 0g cholesterol 125 mg g Total Carbs 14g Total Carbs 14g Dietary Fiber 5g Total Sugar 5g Protein 40g g

408)   *Corn-Crusted Chicken Tenders*
Ingredients:

- (4 Servings)
- 2 chicken breasts, cut into strips
- Salt and black pepper to taste
- 2 eggs
- 1 cup ground cornmeal

Direction:(Prep + Cook Time: 25 minutes)

✓ Preheat the air fryer to 390 F.

✓ In a bowl, mix cornmeal, salt, and black pepper.

✓ In another bowl, beat the eggs; season with salt and pepper.

✓ Dip the chicken in the eggs and then coat in the cornmeal.

✓ Spray the strips with cooking spray and place them in the frying basket in a single layer.

✓ AirFry for 6 minutes, slide the basket out, and flip the sticks.

✓ Cook for 6-8 more minutes until golden brown.

✓ Serve hot.

nutritional value: Calories 368 Total Fat 15g Saturated Fat 5.9g *Trans Fat* 0.2g cholesterol 99 mg g Total Carbs 34g Dietary Fiber 1.3g Sugar 2.4g Protein 24g

409)   *Chicken & Oat Croquettes*
Ingredients:

- (4 Servings)
- 1 lb ground chicken
- 2 eggs
- Salt and black pepper to taste
- 1 cup oats, crumbled
- ½ tsp garlic powder
- 1 tsp dried parsley

Direction:(Prep + Cook Time: 20 minutes)

✓ Preheat the air fryer to 360 F.

✓ Mix the chicken with garlic, parsley, salt, and pepper.

✓ In a bowl, beat the eggs with a pinch of salt.

✓ In a third bowl, add the oats.

✓ Form croquettes out of the chicken mixture.

✓ Dip in the eggs and coat in the oats.

✓ AirFry them in the greased frying basket for 10 minutes, shaking once.

nutritional value: Calories 173.6 Total Fat 4.4 g Saturated Fat 1.7 g g cholesterol 89.1 8 mg Total Carbs 9.2 g Dietary Fiber 0.6 g Sugar 1.7 g Protein 23.8 g

410)   *Crunchy Chicken Egg Rolls*
Ingredients:

- (4 Servings)
- 2 tsp olive oil
- 2 garlic cloves, minced
- ¼ cup soy sauce
- 1 tsp grated fresh ginger
- 1 lb ground chicken

- 2 cups white cabbage, shredded
- 1 onion, chopped
- 1 egg, beaten
- 8 egg roll wrappers

Direction:(Prep + Cook Time: 30 minutes)

✓ Heat olive oil in a pan over medium heat and add garlic, onion, ginger, and ground chicken.

✓ Sauté for 5 minutes until the chicken is no longer pink.

✓ Pour in the soy sauce and shredded cabbage and stir-fry for another 5-6 minutes until the cabbage is tender.

✓ Remove from the heat and let cool slightly.

✓ Fill each egg wrapper with the mixture, arranging it just below the center of the wrappers Fold in both sides and roll up tightly.

✓ Use the beaten egg to seal the edges.

✓ Brush the tops with the remaining beaten egg.

✓ Place the rolls in the greased frying basket, spray them with cooking spray, and AirFry for 12-14 minutes at 370 F until golden, turning once halfway through.

✓ Let cool slightly and serve.

nutritional: Calories 160.1 Total Fat 4g Saturated Fat 1 1 mg Carbs 24g Net carbs 22g Sugar 7g Fiber 2g Protein 6g

411)   *Asian Veggie Spring Rolls*

Ingredients:

- (4 Servings)
- 4 spring roll wrappers
- ½ cup cooked vermicelli noodles
- 1 garlic clove, minced
- 1 tbsp fresh ginger, minced
- 1 tbsp soy sauce
- 2 tsp sesame oil
- ½ red bell pepper, seeds removed, chopped
- ½ cup mushrooms, finely chopped
- ½ cup carrots, finely chopped
- ¼ cup scallions, finely chopped

Direction:(Prep + Cook Time: 30 minutes)

✓ Warm sesame oil in a saucepan over medium heat and add garlic, ginger, soy sauce, bell pepper, mushrooms, carrots, and scallions and stir-fry for 5 minutes.

✓ Stir in vermicelli noodles and set aside.

✓ Place the wrappers onto a working board.

✓ Spoon the veggie-noodle mixture at the center of the roll wrappers.

✓ Roll and tuck in the corners and edges to create neat and secure rolls.

✓ Spray with oil and place them in the frying basket.

✓ AirFry for 12-14 minutes at 340 F, turning once or twice until golden.

nutritional value: Calories 210 Total Fat 7g Saturated Fat 2.5g Carbs 33g Net carbs 31g Fiber 2g Glucose 4g Protein 4g

412)   *Herby Meatballs*

Ingredients:

- (4 Servings)
- 1 lb ground beef
- 1 onion, finely chopped
- 2 garlic cloves, finely chopped
- 1 egg
- 1 cup breadcrumbs
- ½ cup Mediterranean herbs
- Salt and black pepper to taste
- 1 tbsp olive oil.

Direction:(Prep + Cook Time: 30 minutes)

✓ In a bowl, add the ground beef, onion, garlic, egg, breadcrumbs, herbs, salt, and pepper and mix with your hands to combine.

✓ Shape into balls and brush them with olive oil.

✓ Arrange the meatballs in the frying basket and AirFry for 15-16 minutes at 380 F, turning once halfway through.

✓ Serve immediately.

nutritional value: Cals 185 Fat 11.20g Saturated Fat 4.900g Carbs 1.30g Sugar 0.20g Fiber 0.1g Protein 19.60g Salt1.50g

413)   *Chili Cheese Balls*

Ingredients:

- (4 Servings)
- 2 cups cottage cheese, crumbled
- 2 cups Parmesan cheese, grated
- 2 red potatoes, boiled and mashed
- 1 medium onion, finely chopped
- 1 ½ tsp red chili flakes
- 1 green chili, finely chopped
- Salt to taste
- 2 tbsp fresh cilantro, chopped
- 1 cup flour
- 1 cup breadcrumbs

Direction:(Prep + Cook Time: 25 minutes)

✓ In a bowl, combine the cottage and Parmesan cheeses, onion, chili flakes, green chili, salt, cilantro, flour, and mashed potatoes.

✓ Mold balls out of the mixture and roll them in breadcrumbs.

✓ Place them in the greased frying basket and AirFry for 14-16 minutes at 350 F, shaking once or twice.

✓ Serve warm.

nutritional value: Calories 372.25 Kcal Total Fat 29.76g cholesterol 91.85 mg 6 mg 14 mg Total Carbs 3.39g Sugar 1.66g Dietary Fiber 1.1g Protein 23.04g g 3 mg

414)   *Cheesy Sticks with Sweet Thai Sauce*

Ingredients:

- (4 Servings)

- 12 sticks mozzarella cheese
- 2 cups breadcrumbs
- 3 eggs
- 1 cup sweet Thai sauce
- 4 tbsp skimmed milk.

Direction:(Prep + Cook Time: 25 minutes)
- ✓ Pour the breadcrumbs into a bowl.
- ✓ Beat the eggs with milk in another bowl.
- ✓ One after the other, dip the sticks in the egg mixture, in the crumbs, then in the egg mixture again, and lastly in the crumbs again.
- ✓ Freeze for 1 hour.
- ✓ Preheat the air fryer to 380 F.
- ✓ Arrange the sticks in the greased frying basket and AirFry for 10-12 minutes, flipping halfway through. Work in batches.
- ✓ Serve with sweet Thai sauce.

nutritional value: Calories 311 Total Fat 18.3g Saturated Fat 4g Trans Fat 0g cholesterol 53.3 mg mg Total Carbs 17g Dietary Fiber 0.4g Sugar 0g Protein 19.3g

415)   *Potato Chips with Chives*
Ingredients:
- (4 Servings)
- 1 lb potatoes, cut into thin slices
- ¼ cup olive oil
- 1 tbsp garlic paste
- 2 tbsp chives, chopped A
- pinch of salt

Direction:(Prep + Cook Time: 40 minutes)
- ✓ Preheat the air fryer to 390 F.
- ✓ In a bowl, add olive oil, garlic paste, and salt and mix to obtain a marinade.
- ✓ Add the potatoes and let them sit for 30 minutes. Lay the potato slices into the frying basket and AirFry for 20 minutes.
- ✓ At the 10-minute mark, give the chips a turn and sprinkle with freshly chopped chives.

nutritional value: Calories 218 Total Fat 14g Saturated Fat 1.3g Total Carbs 21g Sugar 1g Protein 2.8g

416)   *Quick Pickle Chips*
Ingredients:
- (4 Servings)
- 36 sweet pickle chips, drained 1 cup flour
- ¼ cup cornmeal

Direction:(Prep + Cook Time: 15 minutes)
- ✓ Preheat the air fryer to 400 F.
- ✓ In a bowl, mix flour, cayenne pepper, and cornmeal Dip the pickles in the flour mixture and spritz with cooking spray.
- ✓ AirFry for 10 minutes until golden brown, turning once.

nutritional value: Calories 20.0 Total Fat 0.1 g Saturated Fat 0.0 g g cholesterol 0.0 1 mg Total Carbs 5.8 g Dietary Fiber 0.5 g Sugar 3.7 g Protein 0.5 g %

Copper 2.1 Manganese 9.0 % Niacin 0.7 %

417)   *Garlicky Potato Chips with Herbs*
Ingredients:
- (2 Servings)
- 2 potatoes, thinly sliced
- 1 tbsp olive oil
- 1 garlic cloves, crushed
- 1 tsp each of fresh rosemary, thyme, oregano, chopped
- Salt and black pepper to taste

Direction:(Prep + Cook Time: 40 minutes)
- ✓ In a bowl, mix olive oil, garlic, herbs, salt, and pepper.
- ✓ Coat the potatoes thoroughly in the mixture.
- ✓ Arrange them in the frying basket and AirFry for 18-20 minutes at 360 F, shaking every 4-5 minutes

nutritional value: Calories140 Total Fat 8g Saturated Fat 1g *Trans Fat* 0g cholesterol 0 mg Total Carbs 17g Dietary Fiber 2g Sugar 4g

418)   *Hot Carrot Crisps*
Ingredients:
- (2 Servings)
- 2 large carrots, cut into strips
- ½ tsp oregano
- ½ tsp hot paprika
- ½ tsp garlic powder
- 1 tbsp olive oil
- Salt to taste

Direction:(Prep + Cook Time: 25 minutes)
- ✓ Put the carrots in a bowl and stir in the remaining ingredients; toss to coat Arrange the carrots in the greased frying basket and AirFry for 13-15 minutes at 390 F, shaking once.
- ✓ Serve warm.

nutritional value: 71 Calories, 1 g Fat , 0 g Saturated Fat , 0 mg cholesterol, 213 mg Carbohydrate, 5 g Fiber , 7 g Sugar , 2 g Protein

419)   *Root Vegetable Chips*
Ingredients:
- 4 Servings)
- 1 carrot, sliced
- 1 parsnip, sliced
- 1 potato, sliced
- 1 daikon, sliced
- 2 tbsp olive oil
- 1 tbsp soy sauce

Direction:(Prep + Cook Time: 25 minutes)
- ✓ Preheat the air fryer to 400 F.
- ✓ In a bowl, mix olive oil and soy sauce.
- ✓ Add in the veggies and toss to coat; marinate for 5 minutes.
- ✓ Transfer them to the fryer and AirFry for 15 minutes, tossing once

nutritional: Cal 150 Total Fat 8g cholesterol 0 mg Total Carbs 17g Dietary Fiber 2g Sugar 5g Protein 1g

420) *Mexican-Style Air Fryer Nachos*

Ingredients:

- (4 Servings)
- 8 corn tortillas, cut into wedges
- 1 tbsp olive oil
- ½ tsp ground cumin
- ½ tsp chili powder
- ½ tsp paprika
- ½ tsp cayenne pepper
- ½ tsp salt
- ½ tsp ground coriander

Direction:(Prep + Cook Time: 20 minutes)

- ✓ Preheat the air fryer to 370 F.
- ✓ Brush the tortilla wedges with olive oil and arrange them in the frying basket in an even layer.
- ✓ Mix the spices thoroughly in a small bowl.
- ✓ Sprinkle the tortilla wedges with the spice mixture. AirFry for 2-3 minutes, shake the basket, and fry for another 2-3 minutes until crunchy and nicely browned.
- ✓ Serve the nachos immediately.

nutritional value: Calories: 352kcal | Carbs : 41.7g | Protein : 11.9g | Fat : 16.5g | Saturated Fat : 4.7g | cholesterol: 12 mg | Fiber : 6.1g | Sugar : 1.6g |

421) *Crispy Hasselback Potatoes*

Ingredients:

- 4 Servings)
- 2 tbsp lard, melted
- 1 lb russet potatoes
- 1 tbsp olive oil
- Salt and black pepper to taste
- 1 garlic clove, crushed
- 1 tbsp fresh dill, chopped

Direction:(Prep + Cook Time: 25 minutes)

- ✓ Preheat the air fryer to 400 F.
- ✓ On the potatoes, make thin vertical slits, around 1/5 inch apart.
- ✓ Make sure to cut the potatoes 3/4-the way down so that they can hold together.
- ✓ Mix together the lard, olive oil, and garlic in a bowl Brush the potatoes with some of the mixtures.
- ✓ Season with salt and pepper and place them in the greased frying basket.
- ✓ AirFry for 25-30 minutes, brushing once halfway through so they don't dry during cooking, until golden and crispy around the edges.
- ✓ Sprinkle with dill. Serve and enjoy

nutritional value: Calories 218 Fat 9g Carbs 28g Fiber 4g Sugar 1g Protein 3g

422) *Sweet Potato Boats*

Ingredients:

- (4 Servings)
- 4 sweet potatoes, boiled and halved lengthwise
- 2 tbsp olive oil
- 1 shallot, chopped
- 1 cup canned mixed beans
- ¼ cup mozzarella cheese, grated
- Salt and black pepper to taste

Direction:(Prep + Cook Time: 25 minutes)

- ✓ Preheat the air fryer to 400 F.
- ✓ Grease the frying basket with olive oil.
- ✓ Scoop out the flesh from the potatoes, so shells are formed.
- ✓ Chop the potato flesh and put it in a bowl.
- ✓ Add in shallot, mixed beans, salt, and pepper; mix to combine.
- ✓ Fill the potato shells with the mixture and top with the cheese.
- ✓ Arrange on the basket and place inside the fryer.
- ✓ Bake for 10-12 minutes.

nutritional value: Calories: 173 Protein : 3 g Carbohydrate: 40 g Sugar : 8 g Total Fat : 0.2 g

423) *Thyme & Garlic Sweet Potato Wedges*

Ingredients:

- (2 Servings)
- ½ lb sweet potatoes, cut into wedges
- 1 tbsp coconut oil
- ¼ tsp chili powder
- v¼ tsp salt
- ¼ tsp garlic powder
- ¼ tsp smoked paprika
- ¼ tsp dried thyme
- ¼ tsp cayenne pepper

Direction:(Prep + Cook Time: 30 minutes)

- ✓ In a bowl, mix coconut oil, salt, chili and garlic powders, paprika, thyme, and cayenne pepper.
- ✓ Toss in the potato wedges. Arrange the wedges on the frying basket and AirFry for 23-25 minutes at 380 F, shaking a few times through cooking until golden.
- ✓ Serve and enjoy!

nutritional value: Calories 194 Fat 7g Saturated Fat 1g Carbs 31g Fiber 4g Sugar 6g Protein 2g g

424) *Prosciutto & Cheese Stromboli*

Ingredients:

- (4 Servings)
- 1 (13-oz) pizza crust
- 4 (1-oz) fontina cheese slices
- 8 slices prosciutto
- 12 cherry tomatoes, halved

- 4 fresh basil leaves, chopped
- ½ tsp dried oregano
- Salt and black pepper to taste

Direction:Prep + Cook Time: 30 minutes

✓ Roll out the pizza crust on a lightly floured work surface; slice into 4 squares.
✓ Top each one with a slice of fontina cheese, 2 slices of prosciutto, 3 halved cherry tomatoes, oregano, and basil.
✓ Season with salt and black pepper Close the rectangles by folding in half, press, and seal the edges with a fork.
✓ Spritz with cooking spray and transfer to the greased frying basket.
✓ Bake for 15 minutes, turning once.

nutritional value: Calories 1030 Total Fat 50g Saturated Fat 21g *Trans Fat* 0.5g cholesterol 170 mg Total Carbs 91g Dietary Fiber 5g Sugar 7g Protein 52g

425)   *Fava Bean Falafel Bites*
Ingredients:

- 4 Servings)
- 1 tbsp olive oil
- 1 can (15.5-oz) fava beans, drained
- 1 red onion, chopped
- 2 tsp chopped fresh cilantro
- 1 tsp ground cumin
- Salt to taste
- 1 garlic clove, minced
- 3 tbsp flour
- 4 lemon wedges to serve

Direction:(Prep + Cook Time: 20 minutes)

✓ Preheat the air fryer to 380 F.
✓ In a food processor, pulse all the ingredients until a thick paste is formed.
✓ Shape the mixture into ping pong-sized balls.
✓ Brush with olive oil and insert in the greased frying basket. AirFry for 12 minutes, turning once halfway through.
✓ Plate and serve with lemon wedges.

nutritional value: Calorie 298clCarbs 20 g Dietary Fiber 10 g Sugar 8 g Fat 16 g Saturated 5 g Protein 13 g

426)   *Plum & Pancetta Bombs*
Ingredients:

- (4-6 Servings)
- 1 ¼ cups soft goat cheese, crumbled
- 1 tbsp fresh rosemary, finely chopped
- 1 cup almonds, chopped
- Salt and black pepper to taste
- 15 dried plums, soaked and chopped
- 15 pancetta slices

Direction:(Prep + Cook Time: 20 minutes

✓ Line the frying basket with baking paper.
✓ In a bowl, add goat cheese, rosemary, almonds, salt, black pepper, and plums; stir well.

✓ Roll into balls and wrap with a pancetta slice Place them into the fryer and AirFry for 10 minutes at 400 F, shaking once.
✓ Let cool for a few minutes.
✓ Serve with toothpicks

nutritional value: Calorie 246cl Carbs 0 g Fat 19 g Saturated 0 g Polyunsaturated 0 g Monounsaturated 0 g Trans 0 g Protein 17 g cholesterol 0 mg

427)   *Fried Sausage Ravioli*
Ingredients:

- (6 Servings)
- 2 (18-oz) packages of fresh ravioli
- 1 cup flour
- 1 cup marinara sauce
- 4 eggs, beaten in a bowl
- 2 cups breadcrumbs
- 2 tbsp Parmesan cheese, grated

Direction:(Prep + Cook Time: 15 minutes)

✓ Preheat the air fryer to 400 F.
✓ In a bowl, mix breadcrumbs with Parmesan cheese.
✓ Dip pasta into the flour, then into the eggs, and finally in the breadcrumb mixture.
✓ Arrange the coated ravioli on the greased frying basket in an even layer and spritz them with cooking spray.
✓ AirFry for 10-12 minutes, turning once halfway through cooking until nice and golden.
✓ Serve hot with the marinara sauce.

nutritional value: Calories 98 Total Fat 4.6g Saturated Fat 1g *Trans Fat* 0.1g onounsaturated Fat 1.1g cholesterol 16 mg Total Carbs 11g Dietary Fiber 0.8g Sugar 1.4g Protein 3.2g

428)   *Roasted Hot Chickpeas*
Ingredients:

- (4 Servings)
- 1 (19-oz) can chickpeas, drained and rinsed
- 2 tbsp olive oil
- ½ tsp ground cumin
- ¼ tsp mustard powder
- ¼ tsp onion powder
- ½ tsp chili powder
- ¼ tsp cayenne pepper
- ¼ tsp salt

Direction:(Prep + Cook Time: 25 minutes)

✓ Preheat the air fryer to 385 F.
✓ In a mixing bowl, thoroughly combine the olive oil, cumin, mustard powder, onion powder, chili powder, cayenne pepper, and salt.
✓ Add in the chickpeas.
✓ Toss them until evenly coated.
✓ Transfer the Chickpeas to the frying basket and Air Fry, shaking the basket every 2-3 minutes.
✓ Cook until they're as crunchy as you like them, about 15-20 minutes.

✓ Serve.

nutritional value: Calories 119 Total Fat 3.9g Saturated Fat 0.5g ounsaturated Fat 2.1g cholesterol 0 mg g Total Carbs 16g Dietary Fiber 3.2g Sugar 2.8g Protein 5.3g

429) Paprika Baked Parsnips
Ingredients:

- (4 Servings)
- ½ tbsp paprika
- 1 lb parsnips, peeled and halved
- 4 tbsp avocado oil
- 2 tbsp fresh cilantro, chopped
- 2 tbsp Parmesan cheese, grated
- 1 tsp garlic powder
- Salt and black pepper to taste

Direction:(Prep + Cook Time: 20 minutes)

✓ Preheat the air fryer to 390 F.
✓ In a bowl, mix paprika, avocado oil, garlic, salt, and black pepper.
✓ Toss in the parsnips to coat.
✓ Arrange them on the greased frying basket and Bake for 14-16 minutes, turning once halfway through cooking, until golden and crunchy.
✓ Remove and sprinkle with Parmesan cheese and cilantro.
✓ Serve.

nutritional value: Calories: 237; Total Fat : 8g; Saturated Fat : 1g; cholesterol: 0 mg Carbohydrate: 42g; Dietary Fiber : 12g; Sugar : 11g; Protein : 3g

430) Air-Fried Cheesy Broccoli with Garlic
Ingredients:

- (2 Servings)
- 2 tbsp butter, melted
- 1 egg white
- 1 garlic clove, grated
- Salt and black pepper to taste
- ½ lb broccoli florets
- ⅓ cup grated Parmesan cheese

Direction:Prep + Cook Time: 20 minutes)

✓ In a bowl, whisk together butter, egg white, garlic, salt, and black pepper.
✓ Toss in the broccoli to coat.
✓ Arrange them in a single layer in the greased frying basket and AirFry for 10 minutes at 360 F, shaking once.
✓ Remove to a plate and sprinkle with Parmesan cheese.
✓ Serve immediately.

nutritional value: Calories: 43kcal | Carbs : 8g | Protein : 3g | Fat : 1g | Saturated Fat : 1g | Fiber : 3g | Sugar : 2g

431) Roasted Coconut Carrots
Ingredients:

- (4 Servings)
- 1 tbsp coconut oil, melted
- 1 lb horse carrots, sliced
- Salt and black pepper to taste
- ½ tsp chili powder

Direction:(Prep + Cook Time: 15 minutes)

✓ Preheat the air fryer to 400 F.
✓ In a bowl, mix the carrots with coconut oil, chili powder, salt, and black pepper.
✓ Place them in the fryer and AirFry for 7 minutes.
✓ Shake the basket and cook for another 5 minutes until golden brown. Serve.

nutritional: Calories: 111.3kcal Carbs : 19g Protein : 2g Fat : 3.7g Saturated Fat : 2.9g Fiber : 5.6g Sugar : 9.5g

432) Pumpkin Wedges
Ingredients:

- (4 Servings)
- 1 lb pumpkin, washed and cut into wedges
- 1 tbsp paprika
- 2 tbsp olive oil
- 1 lime, juiced
- 1 tbsp balsamic vinegar
- Salt and black pepper to taste
- 1 tsp turmeric

Direction:(Prep + Cook Time: 20 minutes)

✓ Preheat the air fryer to 400 F.
✓ Add the pumpkin wedges to the greased frying basket and AirFry for 10-12 minutes, flipping once.
✓ In a bowl, mix olive oil, lime juice, balsamic vinegar, turmeric, salt, black pepper, and paprika.
✓ Drizzle the dressing over the pumpkin and fry for 5 more minutes.
✓ Serve warm.

nutritional value: Calories 82.9 Total Fat 1.2 g Saturated Fat 0.0 g g cholesterol 0.0 mg Total Carbs 16.7 g Dietary Fiber 2.4 g Sugar 3.6 g Protein 2.8 g % Copper 0.0 Manganese 0.0 % Niacin 0.0

433) Baked Butternut Squash
Ingredients:

- (4 Servings)
- 2 cups butternut squash, cubed
- 2 tbsp olive oil
- Salt and black pepper to taste
- ¼ tsp dried thyme
- 1 tbsp fresh parsley, finely chopped

Direction:(Prep + Cook Time: 25 minutes

✓ In a bowl, add squash, olive oil, salt, black pepper, and thyme; toss to coat.
✓ Place the squash in the air fryer and AirFry for 12-14 minutes at 360 F, shaking once or twice.
✓ Serve sprinkled with fresh parsley.

nutritional value: 26Kcal/110KJ0.7g Protein 0.1g Fat

5.9g carbohydrate 1.5g Fiber 224 mg

434) *Cheesy Mushrooms*
Ingredients:
- (2 Servings)
- 2 tbsp olive oil Salt and black pepper to taste
- 10 button mushroom caps
- 2 tbsp mozzarella cheese, grated
- 2 tbsp cheddar cheese, grated
- 1 tsp Italian seasoning

Direction:(Prep + Cook Time: 20 minutes)
- ✓ Preheat the air fryer to 390 F.
- ✓ In a bowl, mix olive oil, salt, black pepper, and Italian seasoning.
- ✓ Toss in the mushrooms to coat.
- ✓ Mix the cheeses in a separate bowl. Stuff the mushrooms with the cheese mixture and place them in the frying basket.
- ✓ Bake for 10-12 minutes until golden on top.
- ✓ Serve warm.

nutritional: Calories 53 Total Fat 4.1g Saturated Fat 0.8g *Trans Fat* 0g cholesterol 2 mg Total Carbs 3.1g Dietary Fiber 0.5g Sugar 0.5g Protein 1.4g

435) *Walnut & Cheese Filled Mushrooms*
Ingredients:
- (4 Servings)
- 4 large portobello mushroom caps
- ⅓ cup walnuts, finely chopped
- 1 tbsp canola oil
- ½ cup mozzarella cheese, shredded
- 2 tbsp fresh parsley, chopped

Direction:(Prep + Cook Time: 20 minutes)
- ✓ Preheat the air fryer to 350 F.
- ✓ Grease the frying basket with cooking spray.
- ✓ Rub the mushrooms with canola oil and fill them with mozzarella cheese.
- ✓ Top with walnuts and arrange them in the greased frying basket.
- ✓ Bake for 10-12 minutes or until golden on top.
- ✓ Remove and let cool for a few minutes.
- ✓ Sprinkle with freshly chopped parsley and serve

nutritional value: Calories 55.2 Total Fat 3.3 g Saturated Fat 1.0 g cholesterol 4.1 4 mg Total Carbs 2.3 g Dietary Fiber 0.4 g Sugar 0.5 g Protein 4.6 g %

436) *Paprika Serrano Peppers*
Ingredients:
- (4 Servings)
- 4 serrano peppers, halved and seeds removed
- 3 oz ricotta cheese, crumbled
- 1 cup breadcrumbs
- 1 tsp paprika
- 1 tbsp chives, chopped

- 1 tbsp olive oil

Direction:(Prep + Cook Time: 20 minutes)
- ✓ Preheat the air fryer to 380 F.
- ✓ Grease the frying basket with cooking spray.
- ✓ In a bowl, combine ricotta cheese, paprika, and chives. Spoon the mixture into the pepper halves and top with breadcrumbs.
- ✓ Drizzle with olive oil.
- ✓ Place in the basket and Bake for 10-12 minutes.
- ✓ Serve warm.

nutritional value: Calories: 34 Fat : 0.5g Carbs : 7g Fiber : 3.9g Sugar 4g Protein : 1.8g

437) *Chili Edamame*
Ingredients:
- (4 Servings)
- 1 (16-oz) bag frozen edamame in pods
- 1 red chili, finely chopped
- 1 tbsp olive oil
- ½ tsp garlic salt
- ½ tsp red pepper flakes
- Black pepper to taste

Direction:(Prep + Cook Time: 20 minutes)
- ✓ Preheat the air fryer to 380 F.
- ✓ In a mixing bowl, combine olive oil, garlic salt, red pepper flakes, and black pepper and mix well.
- ✓ Add in the edamame and toss to coat.
- ✓ Transfer to the frying basket in a single layer and AirFry for 10 minutes, shaking once.
- ✓ Cook until lightly browned and just crispy.
- ✓ Work in batches if needed.
- ✓ Serve topped with the red chili.

nutritional: Calories 370 Total Fat 12g Saturated Fat 0g *Trans Fat* 0g cholesterol 0 mg Total Carbs 27g Dietary Fiber 15g Sugar 6gs Protein 32g

438) *Brie Cheese Croutons with Herbs*
Ingredients:
- (2 Servings)
- 2 tbsp olive oil
- 1 tbsp french herbs
- 6 oz brie cheese, chopped
- 2 slices bread, halved

Direction:(Prep + Cook Time: 15 minutes + cooling time)
- ✓ Preheat the air fryer to 340 F.
- ✓ Brush the bread slices with olive oil and sprinkle with herbs.
- ✓ Top with brie cheese Place in the greased frying basket and Bake for 10-12 minutes.
- ✓ Let cool, then cut into cubes.

nutritional value: Calories 100 Total Fat 9g Saturated Fat 4 Carbs 0g Net carbs 0g Sugar 0g Fiber 0g Protein 4g

439)   *Super Cabbage Canapes*
Ingredients:

- (2 Servings)
- 1 whole cabbage, cut into rounds
- ½ cup mozzarella cheese, shredded
- ½ carrot, cubed
- ¼ onion, cubed
- ¼ bell pepper, cubed
- 1 tbsp fresh basil, chopped

Direction:(Prep + Cook Time: 20 minutes)

✓ Preheat the air fryer to 360 F.

✓ In a bowl, mix onion, carrot, bell pepper, and mozzarella cheese.

✓ Toss to coat evenly.

✓ Add the cabbage rounds to the greased frying basket, top with the cheese mixture, and Bake for 5-8 minutes.

✓ Garnish with basil and serve

nutritional value: Calories: 22 Fat : 0.1g Carbs : 5.2g Fiber : 2.2g Sugar 2.9g Protein : 1.1

440)   *Broccoli Cheese Quiche*
Ingredients:

- (3 Servings)
- 1 head broccoli, cut into florets
- ½ cup Parmesan cheese, grated
- ¼ cup heavy cream
- Salt and black pepper to taste 5 eggs

Direction:(Prep + Cook Time: 30 minutes)

✓ Preheat the air fryer to 340 F.

✓ Beat the eggs with the heavy cream.

✓ Season with salt and black pepper.

✓ In a greased baking dish, lay the florets and cover with the egg mixture.

✓ Spread Parmesan cheese on top and place inside the frying basket. Bake for 10-12 minutes until golden brown on top.

✓ Serve warm.

nutritional value: Calories 411 cholesterol 210 mg g Total Carbs 20g Dietary Fiber 2.6g Sugar 4.4g Protein 16g

441)   *Easy Parmesan Sandwich*
Ingredients:

- (1 Serving)
- 4 tbsp Parmesan cheese, shredded
- 2 scallions
- 1 tbsp butter, softened
- 2 bread slices

Direction:(Prep + Cook Time: 20 minutes)

✓ Preheat the air fryer to 360 F.

✓ Spread only one side of the bread slices with butter.

✓ Cover one of the buttered slices with Parmesan and scallions and top with the buttered side of the other slice to form a sandwich.

✓ Place in the frying basket and Bake for 10-12 minutes.

✓ Cut into 4 triangles and serve.

nutritional value: Calories 437.3 Total Fat 13.4 g Saturated Fat 6.9 g cholesterol 90.1 5 mg Total Carbs 34.2 g Dietary Fiber 4.5 g Sugar 8.5 g Protein 44.2 g Copper 2.9 % Manganese 1.3 % Niacin 63.7 %

442)   *Salty Carrot Cookies*
Ingredients:

- (4 Servings)
- 6 carrots, boiled and mashed
- Salt and black pepper to taste
- ½ tsp parsley
- 1 ¼ oz oats
- 1 whole egg, beaten
- ½ tsp thyme

Direction:(Prep + Cook Time: 25 minutes)

✓ Preheat the air fryer to 360 F.

✓ In a bowl, combine carrots, salt, black pepper, egg, oats, thyme, and parsley; mix well to form batter.

✓ Shape into cookie shapes.

✓ Place the cookies in the greased frying basket and Bake for 14-16 minutes, flipping once halfway through.

✓ Serve.

nutritional value: Calories 110.9 Total Fat 5.6 g Saturated Fat 0.6 g g cholesterol 0.0 mg Total Carbs 14.1 g Dietary Fiber 0.5 g Sugar 0.4 Protein 1.4 g % Copper 1.0 Manganese 4.3 % Niacin 3.4 % Pantothenic

443)   *Mini Cheese Scones*
Ingredients:

- (4 Servings)
- 1 cup flour
- A pinch of salt
- 1 tsp baking powder
- 2 oz butter, cubed
- 1 tsp fresh chives, chopped
- 1 egg
- ¼ cup milk
- ½ cup cheddar cheese, shredded

Direction:(Prep + Cook Time: 30 minutes)

✓ Preheat the air fryer to 360 F.

✓ Sith the flour in a bowl and mix in butter, baking powder, and salt until a breadcrumb mixture is formed.

✓ Add cheese, chives, milk, and egg, and mix to get a sticky dough.

✓ Roll the dough into small balls.

✓ Place the balls in the greased frying basket and AirFry for 18-20 minutes, shaking once or twice. Serve warm

nutritional value: Calories 154 Total Fat 9.5g Saturated Fat 5.6g *Trans Fat* 0.3g cholesterol 51 mg Total Carbs 13g Dietary Fiber 0.4g Sugar 0.3g Protein 4.4g

444) *Cheddar Cheese Biscuits*
Ingredients:

- 4 Servings)
- ½ cup butter, softened
- 1 tbsp melted butter.
- 1 tsp salt
- 2 cups flour
- ½ cup buttermilk
- ½ cup cheddar cheese, grated
- 1 egg, beaten

Direction:(Prep + Cook Time: 30 minutes + cooling time)

- ✓ Preheat the air fryer to 360 F.
- ✓ In a bowl, mix salt, flour, butter, cheese, and buttermilk to form a batter.
- ✓ Shape into balls and flatten them into biscuits.
- ✓ Arrange them on a greased frying basket and brush with the beaten egg.
- ✓ Drizzle with melted butter and Bake in the fryer for 18-20 minutes, flipping once.

nutritional value: Calories160 kCal Total Carbs 15 g Net Carbs 14 g Fiber 1 g Sugar 1 g Fat 10 g Saturated Fat 4 g cholesterol 10 mg

445) *Cauliflower & Tofu Croquettes*
Ingredients:

- (4 Servings)
- 1 lb cauliflower florets
- 2 eggs
- ½ cup tofu, crumbled
- ½ cup mozzarella cheese ⅓ cup breadcrumbs
- 1 tsp dried thyme
- ¼ tsp ground cumin
- ½ tsp onion powder
- Salt and black pepper to taste
- 1 cup chipotle aioli

Direction:(Prep + Cook Time: 30 minutes)

- ✓ Place the cauliflower florets in your food processor and pulse until it resembles rice.
- ✓ Microwave the resulting "rice" in a heatproof dish for 4-6 minutes until it have softened completely.
- ✓ Let cool.
- ✓ Preheat the air fryer to 390 F.
- ✓ Add the eggs, tofu, mozzarella cheese, breadcrumbs, thyme, cumin, onion powder, salt, and pepper to the cauliflower rice and mix to combine.
- ✓ Form the mixture into croquettes and arrange them on the greased frying basket.
- ✓ Spritz with cooking spray.
- ✓ AirFry for 14-16 minutes, turning once, until golden brown.
- ✓ Serve warm with the chipotle aioli.

nutritional value: Kcal 155 Fat 9g Saturates 3g Carbs 12g Sugar 2g Fiber 1g Protein 5g Salt 0.23g

446) *Cheesy Mushroom & Cauliflower Balls*
Ingredients:

- (4 Servings)
- ½lb mushrooms, diced
- 3 tbsp olive oil + some more for brushing
- 1 small red onion, chopped
- 3 garlic cloves, minced
- 3 cups cauliflower, chopped
- 1 cup breadcrumbs
- 1 cup Grana Padano cheese, grated
- 2 sprigs fresh thyme, chopped
- Salt and black pepper to taste

Direction:(Prep + Cook Time: 25 minutes + cooling time)

- ✓ Heat 3 tbsp olive oil in a skillet over medium heat and sauté garlic and onion for 3 minutes.
- ✓ Add in mushrooms and cauliflower and stir-fry for 5 minutes.
- ✓ Add in Grana Padano cheese, black pepper, thyme, and salt.
- ✓ Turn off and let cool.
- ✓ Make small balls out of the mixture and refrigerate for 30 minutes.
- ✓ Preheat the air fryer to 350 F.
- ✓ Remove the balls from the refrigerator and roll in the breadcrumbs.
- ✓ Brush with olive oil and place in the frying basket without overcrowding. Bake for 14-16 minutes, tossing every 4-5 minutes.
- ✓ Serve with sautéed zoodles and tomato sauce, if desired.

nutritional value: Cal 395.6 Total Fat 33.3g Saturated Fat 12.8g g rans- Fat 0.7g cholesterol 57.6 Carbs 10.3g Net carbs 6.7g Sugar 4g Fiber 3.6g Glucose 3.1g Fructose 0.7g Protein 16.4g

447) *Spicy Cheese Lings*
Ingredients:

- (4 Servings)
- ½ cup grated cheddar cheese + extra for rolling
- 1 cup flour + extra for kneading
- ¼ tsp chili powder
- ½ tsp baking powder
- 3 tsp butter, melted
- A pinch of salt

Direction:(Prep + Cook Time: 20 minutes)

- ✓ In a bowl, mix the cheese, flour, baking powder, chili powder, butter, and salt.
- ✓ Add some Water and mix well to get a dough.
- ✓ Remove the dough onto a flat, floured surface.
- ✓ Using a rolling pin, roll out into a thin sheet and
- ✓ cut into lings' shape.
- ✓ Add the cheese lings to the greased frying basket and AirFry for 10-12 minutes at 350 F, flipping once halfway through.

✓ Serve with ketchup if desired
nutritional value: Calories 20 Total Fat 1.5g Carbs 2g Net carbs 2g Fiber 0g Protein 0g

448) *Cocktail Meatballs*
Ingredients:
- (4 Servings)
- ½ lb ground beef
- ½ lb ground pork
- 2 oz bacon, chopped
- 1 cup jalapeño tomato ketchup 1 egg
- Salt and black pepper to taste
- ¼ tsp cayenne pepper
- 2 oz cheddar cheese, shredded

Direction:(Prep + Cook Time: 30 MINUTES)
✓ Preheat the air fryer to 400 F.
✓ In a bowl, thoroughly mix all ingredients.
✓ Form the mixture into 1-inch balls using an ice cream scoop.
✓ Place them into the greased frying basket and spray with cooking oil.
✓ AirFry for 8-10 minutes, turning once.
✓ Serve with toothpicks and jalapeño tomato ketchup on the side.
nutritional value: Calories 56c Total Fat 2.4g Saturated Fat 0.7g *Trans Fat* 0.1g onounsaturated Fat 1.1g cholesterol 8.7 mg Total Carbs 5.3g Dietary Fiber 0.2g Sugar 1.7g Protein 3.2g

449) *French Beans with Toasted Almonds*
Ingredients:
- (4 Servings)
- 1 lb French beans, trimmed
- Salt and black pepper to taste
- ½ tbsp onion powder
- 2 tbsp olive oil
- ½ cup toasted almonds, chopped

Direction:(Prep + Cook Time: 15 minutes)
✓ Preheat air fryer to 400 F.
✓ In a bowl, drizzle the beans with olive oil.
✓ Add onion powder, salt, and pepper and toss to coat.
✓ AirFry for 10-12 minutes, shaking once.
✓ Sprinkle with almonds and serve.
nutritional value: 68 calories; Protein 2.2g; Carbs 5g; Dietary Fiber 2.5g; Sugar 1g; Fat 5.1g; saturated Fat 0.5g;

450) *Cheddar Black Bean Burritos*
Ingredients:
- (4 Servings)
- 4 tortillas
- 1 cup cheddar cheese, grated
- 1 can (8 oz) black beans, drained

- 1 tsp taco seasoning
Direction:(Prep + Cook Time: 10 minutes)
✓ Preheat the air fryer to 350 F.
✓ Mix the beans with the taco seasoning.
✓ Divide the bean mixture between the tortillas and top with cheddar cheese.
✓ Roll the burritos and arrange them on the greased frying basket.
✓ Place in the air fryer and Bake for 4-5 minutes, flip, and cook for 3 more minutes.
✓ Serve warm.
nutritional value: Calories 377.6 Total Fat 14.6 g Saturated Fat 7.2 g g cholesterol 35.5 3 mg Total Carbs 45.4 g Dietary Fiber 11.5 g Sugar 1.0 g Protein 19.1 g Calciu 24.3 % Copper 9.5 % 7 %

451) *Smoky Hazelnuts*
Ingredients:
- (4-6 Servings)
- 2 cups almonds
- 2 tbsp liquid smoke
- Salt to taste
- 1 tbsp molasses

Direction:(Prep + Cook Time: 20 minutes)
✓ Preheat the air fryer to 360 F.
✓ In a bowl, add salt, liquid smoke, molasses, and almonds; toss to coat.
✓ Place the hazelnuts in the greased frying basket and Bake for 5-8 minutes, shaking once.
✓ Serve warm.
nutritional value: calories: 176 total fat : 17 grams protein : 4.2 grams carbs: 4.7 grams fiber : 2.7 grams ,

452) *Spiced Almonds*
Ingredients:
- (4 Servings)
- ½ tsp ground cinnamon
- ½ tsp smoked paprika
- 1 cup almonds
- 1 egg white
- Sea salt to taste

Direction:(Prep + Cook Time: 15 minutes)
✓ Preheat the air fryer to 310 F.
✓ Grease the frying basket with cooking spray.
✓ In a bowl, whisk the egg white with cinnamon and paprika and stir in the almonds.
✓ Spread the almonds in the frying basket and AirFry for 12-14 minutes, shaking once or twice.
✓ Remove and sprinkle with sea salt to serve.
nutritional value: Calories 7.7 Total Fat 0.7g Saturated Fat 0.1g *Trans Fat* 0g ams cholesterol 0 mg g Total Carbs 0.3g Dietary Fiber 0.1g Sugar 0.1g Protein 0.3g

453) *Roasted Pumpkin Seeds with Cardamom*
Ingredients:
- (4 Servings)

- 1 cup pumpkin seeds, pulp removed, rinsed
- 1 tbsp butter, melted
- 1 tbsp brown Sugar
- 1 tsp orange zest
- ½ tsp cardamom
- ½ tsp salt

Direction:(Prep + Cook Time: 25 minutes)
- ✓ Preheat air fryer to 320 F.
- ✓ Place the pumpkin seeds in a greased baking dish and place the dish in the fryer.
- ✓ AirFry for 4-5 minutes to avoid moisture.
- ✓ In a bowl, whisk butter, Sugar , zest, cardamom, and salt.
- ✓ Add the seeds to the bowl and toss to coat well.
- ✓ Transfer the seeds to the baking dish inside the fryer and Bake for 13-15 minutes, shaking the basket every 5 minutes, until lightly browned.
- ✓ Serve warm.

nutritional: Calories 169 Total Fat 14g Trans Fat 0g onounsaturated Fat 4.6g cholesterol 0 mg g Total Carbs 4.3g Dietary Fiber 1.9g Sugar 0.4g Protein 8.8g

399) *Masala Cashew Nuts*
Ingredients:
- (2 Servings)
- 1 cup cashew nuts
- Salt and black pepper to taste
- ½ tsp ground coriander
- 1 tsp garam masala

Direction:(Prep + Cook Time: 10 minutes)
- ✓ Preheat the air fryer to 360 F.
- ✓ In a bowl, mix coriander, garam masala, salt, and pepper. Add cashews and toss to coat.
- ✓ Place in a greased baking dish and AirFry in the fryer for 5-8 minutes, shaking once.

nutrition: 157 calories8.56 grams g carbohydrate1.68 g Sugar 0.9 g of Fiber 5.17 g Protein 12.43 g

454) *Sweet Mixed Nuts*
Ingredients:
- (5 Servings)
- ½ cup pecans
- ½ cup walnuts
- ½ cup almonds
- A pinch of cayenne pepper
- 1 tbsp Sugar
- 2 tbsp egg whites
- 2 tsp ground cinnamon
- Cooking spray

Direction:(Prep + Cook Time: 15 minutes)
- ✓ Add cayenne pepper, Sugar , and cinnamon to a bowl and mix well; set aside.
- ✓ In another bowl, mix pecans, walnuts, almonds, and egg whites.
- ✓ Add in the spice mixture and stir.

- ✓ Grease a baking dish with cooking spray.
- ✓ Pour in the nuts and place the dish in the fryer.
- ✓ Bake for 5-7 minutes.
- ✓ Stir the nuts using a wooden spoon and cook for 4-5 more minutes.
- ✓ Pour the nuts into the bowl and let cool slightly.

nutritional value: Calories 150 Total Fat 11g Saturated Fat 1.5g Trans Fat 0g cholesterol 0 mg Total Carbs 11g Dietary Fiber 2g Sugar 7g Protein 4g

400) *Char Siew Pork Ribs*
Ingredients:
- (4 Servings)
- 2 lb pork ribs
- 2 tbsp char siew sauce
- 2 tbsp minced ginger
- 1 tbsp soy sauce
- 2 tbsp hoisin sauce
- 2 tbsp sesame oil
- 1 tsp honey
- 4 garlic cloves, minced

Direction:(Prep + Cook Time: 35 minutes + marinating time)
- ✓ Whisk together all the ingredients, except for the ribs, in a large bowl.
- ✓ Add in the ribs and toss to coat.
- ✓ Cover with a lid. Place the bowl in the fridge to marinate for 2 hours.
- ✓ Preheat the air fryer to 390 F. Put the ribs in the greased frying basket and place in the fryer; do not throw away the liquid from the bowl. Bake for 15 minutes. Pour in the marinade and cook for 10-12 more minutes. Serve hot.

nutritional value: Calories 449 Total Fat 27gSaturated Fat 12g Total Carbs 16gTotal Sugar 16g Protein 36g

401) *Cornbread with Pulled Pork*
Ingredients
- 2 ½ cups pulled pork, leftover works well too
- 1 teaspoon dried rosemary
- 1/2 teaspoon chili powder
- 3 cloves garlic, peeled and pressed
- 1/2 recipe cornbread
- 1/2 tablespoon brown sugar
- 1/3 cup scallions, thinly sliced
- 1 teaspoon sea salt

Directions (Ready in about 24 minutes | Servings 2)
- ✓ Preheat a large-sized nonstick skillet over medium heat; now, cook the scallions together with the garlic and pulled pork.
- ✓ Next, add the sugar, chili powder, rosemary, and salt. Cook, stirring occasionally, until the mixture is thickened.
- ✓ Preheat your air fryer to 335 degrees F. Now, coat two mini loaf pans with a cooking spray. Add the pulled pork mixture and spread over the bottom

using a spatula.

✓ Spread the previously prepared cornbread batter over top of the spiced pulled pork mixture.

✓ Bake this cornbread in the preheated air fryer until a tester inserted into the center of it comes out clean, or for 18 minutes. Bon appétit!

Nutritions: 239 Calories; 7.6g Fat; 6.3g Carbs; 34.6g Protein; 4g Sugars

402) *Famous Cheese and Bacon Rolls*

Ingredients

- 1/3 cup Swiss cheese, shredded
- 10 slices of bacon
- 10 ounces canned crescent rolls
- 2 tablespoons yellow mustard 6

Directions (Ready in about 10 minutes | Servings 6)

✓ Start by preheating your air fryer to 325 degrees F.

✓ Then, form the crescent rolls into "sheets". Spread mustard over the sheets. Place the chopped Swiss cheese and bacon in the middle of each dough sheet.

✓ Create the rolls and bake them for about 9 minutes.

✓ Then, set the machine to 385 degrees F; bake for an additional 4 minutes in the preheated air fryer. Eat warm with some extra yellow mustard.

Nutritions: 386 Calories; 16.2g Fat; 29.7g Carbs; 14.7g Protein; 4g Sugars

403) *Baked Eggs with Kale and Ham*

Ingredients

- 2 eggs
- 1/4 teaspoon dried or fresh marjoram
- 2 teaspoons chili powder
- 1/3 teaspoon kosher salt
- ½ cup steamed kale
- 1/4 teaspoon dried or fresh rosemary
- 4 pork ham slices
- 1/3 teaspoon ground black pepper, or more to taste

Directions (Ready in about 15 minutes | Servings 2)

✓ Divide the kale and ham among 2 ramekins; crack an egg into each ramekin. Sprinkle with seasonings.

✓ Cook for 15 minutes at 335 degrees F or until your eggs reach desired texture.

✓ Serve warm with spicy tomato ketchup and pickles. Bon appétit!

Nutritions: 417 Calories; 17.8g Fat; 3g Carbs; 61g **Protein**; 0.9g Sugars

404) *Easiest Pork Chops Ever*

Ingredients

- 1/3 cup Italian breadcrumbs
- Roughly chopped fresh cilantro, to taste
- 2 teaspoons Cajun seasonings
- Nonstick cooking spray
- 2 eggs, beaten

- 3 tablespoons white flour
- 1 teaspoon seasoned salt
- Garlic & onion spice blend, to taste
- 6 pork chops
- 1/3 teaspoon freshly cracked black pepper

Directions (Ready in about 22 minutes | Servings 6)

✓ Coat the pork chops with Cajun seasonings, salt, pepper, and the spice blend on all sides.

✓ Then, add the flour to a plate. In a shallow dish, whisk the egg until pale and smooth. Place the Italian breadcrumbs in the third bowl.

✓ Dredge each pork piece in the flour; then, coat them with the egg; finally, coat them with the breadcrumbs. Spritz them with cooking spray on both sides.

✓ Now, air-fry pork chops for about 18 minutes at 345 degrees F; make sure to taste for doneness after first 12 minutes of cooking. Lastly, garnish with fresh cilantro. Bon appétit!

Nutritions: 398 Calories; 21g Fat; 4.7g Carbs; 44.2g Protein; 0.5g Sugars

405) *Onion Rings Wrapped in Bacon*

Ingredients

- 12 rashers back bacon
- 1/2 teaspoon ground black pepper
- Chopped fresh parsley, to taste
- 1/2 teaspoon paprika
- 1/2 teaspoon chili powder
- 1/2 tablespoon soy sauce
- ½ teaspoon salt

Directions (Ready in about 25 minutes | Servings 4)

✓ Start by preheating your air fryer to 355 degrees F.

✓ Season the onion rings with paprika, salt, black pepper, and chili powder. Simply wrap the bacon around the onion rings; drizzle with soy sauce.

✓ Bake for 17 minutes, garnish with fresh parsley and serve. Bon appétit!

Nutritions: 317 Calories; 16.8g Fat; 22.7g Carbs; 20.2g Protein; 2.7g Sugars

406) *Easy Pork Burgers with Blue Cheese*

Ingredients

- 1/3 cup blue cheese, crumbled
- 6 hamburger buns, toasted
- 2 teaspoons dried basil
- 1/3 teaspoon smoked paprika
- 1 pound ground pork
- 2 tablespoons tomato puree
- 2 small-sized onions, peeled and chopped
- 1/2 teaspoon ground black pepper
- 3 garlic cloves, minced
- 1 teaspoon fine sea salt

Directions (Ready in about 44 minutes | Servings 6)

✓ Start by preheating your air fryer to 385 degrees F.

✓ In a mixing dish, combine the pork, onion, garlic, tomato puree, and seasonings; mix to combine well.

✓ Form the pork mixture into six patties; cook the burgers for 23 minutes. Pause the machine, turn the temperature to 365 degrees F and cook for 18 more minutes.

✓ Place the prepared burger on the bottom bun; top with blue cheese; assemble the burgers and serve warm.

Nutritions: 383 Calories; 19.5g Fat; 24.7g Carbs; 25.7g Protein; 4g Sugars

407) *Sausage, Pepper and Fontina Frittata*

Ingredients

- 3 pork sausages, chopped
- 5 well-beaten eggs
- 1 ½ bell peppers, seeded and chopped
- 1 teaspoon smoked cayenne pepper
- 2 tablespoons Fontina cheese
- 1/2 teaspoon tarragon
- 1/2 teaspoon ground black pepper
- 1 teaspoon salt

Directions(Ready in about 14 minutes | Servings 5)

✓ In a cast-iron skillet, sweat the bell peppers together with the chopped pork sausages until the peppers are fragrant and the sausage begins to release liquid.

✓ Lightly grease the inside of a baking dish with pan spray.

✓ Throw all of the above ingredients into the prepared baking dish, including the sautéed mixture; stir to combine.

✓ Bake at 345 degrees F approximately 9 minutes. Serve right away with the salad of choice.

Nutritions: 420 Calories; 19.6g Fat; 3.7g Carbs; 41g Protein; 2g Sugars

408) *Ground Pork and Wild Rice Casserole*

Ingredients

- 1 teaspoon olive oil
- 1 small-sized yellow onion, chopped
- 1 pound ground pork (84% lean)
- Salt and black pepper, to taste
- 1/2 cups cooked wild rice, uncooked
- 1/2 cup cream of mushroom soup
- 1/2 tomato paste
- 1 jalapeno pepper, minced
- 1 teaspoon Italian spice mix
- 1/2 cup Asiago cheese, shredded

Directions (Ready in about 25 minutes | Servings 3)

✓ Start by preheating your Air Fryer to 350 degrees F.

✓ Heat the olive oil in a nonstick over medium-high heat. Then, sauté the onion and ground pork for 6

to 7 minutes, crumbling with a spatula. Season with salt and black pepper to your liking.

✓ Spoon the pork mixture into a lightly greased baking dish.

✓ Spoon the cooked rice over the pork layer. In a mixing dish, thoroughly combine the remaining ingredients.

✓ Bake for 15 minutes or until bubbly and heated through.

Nutritions: 506 Calories; 34.7g Fat; 13.4g Carbs; 34.7g Protein; 2.3g Sugars

409) *Dijon Mustard and Honey Roasted Pork Cutlets*

Ingredients

- 1 pound pork cutlets
- 1 teaspoon cayenne pepper
- Kosher salt and ground black pepper, to season
- 1/2 teaspoon garlic powder
- 1 tablespoon honey
- 1 teaspoon Dijon mustard

Directions (Ready in about 15 minutes | Servings 2)

✓ Spritz the sides and bottom of the cooking basket with a nonstick cooking spray.

✓ Place the pork cutlets in the cooking basket; sprinkle with cayenne pepper, salt, black pepper and garlic powder.

✓ In a mixing dish, thoroughly combine the honey and Dijon mustard.

✓ Cook the pork cutlets at 390 degrees F for 6 minutes. Flip halfway through, rub with the honey mixture and continue to cook for 6 minutes more. Serve immediately.

Nutritions: 326 Calories; 12.7g Fat; 15.1g Carbs; 38.7g Protein; 13g Sugars

410) *Fried Pork Loin Chops*

Ingredients

- 1 egg
- 1/4 cup cornmeal
- 1/4 cup crackers, crushed
- 1/2 teaspoon garlic powder
- 1/2 teaspoon cayenne pepper
- Salt and black pepper, to taste
- 2 boneless pork loin chops, about 1-inch thick, 6 ounces each

Directions (Ready in about 15 minutes | Servings 2)

✓ In a shallow mixing bowl, whisk the egg until pale and frothy.

✓ In another bowl, mix the cornmeal, crushed crackers, garlic powder, cayenne pepper, salt and black pepper.

✓ Dip each pork loin chop in the beaten egg. Then, roll them over the cornmeal mixture.

✓ Spritz the bottom of the cooking basket with cooking oil. Add the breaded pork cutlets and cook at 395 degrees F for 6 minutes.

✓ Flip and cook for 6 minutes on the other side. Serve

warm.
Nutritions: 379 Calories; 12g Fat; 19.1g Carbs; 45.5g Protein; 2.3g Sugars

411)   *Pork Loin with Roasted Peppers*
Ingredients

- 3 red bell peppers
- 1 ½ pounds pork loin
- 1 garlic clove, halved
- 1 teaspoon lard, melted
- 1/2 teaspoon cayenne pepper
- 1/4 teaspoon cumin powder
- 1/4 teaspoon ground bay laurel
- Kosher salt and ground black pepper, to taste

Directions (Ready in about 55 minutes | Servings 3)

- ✓ Roast the peppers in the preheated Air Fryer at 395 degrees F for 10 minutes, flipping them halfway through the cooking time.
- ✓ Let them steam for 10 minutes; then, peel the skin and discard the stems and seeds. Slice the peppers into halves and add salt to taste.
- ✓ Rub the pork with garlic; brush with melted lard and season with spices until well coated on all sides.
- ✓ Place in the cooking basket and cook at 360 digress F for 25 minutes. Turn the meat over and cook an additional 20 minutes. Serve with roasted peppers.

Nutritions: 409 Calories; 20.1g Fat; 4.3g Carbs; 49g Protein; 2.4g Sugars

412)   *BBQ-Glazed Meatloaf Muffins*
Ingredients

- 1 pound lean ground pork
- 1 small onion, chopped
- 2 cloves garlic, crushed
- 1/4 cup carrots, grated
- 1 serrano pepper, seeded and minced
- 1 teaspoon stone-ground mustard
- 1/4 cup crackers, crushed
- 1 egg, lightly beaten
- Sea salt and ground black pepper, to taste
- 1/2 cup BBQ sauce

Directions (Ready in about 45 minutes | Servings 3)

- ✓ Mix all ingredients, except for the BBQ sauce, until everything is well incorporated.
- ✓ Brush a muffin tin with vegetable oil. Use an ice cream scoop to spoon the meat mixture into the cups. Top each meatloaf cup with a spoonful of BBQ sauce.
- ✓ Bake in the preheated Air Fryer at 395 degrees F for about 40 minutes. Transfer to a cooling rack.
- ✓ Wait for a few minutes before unmolding and serving.

Nutritions: 269 Calories; 9.7g Fat; 9.1g Carbs; 36.6g Protein; 4.4g Sugars

413)   *Pork Tenderloin with Brussels Sprouts*
Ingredients

- 1 pound Brussels sprouts, halved
- 1 ½ pounds tenderloin
- 1 teaspoon peanut oil
- 1 teaspoon garlic powder
- 1 tablespoon coriander, minced
- 1 teaspoon smoked paprika
- Sea salt and ground black pepper, to taste

Directions (Ready in about 20 minutes | Servings 3)

- ✓ Toss the Brussels sprouts and pork with oil and spices until well coated.
- ✓ Place in the Air Fryer cooking basket. Cook in the preheated Air Fryer at 370 degrees F for 15 minutes.
- ✓ Taste and adjust seasonings. Eat warm.

Nutritions: 381 Calories; 11.7g Fat; 14.1g Carbs; 56g Protein; 3.4g Sugars

414)   *Meatballs with Sweet and Sour Sauce*
Ingredients

- Meatballs:
- 1/2 pound ground pork
- 1/4 pound ground turkey
- 2 tablespoons scallions, minced
- 1/2 teaspoon garlic, minced
- 4 tablespoons tortilla chips, crushed
- 4 tablespoons parmesan cheese, grated
- 1 egg, beaten
- Salt and red pepper, to taste
- Sauce:
- 6 ounces jellied cranberry
- 2 ounces hot sauce
- 2 tablespoons molasses
- 1 tablespoon wine vinegar

Directions (Ready in about 20 minutes | Servings 3)

- ✓ In a mixing bowl, thoroughly combine all ingredients for the meatballs. Stir to combine well and roll the mixture into 8 equal meatballs.
- ✓ Cook in the preheated Air Fryer at 400 degrees F for 7 minutes. Shake the basket and continue to cook for 7 minutes longer.
- ✓ Meanwhile, whisk the sauce ingredients in a nonstick skillet over low heat; let it simmer, partially covered, for about 20 minutes. Fold in the prepared meatballs and serve immediately.

Nutritions: 486 Calories; 14.8g Fat; 54.1g Carbs; 33.6g Protein; 20.4g Sugars

415)   *Perfect Pork Wraps*
Ingredients

- 1/2 pound pork loin
- 1 teaspoon butter, melted
- Salt and black pepper, to season

- 1/2 teaspoon marjoram
- 1/2 teaspoon hot paprika
- 2 tortillas
- Sauce:
- 2 tablespoons tahini
- 1 tablespoon sesame oil
- 2 tablespoons soy sauce
- 1 tablespoon lime juice
- 1 tablespoon white vinegar
- 1 teaspoon fresh ginger, peeled and grated
- 2 garlic cloves, pressed
- 1 teaspoon honey

Directions (Ready in about 55 minutes | Servings 2)

✓ Rub the pork with melted butter and season with salt, pepper, marjoram and hot paprika.

✓ Place in the cooking basket and cook at 360 digress F for 25 minutes. Turn the meat over and cook an additional 20 minutes.

✓ Place the roasted pork loin on a cutting board. Slice the roasted pork loin into strips using a sharp kitchen knife.

✓ In the meantime, mix the sauce ingredients with a wire whisk.

✓ Turn the temperature to 390 degrees F. Spoon the pork strips and sauce onto each tortilla; wrap them tightly.

✓ Drizzle with a nonstick cooking spray and bake about 6 minutes. Serve warm.

Nutritions: 558 Calories; 25.7g Fat; 44.1g Carbs; 34.3g Protein; 7.2g Sugars

416) *Easy Munchy Pork Bites*
Ingredients

- 1 pound pork stew meat, cubed
- 2 garlic cloves, crushed
- 1/4 cup dark rum
- 1/4 cup soy sauce
- 1 tablespoon lemon juice
- 1 tablespoon white vinegar
- 1 tablespoon olive oil
- 1/2 teaspoon sea salt
- 1 teaspoon mixed peppercorns
- 1/2 cup corn flakes, crushed

Directions (Ready in about 15 minutes + marinating time | Servings 2)

✓ Place all ingredients, except for the cornflakes, in a ceramic dish. Stir to combine, cover and transfer to your refrigerator. Let it marinate at least 3 hours in your refrigerator.

✓ Discard the marinade and dredge the pork cubes in the crushed cornflakes, shaking off any residual coating.

✓ Now, cook the pork in your Air Fryer at 400 degrees F for 12 minutes. Shake the basket halfway through the cooking time.

Nutritions: 612 Calories; 24.4g Fat; 35.1g Carbs; 54.3g Protein; 6.4g Sugars

417) *Authentic Balkan-Style Cevapi*
Ingredients

- 1/2 pound lean ground pork
- 1/2 pound ground chuck
- 2 cloves garlic, minced
- 2 tablespoons green onions, chopped
- 1 tablespoon parsley, finely chopped
- 1 tablespoon coriander, finely chopped
- 1/2 teaspoon smoked paprika
- Sea salt and ground black pepper, to taste
- 2 ciabatta bread

Directions (Ready in about 55 minutes | Servings 3)

✓ Mix the ground meat with the garlic, green onion, herbs and spices.

✓ Roll the mixture into small sausages, about 3 inches long.

✓ Spritz a cooking basket with a nonstick cooking spray. Cook cevapi at 380 degrees F for 10 minutes, shaking the basket periodically to ensure even cooking.

✓ Serve in ciabatta bread with some extra onions, mustard or ketchup. Bon appétit!

Nutritions: 278 Calories; 7.4g Fat; 23.1g Carbs; 27.5g Protein; 2.6g Sugars

418) *Rustic Ground Pork-Stuffed Peppers*
Ingredients

- 1 pound lean ground pork
- 1 small-sized shallot, chopped
- 2 cloves garlic, minced
- 2 tablespoons ketchup
- Sea salt and ground black pepper, to season
- 1/2 teaspoon cayenne pepper
- 4 bell peppers, tops and cores removed
- 1 teaspoon olive oil
- 1/2 cup Colby cheese, shredded

Directions (Ready in about 20 minutes | Servings 4)

✓ Preheat a nonstick skillet over medium-high flame. Then, cook the pork and shallot for 3 minutes or until the meat is no longer pink.

✓ Add in the garlic and continue to cook until fragrant for 1 minute or so. Stir the ketchup into the skillet; season the meat mixture with salt, black pepper and cayenne pepper.

✓ Place the bell peppers cut side-up in the Air Fryer cooking basket and drizzle with oil. Spoon the meat mixture into each pepper.

✓ Cook in your Air Fryer at 360 degrees F for 12 minutes. Top with cheese and continue to bake for 4 minutes longer. Enjoy!

Nutritions: 258 Calories; 11.4g Fat; 9.3g Carbs; 25g Protein; 5g Sugars

419) *Sunday Meatball Sliders*
Ingredients

- 1/2 pound lean ground pork

- 1 shallot, chopped
- 1 teaspoon garlic, pressed
- 1 tablespoon soy sauce
- 1/2 cup quick-cooking oats
- 1 tablespoon Italian parsley, minced
- 1/2 teaspoon fresh ginger, ground
- 1/4 teaspoon ground bay laurel
- 1/2 teaspoon red pepper flakes, crushed
- Sea salt and ground black pepper, to taste
- 4 dinner rolls

Directions (Ready in about 15 minutes | Servings 2)

✓ In a mixing bowl, thoroughly combine the ground pork, shallot, garlic, soy sauce, oats, parsley, ginger and spices; stir until everything is well incorporated.

✓ Shape the mixture into 4 meatballs.

✓ Add the meatballs to the cooking basket and cook them at 360 degrees for 10 minutes. Check the meatballs halfway through the cooking time.

✓ Place one meatball on top of the bottom half of one roll. Top with the other half of the roll and serve immediately. Bon appétit!

Nutritions: 413 Calories; 11.1g Fat; 48.3g Carbs; 33.5g Protein; 6.3g Sugars

420) *Country-Style Pork Goulash*

Ingredients

- 1/2 pound pork stew meat, cut into bite-sized chunks
- 2 pork good quality sausages, sliced
- 1 small onion, sliced into rings
- 2 Italian peppers, sliced
- 1 Serrano pepper, sliced
- 2 garlic cloves, minced
- 1 tablespoon soy sauce
- 1/2 teaspoon ground cumin
- 1 bay leaf
- Salt and black pepper, to taste
- 1 cup beef stock

Directions (Ready in about 45 minutes | Servings 2)

✓ Place the pork and sausage in the Air Fryer cooking basket. Cook the meat at 380 degrees F for 15 minutes, shaking the basket once or twice; place in a heavy-bottomed pot.

✓ Now, add the onion and peppers to the cooking basket; cook your vegetables at 400 degrees F for 10 minutes and transfer to the pot with the pork and sausage.

✓ Add in the remaining ingredients and cook, partially covered, for 15 to 20 minutes until everything is cooked through.

✓ Spoon into individual bowls and serve. Enjoy!

Nutritions: 474 Calories; 27.1g Fat; 10g Carbs; 44.5g Protein; 5.7g Sugars

421) *Korean Pork Bulgogi Bowl*

Ingredients

- 2 pork loin chops
- 1 teaspoon stone-ground mustard
- 1 teaspoon cayenne pepper
- Kosher salt and ground black pepper, to taste
- 2 stalks green onion
- 1/2 teaspoon fresh ginger, grated
- 1 garlic clove, pressed
- 1 tablespoon rice wine
- 2 tablespoons gochujang chili paste
- 1 teaspoon sesame oil
- 1 tablespoon sesame seeds, lightly toasted

Directions (Ready in about 20 minutes | Servings 2)

✓ Toss the pork loin chops with the mustard, cayenne pepper, salt and black pepper.

✓ Cook in the preheated Air Fryer at 400 degrees F for 10 minutes. Check the pork chops halfway through the cooking time.

✓ Add the green onions to the cooking basket and continue to cook for a further 5 minutes.

✓ In the meantime, whisk the fresh ginger, garlic, wine, gochujang chili paste and sesame oil. Simmer the sauce for about 5 minutes until thoroughly warmed.

✓ Slice the pork loin chops into bite-sized strips and top with green onions and sauce. Garnish with sesame seeds. Enjoy!

Nutritions: 317 Calories; 13.1g Fat; 8.7g Carbs; 42.1g Protein; 2.4g Sugars

422) *Mexican Pork Quesadillas*

Ingredients

- 1/2 pound pork tenderloin, cut into strips
- 1 teaspoon peanut oil
- 1/2 teaspoon onion powder
- 1/2 teaspoon garlic powder
- 1/2 teaspoon red pepper flakes
- 1/4 teaspoon dried basil
- 1/2 teaspoon Mexican oregano
- 1/2 teaspoon dried marjoram
- Sea salt and ground black pepper, to taste
- 2 flour tortillas
- Pico de Gallo:
- 1 tomato, diced
- 3 tablespoons onion, chopped
- 3 tablespoons cilantro, chopped
- 3 tablespoons lime juice

Directions (Ready in about 25 minutes | Servings 2)

✓ Toss the pork tenderloin strips with peanut oil and spices.

✓ Cook in the preheated Air Fryer at 370 degrees F for 15 minutes, shaking the cooking basket halfway through the cooking time.

✓ Meanwhile, make the Pico de Gallo by whisking the

ingredients or it.

- ✓ Assemble your tortillas with the meat mixture and Pico de Gallo; wrap them tightly. Turn the temperature to 390 degrees F.
- ✓ Drizzle the tortillas with a nonstick cooking spray and bake about 6 minutes. Eat warm.

Nutritions: 517 Calories; 11.8g Fat; 67g Carbs; 34.5g Protein; 7.8g Sugars

423) Pork and Mushroom Kabobs

Ingredients

- 1 pound pork butt, cut into bite-sized cubes
- 8 button mushrooms
- 1 red bell pepper, sliced
- 1 green bell pepper, sliced
- 2 tablespoons soy sauce
- 2 tablespoons lime juice
- Salt and black pepper, to taste

Directions (Ready in about 20 minutes | Servings 2)

- ✓ Toss all ingredients in a bowl until well coated.
- ✓ Thread the pork cubes, mushrooms and peppers onto skewers.
- ✓ Cook in the preheated Air Fryer at 395 degrees F for 12 minutes, flipping halfway through the cooking time.

Nutritions: 385 Calories; 16.2g Fat; 11.9g Carbs; 47.5g Protein; 7.2g Sugars

424) Warm Pork Salad

Ingredients

- 1 pound pork shoulder, cut into strips
- 1/4 teaspoon fresh ginger, minced
- 1 teaspoon garlic, pressed
- 1 tablespoon olive oil
- 1 tablespoon honey
- 2 teaspoons fresh cilantro, chopped
- 1 tablespoon Worcestershire sauce
- 1 medium-sized cucumber, sliced
- 1 cup arugula
- 1 cup baby spinach
- 1 cup Romaine lettuce
- 1 tomato, diced
- 1 shallot, sliced

Directions (Ready in about 20 minutes | Servings 3)

- ✓ Spritz the Air Fryer cooking basket with a nonstick spray. Place the pork in the Air Fryer cooking basket.
- ✓ Cook at 400 degrees F for 13 minutes, shaking the basket halfway through the cooking time.
- ✓ Transfer the meat to a serving bowl and toss with the remaining ingredients.

Nutritions: 315 Calories; 13.3g Fat; 15.5g Carbs; 30.5g Protein; 10.2g Sugars

425) Delicious Chifa Chicharonnes

Ingredients

- 1/2 pound pork belly
- 2 cloves garlic, chopped
- 1 rosemary sprig, crushed
- 1 thyme sprig, crushed
- 1 teaspoon coriander
- 3 tablespoons kecap manis
- Salt and red pepper, to taste

Directions (Ready in about 1 hour 10 minutes | Servings 3)

- ✓ Put the pork belly, rind side up, in the cooking basket; add in the garlic, rosemary, thyme and coriander.
- ✓ Cook in the preheated Air Fryer at 350 degrees F for 20 minutes; turn it over and cook an additional 20 minutes.
- ✓ Turn the temperature to 400 degrees F, rub the pork belly with the kecap manis and sprinkle with salt and red pepper. Continue to cook for 15 to 20 minutes more.
- ✓ Let it rest on a wire rack for 10 minutes before slicing and serving. Enjoy!

Nutritions: 415 Calories; 40g Fat; 5.3g Carbs; 7.3g Protein; 3.6g Sugars

426) Classic Fried Bacon

Ingredients

- 1/2 pound bacon slices
- 1/2 cup tomato ketchup
- 1/4 teaspoon cayenne pepper
- 1/4 teaspoon dried marjoram
- 1 teaspoon Sriracha sauce

Directions (Ready in about 10 minutes | Servings 4)

- ✓ Place the bacon slices in the cooking basket.
- ✓ Cook the bacon slices at 400 degrees F for about 8 minutes.
- ✓ Meanwhile, make the sauce by mixing the remaining ingredients. Serve the warm bacon with the sauce on the side. Bon appétit!

Nutritions: 235 Calories; 23g Fat; 1.3g Carbs; 7.3g Protein; 1.1g Sugars

427) Chinese Five-Spice Pork Ribs

Ingredients

- 2 ½ pounds country-style pork ribs
- 1 teaspoon mustard powder
- 1 teaspoon cumin powder
- 1 teaspoon shallot powder
- 1 tablespoon Five-spice powder
- Coarse sea salt and ground black pepper
- 1 teaspoon sesame oil
- 2 tablespoons soy sauce

Directions (Ready in about 35 minutes | Servings 3)

- ✓ Toss the country-style pork ribs with spices and sesame oil and transfer them to the Air Fryer cooking basket.

✓ Cook at 360 degrees F for 20 minutes; flip them over and continue to cook an additional 14 to 15 minutes.

✓ Drizzle with soy sauce just before serving.

Nutritions: 591 Calories; 25g Fat; 6.3g Carbs; 73g Protein; 3.1g Sugars

428) *Honey and Herb Roasted Pork Tenderloin*

Ingredients

- 1 garlic clove, pressed
- 2 tablespoons honey
- 2 tablespoons Worcestershire sauce
- 2 tablespoons tequila
- 2 tablespoons yellow mustard
- 1 pound pork tenderloin, sliced into 3 pieces
- 1 teaspoon rosemary
- 1 teaspoon basil
- 1/2 teaspoon oregano
- 1/2 teaspoon parsley flakes
- Salt and black pepper, to taste

Directions (Ready in about 20 minutes + marinating time | Servings 3)

✓ In a glass bowl, thoroughly combine the garlic, honey, Worcestershire sauce, tequila and mustard.

✓ Add in the pork tenderloin pieces, cover and marinate in your refrigerator for about 1 hour.

✓ Transfer the pork tenderloin to the cooking basket, discarding the marinade. Sprinkle the pork tenderloin with herbs, salt and black pepper.

✓ Cook in your Air Fryer at 370 degrees F for 15 minutes, checking periodically and basting with the reserved marinade. Serve warm.

Nutritions: 231 Calories; 3.6g Fat; 15.3g Carbs; 32.2g Protein; 13.4g Sugars

429) *Pork Loin with Greek-Style Sauce*

Ingredients

- 1/2 pound boneless pork loin, well-trimmed
- 1 garlic clove, halved
- 1 teaspoon grainy mustard
- Kosher salt and ground black pepper, to taste
- 1/2 teaspoon lard, melted
- 1/4 cup mayonnaise
- 1/4 cup Greek-style yogurt
- 1/4 teaspoon dried dill
- 1/2 teaspoon garlic, pressed

Directions (Ready in about 55 minutes | Servings 2)

✓ Rub the pork with garlic halves on all sides; then, rub the pork with mustard. Season it with salt and pepper and drizzle with melted lard.

✓ Transfer to the Air Fryer cooking basket and cook at 360 degrees F for 45 minutes, turning over halfway through the cooking time.

✓ In the meantime, make the sauce by whisking all ingredients.

✓ Let it rest for 8 to 10 minutes before carving and serving. Serve the warm pork loin with the sauce on the side.

Nutritions: 361 Calories; 26.4g Fat; 3.3g Carbs; 26.3g Protein; 1.4g Sugars

430) *Pork Cutlets with Pearl Onions*

Ingredients

- 2 pork cutlets
- 1 teaspoon onion powder
- 1/2 teaspoon cayenne pepper
- Sea salt and black pepper, to taste
- 1/4 cup flour
- 1/4 cup Pecorino Romano cheese, grated
- 1 cup pearl onions

Directions (Ready in about 20 minutes | Servings 2)

✓ Toss the pork cutlets with the onion powder, cayenne pepper, salt, black pepper, flour and cheese.

✓ Transfer the pork cutlets to the lightly oiled cooking basket. Scatter pearl onions around the pork.

✓ Cook in the preheated Air Fryer at 360 degrees for 15 minutes, turning over halfway through the cooking time.

Nutritions: 292 Calories; 6.4g Fat; 20.3g Carbs; 36.4g Protein; 3.7g Sugars

431) *German-Style Pork with Sauerkraut*

Ingredients

- 1 pound pork butt
- 2 teaspoons olive oil
- 1 teaspoon dried thyme
- Salt and black pepper, to taste
- 1 tart apple, thinly sliced
- 1 onion, thinly sliced
- 2 garlic cloves, minced
- 1 bay leaf
- 1/2 teaspoon cayenne pepper
- 1 pound sauerkraut, drained

Directions (Ready in about 15 minutes | Servings 3)

✓ Toss the pork butt with 1 teaspoon of olive oil, thyme, salt and black pepper. Place the pork in the Air Fryer cooking basket.

✓ Cook the pork at 400 degrees F for 7 minutes. Top with apple slices and cook for a further 7 minutes.

✓ Meanwhile, heat the olive oil in a large saucepan over medium-high heat. Now, sauté the onion for 2 to 3 minutes or until just tender and translucent.

✓ Add in the garlic, bay leaf, cayenne pepper and sauerkraut and continue to cook for 10 minutes more or until cooked through.

✓ Slice the pork into 3 portions; top the warm sauerkraut with the pork. Bon appétit!

Nutritions: 298 Calories; 12g Fat; 17.5g Carbs; 30.2g Protein; 10.2g Sugars

432) *Pineapple Pork Carnitas*

Ingredients

- 1/2 pound pork loin
- 1/2 teaspoon paprika
- Kosher salt and ground black pepper, to taste
- 4 ounces fresh pineapple, crushed
- 1/4 cup water
- 1/4 cup tomato paste
- 1 tablespoon soy sauce
- 1 teaspoon brown mustard
- 1 garlic clove, minced
- 1 shallot, minced
- 1 green chili pepper, minced
- 4 (6-inch) corn tortillas, warmed

Directions (Ready in about 55 minutes | Servings 2)

- ✓ Pat the pork loin dry and season it with paprika, salt and black pepper. Then, cook the pork in your Air Fryer at 360 degrees F for 20 minutes; turn it over and cook an additional 25 minutes.
- ✓ Then, preheat a sauté pan over a moderately high heat. Combine the pineapple, water, tomato paste, soy sauce, mustard, garlic, shallot and green chili, bringing to a rolling boil.
- ✓ Turn the heat to simmer; continue to cook until the sauce has reduced by half, about 15 minutes.
- ✓ Let the pork rest for 10 minutes; then, shred the pork with two forks. Spoon the sauce over the pork and serve in corn tortillas. Enjoy!

Nutritions: 356 Calories; 7.4g Fat; 43.5g Carbs; 31.1g Protein; 16.5g Sugars

433) *Tacos Al Pastor*

Ingredients

- Pork:
- 1 pound pork loin
- 1 tablespoon honey
- Sea salt and ground black pepper, to taste
- 1/2 teaspoon cayenne pepper
- 1/2 teaspoon garlic powder
- 1/2 teaspoon thyme
- 1 teaspoon olive oil
- Tacos:
- 1 tablespoon annatto seeds
- 1 tablespoon olive oil
- 1/2 teaspoon coriander seeds
- 1 clove garlic, crushed
- 1 tablespoon apple cider vinegar
- 1 dried guajillo chili, deseeded and crushed
- 3 corn tortillas

Directions (Ready in about 50 minutes | Servings 3)

- ✓ Pat dry pork loin; toss the pork with the remaining ingredients until well coated on all sides.
- ✓ Cook in the preheated Air Fryer at 360 degrees F for 45 minutes, turning over halfway through the cooking time.
- ✓ In the meantime, make the achiote paste by mixing the annatto seeds, olive oil, coriander seeds, garlic, apple cider vinegar and dried guajillo chili in your blender.
- ✓ Slice the pork into bite-sized pieces. Spoon the pork and achiote onto warmed tortillas. Enjoy!

Nutritions: 356 Calories; 14.4g Fat; 19.6g Carbs; 36.3g Protein; 6.8g Sugars

434) *Italian Nonna's Polpette*

Ingredients

- 1 teaspoon olive oil
- 2 tablespoons green onions, chopped
- 1/2 teaspoon garlic, pressed
- 1/2 pound sweet Italian pork sausage, crumbled
- 1 tablespoon parsley, chopped
- 1/2 teaspoon cayenne pepper
- Sea salt and ground black pepper, to taste
- 1 egg
- 2 tablespoons milk
- 1 crustless bread slice

Directions (Ready in about 15 minutes | Servings 3)

- ✓ Mix the olive oil, green onions, garlic, sausage, parsley, cayenne pepper, salt and black pepper in a bowl.
- ✓ Whisk the egg and milk until pale and frothy. Soak the bread in the milk mixture. Add the soaked bread to the sausage mixture. Mix again to combine well.
- ✓ Shape the mixture into 8 meatballs.
- ✓ Add the meatballs to the cooking basket and cook them at 360 degrees for 5 minutes. Then, turn them and cook the other side for 5 minutes more. You can serve these meatballs over spaghetti. Bon appétit!

Nutritions: 356 Calories; 14.4g Fat; 19.6g Carbs; 36.3g Protein; 6.8g Sugars

435) *Pork Sausage with Baby Potatoes*

Ingredients

- 1 pound pork sausage, uncooked
- 1 pound baby potatoes
- 1/4 teaspoon paprika
- 1/2 teaspoon dried rosemary leaves, crushed
- Himalayan salt and black pepper, to taste

Direction(Ready in about 35 minutes | Servings 3)

- ✓ Put the sausage into the Air Fryer cooking basket.
- ✓ Cook in the preheated Air Fryer at 380 degrees F for 15 minutes; reserve.
- ✓ Season the baby potatoes with paprika, rosemary, salt and black pepper. Add the baby potatoes to the cooking basket.
- ✓ Cook the potatoes at 400 degrees F for 15 minutes, shaking the basket once or twice. Serve warm sausages with baby potatoes and enjoy!

Nutritions: 640 Calories; 47.5g Fat; 27.4g Carbs; 24.3g Protein; 1.1g Sugars

436) *Caprese Pork Chops*

Ingredients

- 1 pound center-cut pork chops, boneless
- 1/4 cup balsamic vinegar
- 1 tablespoon honey
- 1 tablespoon whole-grain mustard
- 1/2 teaspoon olive oil
- 1/2 teaspoon smoked paprika
- Salt and black pepper, to taste
- 1/2 teaspoon shallot powder
- 1/2 teaspoon porcini powder
- 1/2 teaspoon granulated garlic
- 3 slices fresh mozzarella
- 3 thick slices tomatoes
- 2 tablespoons fresh basil leaves, chopped

Directions (Ready in about 15 minutes + marinating time | Servings 3)

- ✓ Place the pork chops, balsamic vinegar, honey, mustard, olive oil and spices in a bowl. Cover and let it marinate in your refrigerator for 1 hour.
- ✓ Cook in the preheated Air Fryer at 400 degrees F for 7 minutes. Top with cheese and continue to cook for 5 minutes more.
- ✓ Top with sliced tomato and basil and serve immediately.

Nutritions: 345 Calories; 12.9g Fat; 14.7g Carbs; 40.3g Protein; 10.8g Sugars

437) *Keto Crispy Pork Chops*

Ingredients

- 3 center-cut pork chops, boneless
- 1/2 teaspoon paprika
- Sea salt and ground black pepper, to taste
- 1/4 cup Romano cheese, grated
- 1/4 cup crushed pork rinds
- 1/2 teaspoon garlic powder
- 1/2 teaspoon mustard seeds
- 1/2 teaspoon dried marjoram
- 1 egg, beaten
- 1 tablespoon buttermilk
- 1 teaspoon peanut oil

Directions (Ready in about 20 minutes | Servings 3)

- ✓ Pat the pork chops dry with kitchen towels. Season them with paprika, salt and black pepper.
- ✓ Add the Romano cheese, crushed pork rinds, garlic powder, mustard seeds and marjoram to a rimmed plate.
- ✓ Beat the egg and buttermilk in another plate. Now, dip the pork chops in the egg, then in the cheese/pork rind mixture.
- ✓ Drizzle the pork with peanut oil. Cook in the preheated Air Fryer at 400 degrees F for 12 minutes, flipping pork chops halfway through the cooking time.
- ✓ Serve with keto-friendly sides such as cauliflower

rice. Bon appétit!

Nutritions: 467 Calories; 26.8g Fat; 2.7g Carbs; 50.3g Protein; 1.3g Sugars

438) *The Best BBQ Ribs Ever*

Ingredients

- 1/2 pound ribs
- Sea salt and black pepper, to taste
- 1/2 teaspoon red chili flakes
- 1 tablespoon agave syrup
- 1/2 teaspoon garlic powder
- 1/2 cup tomato paste
- 1 teaspoon brown mustard
- 1 tablespoon balsamic vinegar
- 1 tablespoon Worcestershire sauce

Directions (Ready in about 40 minutes | Servings 2)

- ✓ Place the pork ribs, salt, black pepper and red pepper flakes in a Ziplock bag; shake until the ribs are coated on all sides.
- ✓ Roast in the preheated Air Fryer at 350 degrees F for 35 minutes.
- ✓ In a saucepan over medium heat, heat all sauce ingredients, bringing to a boil. Turn the heat to a simmer until the sauce has reduced by half.
- ✓ Spoon the sauce over the ribs and serve warm. Bon appétit!

Nutritions: 492 Calories; 33.5g Fat; 26.8g Carbs; 22.5g Protein; 19.7g Sugars

439) *Easy Pork Pot Stickers*

Ingredients

- 1/2 pound lean ground pork
- 1/2 teaspoon fresh ginger, freshly grated
- 1 teaspoon chili garlic sauce
- 1 tablespoon soy sauce
- 1 tablespoon rice wine
- 1/4 teaspoon Szechuan pepper
- 2 stalks scallions, chopped
- 1 tablespoon sesame oil
- 8 (3-inch) round wonton wrappers

Directions (Ready in about 10 minutes | Servings 2)

- ✓ Cook the ground pork in a preheated skillet until no longer pink, crumbling with a fork. Stir in the other ingredients, except for the wonton wrappers; stir to combine well.
- ✓ Place the wonton wrappers on a clean work surface. Divide the pork filling between the wrappers. Wet the edge of each wrapper with water, fold the top half over the bottom half and pinch the border to seal.
- ✓ Place the pot stickers in the cooking basket and brush them with a little bit of olive oil. Cook the pot sticker at 400 degrees F for 8 minutes. Serve immediately.

Nutritions: 352 Calories; 13.5g Fat; 27.8g Carbs; 31.2g Protein; 2.2g Sugars

440) *Chinese Char Siu Pork*

Ingredients

- 1 pound pork shoulder, cut into long strips
- 1/2 teaspoon Chinese five-spice powder
- 1/4 teaspoon Szechuan pepper
- 1 tablespoon hoisin sauce
- 2 tablespoons hot water
- 1 teaspoon sesame oil
- 1 tablespoon Shaoxing wine
- 1 tablespoon molasses

Directions (Ready in about 25 minutes + marinating time | Servings 3)

- ✓ Place all ingredients in a ceramic dish and let it marinate for 2 hours in the refrigerator.
- ✓ Cook in the preheated Air Fryer at 390 degrees F for 20 minutes, shaking the basket halfway through the cooking time.
- ✓ Heat the reserved marinade in a wok for about 15 minutes or until the sauce has thickened. Spoon the sauce over the warm pork shoulder and serve with rice if desired. Enjoy!

Nutritions: 246 Calories; 10.3g Fat; 7.8g Carbs; 28.6g Protein; 6.7g Sugars

441) *Texas Pulled Pork*

Ingredients

- 1 pound pork shoulder roast
- 1 teaspoon butter, softened
- 1 teaspoon Italian seasoning mix
- 1/2 cup barbecue sauce
- 1/4 cup apple juice
- 1 teaspoon garlic paste
- 2 tablespoons soy sauce
- 2 hamburger buns, split

Directions (Ready in about 1 hour | Servings 3)

- ✓ Brush the pork shoulder with butter and sprinkle with Italian seasoning mix on all sides.
- ✓ Cook in the preheated Air Fryer at 360 degrees F for 1 hour, shaking the basket once or twice.
- ✓ Meanwhile, warm the barbecue sauce, apple juice, garlic paste and soy sauce in a small saucepan.
- ✓ Remove the pork shoulder from the basket and shred the meat with two forks. Spoon the sauce over the pork and stir to combine well.
- ✓ Spoon the pork into the toasted buns and eat warm. Bon appétit!

Nutritions: 415 Calories; 10.7g Fat; 39.3g Carbs; 37.9g Protein; 21.7g Sugars

442) *Herb-Crusted Pork Roast*

Ingredients

- 1/2 pound pork loin
- Salt and black pepper, to taste
- 1/2 teaspoon onion powder
- 1/2 teaspoon parsley flakes
- 1/2 teaspoon oregano
- 1/2 teaspoon thyme
- 1/2 teaspoon grated lemon peel
- 1 teaspoon garlic, minced
- 1 teaspoon butter, softened

Directions (Ready in about 1 hour | Servings 2)

- ✓ Pat the pork loin dry with kitchen towels. Season it with salt and black pepper.
- ✓ In a bowl, mix the remaining ingredients until well combined.
- ✓ Coat the pork with the herb rub, pressing to adhere well.
- ✓ Cook in the preheated Air Fryer at 360 degrees F for 30 minutes; turn it over and cook on the other side for 25 minutes more.

Nutritions: 220 Calories; 11.4g Fat; 3.3g Carbs; 24.9g Protein; 1.7g Sugars

443) *Perfect Meatball Hoagies*

Ingredients

- 1/2 pound lean ground pork
- 1 teaspoon fresh garlic, minced
- 2 tablespoons fresh scallions, chopped
- 1 teaspoon dried basil
- 1/2 teaspoon dried oregano
- 1/2 teaspoon dried parsley flakes
- Sea salt and ground black pepper, to taste
- 1 tablespoon soy sauce
- 1 egg, beaten
- 1/4 cup Pecorino Romano cheese, grated
- 1/2 cup quick-cooking oats
- 2 hoagie rolls
- 1 medium-sized tomato, sliced
- 2 pickled cherry peppers

Directions(Ready in about 15 minutes | Servings 2)

- ✓ In a mixing bowl, thoroughly combine the ground pork, garlic, scallions, basil, oregano, parsley, salt, black pepper, soy sauce, eggs, cheese and quick-cooking oats. Mix until well incorporated.
- ✓ Shape the mixture into 6 meatballs.
- ✓ Add the meatballs to the cooking basket and cook them at 360 degrees for 10 minutes. Turn the meatballs halfway through the cooking time.
- ✓ Cut the hoagie rolls lengthwise almost entirely through. Layer the meatballs onto the bottom of the roll.
- ✓ Top with the tomato and peppers. Close the rolls, cut in half and serve immediately.

Nutritions: 433 Calories; 16.4g Fat; 33g Carbs; 39.7g Protein; 7g Sugars

444) *Balsamic Pork Chops with Asparagus*

Ingredients

- 2 pork loin chops
- 1 pound asparagus spears, cleaned and trimmed
- 1 teaspoon sesame oil

- 2 tablespoons balsamic vinegar
- 1 teaspoon yellow mustard
- 1/2 teaspoon garlic, minced
- 1/2 teaspoon smoked pepper
- 1/4 teaspoon dried dill
- Salt and black pepper, to taste

Directions (Ready in about 15 minutes | Servings 2)

✓ Toss the pork loin chops and asparagus with the other ingredients until well coated on all sides.

✓ Place the pork in the Air Fryer cooking basket and cook at 400 degrees F for 7 minutes; turn them over, top with the asparagus and continue to cook for a further 5 minutes.

✓ Serve warm with mayo, sriracha sauce, or sour cream if desired. Bon appétit!

Nutritions: 308 Calories; 9.4g Fat; 11.9g Carbs; 44.3g Protein; 6.6g Sugars

445) *Bacon with Onions Rings and Remoulade Sauce*

Ingredients

- 2 thick bacon slices
- 8 ounces onion rings, frozen
- 1 teaspoon yellow mustard
- 2 tablespoons mayonnaise
- 1/4 teaspoon paprika
- 1 teaspoon hot sauce
- Salt and black pepper, to taste

Directions (Ready in about 15 minutes | Servings 2)

✓ Place the slices of bacon and onion rings in the Air Fryer cooking basket.

✓ Cook the bacon and onion rings at 400 degrees F for 4 minutes; shake the basket and cook for a further 4 minutes or until cooked through.

✓ Meanwhile, make the Remoulade sauce by whisking the remaining ingredients. Arrange the bacon and onion rings on plates and garnish with Remoulade sauce.

Nutritions: 371 Calories; 32.7g Fat; 11.2g Carbs; 8.5g Protein; 5.3g Sugars

446) *Authentic Greek Pork Gyro*

Ingredients

- 3/4 pound pork butt
- Sea salt and ground black pepper, to taste
- 1/2 teaspoon red pepper flakes, crushed
- 1 teaspoon ground coriander
- 1/2 teaspoon mustard seeds
- 1/2 teaspoon granulated garlic
- 1/2 teaspoon oregano
- 1/2 teaspoon basil
- 1 teaspoon olive oil
- 2 pita bread, warmed
- 4 lettuce leaves
- 1 small tomato, diced

- 2 tablespoons red onion, chopped
- Tzatziki:
- 1/2 cup Greek-style yogurt
- 1 tablespoon cucumber, minced and drained
- 1 teaspoon fresh lemon juice
- 1 teaspoon fresh dill, minced
- 1/4 teaspoon fresh garlic, pressed

Directions (Ready in about 20 minutes | Servings 2)

✓ Toss the pork butt with salt, black pepper, red pepper flakes, coriander, mustard seeds, granulated garlic, oregano, basil and olive oil.

✓ Transfer the pork butt to the Air Fryer cooking basket.

✓ Cook the pork at 400 degrees F for 7 minutes. Turn the pork over and cook for a further 7 minutes. Shred the meat with two forks.

✓ In the meantime, make the Tzatziki sauce by whisking all ingredients until everything is well combined.

✓ Spoon the pork onto each pita bread; top with Tzatziki, lettuce, tomato and red onion. Serve immediately and enjoy!

Nutritions: 493 Calories; 26.2g Fat; 26.9g Carbs; 36.2g Protein; 7.5g Sugars

447) *Autumn Boston Butt with Acorn Squash*

Ingredients

- 1 pound Boston butt
- 1 garlic clove, pressed
- 1/4 cup rice wine
- 1 teaspoon molasses
- 1 tablespoon Hoisin sauce
- 1/2 teaspoon red pepper flakes
- 1 teaspoon Sichuan pepper
- 1/2 teaspoon Himalayan salt
- 1/2 pound acorn squash, cut into 1/2-inch cubes

Directions (Ready in about 25 minutes + marinating time | Servings 3)

✓ Place the Boston butt, garlic, rice wine, molasses, Hoisin sauce, red pepper flakes, Sichuan pepper and Himalayan salt in a ceramic dish.

✓ Cover and allow it to marinate for 2 hours in your refrigerator.

✓ Cook in the preheated Air Fryer at 400 degrees F for 10 minutes. Turn the Boston butt over and baste with the reserved marinade.

✓ Stir the squash cubes into the cooking basket and cook for 10 minutes on the other side. Taste, adjust seasonings and serve immediately.

Nutritions: 396 Calories; 13.3g Fat; 20.9g Carbs; 44.2g Protein; 6.3g Sugars

448) *Rustic Pizza with Ground Pork*

Ingredients

- 1 (10-count) can refrigerator biscuits
- 4 tablespoons tomato paste

- 1 tablespoon tomato ketchup
- 2 teaspoons brown mustard
- 1/2 cup ground pork
- 1/2 cup ground beef sausage
- 1 red onion, thinly sliced
- 1/2 cup mozzarella cheese, shredded

Directions (Ready in about 30 minutes | Servings 4)

✓ Spritz the sides and bottom of a baking pan with a nonstick cooking spray.

✓ Press five biscuits into the pan. Brush the top of biscuit with 2 tablespoons of tomato paste.

✓ Add 1/2 tablespoon of ketchup, 1 teaspoon of mustard, 1/4 cup of ground pork, 1/4 cup of beef sausage. Top with 1/2 of the red onion slices.

✓ Bake in the preheated Air Fryer at 360 degrees F for 10 minutes. Top with 1/4 cup of mozzarella cheese and bake another 5 minutes.

✓ Repeat the process with the second pizza. Slice the pizza into halves, serve and enjoy!

Nutritions: 529 Calories; 9.6g Fat; 65.5g Carbs; 37.9g Protein; 0.9g Sugars

449)   *Pork Koftas with Yoghurt Sauce*

Ingredients

- 2 teaspoons olive oil
- 1/2 pound ground pork
- 1/2 pound ground beef
- 1 egg, whisked
- Sea salt and ground black pepper, to taste
- 1 teaspoon paprika
- 2 garlic cloves, minced
- 1 teaspoon dried marjoram
- 1 teaspoon mustard seeds
- 1/2 teaspoon celery seeds
- Yogurt Sauce:
- 2 tablespoons olive oil
- 2 tablespoons fresh lemon juice
- Sea salt, to taste
- 1/4 teaspoon red pepper flakes, crushed
- 1/2 cup full-fat yogurt
- 1 teaspoon dried dill weed

Directions (Ready in about 25 minutes | Servings 4)

✓ Spritz the sides and bottom of the cooking basket with 2 teaspoons of olive oil.

✓ In a mixing dish, thoroughly combine the ground pork, beef, egg, salt, black pepper, paprika, garlic, marjoram, mustard seeds, and celery seeds.

✓ Form the mixture into kebabs and transfer them to the greased cooking basket. Cook at 365 degrees F for 11 to 12 minutes, turning them over once or twice.

✓ In the meantime, mix all the sauce ingredients and place in the refrigerator until ready to serve. Serve the pork koftas with the yogurt sauce on the side. Enjoy!

Nutritions: 407 Calories; 28.5g Fat; 3.4g Carbs; 32.9g

Protein; 1.3g Sugars

450)   *Spicy Bacon-Wrapped Tater Tots*

Ingredients

- 10 thin slices of bacon
- 10 tater tots, frozen
- 1 teaspoon cayenne pepper
- Sauce:
- 1/4 cup mayo
- 4 tablespoons ketchup
- 1 teaspoon rice vinegar
- 1 teaspoon chili powder

Directions (Ready in about 25 minutes | Servings 5)

✓ Lay the slices of bacon on your working surface. Place a tater tot on one end of each slice; sprinkle with cayenne pepper and roll them over.

✓ Cook in the preheated Air Fryer at 390 degrees F for 15 to 16 minutes.

✓ Whisk all ingredients for the sauce in a mixing bowl and store in your refrigerator, covered, until ready to serve.

✓ Serve Bacon-Wrapped Tater Tots with the sauce on the side. Enjoy!

Nutritions: 297 Calories; 26.1g Fat; 9.3g Carbs; 7.1g Protein; 3.2g Sugars

451)   *Pork Cutlets with a Twist*

Ingredients

- 1 cup water
- 1 cup red wine
- 1 tablespoon sea salt
- 2 pork cutlets
- 1/2 cup all-purpose flour
- 1 teaspoon shallot powder
- 1/2 teaspoon porcini powder
- Sea salt and ground black pepper, to taste
- 1 egg
- 1/4 cup yogurt
- 1 teaspoon brown mustard
- 1 cup tortilla chips, crushed

Directions(Ready in about 1 hour 20 minutes | Servings 2)

✓ In a large ceramic dish, combine the water, wine and salt. Add the pork cutlets and put for 1 hour in the refrigerator.

✓ In a shallow bowl, mix the flour, shallot powder, porcini powder, salt, and ground pepper. In another bowl, whisk the eggs with yogurt and mustard.

✓ In a third bowl, place the crushed tortilla chips.

✓ Dip the pork cutlets in the flour mixture and toss evenly; then, in the egg mixture. Finally, roll them over the crushed tortilla chips.

✓ Spritz the bottom of the cooking basket with cooking oil. Add the breaded pork cutlets and cook at 395 degrees F and for 10 minutes.

✓ Flip and cook for 5 minutes more on the other side.

Serve warm.

Nutritions: 579 Calories; 19.4g Fat; 50g Carbs; 49.6g Protein; 2.2g Sugars

452) *Cheesy Creamy Pork Casserole*

Ingredients

- 2 tablespoons olive oil
- 2 pounds pork tenderloin, cut into serving-size pieces
- 1 teaspoon coarse sea salt
- 1/2 teaspoon freshly ground pepper
- 1/4 teaspoon chili powder
- 1 teaspoon dried marjoram
- 1 tablespoon mustard
- 1 cup Ricotta cheese
- 1 ½ cups chicken broth

Directions (Ready in about 25 minutes | Servings 4)

- ✓ Start by preheating your Air Fryer to 350 degrees F.
- ✓ Heat the olive oil in a pan over medium-high heat. Once hot, cook the pork for 6 to 7 minutes, flipping it to ensure even cooking.
- ✓ Arrange the pork in a lightly greased casserole dish. Season with salt, black pepper, chili powder, and marjoram.
- ✓ In a mixing dish, thoroughly combine the mustard, cheese, and chicken broth. Pour the mixture over the pork chops in the casserole dish.
- ✓ Bake for another 15 minutes or until bubbly and heated through.

Nutritions: 433 Calories; 20.4g Fat; 2.6g Carbs; 56.5g Protein; 0.3g Sugars

453) *Herbed Pork Loin with Carrot Chips*

Ingredients

- 1 tablespoon peanut oil
- 1 ½ pounds pork loin, cut into 4 pieces
- Coarse sea salt and ground black pepper, to taste
- 1/2 teaspoon onion powder
- 1 teaspoon garlic powder
- 1/2 teaspoon cayenne pepper
- 1/2 teaspoon dried rosemary
- 1/2 teaspoon dried basil
- 1/2 teaspoon dried oregano
- 1 pound carrots, cut into matchsticks
- 1 tablespoon coconut oil, melted

Directions(Ready in about 1 hour 15 minutes | Servings 4)

- ✓ Drizzle 1 tablespoon of peanut oil all over the pork loin. Season with salt, black pepper, onion powder, garlic powder, cayenne pepper, rosemary, basil, and oregano.
- ✓ Cook in the preheated Air Fryer at 360 degrees F for 55 minutes; make sure to turn the pork over every 15 minutes to ensure even cooking.

- ✓ Test for doneness with a meat thermometer.
- ✓ Toss the carrots with melted coconut oil; season to taste and cook in the preheated Air Fryer at 380 degrees F for 15 minutes.
- ✓ Serve the warm pork loin with the carrots on the side. Enjoy!

Nutritions: 461 Calories; 25.8g Fat; 10.8g Carbs; 44g Protein; 5.3g Sugars

454) *Easy Pork & Parmesan Meatballs*

Ingredients

- 1 pound ground pork
- 2 tablespoons tamari sauce
- 1 teaspoon garlic, minced
- 2 tablespoons spring onions, finely chopped
- 1 tablespoon brown sugar
- 1 tablespoon olive oil
- 1/2 cup breadcrumbs
- 2 tablespoons parmesan cheese, preferably freshly grated

Directions (Ready in about 15 minutes | Servings 3)

- ✓ Combine the ground pork, tamari sauce, garlic, onions, and sugar in a mixing dish. Mix until everything is well incorporated.
- ✓ Form the mixture into small meatballs.
- ✓ In a shallow bowl, mix the olive oil, breadcrumbs, and parmesan. Roll the meatballs over the parmesan mixture.
- ✓ Cook at 380 degrees F for 3 minutes; shake the basket and cook an additional 4 minutes or until meatballs are browned on all sides.

Nutritions: 539 Calories; 38.4g Fat; 17.5g Carbs; 29.2g Protein; 4.3g Sugars

455) *Italian-Style Honey Roasted Pork*

Ingredients

- 1 teaspoon Celtic sea salt
- 1/2 teaspoon black pepper, freshly cracked
- 1/4 cup red wine
- 2 tablespoons mustard
- 2 tablespoons honey
- 2 garlic cloves, minced
- 1 pound pork top loin
- 1 tablespoon Italian herb seasoning blend

Directions (Ready in about 50 minutes | Servings 3)

- ✓ In a ceramic bowl, mix the salt, black pepper, red wine, mustard, honey, and garlic. Add the pork top loin and let it marinate at least 30 minutes.
- ✓ Spritz the sides and bottom of the cooking basket with a nonstick cooking spray.
- ✓ Place the pork top loin in the basket; sprinkle with the Italian herb seasoning blend.
- ✓ Cook the pork tenderloin at 370 degrees F for 10 minutes. Flip halfway through, spraying with cooking oil and cook for 5 to 6 minutes more. Serve immediately.

Nutritions: 314 Calories; 9.8g Fat; 13g Carbs; 41.8g

Protein; 11.8g Sugars

456)   *Ground Pork and Cheese Casserole*

Ingredients

- 1 tablespoon olive oil
- 1 ½ pounds pork, ground
- Sea salt and ground black pepper, to taste
- 1 medium-sized leek, sliced
- 1 teaspoon fresh garlic, minced
- 2 carrots, trimmed and sliced
- 1 (2-ounce) jar pimiento, drained and chopped
- 1 can (10 ¾-ounces) condensed cream of mushroom soup
- 1 cup water
- 1/2 cup ale
- 1 cup cream cheese
- 1/2 cup soft fresh breadcrumbs
- 1 tablespoon fresh cilantro, chopped

Directions (Ready in about 45 minutes | Servings 4)

✓ Start by preheating your Air Fryer to 320 degrees F.

✓ Add the olive oil to a baking dish and heat for 1 to 2 minutes. Add the pork, salt, pepper and cook for 6 minutes, crumbling with a fork.

✓ Add the leeks and cook for 4 to 5 minutes, stirring occasionally.

✓ Add the garlic, carrots, pimiento, mushroom soup, water, ale, and cream cheese. Gently stir to combine.

✓ Turn the temperature to 370 degrees F.

✓ Top with the breadcrumbs. Place the baking dish in the cooking basket and cook approximately 30 minutes or until everything is thoroughly cooked. Serve garnished with fresh cilantro.

Nutritions: 561 Calories; 28g Fat; 22.2g Carbs; 52.5g Protein; 7.7g Sugars

457)   *Mexican-Style Ground Pork with Peppers*

Ingredients

- 2 chili peppers
- 1 red bell pepper
- 2 tablespoons olive oil
- 1 large-sized shallot, chopped
- 1 pound ground pork
- 2 garlic cloves, minced
- 2 ripe tomatoes, pureed
- 1 teaspoon dried marjoram
- 1/2 teaspoon mustard seeds
- 1/2 teaspoon celery seeds
- 1 teaspoon Mexican oregano
- 1 tablespoon fish sauce
- 2 tablespoons fresh coriander, chopped
- Salt and ground black pepper, to taste

- 2 cups water
- 1 tablespoon chicken bouillon granules
- 2 tablespoons sherry wine
- 1 cup Mexican cheese blend

Directions (Ready in about 40 minutes | Servings 4)

✓ Roast the peppers in the preheated Air Fryer at 395 degrees F for 10 minutes, flipping them halfway through cook time.

✓ Let them steam for 10 minutes; then, peel the skin and discard the stems and seeds. Slice the peppers into halves.

✓ Heat the olive oil in a baking pan at 380 degrees F for 2 minutes; add the shallots and cook for 4 minutes. Add the ground pork and garlic; cook for a further 4 to 5 minutes.

✓ After that, stir in the tomatoes, marjoram, mustard seeds, celery seeds, oregano, fish sauce, coriander, salt, and pepper. Add a layer of sliced peppers to the baking pan.

✓ Mix the water with the chicken bouillon granules and sherry wine. Add the mixture to the baking pan.

✓ Cook in the preheated Air Fryer at 395 degrees F for 10 minutes. Top with cheese and bake an additional 5 minutes until the cheese has melted. Serve immediately.

Nutritions: 505 Calories; 39.4g Fat; 9.9g Carbs; 28g Protein; 5.1g Sugars

458)   *Pork Shoulder with Molasses Sauce*

Ingredients

- 2 tablespoons molasses
- 2 tablespoons soy sauce
- 2 tablespoons Shaoxing wine
- 2 garlic cloves, minced
- 1 teaspoon fresh ginger, minced
- 1 tablespoon cilantro stems and leaves, finely chopped
- 1 pound boneless pork shoulder
- 2 tablespoons sesame oil

Directions (Ready in about 25 minutes + marinating time | Servings 3)

✓ In a large-sized ceramic dish, thoroughly combine the molasses, soy sauce, wine, garlic, ginger, and cilantro; add the pork shoulder and allow it to marinate for 2 hours in the refrigerator.

✓ Then, grease the cooking basket with sesame oil. Place the pork shoulder in the cooking basket; reserve the marinade.

✓ Cook in the preheated Air Fryer at 395 degrees F for 14 to 17 minutes, flipping and basting with the marinade halfway through. Let it rest for 5 to 6 minutes before slicing and serving.

✓ While the pork is roasting, cook the marinade in a preheated skillet over medium heat; cook until it has thickened.

✓ Brush the pork shoulder with the sauce and enjoy!

Nutritions: 353 Calories; 19.6g Fat; 13.5g Carbs; 29.2g Protein; 12.2g Sugars

459) *Tender Spare Ribs*
Ingredients
- 1 rack pork spareribs, fat trimmed and cut in half
- 2 tablespoons fajita seasoning
- 2 tablespoons smoked paprika
- Sea salt and pepper, to taste
- 1 tablespoon prepared brown mustard
- 3 tablespoons Worcestershire sauce
- 1/2 cup beer
- 1 tablespoon peanut oil

Directions (Ready in about 35 minutes + marinating time | Servings 4)
✓ Toss the spareribs with the fajita seasoning, paprika, salt, pepper, mustard, and Worcestershire sauce. Pour in the beer and let it marinate for 1 hour in your refrigerator.
✓ Rub the sides and bottom of the cooking basket with peanut oil.
✓ Cook the spareribs in the preheated Air Fryer at 365 degrees for 17 minutes. Turn the ribs over and cook an additional 14 to 15 minutes. Serve warm. Bon appétit!

Nutritions: 443 Calories; 35.2g Fat; 10g Carbs; 20.5g Protein; 3.1g Sugars

460) *Pork Belly with New Potatoes*
Ingredients
- 1 ½ pounds pork belly, cut into 4 pieces
- Kosher salt and ground black pepper, to taste
- 1 teaspoon smoked paprika
- 1/2 teaspoon turmeric powder
- 2 tablespoons oyster sauce
- 2 tablespoons green onions
- 4 cloves garlic, sliced
- 1 pound new potatoes, scrubbed

Directions(Ready in about 50 minutes | Servings 4)
✓ Preheat your Air Fryer to 390 degrees F. Pat dry the pork belly and season with all spices listed above.
✓ Add the oyster sauce and spritz with a nonstick cooking spray on all sides. Now, cook in the preheated Air Fryer for 30 minutes. Turn them over every 10 minutes.
✓ Increase the temperature to 400 degrees F. Add the green onions, garlic, and new potatoes.
✓ Cook another 15 minutes, shaking occasionally. Serve warm.

Nutritions: 547 Calories; 30.2g Fat; 20.9g Carbs; 45.1g Protein; 1.1g Sugars

461) *Smoky Mini Meatloaves with Cheese*
Ingredients
- 1 pound ground pork
- 1/2 pound ground beef
- 1 package onion soup mix
- 1/2 cup seasoned bread crumbs
- 4 tablespoons Romano cheese, grated
- 2 eggs
- 1 carrot, grated
- 1 bell pepper, chopped
- 1 serrano pepper, minced
- 2 scallions, chopped
- 2 cloves garlic, finely chopped
- 2 tablespoons soy sauce sauce
- Sea salt and black pepper, to your liking
- Glaze:
- 1/2 cup tomato paste
- 2 tablespoons ketchup
- 1 tablespoon brown mustard
- 1 teaspoon smoked paprika
- 1 tablespoon honey

Directions (Ready in about 50 minutes | Servings 4)
✓ In a large mixing bowl, thoroughly combine all ingredients for the meatloaf. Mix with your hands until everything is well incorporated.
✓ Then, shape the mixture into four mini loaves. Transfer them to the cooking basket previously generously greased with cooking oil.
✓ Cook in the preheated Air Fryer at 385 degrees F approximately 43 minutes.
✓ Mix all ingredients for the glaze. Spread the glaze over mini meatloaves and cook for another 6 minutes. Bon appétit!

Nutritions: 585 Calories; 38.4g Fat; 22.2g Carbs; 38.5g Protein; 14.6g Sugars

462) *Asian Sticky Ribs*
Ingredients
- 1 teaspoon salt
- 1 teaspoon cayenne pepper
- 1/2 teaspoon ground black pepper
- 2 teaspoons raw honey
- 2 garlic cloves, minced
- 1 (1-inch) piece ginger, peeled and grated
- 1/2 teaspoon onion powder
- 1/2 teaspoon porcini powder
- 1 teaspoon mustard seeds
- 1 tablespoon sweet chili sauce
- 1 tablespoon balsamic vinegar
- 1 ½ pounds pork country-style ribs

Directions (Ready in about 40 minutes | Servings 4)
✓ In a mixing bowl, combine the salt, cayenne pepper, black pepper, honey, garlic, ginger, onion powder, porcini powder, mustard seeds, sweet chili sauce, and balsamic vinegar.
✓ Toss and rub the seasoning mixture all over the pork ribs.
✓ Cook the country-style ribs at 360 degrees F for 15 minutes; flip the ribs and cook an additional 20

minutes or until they are tender inside and crisp on the outside.

✓ Serve warm, garnished with fresh chives if desired.
Nutritions: 446 Calories; 29.6g Fat; 5.5g Carbs; 45.1g Protein; 4.1g Sugars

463)   *Country-Style Pork Meatloaf*
Ingredients

- 1/2 pound lean minced pork
- 1/3 cup breadcrumbs
- 1/2 tablespoons minced green garlic
- 1½ tablespoon fresh cilantro, minced
- 1/2 tablespoon fish sauce
- 1/3 teaspoon dried basil
- 2 leeks, chopped
- 2 tablespoons tomato puree
- 1/2 teaspoons dried thyme
- Salt and ground black pepper, to taste

Directions (Ready in about 25 minutes | Servings 4)

✓ Add all ingredients, except for breadcrumbs, to a large-sized mixing dish and combine everything using your hands.

✓ Lastly, add the breadcrumbs to form a meatloaf.

✓ Bake for 23 minutes at 365 degrees F. Afterward, allow your meatloaf to rest for 10 minutes before slicing and serving. Bon appétit!

Nutritions:460 Calories; 26.6g Carbs; 48.9g Protein;

464)   *Grilled Lemony Pork Chops*
Ingredients

- 5 pork chops
- 1/3 cup vermouth
- 1/2 teaspoon paprika
- 2 sprigs thyme, only leaves, crushed
- 1/2 teaspoon dried oregano
- Fresh parsley, to serve
- 1 teaspoon garlic salt½ lemon, cut into wedges
- 1 teaspoon freshly cracked black pepper
- 3 tablespoons lemon juice
- 3 cloves garlic, minced
- 2 tablespoons canola oil

Directions (Ready in about 34 minutes | Servings 5)

✓ Firstly, heat the canola oil in a sauté pan over a moderate heat. Now, sweat the garlic until just fragrant.

✓ Remove the pan from the heat and pour in the lemon juice and vermouth. Now, throw in the seasonings. Dump the sauce into a baking dish, along with the pork chops.

✓ Tuck the lemon wedges among the pork chops and air-fry for 27 minutes at 345 degrees F. Bon appétit!

Nutritions: 400 Calories; 23g Fat; 4.1g Carbs; 40.5g Protein; 1.5g Sugars

465)   *Herbed Crumbed Filet Mignon*
Ingredients

- 1/2 pound filet mignon
- Sea salt and ground black pepper, to your liking
- 1/2 teaspoon cayenne pepper
- 1 teaspoon dried basil
- 1 teaspoon dried rosemary
- 1 teaspoon dried thyme
- 1 tablespoon sesame oil
- 1 small-sized egg, well-whisked
- 1/2 cup seasoned breadcrumbs

Directions (Ready in about 20 minutes | Servings 4)

✓ Season the filet mignon with salt, black pepper, cayenne pepper, basil, rosemary, and thyme. Brush with sesame oil.

✓ Put the egg in a shallow plate. Now, place the breadcrumbs in another plate.

✓ Coat the filet mignon with the egg; then, lay it into the crumbs. Set your Air Fryer to cook at 360 degrees F.

✓ Cook for 10 to 13 minutes or until golden. Serve with mixed salad leaves and enjoy!

Nutritions: 268 Calories; 14.5g Fat; 1.0g Carbs; 32.0g Protein; 0.0g Sugars

466)   *The Best London Broil Ever*
Ingredients

- 2 pounds London broil
- 3 large garlic cloves, minced
- 3 tablespoons balsamic vinegar
- 3 tablespoons whole-grain mustard
- 2 tablespoons olive oil
- Sea salt and ground black pepper, to taste
- 1/2 teaspoon dried hot red pepper flakes

Directions (Ready in about 30 minutes + marinating time | Servings 8)

✓ Score both sides of the cleaned London broil.

✓ Thoroughly combine the remaining ingredients; massage this mixture into the meat to coat it on all sides. Let it marinate for at least 3 hours.

✓ Set the Air Fryer to cook at 400 degrees F; Then cook the London broil for 15 minutes. Flip it over and cook another 10 to 12 minutes. Bon appétit!

Nutritions: 257 Calories; 9.2g Fat; 0.1g Carbs; 41.0g Protein; 0.4g Sugars

467)   *Memphis-Style Pork Ribs*
Ingredients:

- (4 Servings)
- 1 ½ lb St. Louis–style pork spareribs
- Salt and black pepper to taste
- ½ tsp sweet paprika
- ½ tsp dry mustard
- 1 tbsp brown Sugar
- 1 tbsp cayenne pepper
- 1 tsp poultry seasoning
- 1 tsp shallot powder

- 1 tsp garlic powder
- ½ cup hot sauce

Direction:(Prep + Cook Time: 40 minutes)

✓ Preheat the air fryer to 370 F.

✓ Cut the ribs individually. In a bowl, mix all the remaining ingredients, except for the hot sauce.

✓ Add the ribs to the bowl and rub the seasoning onto the meat.

✓ Place the ribs in the greased frying basket and Bake for 20 minutes, turn them over, and cook for 10 more minutes or until the ribs are tender inside and golden brown and crisp on the outside.

✓ Serve with hot sauce.

nutritional value: Calories 430 kCal Total Carbs 7 g Net Carbs 5 g Fiber 2 g Sugar 5 g Protein 32 g Fat 31 g Monounsat. Fat 13 g Polyunsat. Fat 6 g Saturated Fat 11 g cholesterol 120 mg

468) *Roasted Pork Rack with Macadamia Nuts*

Ingredients:

- (2 Servings)
- 1 lb pork rack
- 2 tbsp olive oil
- 1 clove garlic, minced
- 1 tbsp rosemary, chopped
- Salt and black pepper to taste
- 1 cup macadamia nuts, finely chopped
- 1 tbsp breadcrumbs
- 1 egg, beaten in a bowl

Direction:(Prep + Cook Time: 65 minutes)

✓ Mix the olive oil and garlic vigorously in a bowl to make garlic oil.

✓ Place the rack of pork on a chopping board and brush with the garlic oil.

✓ Sprinkle with salt and pepper.

✓ Preheat the fryer to 370 F.

✓ In a bowl, add breadcrumbs, macadamia nuts, and rosemary.

✓ Brush the meat with the beaten egg on all sides and generously sprinkle with the nut mixture.

✓ Place the coated pork in the frying basket and Bake for 30 minutes.

✓ Flip over and cook further for 5-8 minutes.

✓ Remove the meat onto a chopping board and let it rest for 10 minutes before slicing.

✓ Serve with a salad or steamed rice.

nutritional value: CALORIES 1201ENERGY 5027 kj FAT 71gSATURATES 22g FIBER 7g PROTEIN 101g gCARBS 36g SUGAR 16g

469) *Chinese Sticky Ribs*

Ingredients:

- (4 Servings)
- 1 tbsp sesame oil
- 1 ½ lb pork ribs
- ½ tsp red chili flakes

- 2 tbsp light brown Sugar
- 1-inch piece ginger, grated
- 2 scallions, chopped 2 garlic cloves, minced
- 1 tbsp balsamic vinegar
- ½ tsp onion powder
- ½ tsp Chinese Five spice powder
- 1 tbsp sweet chili sauce
- Salt and black pepper to taste

Direction:(Prep + Cook Time: 45 minutes + marinating time)

✓ In a bowl, mix the red chili flakes, brown Sugar, ginger, garlic, vinegar, onion powder, Five spice powder, chili sauce, salt, and black pepper.

✓ Add in the ribs and toss to coat.

✓ Chill for at least 1 hour.

✓ Preheat the air fryer to 370 F.

✓ Remove the ribs from the fridge and place them in the greased frying basket.

✓ Brush with sesame oil and Bake for 25-30 minutes, flipping once.

✓ Serve topped with scallions.

nutritional value: Calories 423 Total Fat 28g Saturated Fat 8.5g Trans Fat 0.2g cholesterol 95 mg g g Total Carbs 21g Dietary Fiber 2.8g Sugar 6.2g Protein 22g

470) *Pork Sausage with Butter Bean Ratatouille*

Ingredients:

- (4 Servings)
- 4 pork sausages For Ratatouille
- 1 red bell pepper, chopped
- 2 zucchinis, chopped
- 1 eggplant, chopped
- 1 medium red onion, chopped
- 2 tbsp olive oil
- 1 cup canned butter beans, drained
- 15 oz canned tomatoes, chopped
- 1 tbsp balsamic vinegar
- 2 garlic cloves, minced
- 1 red chili, minced

Direction:(Prep + Cook Time: 45 minutes)

✓ Preheat the air fryer to 390 F.

✓ Add the sausages to the greased frying basket and AirFry for 12-15 minutes, turning once halfway through.

✓ Cover with foil to keep warm.

✓ Mix all ratatouille ingredients in the frying basket and Bake for 15-18 minutes, shaking once.

✓ Serve the sausages with ratatouille.

nutritional value: Calories 540 Total Fat 24g Saturated Fat 8g cholesterol60 mg g Total Carbohydrate54g Dietary Fiber 9g Sugar s7g Protein 27g

471) *Maple Mustard Pork Balls*

Ingredients:

- (4 Servings)
- 1 lb ground pork
- 1 large onion, chopped
- ½ tsp maple syrup
- 1 tsp yellow mustard
- ½ cup basil leaves, chopped
- Salt and black pepper to taste
- 2 tbsp cheddar cheese, grated
- 1 cup marinara sauce

Direction:(Prep + Cook Time: 25 minutes)

- ✓ In a bowl, add the ground pork, onion, maple syrup, mustard, basil leaves, salt, pepper, and cheddar cheese; mix well and form small balls.
- ✓ Place in the greased air fryer and AirFry for 12 minutes at 400 F.
- ✓ Slide the basket out and shake the meatballs. Cook further for 5 minutes.
- ✓ Serve with marinara sauce.

nutritional value: Calories: 188.4 Protein : 12.1g Carbs : 12.3g Dietary Fiber : 0.6g Sugar 8.1g Fat : 9.9gSaturated Fat : 4.1g cholesterol: 68.2 mg

472) *Pork Meatball Noodle Bowl*

Ingredients:

- (4 Servings)
- 2 lb ground pork
- 2 eggs, beaten
- 1 tbsp cooking oil, for greasing
- 1cup panko breadcrumbs
- 1 shallot, chopped
- 2 tsp soy sauce
- 2 garlic cloves, minced
- ½ tsp ground ginger
- 2 cups rice noodles, cooked
- 1 gem lettuce, torn
- 1 carrot, shredded
- 1 cucumber, peeled, thinly sliced
- 1 cup Asian sesame dressing
- 1 lime, cut into wedges

Direction:(Prep + Cook Time: 30 minutes)

- ✓ Preheat the air fryer to 390 F.
- ✓ Mix the ground pork, eggs, breadcrumbs, shallot, soy sauce, garlic, and ginger in a mixing bowl.
- ✓ Divide the mixture into 24 balls.
- ✓ Place them into the greased frying basket.
- ✓ AirFry for 12-15 minutes, shaking the basket every 5 minutes to ensure even cooking. Cook until the meatballs are golden brown.
- ✓ Divide the rice noodles, lettuce, carrot, and cucumber between 4 bowls.
- ✓ Top with meatballs and drizzle with the sesame dressing.

- ✓ Serve with lime wedges and enjoy.

nutritional value:Carbs52 g Dietary Fiber 3 g Sugar 4 g Fat 31 gSaturated19 g Protein 27 g

473) *Traditional Swedish Meatballs*

Ingredients:

- (4 Servings)
- 1 lb ground pork
- 1 tbsp fresh dill, chopped
- ½ tsp nutmeg
- ⅓ cup seasoned breadcrumbs
- 1 egg, beaten
- Salt and white pepper to taste 2
- tbsp butter
- ⅓ cup sour cream
- 2 tbsp flour

Direction:(Prep + Cook Time: 25 minutes)

- ✓ Preheat the air fryer to 360 F. In a bowl, combine the ground pork, dill, nutmeg, breadcrumbs, egg, salt, and pepper and mix well.
- ✓ Shape the mixture into small balls.
- ✓ AirFry them in the greased frying basket for 12-14 minutes, flipping once.
- ✓ Meanwhile, melt butter in a saucepan over medium heat and stir in the flour until lightly browned, about 2 minutes.
- ✓ Gradually pour 1 cup of Water and whisk until the sauce thickens.
- ✓ Stir in sour cream and cook for 1 minute. Pour the sauce over the meatballs to serve.

nutritional value: Calories: 370 Total Fat : 17 g Saturated Fat : 6 g Trans Fat : 0 g cholesterol: 90 mg Total Carbs : 39 g Dietary Fiber : 4 g Sugar 1 g Protein : 16 g

474) *Best Ever Pork Burgers*

Ingredients:

- (2 Servings)
- ½ lb ground pork
- ½ medium onion, chopped
- ½ tsp herbs de Provence
- ½ tsp garlic powder
- ½ tsp dried basil
- 4 slices cheddar cheese
- ½ tsp mustard
- Salt and black pepper to taste
- 2 bread buns, halved.
- ½ red onion, sliced in 2-inch rings
- 1 large tomato, sliced in 2-inch rings
- ½ lettuce leaves, torn

Direction:(Prep + Cook Time: 30 minutes)

- ✓ In a bowl, combine the ground pork, onion, herbs de Provence, garlic powder, basil, mustard, salt, and pepper and mix evenly.
- ✓ Form 2 patties out of the mixture and place on a flat

plate. Preheat the air fryer to 370 F.

✓ Place the pork patties in the greased frying basket and Bake for 10-12 minutes.

✓ Slid the basket out and turn the patties. Continue cooking for 5 more minutes.

✓ Lay lettuce on bun bottoms, add the patties, followed by a slice of onion, tomato, and cheddar cheese, and cover with the bun tops.

✓ Serve with ketchup and french fries if desired.

nutritional value: Calories 301 Total Fat 21g Saturated Fat 7.8g Trans Fat 0g cholesterol 95 mg g Total Carbs 0.1g Dietary Fiber 0.1g Sugar 0g Protein 26g

475) *Pork & Pear Blue Cheese Patties*

Ingredients:

* (2 Servings)
* ½ lb ground pork
* 1 pear, peeled and grated
* 1 cup breadcrumbs
* 2 oz blue cheese, crumbled
* ½ tsp ground cumin
* Salt and black pepper to taste.

Direction:(Prep + Cook Time: 20 minutes)

✓ In a bowl, add the ground pork, pear, breadcrumbs, cumin, blue cheese, salt, and black pepper, and mix with your hands.

✓ Shape into 2 even-sized burger patties.

✓ Arrange the patties on the greased frying basket and AirFry for 12-14 minutes at 380 F, turning once halfway through.

✓ Serve warm.

nutritional: Energy (kJ)3410 kJ Energy (kcal)815 kcal Fat 31.0 go saturates10.0 gCarbohydrate96 g Sugar s14.0 g Protein 42 g Salt 1.0 g

476) *Serbian Pork Skewers with Yogurt Sauce*

Ingredients:

* (4 Servings)
* 1 lb pork sausage meat
* Salt and black pepper to taste
* 1 onion, chopped
* ½ tsp garlic puree
* 1 tsp ground cumin
* 1 cup Greek yogurt
* 2 tbsp walnuts, finely chopped
* 1 tbsp fresh dill, chopped

Direction:(Prep + Cook Time: 25 minutes)

✓ Preheat the air fryer to 340 F.

✓ In a bowl, mix the sausage meat, onion, garlic puree, ground cumin, salt, and pepper.

✓ Knead until everything is well incorporated.

✓ Form patties out the mixture, about ½ inch thick, and thread them onto flat skewers.

✓ Lay them on the greased frying basket.

✓ AirFry for 14-16 minutes, turning them over once or twice until golden.

✓ Whisk the yogurt, walnuts, garlic, dill, and salt in a small bowl to obtain a sauce.

✓ Serve the skewers with the yogurt sauce.

nutritional value: Calories: 314Total Fat : 14g cholesterol: 94 mg g Carbs : 10g Fiber : 1g Sugar : 5g Protein : 37g

477) *Italian Fennel & Pork Balls*

Ingredients:

* (4 Servings)
* 1 lb pork sausage meat
* 1 whole egg, beaten
* 1 onion, chopped
* 2 tbsp fresh sage, chopped
* 2 tbsp ground almonds
* ¼ head fennel bulb, chopped
* 1 cup passata di Pomodoro (tomato sauce)
* Salt and black pepper to taste

Direction:(Prep + Cook Time: 30 minutes)

✓ Preheat the air fryer to 350 F.

✓ Place the sausage meat, onion, almonds, fennel, egg, salt, and pepper in a bowl.

✓ Mix with hands until well combined.

✓ Shape the mixture into balls.

✓ Add them to the greased frying basket and Bake for 14-16 minutes, shaking once.

✓ Top with sage and serve with passata sauce.

nutritional value: Calories 429.4 Total Fat 16.1 g Saturated Fat 7.1 g cholesterol0.0 5 mg Total Carbs 29.4 g Dietary Fiber 1.1 g Sugar 6.8 g Protein 38.1 g % C

478) *Mediterranean Pork Kabobs*

Ingredients:

* (4 Servings)
* Salt and black pepper to taste
* 1 green bell pepper, cut into chunks
* 1 lb pork tenderloin, cubed
* 8 pearl onions, halved
* ½ tsp Italian seasoning mix
* ½ tsp smoked paprika
* 1 zucchini, cut into chunks

Direction:(Prep + Cook Time: 30 minutes)

✓ Preheat the air fryer to 350 F.

✓ In a bowl, mix the pork, paprika, salt, and pepper.

✓ Thread alternating the vegetables and the pork cubes onto bamboo skewers.

✓ Spray with cooking spray and transfer to the frying basket.

✓ Bake for 15-18 minutes, flipping once halfway through.

✓ Serve sprinkled with Italian mix.

nutritional value: Calories

260 Total Fat 7gSaturated Fat 1.5g Trans Fat 0g cholesterol 60 mg Total Carbs 21g Dietary Fiber

3gTotal Sugar 2g Protein 28g

479) *Sausage Sticks Rolled in Bacon*
Ingredients:

- (4 Servings)
- Sausage: 8 bacon strips
- 8 pork sausages Relish:
- 8 large tomatoes, chopped
- 1 clove garlic, peeled
- 1 small onion, peeled
- 3 tbsp fresh parsley, chopped
- Salt and black pepper to taste
- 2 tbsp Sugar
- 1 tsp smoked paprika
- 1 tbsp white wine vinegar

Direction:(Prep + Cook Time: 40 minutes + chilling time)

✓ Pulse the tomatoes, garlic, and onion in a food processor until the mixture is pulpy.

✓ Transfer to a saucepan over medium heat and add vinegar, salt, and pepper; simmer for 10 minutes. Stir in the smoked paprika, parsley, and Sugar Let cool for 1 hour. Neatly wrap each sausage in a bacon strip and stick it in a bamboo skewer at the end of the sausage to secure the bacon ends.

✓ Place in a greased frying basket and AirFry for 12-14 minutes at 350 F, turning once halfway through.

✓ Serve the sausages with the cooled relish.

nutritional: Cals 438 Fat 19.00g Saturated Fat 6.600g Carbs 43.00g Sugar 1.10g Protein 22.00g Salt 6.75g

480) *Veggies & Pork Pinchos*
Ingredients:

- (4 Servings)
- 1 lb pork tenderloin, cubed
- 2 tbsp olive oil
- 1 lime, juiced and zested
- 2 cloves garlic, minced
- 1 tsp chili powder
- 1 tsp ground fennel seeds
- ½ tsp ground cumin
- Salt and white pepper to taste
- 1 red pepper, cut into chunks
- ½ cup mushrooms, quartered

Direction:(Prep + Cook Time: 25 minutes+ marinating time)

✓ In a bowl, mix half of the olive oil, lime zest and juice, garlic, chili, ground fennel, cumin, salt, and white pepper.

✓ Add in the pork and stir to coat.

✓ Cover with cling film and place in the fridge for 1 hour. Preheat the air fryer to 380 F.

✓ Season the mushrooms and red pepper with salt and black pepper and drizzle with the remaining olive oil.

✓ Thread alternating the pork, mushroom, and red pepper pieces onto short skewers.

✓ Place in the greased frying basket and AirFry for 15 minutes, turning once.

✓ Serve hot.

nutritional value: Calorie 150cal Fat 5 g Saturated0 g Polyunsaturated 0 g Monounsaturated 0 g Trans 0 g Protein 21 g

481) *Spicy Tricolor Pork Kebabs*
Ingredients:

- (4 Servings)
- 1 lb pork steak, cut into cubes
- ¼ cup soy sauce
- 2 tsp smoked paprika
- 1 tsp chili powder
- 1 tsp garlic salt
- 1 tsp red chili flakes
- 1 green squash, seeded and cut into cubes
- 1 tbsp white wine vinegar
- 3 tbsp steak sauce Skewing:
- 1 green pepper, cut into cubes
- 1 red pepper, cut into cubes
- 1 yellow squash, seeded and cut into cubes
- Salt and black pepper to taste A bunch of skewers

Direction:(Prep + Cook Time: 25 minutes + marinating time)

✓ In a mixing bowl, add the pork cubes, soy sauce, smoked paprika, chili powder, garlic salt, red chili flakes, wine vinegar, and steak sauce.

✓ Mix with a spoon and marinate for 1 hour in the fridge.

✓ Preheat the air fryer to 370 F.

✓ On each skewer, stick the pork cubes and vegetables, alternating them.

✓ Arrange the skewers on the greased frying basket and Bake them for 12-14 minutes, flipping once.

nutritional value: Calories: 122 Fat : 3g Carbs : 0g Fiber : 0g Sugar 0g Protein : 22g

482) *Sweet Pork Tenderloin*
Ingredients:

- (4 Servings)
- 1 lb pork tenderloin, sliced
- 2 tbsp quince preserve
- 1 orange, juiced and zested
- 2 tbsp olive oil
- 1 tbsp soy sauce
- Salt and black pepper to taste

Direction:(Prep + Cook Time: 30 minutes)

✓ Brush the sliced tenderloin with 1 tbsp of olive oil and season with salt and black pepper.

✓ Put them into the greased frying basket and Bake for 13-15 minutes at 380 F, turning once halfway through.

✓ Heat the remaining olive oil in a skillet over low heat

and add in orange juice, soy sauce, orange zest, and quince preserve.

✓ Simmer until the sauce thickens slightly, about 2-3 minutes. Season to taste.

✓ Arrange the sliced pork on a platter and pour the quince sauce over. Serve immediately.

nutritional: Calories259.4 Total Fat 8.2 g Saturated Fat 3.0 g g cholesterol 88.4 Potassiu 434.1 mg Total Carbs 9.6 g Dietary Fiber 0.5 g Sugar 8.4 g Protein 34.5 g

483) *Stuffed Pork Tenderloin*

Ingredients:

- (4 Servings)
- 1 lb pork tenderloin, butterflied
- Salt and black pepper to taste
- 1 cup spinach 3 oz cream cheese
- 16 bacon slices
- 1 small onion, sliced
- 1 tbsp olive oil
- 1 clove garlic, minced
- ½ tsp dried thyme
- ½ tsp dried rosemary

Direction:(Prep + Cook Time: 45 minutes)

✓ Place the tenderloin on a chopping board, cover it with plastic wrap and pound it using a kitchen hammer to a 2-inches flat and square piece.

✓ Trim the uneven sides with a knife to have a perfect square; transfer to a plate. On the same chopping board, place and weave the bacon slices into a square of the pork's size.

✓ Place the pork on the bacon weave and set aside.

✓ Heat olive oil in a skillet over medium heat and sauté onion and garlic until transparent, 3 minutes.

✓ Add in the spinach, rosemary, thyme, salt, and pepper, and cook until the spinach wilts.

✓ Stir in the cream cheese until the mixture is even.

✓ Turn the heat off.

✓ Preheat the air fryer to 360 F.

✓ Spread the spinach mixture onto the pork loin.

✓ Roll up the bacon and the pork over the spinach stuffing.

✓ Secure the ends with toothpicks and place in the greased air fryer.

✓ Bake for 15 minutes, turn them over, and cook for 5 more minutes or until golden.

✓ Let cool slightly before slicing.

nutritional value: Calorie 296cal Carbs4 g Dietary Fiber 1 g Fat 16 g Protein 32 g cholesterol89 mg

484) *Pork Lettuce Cups*

Ingredients:

- (4 Servings)
- 1 tbsp sesame oil
- 1 lb pork tenderloin, sliced
- ½ white onion, sliced

- 2 tbsp sesame seeds, toasted
- 2 Little Gem lettuces, leaves separated
- 1 cup radishes, cut into matchsticks
- 1 tsp red chili flakes
- 2 tbsp teriyaki sauce
- 1 tsp honey
- Salt and black pepper to taste

Direction:(Prep + Cook Time: 30 minutes + marinating time)

✓ In a bowl, whisk teriyaki sauce, red chili flakes, honey, sesame oil, salt, and black pepper.

✓ Add in the pork and toss to coat.

✓ Cover with a lid and leave in the fridge to marinate for 30 minutes.

✓ Preheat the air fryer to 360 F.

✓ Remove the pork from the marinade and place it in the greased frying basket, reserving the marinade liquid.

✓ AirFry for 11-13 minutes, turning once halfway through.

✓ Arrange the lettuce leaves on a serving platter and divide the pork between them.

✓ Top with onion, radishes, and sesame seeds.

✓ Drizzle with the reserved marinade and serve.

nutritional: Calories 175.9 Total Fat 5.0 g Saturated Fat 1.4 g gCholesterol48.3 9 mg Total Carbs 13.7 g Dietary Fiber 1.5 g Sugar 3.3 g Protein 18.5 g % Copper 5.4

485) *Sage-Rubbed Pork Tenderloin*

Ingredients:

- 4 Servings)
- 1 lb boneless pork tenderloin
- 1 tbsp lime juice
- ½ tbsp soy sauce
- 1 tbsp olive oil
- ½ tbsp chili powder
- 1 garlic clove, minced
- 2 tbsp fresh sage, minced
- ½ tsp ground coriander

Direction:(Prep + Cook Time: 45 minutes + marinating time)

✓ Combine the lime juice, olive oil, soy sauce, chili powder, garlic, sage, and ground coriander in a bowl.

✓ Add in the pork and toss to coat.

✓ Cover with foil and refrigerate for at least 1 hour.

✓ Preheat the air fryer to 390 F.

✓ Remove the pork from the bag, shaking off any extra marinade.

✓ Place in the greased frying basket and AirFry for 15 minutes.

✓ Flip it over and cook for another 5-7 minutes. Remove and let sit for 10 minutes so before cutting.

✓ Serve warm with steamed veggies or rice.

nutritional value: 256 calories; calories from Fat 67 % ; Protein 20g; Fat 19g; saturated Fat 7.8g; Carbs 1.9g; Fiber 0.1g; ; cholesterol 86 mg .

486) *Zesty Breaded Pork Chops*

Ingredients:

- (4 Servings)
- Salt and black pepper to taste
- 2 eggs 1 cup breadcrumbs
- ½ tsp garlic powder
- 4 lean pork chops 1 tsp paprika
- ½ tsp dried oregano
- ½ tsp cayenne pepper
- ¼ tsp dry mustard 1 lemon, zested.

Direction:(Prep + Cook Time: 30 minutes)

- ✓ In a bowl, whisk the eggs with 1 tbsp of Water .
- ✓ In another bowl, add the breadcrumbs, salt, black pepper, garlic powder, paprika, oregano, cayenne pepper, lemon zest, and dry mustard and mix evenly.
- ✓ Preheat the air fryer to 380 F.
- ✓ In the egg mixture, dip each pork chop and then dip in the crumb mixture.
- ✓ Place in a greased frying basket and AirFry for 10 minutes.
- ✓ Flip and cook for another 5 minutes or until golden.
- ✓ Remove the chops to a chopping board and let them rest for 3 minutes before slicing.

nutritional: Calories 400 Total Fat 22g Saturated Fat 4.5g Trans Fat 0.3g cholesterol 124 mg g Total Carbs 22g Dietary Fiber 1.5g Sugar 1.7g Protein 26g

487) *Hungarian-Style Pork Chops*

Ingredients:

- (4 Servings)
- 1 lb pork chops, boneless
- 2 tbsp olive oil
- 2 tsp Hungarian paprika
- ¼ tsp ground bay leaf
- ½ tsp dried thyme
- 1 tsp garlic powder
- Salt and black pepper to taste
- ¼ cup yogurt 2 garlic cloves, minced

Direction:(Prep + Cook Time: 30 minutes)

- ✓ Preheat the air fryer to 380 F.
- ✓ Spray the frying basket with non-stick cooking spray.
- ✓ Mix the Hungarian paprika, ground bay leaf, thyme, garlic powder, salt, and black pepper in a bowl.
- ✓ Rub the pork with the mixture, drizzle with some olive oil, and place the chops in the fryer to AirFry for 14-16 minutes, turning once.
- ✓ Mix yogurt with the remaining oil, garlic, and salt. Serve the chops drizzled with the sauce.

nutritional: Calories 209.1 Total Fat 11.8 g Saturated Fat 5.5 g g cholesterol 66.7 9 mg Total Carbs 3.4 g Dietary Fiber 0.4 g Sugar 0.4 g Protein 22.5 g %

488) *Pork Chops with Mustard-Apricot Glaze*

Ingredients:

- (4 Servings)
- 4 pork chops, ½-inch thick
- Salt and black pepper to taste
- 1 tbsp apricot jam
- 1 ½ tbsp minced, finely chopped
- 2 tbsp wholegrain mustard

Direction:(Prep + Cook Time: 25 minutes

- ✓ In a bowl, add apricot jam, garlic, mustard, salt, and black pepper; mix well.
- ✓ Add the pork chops and toss to coat.
- ✓ Place the chops in the greased frying basket and Bake for 10 minutes at 350 F.
- ✓ Turn the chops with a spatula and cook further for 6-8 minutes until golden and crispy.
- ✓ Once ready, remove the chops to a serving platter and serve with a side of steamed green veggies if desired.

nutritional value: calories 408kcal fat 23.5g saturated fat 6.5g carbs 5.7g 3.5g sugar 0.3g fiber 38.6g protein 128 mg cholesterol

489) *Southeast-Asian Pork Chops*

Ingredients:

- (4 Servings)
- 4 pork chops
- 2 garlic cloves, minced
- ½ tbsp Sugar
- 4 stalks lemongrass, trimmed and chopped
- 2 shallots, chopped
- 2 tbsp olive oil
- 1 ¼ tsp soy sauce
- 1 ¼ tsp fish sauce
- Salt and black pepper to taste.

Direction:(Prep + Cook Time: 25 minutes + marinating time)

- ✓ In a bowl, add garlic, Sugar , lemongrass, shallots, olive oil, soy sauce, fish sauce, salt, and pepper; mix well.
- ✓ Add in the pork chops, coat them with the mixture and marinate for 2 hours in the fridge.
- ✓ Preheat the air fryer to 400 F.
- ✓ Remove the chops from the marinade and place them in the frying basket.
- ✓ Bake for 14-16 minutes, flipping once, until golden.
- ✓ Serve with sautéed asparagus if desired.

nutritional value: Calorie 238 kcal Protein 33.14 g Fat 9.74 g Carbs 8.28 g Sugar added 0 g Roughage 0.76 g Niacin 0.37 mg

490) *Mexican Pork Chops with Black Beans*

Ingredients:

- (4 Servings)

- 4 pork chops
- 1 lime, juiced
- Salt and black pepper to taste
- 1 tsp garlic powder
- 1 tsp onion powder
- ½ cup tomato sauce
- 2 tbsp olive oil
- 1 onion, chopped
- 3 garlic cloves, minced
- ½ tsp oregano
- 1 tsp chipotle chili pepper
- 1 cup long-grain rice
- 2 tbsp butter
- 1 cup canned black beans, drained

Direction:(Prep + Cook Time: 45 minutes + marinating time)

✓ In a bowl, whisk the onion powder, garlic powder, chipotle pepper, oregano, lime juice, olive oil, salt, and pepper.
✓ Coat the pork with the mixture.
✓ Cover and place in fridge and marinate for at least 1 hour.
✓ Melt the butter in a saucepan over medium heat.
✓ Sauté the onion and garlic for 3 minutes.
✓ Stir in the rice for 1 minute and pour in the tomato sauce and 2 cups of Water .
✓ Season with salt and pepper and bring to a boil.
✓ Reduce the heat and simmer for 16 minutes or until the rice is tender.
✓ Stir in the beans. Preheat the air fryer to 350 F.
✓ Remove the meat from the marinade and place the chops in the greased air fryer.
✓ Bake for 15-18 minutes, flipping once halfway through.
✓ Serve with rice and black beans.

Nutritional: Calories Per Serving370 Total Fat G 10saturated Fat G 2 Cholesterol (Mg)95 10total Carbs G 24 Dietary Fiber G 8 Protein G 49 55 2.9

491) Roasted Pork Chops with Mushrooms

Ingredients:

- (4 Servings)
- 1 lb boneless pork chops
- 2 carrots, cut into sticks
- 1 cup mushrooms, sliced
- 2 tbsp olive oil
- 2 garlic cloves, minced
- 1 tsp cayenne pepper
- 1 tsp dried thyme
- Salt and black pepper to taste

Direction:(Prep + Cook Time: 25 minutes)

✓ Preheat the air fryer to 360 F.
✓ Season the hops with cayenne pepper, thyme, salt, and black pepper.
✓ In a bowl, combine carrots, garlic, olive oil, mushrooms, and salt.
✓ Place the veggies in the greased frying basket, top with the pork chops, and Bake for 15-18 minutes, turning the chops once.
✓ Serve hot.

nutritional value: Calories 662 Total Fat 38.2g Saturated Fat 6.5g g rans- Fat 0.1g cholesterol 186 mg Carbs 13.9g Net carbs 12.6g Sugar 2.6g Fiber 1.3g Glucose 0.7 Fructose 0.5g Sucrose 0.4g Protein 62.7g Copper 0.5 mg Fluoride 0.4µg

492) Italian-Style Apple Pork Chops

Ingredients:

- (4 Servings)
- 1 small onion, sliced
- 3 tbsp olive oil
- 2 tbsp apple cider vinegar
- ¼ tsp brown Sugar
- ½ tsp thyme
- 1 apple, sliced
- ½ tsp rosemary
- ¼ tsp smoked paprika
- 4 pork chops
- Salt and black pepper to taste.

Direction:(Prep + Cook Time: 30 minutes)

✓ Preheat the air fryer to 350.
✓ Heat 2 tbsp olive oil in a skillet over medium heat and stir-fry onion, apple slices, 1 tbsp apple cider vinegar, brown Sugar , thyme, and rosemary for 4 minutes; set aside.
✓ In a bowl, mix remaining olive oil, remaining vinegar, paprika, salt, and pepper.
✓ Add in the chops and toss to coat.
✓ Place them in the air fryer and Bake for 10 minutes, flipping once halfway through.
✓ When cooked, top with the sautéed apples, return to the fryer, and cook for 5 more minutes.
✓ Serve warm.

nutritional value: Calories 292.8 Total Fat 15.3 g Saturated Fat 6.0 g g cholesterol 76.2 5 mg Total Carbs 11.9 g Dietary Fiber 2.1 g Sugar 0.2 g Protein 26.5 g % Copper 4.2 Manganese 7.3 %

493) Sweet French Pork Chops with Blue Cheese

Ingredients:

- (4 Servings)
- 2 tsp olive oil
- 1 tsp butter, softened
- 4 thin-cut pork chops
- ¼ cup blue cheese, crumbled
- 2 tbsp hot mango chutney
- 1 tbsp fresh thyme, chopped

Direction:(Prep + Cook Time: 30 minutes+ marinating time)

- ✓ Preheat the air fryer to 390 F.
- ✓ In a bowl, whisk together butter, mango chutney, and blue cheese; set aside.
- ✓ Season the chops with salt and pepper and drizzle with olive oil.
- ✓ Place the chops in the frying basket and AirFry for 14-16 minutes, flipping once.
- ✓ Remove to a plate and spread the blue cheese mixture on each pork chop.
- ✓ Let sit covered with foil for 5 minutes. Sprinkle with fresh thyme and serve.

nutritional: Cal 541.0 cholesterol 196.9 Total Carbs 3.2 g Dietary Fiber 0.1 g Sugar 2.6 g Protein 68.5 g

494) *Spicy-Sweet Pork Chops*
Ingredients:

- (4 Servings)
- 4 thin boneless pork chops
- 3 tbsp brown Sugar
- ½ tsp cayenne pepper
- ½ tsp ancho chili powder
- ½ tsp garlic powder
- 1 tbsp olive oil
- ½ cup Cholula hot sauce
- Salt and black pepper to taste.

Direction:(Prep + Cook Time: 25 minutes)

- ✓ Preheat your Air Fryer to 375 F.
- ✓ To make the marinade, mix brown Sugar , olive oil, cayenne pepper, garlic powder, salt, and pepper in a small bowl.
- ✓ Dip each pork chop into the marinade, shaking off, and placing them in the frying basket in a single layer.
- ✓ AirFry for 7 minutes Slide the basket out, turn the chops, and brush them with marinade.
- ✓ Cook for another 5 to 8 minutes until golden brown.
- ✓ Plate and top with hot sauce to serve.

nutritional: Cal 228clCarbs1 g Dietary Fat 9 g Protein 31 g

495) *Juicy Double Cut Pork Chops*
Ingredients:

- (4 Servings)
- 4 pork chops
- ½ cup green mole sauce
- 2 tbsp tamarind paste
- 1 garlic clove, minced
- 2 tbsp corn syrup
- 1 tbsp olive oil
- 2 tbsp molasses
- 4 tbsp southwest seasoning
- 2 tbsp ketchup 2 tbsp Water

Direction:(Prep + Cook Time: 25 minutes + marinating time)

- ✓ In a bowl, mix all ingredients, except for the pork chops and mole sauce.
- ✓ Add in the pork chops and toss to coat.
- ✓ Let them marinate for 30 minutes.
- ✓ Preheat the air fryer to 350 F.
- ✓ Place the chops in the greased frying basket.
- ✓ Bake for 16-18 minutes, turning once.
- ✓ Serve the chops drizzled with mole sauce.

nutritional value: Calories 1070 Total Fat 58g Saturated Fat 22g cholesterol 190 mg g Carbs 60g Net carbs 53g Sugar 25g Fiber 7g Protein 61g

496) *Stuffed Pork Chops*
Ingredients:

- (4 Servings)
- 4 thick pork chops
- ½ cup mushrooms, sliced
- 1 shallot, chopped
- Salt and black pepper to taste
- 1 tbsp olive oil
- 2 tbsp butter
- 2 garlic cloves, minced
- 2 tbsp sage, chopped

Direction:(Prep + Cook Time: 35 minutes)

- ✓ Melt the butter in a skillet over medium heat.
- ✓ Add and sauté the shallot, garlic, mushrooms, sage, salt, and black pepper for 4-5 minutes until tender.
- ✓ Preheat the air fryer to 350 F.
- ✓ Cut a pocket into each pork chop to create a cavity.
- ✓ Fill the chops with the mushroom mixture and secure with toothpicks.
- ✓ Season the stuffed chops with salt and pepper and brush with olive oil.
- ✓ Place them in the frying basket and Bake for 18-20 minutes, turning once.
- ✓ Remove the toothpicks and serve.

nutritional value: Calories 616 Total Fat 41gSaturated Fat 14g Trans Fat 0.3g nounsaturated Fat 17g cholesterol 229 mg Total Carbs 3.7g Dietary Fiber 1.1g Sugar 0.7g Protein 57g

497) *Pork Escalopes with Beet & Cabbage Salad*
Ingredients:

- (4 Servings)
- 2 eggs, beaten
- 4 boneless pork chops
- 1 tbsp olive oil
- ½ cup panko breadcrumbs
- ½ tsp garlic powder
- Salt and black pepper to taste
- 1 cup white cabbage, shredded
- 1 red beet, grated
- 1 apple, sliced into matchsticks
- 2 tbsp Italian dressing

Direction:(Prep + Cook Time: 35 minutes)

✓ In a mixing bowl, combine the cabbage, beet, and apple.

✓ Pour the Italian dressing all over and toss to coat.

✓ Keep in the fridge until ready to use.

✓ Preheat the air fryer to 390 F.

✓ Divide the pork chops between two sheets of plastic wrap.

✓ Pound with a meat mallet or rolling pin until thin, about ¼ inch in thickness.

✓ In a shallow bowl, combine the breadcrumbs and garlic powder.

✓ In a second shallow bowl, whisk the eggs with salt and black pepper.

✓ First, coat the pork chop in the egg mixture. Shake off, dredge in the breadcrumbs.

✓ Lay the chops in a single layer in the greased frying basket, spray them with a little bit of olive oil, and AirFry for 8 minutes.

✓ Turn the chops over, spray again with some oil, and cook for another 4-7 minutes.

✓ Serve with the beet-cabbage salad.

nutritional value: Calories 82.5 Total Fat 3.6 g Saturated Fat 0.5 g g cholesterol 0.0 mg mg 2 mg Total Carbs 13.1 g Dietary Fiber 2.4 g Sugar 0.0 g Protein 1.1 g % Copper 4.3 Manganese 11.1 %

498)   *Bavarian-Style Crispy Pork Schnitzel*

Ingredients:

• 4 Servings)

• 4 pork chops, center-cut

• 1 egg, beaten

• 1 tsp chili powder

• 2 tbsp flour

• 2 tbsp sour cream

• Salt and black pepper to taste

• ½ cup breadcrumbs

• 2 tbsp olive oil

Direction:(Prep + Cook Time: 25 minutes)

✓ Preheat the air fryer to 380 F.

✓ Using a meat tenderizer, pound the chops until ¼-inch thickness.

✓ Whisk the egg and sour cream in a bowl.

✓ Mix the breadcrumbs with chili powder, salt, and pepper in another bowl.

✓ Coat the chops with flour, then egg mixture, and finally in breadcrumbs.

✓ Brush with olive oil and arrange them on the frying basket.

✓ AirFry for 13-15 minutes, turning once until golden brown.

✓ Serve.

nutritional: Calorie 118clCarbs8 g Dietary Fiber 1 g Sugar Fat 2 gSaturated0 g Polyunsaturated 0 g Protein 17 g cholesterol 65 mg

499)   *Italian Pork Scallopini*

Ingredients:

• (4 Servings)

• 4 pork loin thin steaks

• Salt and black pepper to taste

• ¼ cup Parmesan cheese, grated

• 2 tbsp Italian breadcrumbs

Direction:(Prep + Cook Time: 20 minutes)

✓ Preheat the air fryer to 390 F.

✓ Spritz the frying basket with cooking spray.

✓ In a bowl, mix Italian breadcrumbs and Parmesan cheese.

✓ Season the pork steaks with salt and black pepper.

✓ Roll them in the breadcrumb mixture and spray them with cooking spray.

✓ Transfer to the frying basket and AirFry for 14-16 minutes, turning once halfway through.

✓ Serve immediately.

nutritional value: Calories 200 Total Fat 8g Saturated Fat 4.5g cholesterol 60 mg Total Carbs 12g Dietary Fiber 1gTotal Sugar 3g Protein 19g

500)   *Provençal Pork Medallions*

Ingredients:

• (4 Servings)

• 1 lb pork medallions

• 1 tbsp olive oil

• 1 tbsp herbs de Provence

• ½ cup dry white wine

• ½ lemon, juiced and zested

• Salt and black pepper to taste.

Direction:(Prep + Cook Time: 30 minutes + marinating time)

✓ Preheat the air fryer to 360 F.

✓ Season the pork medallions with salt and black pepper and drizzle with olive oil.

✓ Place them in the frying basket and AirFry for 12-14 minutes, flipping once.

✓ Place a saucepan over medium heat and add white wine and 2 tbsp of Water ; bring to a boil. Reduce the heat and add in the lemon zest and juice and herbs de Provence; season with salt and pepper.

✓ Simmer until the sauce thickens, about 2-3 minutes.

✓ Pour the sauce over the medallions and serve.

nutritional:Calories 120 Saturated Fat 1 g Total Fat 2 g cholesterol 74 mg Dietary Fiber Trace Protein 24 g

501)   *Thyme Pork Escalopes*

Ingredients:

• (4 Servings)

• 4 pork loin steaks

• 2 tbsp olive oil

• Salt and black pepper to taste

• 2 eggs 1 cup breadcrumbs

• 1 tbsp fresh thyme, chopped

Direction:Prep + Cook Time: 30 minutes + marinating

time)
- ✓ In a bowl, mix olive oil, salt, and pepper to form a marinade.
- ✓ Place the pork in the marinade and let sit for 15 minutes.
- ✓ Preheat the fryer to 400 F.
- ✓ Beat the eggs in a separate bowl and add the breadcrumbs to a plate.
- ✓ Dip the meat into the eggs and then roll in the crumbs.
- ✓ Place the steaks in the greased frying basket and Bake for 16-18 minutes, shaking every 5 minutes.
- ✓ Sprinkle with thyme to serve.

nutritional value: Calories 344 Total Fat 29.9g Tot. Carb. 1.3g Sat. Fat 6.6g Dietary Fiber 0.1g Trans Fat 0g Sugar 0g cholesterol 50.4 mg Protein 17g

502) *Pork Belly the Philippine Style*

Ingredients:
- • (4 Servings)
- • 2 lb pork belly, cut in half, blanched
- • 1 bay leaf, crushed
- • 2 tbsp soy sauce
- • 3 garlic cloves, minced
- • 1 tbsp peppercorns
- • 1 tbsp peanut oil
- • ½ tsp salt

Direction:(Prep + Cook Time: 50 minutes + marinating time)
- ✓ Take a mortar and pestle and place in the bay leaf, garlic, salt, peppercorns, and peanut oil.
- ✓ Smash until paste-like consistency forms.
- ✓ Whisk the paste with soy sauce.
- ✓ Pierce the belly skin with a fork.
- ✓ Rub the mixture onto the meat, wrap the pork with a plastic foil and refrigerate for 2 hours.
- ✓ Preheat the fryer to 350 F and grease the basket.
- ✓ AirFry the pork for 30 minutes, flipping once halfway through.

nutritional: Calorie 320cl Fat 23 g Protein 27 g cholesterol 97 mg

503) *Pork Sandwiches with Bacon & Cheddar*

Ingredients:
- • 2 Servings)
- • ½ lb pork steak
- • 1 tsp steak seasoning
- • Salt and black pepper to taste
- • 5 thick bacon slices
- • ½ cup cheddar cheese, grated
- • ½ tbsp Worcestershire sauce
- • 2 burger buns, halved

Direction:(Prep + Cook Time: 40 minutes)
- ✓ Preheat the air fryer to 400 F.
- ✓ Season the pork steak with black pepper, salt, and

steak seasoning.
- ✓ Place in the greased frying basket and Bake for 20 minutes, turning at the 14-minute mark.
- ✓ Remove the steak to a chopping board, let cool slightly, and using two forks, shred into small pieces.
- ✓ Place the bacon in the frying basket and AirFry at 370 F for 5-8 minutes.
- ✓ Chop the bacon and transfer to a bowl.
- ✓ Mix in the pulled pork, Worcestershire sauce, and cheddar cheese.
- ✓ Adjust the seasoning and spoon the mixture into the halved buns.
- ✓ Serve and enjoy.

nutritional value: Calories 330 Total Fat 23gSaturated Fat 10g cholesterol 90 mg Total Carbs 2g Dietary Fiber 0g Sugar 0g Protein 28g

504) *Homemade Chicken Burgers*

Ingredients
- • 1 ¼ pounds chicken white meat, ground
- • 1/2 white onion, finely chopped
- • 1 teaspoon fresh garlic, finely chopped
- • Sea salt and ground black pepper, to taste
- • 1 teaspoon paprika
- • 1/2 cup cornmeal
- • 1 ½ cups breadcrumbs
- • 4 burger buns
- • 4 lettuce leaves
- • 2 small pickles, sliced
- • 2 tablespoons ketchup
- • 1 teaspoon yellow mustard

Directions:(Prep + Cook Time: 30 minutes)
- ✓ Thoroughly combine the chicken, onion, garlic, salt and black pepper in a mixing dish. Form the mixture into 4 equal patties.
- ✓ In a shallow bowl, mix paprika with cornmeal and breadcrumbs. Dip each patty in this mixture, pressing to coat well on both sides.
- ✓ Spritz a cooking basket with a nonstick cooking spray. Air fry the burgers at 370 degrees F for about 11 minutes or to your desired degree of doneness. Place your burgers on burger buns and serve with toppings. Bon appétit!

Nutritional: 238 calories; protein 28.8g; carbohydrates 11.5g; fat 7.8g; cholesterol 110.1mg; sodium 174.9mg.

505) *Chicken Drumsticks with Ketchup-Lemon Sauce*

Ingredients
- • 3 tablespoons lemon juice
- • 1 cup tomato ketchup
- • 1 ½ tablespoons fresh rosemary, chopped
- • 6 skin-on chicken drumsticks, boneless
- • 1/2 teaspoon ground black pepper
- • 2 teaspoons lemon zest, grated

- 1/3 cup honey
- 3 cloves garlic, minced

Directions (Ready in about 20 minutes + marinating time | Servings 6)

✓ Dump the chicken drumsticks into a mixing dish. Now, add the other items and give it a good stir; let it marinate overnight in your refrigerator.

✓ Discard the marinade; roast the chicken legs in your air fryer at 375 degrees F for 22 minutes, turning once.

✓ Now, add the marinade and cook an additional 6 minutes or until everything is warmed through.

Nutritions:274 Calories; 12g Fat; 17.3g Carbs; 23.3g Protein; 16.2g Sugars

506)   *Creamed Cajun Chicken*

Ingredients

- 3 green onions, thinly sliced
- ½ tablespoon Cajun seasoning
- 1 ½ cup buttermilk
- 2 large-sized chicken breasts, cut into strips
- 1/2 teaspoon garlic powder
- 1 teaspoon salt
- 1 cup cornmeal mix
- 1 teaspoon shallot powder
- 1 ½ cup flour
- 1 teaspoon ground black pepper, or to taste

Directions (Ready in about 10 minutes | Servings 6)

✓ Prepare three mixing bowls. Combine 1/2 cup of the plain flour together with the cornmeal and Cajun seasoning in your bowl. In another bowl, place the buttermilk.

✓ Pour the remaining 1 cup of flour into the third bowl.

✓ Sprinkle the chicken strips with all the seasonings. Then, dip each chicken strip in the 1 cup of flour, then in the buttermilk; finally, dredge them in the cornmeal mixture.

✓ Cook the chicken strips in the air fryer baking pan for 16 minutes at 365 degrees F. Serve garnished with green onions. Bon appétit!

Nutritions:400 Calories; 10.2g Fat; 48.2g Carbs; 27.3g Protein; 3.5g Sugars

507)   *Chive, Feta and Chicken Frittata*

Ingredients

- 1/3 cup Feta cheese, crumbled
- 1 teaspoon dried rosemary
- ½ teaspoon brown sugar
- 2 tablespoons fish sauce
- 1 ½ cup cooked chicken breasts, boneless and shredded
- 1/2 teaspoon coriander sprig, finely chopped
- 3 medium-sized whisked eggs
- 1/3 teaspoon ground white pepper
- 1 cup fresh chives, chopped

- 1/2 teaspoon garlic paste
- Fine sea salt, to taste
- Nonstick cooking spray

Directions (Ready in about 10 minutes | Servings 4)

✓ Grab a baking dish that fit in your air fryer.

✓ Lightly coat the inside of the baking dish with a nonstick cooking spray of choice. Stir in all ingredients, minus Feta cheese. Stir to combine well.

✓ Set your machine to cook at 335 degrees for 8 minutes; check for doneness. Scatter crumbled Feta over the top and eat immediately!

Nutritions:176 Calories; 7.7g Fat; 2.4g Carbs; 22.8g Protein; 1.5g Sugars

508)   *Grilled Chicken Tikka Masala*

Ingredients

- 1 teaspoon Tikka Masala
- 1 teaspoon fine sea salt
- 2 heaping teaspoons whole grain mustard
- 2 teaspoons coriander, ground
- 2 tablespoon olive oil
- 2 large-sized chicken breasts, skinless and halved lengthwise
- 2 teaspoons onion powder
- 1 ½ tablespoons cider vinegar
- Basmati rice, steamed
- 1/3 teaspoon red pepper flakes, crushed

Directions (Ready in about 35 minutes + marinating time | Servings 4)

✓ Preheat the air fryer to 335 degrees for 4 minutes.

✓ Toss your chicken together with the other ingredients, minus basmati rice. Let it stand at least 3 hours.

✓ Cook for 25 minutes in your air fryer; check for doneness because the time depending on the size of the piece of chicken.

✓ Serve immediately over warm basmati rice. Enjoy!

Nutritions:319 Calories; 20.1g Fat; 1.9g Carbs; 30.5g Protein; 0.1g Sugars

509)   *Award Winning Breaded Chicken*

Ingredients

For the Marinade:

- 1 1/2 teaspoons olive oil
- 1 teaspoon red pepper flakes, crushed
- 1/3 teaspoon chicken bouillon granules
- 1/3 teaspoon shallot powder
- 1 1/2 tablespoons tamari soy sauce
- 1/3 teaspoon cumin powder
- 1 ½ tablespoons mayo
- 1 teaspoon kosher salt

For the chicken:

- 2 beaten eggs
- Breadcrumbs
- 1 ½ chicken breasts, boneless and skinless

- 1 ½ tablespoons plain flour

Directions (Ready in about 10 minutes + marinating time | Servings 4)

✓ Butterfly the chicken breasts, and then, marinate them for at least 55 minutes.

✓ Coat the chicken with plain flour; then, coat with the beaten eggs; finally, roll them in the breadcrumbs.

✓ Lightly grease the cooking basket. Air-fry the breaded chicken at 345 degrees F for 12 minutes, flipping them halfway

Nutritions:262 Calories; 14.9g Fat; 2.7g Carbs; 27.5g Protein; 0.3g Sugars

510)   *Cheese and Garlic Stuffed Chicken Breasts*

Ingredients

- 1/2 cup Cottage cheese
- 2 eggs, beaten
- 2 medium-sized chicken breasts, halved
- 2 tablespoons fresh coriander, chopped
- 1teaspoon fine sea salt
- Seasoned breadcrumbs
- 1/3teaspoon freshly ground black pepper, to savor
- 3 cloves garlic, finely minced

Directions (Ready in about 20 minutes | Servings 2)

✓ Firstly, flatten out the chicken breast using a meat tenderizer.

✓ In a medium-sized mixing dish, combine the Cottage cheese with the garlic, coriander, salt, and black pepper.

✓ Spread 1/3 of the mixture over the first chicken breast. Repeat with the remaining ingredients. Roll the chicken around the filling; make sure to secure with toothpicks.

✓ Now, whisk the egg in a shallow bowl. In another shallow bowl, combine the salt, ground black pepper, and seasoned breadcrumbs.

✓ Coat the chicken breasts with the whisked egg; now, roll them in the breadcrumbs.

✓ Cook in the air fryer cooking basket at 365 degrees F for 22 minutes. Serve immediately.

Nutritions:424 Calories; 24.5g Fat; 7.5g Carbs; 43.4g Protein; 5.3g Sugars

511)   *Dinner Avocado Chicken Sliders*

Ingredients

- ½ pounds ground chicken meat
- 4 burger buns
- 1/2 cup Romaine lettuce, loosely packed
- ½ teaspoon dried parsley flakes
- 1/3 teaspoon mustard seeds
- 1 teaspoon onion powder
- 1 ripe fresh avocado, mashed
- 1 teaspoon garlic powder
- 1 ½ tablespoon extra-virgin olive oil

- 1 cloves garlic, minced
- Nonstick cooking spray
- Salt and cracked black pepper (peppercorns), to taste

Directions (Ready in about 10 minutes | Servings 4)

✓ Firstly, spritz an air fryer cooking basket with a nonstick cooking spray.

✓ Mix ground chicken meat, mustard seeds, garlic powder, onion powder, parsley, salt, and black pepper until everything is thoroughly combined. Make sure not to overwork the meat to avoid tough chicken burgers.

✓ Shape the meat mixture into patties and roll them in breadcrumbs; transfer your burgers to the prepared cooking basket. Brush the patties with the cooking spray.

✓ Air-fry at 355 F for 9 minutes, working in batches. Slice burger buns into halves. In the meantime, combine olive oil with mashed avocado and pressed garlic.

✓ To finish, lay Romaine lettuce and avocado spread on bun bottoms; now, add burgers and bun tops. Bon appétit!

Nutritions: 321 Calories; 18.7g Fat; 15.8g Carbs; 23.5g Protein; 1.2g Sugars

512)   *Peanut Butter and Chicken Bites*

Ingredients

- 1 ½ tablespoons soy sauce
- 1/2 teaspoon smoked cayenne pepper
- 8 ounces soft cheese
- 1 1/2 tablespoons peanut butter
- 1/3 leftover chicken
- 1 teaspoon sea salt
- 32 wonton wrappers
- 1/3 teaspoon freshly cracked mixed peppercorns
- 1/2 tablespoon pear cider vinegar

Directions (Ready in about 10 minutes | Servings 8)

✓ Combine all of the above ingredients, minus the wonton wrappers, in a mixing dish.

✓ Lay out the wrappers on a clean surface. Now, spread the wonton wrappers with the prepared chicken filling.

✓ Fold the outside corners to the center over the filling; after that, roll up the wrappers tightly; you can moisten the edges with a little water.

✓ Set the air fryer to cook at 360 degrees F. Air fry the rolls for 6 minutes, working in batches. Serve with marinara sauce. Bon appétit!

Nutritions: 150 Calories; 9.7g Fat; 2.1g Carbs; 12.9g Protein; 1.6g Sugars

513)   *Tangy Paprika Chicken*

Ingredients

- 1 ½ tablespoons freshly squeezed lemon juice
- 2 small-sized chicken breasts, boneless
- 1/2 teaspoon ground cumin

- 1 teaspoon dry mustard powder
- 1 teaspoon paprika
- 2 teaspoons cup pear cider vinegar
- 1 tablespoon olive oil
- 2 garlic cloves, minced
- Kosher salt and freshly ground mixed peppercorns, to savor

Directions (Ready in about 30 minutes | Servings 4)
- ✓ Warm the olive oil in a nonstick pan over a moderate flame. Sauté the garlic for just 1 minutes.
- ✓ Remove your pan from the heat; add cider vinegar, lemon juice, paprika, cumin, mustard powder, kosher salt, and black pepper. Pour this paprika sauce into a baking dish.
- ✓ Pat the chicken breasts dry; transfer them to the prepared sauce. Bake in the preheated air fryer for about 28 minutes at 335 degrees F; check for doneness using a thermometer or a fork.
- ✓ Allow to rest for 8 to 9 minutes before slicing and serving. Serve with dressing.

Nutritions: 312 Calories; 17.6g Fat; 2.6g Carbs; 30.4g Protein; 1.2g Sugars

514) *Super-Easy Chicken with Tomato Sauce*

Ingredients
- 1 tablespoon balsamic vinegar
- ½ teaspoon red pepper flakes, crushed
- 1 fresh garlic, roughly chopped
- 2 ½ large-sized chicken breasts, cut into halves
- 1/3 handful fresh cilantro, roughly chopped
- 2 tablespoons olive oil
- 4 Roma tomatoes, diced
- 1 ½ tablespoons butter
- 1/3 handful fresh basil, loosely packed, sniped
- 1 teaspoon kosher salt
- 2 cloves garlic, minced
- Cooked bucatini, to serve

Directions (Ready in about 20 minutes + marinating time | Servings 4)
- ✓ Place the first seven ingredients in a medium-sized bowl; let it marinate for a couple of hours.
- ✓ Preheat the air fryer to 325 degrees F. Air-fry your chicken for 32 minutes and serve warm.
- ✓ In the meantime, prepare the tomato sauce by preheating a deep saucepan. Simmer the tomatoes until you make a chunky mixture. Throw in the garlic, basil, and butter; give it a good stir.
- ✓ Serve the cooked chicken breasts with the tomato sauce and the cooked bucatini. Bon appétit!

Nutritions: 377 Calories; 24.8g Fat; 6.5g Carbs; 31.6g Protein; 4.1g Sugars

515) *Cheesy Pasilla Turkey*
Ingredients
- 1/3 cup Parmesan cheese, shredded

- 2 turkey breasts, cut into four pieces
- 1/3 cup mayonnaise
- 1 ½ tablespoons sour cream
- 1/2 cup crushed crackers
- 1 dried Pasilla peppers
- 1 teaspoon onion salt
- 1/3 teaspoon mixed peppercorns, freshly cracked

Directions(Ready in about 30 minutes | Servings 2)
- ✓ In a shallow bowl, mix the crushed crackers, Parmesan cheese, onion salt, and the cracked mixed peppercorns together.
- ✓ In a food processor, blitz the mayonnaise, along with the cream and dried Pasilla peppers until there are no lumps.
- ✓ Coat the turkey breasts with this mixture, ensuring that all sides are covered.
- ✓ Then, coat each piece of turkey in the Parmesan/cracker mix.
- ✓ Now, preheat the air fryer to 365 degrees F; cook for 28 minutes until thoroughly cooked.

Nutritions: 259 Calories; 19.1g Fat; 7.6g Carbs; 14g Protein; 1.5g Sugars

516) *Festive Turkey Drumsticks with Gala Apples*

Ingredients
- 3 Gala apples, cored and diced
- 1/2 tablespoon Dijon mustard
- 2 sprigs rosemary, chopped
- 3 turkey drumsticks
- 1/3 cup cider vinegar
- 2 teaspoons olive oil
- 1/2cup tamari sauce
- 1/2 teaspoon smoked cayenne pepper
- Kosher salt and ground black pepper, to taste

Directions (Ready in about 30 minutes + marinating time | Servings 6)
- ✓ Dump drumsticks, along with cider vinegar, tamari, and olive oil, into a mixing dish. Let it marinate overnight or at least 3 hours.
- ✓ Set your air fryer to cook at 355 degrees F. Spread turkey drumsticks with Dijon mustard.
- ✓ Season turkey drumsticks with salt, black pepper, smoked cayenne pepper, and rosemary;
- ✓ Place the prepared drumstick in a lightly greased baking dish; scatter diced apples over them; work in batches, one drumstick at a time.
- ✓ Pause the machine after 13 minutes; flip turkey drumstick and continue to cook for a further 10 minutes. Bon appétit!

Nutritions: 100 Calories; 3.6g Fat; 14.7g Carbs; 4.9g Protein; 10.4g Sugars

517) *Roasted Turkey Sausage with Potatoes*
Ingredients
- 1/2 pound red potatoes, peeled and diced

- 1/2 teaspoon onion salt
- 1/2 teaspoon dried sage
- 1/2pound ground turkey
- 1/3 teaspoon ginger, ground
- 1 sprig rosemary, chopped
- 1 ½ tablespoons olive oil
- 1/2 teaspoon paprika
- 2 sprigs thyme, chopped
- 1 teaspoon ground black pepper

Directions (Ready in about 40 minutes | Servings 6)

✓ In a bowl, mix the first six ingredients; give it a good stir. Heat a thin layer of vegetable oil in a nonstick skillet that is placed over a moderate flame.

✓ Form the mixture into patties; fry until they're browned on all sides, or about 12 minutes.

✓ Arrange the potatoes at the bottom of a baking dish. Sprinkle with the rosemary and thyme; add a drizzle of olive oil. Top with the turkey.

✓ Roast for 32 minutes at 365 degrees F, turning once halfway through. Eat warm.

Nutritions: 212 Calories; 17.1g Fat; 6.3g Carbs; 8g Protein; 0.5g Sugars

518)   *Dinner Turkey Sandwiches*

Ingredients

- 1/2 pound turkey breast
- 1 teaspoon garlic powder
- 7 ounces condensed cream of onion soup
- 1/3 teaspoon ground allspice
- BBQ sauce, to savor

Directions (Ready in about 4 hours 30 minutes | Servings 4)

✓ Simply dump the cream of onion soup and turkey breast into your crock-pot. Cook on HIGH heat setting for 3 hours.

✓ Then, shred the meat and transfer to a lightly greased baking dish.

✓ Pour in your favorite BBQ sauce. Sprinkle with ground allspice and garlic powder. Air-fry an additional 28 minutes.

✓ To finish, assemble the sandwiches; add toppings such as pickled or fresh salad, mustard, etc.

Nutritions: 114 Calories; 5.6g Fat; 3.6g Carbs; 13.1g Protein; 0.2g Sugars

519)   *Dijon and Curry Turkey Cutlets*

Ingredients

- 1/2 tablespoon Dijon mustard
- 1/2 teaspoon curry powder
- Sea salt flakes and freshly cracked black peppercorns, to savor
- 1/3pound turkey cutlets
- 1/2 cup fresh lemon juice
- 1/2 tablespoons tamari sauce

Directions (Ready in about 30 minutes + marinating time | Servings 4)

✓ Set the air fryer to cook at 375 degrees. Then, put the turkey cutlets into a mixing dish; add fresh lemon juice, tamari, and mustard; let it marinate at least 2 hours.

✓ Coat each turkey cutlet with the curry powder, salt, and freshly cracked black peppercorns; roast for 28 minutes; work in batches. Bon appétit!

Nutritions: 190 Calories; 16.8g Fat; 2.5g Carbs; 7.4g Protein; 0.8g Sugars

520)   *Super Easy Sage and Lime Wings*

Ingredients

- 1 teaspoon onion powder
- 1/3 cup fresh lime juice
- 1/2 tablespoon corn flour
- 1/2 heaping tablespoon fresh chopped parsley
- 1/3 teaspoon mustard powder
- 1/2 pound turkey wings, cut into smaller pieces
- 2 heaping tablespoons fresh chopped sage
- 1/2 teaspoon garlic powder
- 1/2 teaspoon seasoned salt
- 1 teaspoon freshly cracked black or white peppercorns

Directions (Ready in about 30 minutes + marinating time | Servings 4)

✓ Simply dump all of the above ingredients into a mixing dish; cover and let it marinate for about 1 hours in your refrigerator.

✓ Air-fry turkey wings for 28 minutes at 355 degrees F. Bon appétit!

Nutritions: 127 Calories; 7.6g Fat; 3.7g Carbs; 11.9g Protein; 0.2g Sugars

521)   *Creamy Lemon Turkey!!*

Ingredients

- 1/3 cup sour cream
- 2 cloves garlic, finely minced
- 1/3 teaspoon lemon zest
- 2 small-sized turkey breasts, skinless and cubed
- 1/3 cup thickened cream
- 2 tablespoons lemon juice
- 1 teaspoon fresh marjoram, chopped
- Salt and freshly cracked mixed peppercorns, to taste
- 1/2 cup scallion, chopped
- 1/2 can tomatoes, diced
- 1 ½ tablespoons canola oil

Directions (Ready in about 2 hours 25 minutes | Servings 4)

✓ Firstly, pat dry the turkey breast. Mix the remaining items; marinate the turkey for 2 hours.

✓ Set the air fryer to cook at 355 degrees F. Brush the turkey with a nonstick spray; cook for 23 minutes, turning once. Serve with naan and enjoy!

Nutritions: 260 Calories; 15.3g Fat; 8.9g Carbs; 28.6g Protein; 1.9g Sugars

522)   *Turkey Wontons with Garlic-Parmesan Sauce*

Ingredients

- 8 ounces cooked turkey breasts, shredded
- 16 wonton wrappers
- 1 ½ tablespoons butter, melted
- 1/3 cup cream cheese, room temperature
- 8 ounces Asiago cheese, shredded
- 3 tablespoons Parmesan cheese, grated
- 1 teaspoon garlic powder
- Fine sea salt and freshly ground black pepper, to taste

Directions (Ready in about 15 minutes | Servings 8)

✓ In a small-sized bowl, mix the butter, Parmesan, garlic powder, salt, and black pepper; give it a good stir.

✓ Lightly grease a mini muffin pan; lay 1 wonton wrapper in each mini muffin cup. Fill each cup with the cream cheese and turkey mixture.

✓ Air-fry for 8 minutes at 335 degrees F. Immediately top with Asiago cheese and serve warm. Bon appétit!

Nutritions: 362 Calories; 13.5g Fat; 40.4g Carbs; 18.5g Protein; 1.2g Sugars

523)   *Cajun Turkey Meatloaf*

Ingredients

- 1 1/3 pounds turkey breasts, ground
- ½ cup vegetable stock
- 2 eggs, lightly beaten
- 1/2 sprig thyme, chopped
- 1/2 teaspoon Cajun seasonings
- 1/2 sprig coriander, chopped
- ½ cup seasoned breadcrumbs
- 2 tablespoons butter, room temperature
- 1/2 cup scallions, chopped
- 1/3 teaspoon ground nutmeg
- 1/3 cup tomato ketchup
- 1/2 teaspoon table salt
- 2 teaspoons whole grain mustard
- 1/3 teaspoon mixed peppercorns, freshly cracked

Directions (Ready in about 45 minutes | Servings 6)

✓ Firstly, warm the butter in a medium-sized saucepan that is placed over a moderate heat; sauté the scallions together with the chopped thyme and coriander leaves until just tender.

✓ While the scallions are sautéing, set your air fryer to cook at 365 degrees F.

✓ Combine all the ingredients, minus the ketchup, in a mixing dish; fold in the sautéed mixture and mix again.

✓ Shape into a meatloaf and top with the tomato ketchup. Air-fry for 50 minutes. Bon appétit!

Nutritions: 429 Calories; 31.6g Fat; 8.3g Carbs; 25.3g

Protein; 2.2g Sugars

524)   *Wine-Braised Turkey Breasts*

Ingredients

- 1/3 cup dry white wine
- 1½ tablespoon sesame oil
- 1/2 pound turkey breasts, boneless, skinless and sliced
- 1/2 tablespoon honey
- 1/2 cup plain flour
- 2 tablespoons oyster sauce
- Sea salt flakes and cracked black peppercorns, to taste

Directions (Ready in about 30 minutes + marinating time | Servings 4)

✓ Set the air fryer to cook at 385 degrees. Pat the turkey slices dry and season with the sea salt flakes and the cracked peppercorns.

✓ In a bowl, mix the other ingredients together, minus the flour; rub your turkey with this mixture. Set aside to marinate for at least 55 minutes.

✓ Coat each turkey slice with the plain flour. Cook for 27 minutes; make sure to flip once or twice and work in batches. Bon appétit!

Nutritions: 230 Calories; 11.6g Fat; 15.2g Carbs; 16.1g Protein; 2.2g Sugars

525)   *Italian-Style Turkey Meatballs*

Ingredients

- 1 ½ pounds ground turkey
- 1/2 cup parmesan cheese, grated
- 1/2 cup tortilla chips, crumbled
- 1 yellow onion, finely chopped
- 2 tablespoons Italian parsley, finely chopped
- 1 egg, beaten
- 2 cloves garlic, minced
- 1 tablespoon soy sauce
- 1 teaspoon Italian seasoning mix
- 1 teaspoon olive oil

Directions :(Prep + Cook Time: 30 minutes)

✓ Thoroughly combine all of the above ingredients until well incorporated.

✓ Shape the mixture into 10 equal meatballs.

✓ Spritz a cooking basket with a nonstick cooking spray. Cook at 360 degrees F for about 10 minutes or to your desired degree of doneness.

Nutrition:Calories: 253kcal (13%)Carbohydrates: 7g (2 %)Protein: 26g (52%)Fat: 14g (22%)Saturated Fat: 4g (25%) Fat: 4gMonounsaturated Fat: 0 Cholesterol: 129mg Fiber: 1g (4%)Sugar: 2g

526)   *Hot Chicken Drumettes with Peppers*

Ingredients

- 1/2 cup all-purpose four
- 1 teaspoon kosher salt
- 1 teaspoon shallot powder

- 1/2 teaspoon dried basil
- 1/2 teaspoon dried oregano
- 1/2 teaspoon smoked paprika
- 1 tablespoon hot sauce
- 1/4 cup mayonnaise
- 1/4 cup milk
- 1 pound chicken drumettes
- 2 bell peppers, sliced

Directions :(Prep + Cook Time: 30 minutes)

✓ In a shallow bowl, mix the flour, salt, shallot powder, basil, oregano and smoked paprika.

✓ In another bowl, mix the hot sauce, mayonnaise and milk.

✓ Dip the chicken drumettes in the flour mixture, then, coat them with the milk mixture; make sure to coat well on all sides.

✓ Cook in the preheated Air Fryer at 380 degrees F for 28 to 30 minutes; turn them over halfway through the cooking time. Reserve chicken drumettes, keeping them warm.

✓ Then, cook the peppers at 400 degrees F for 13 to 15 minutes, shaking the basket once or twice. Eat warm.

Nutritional Value: Calories: 47.3 g Fat: 1.5 g Carbohydrates: 0 Sugar: 0 Sodium: 115 g Fiber: 0 Protein: 6.4 g Cholesterol: 17.8 mg

527)   *Chicken Nuggets with Turnip Chips*

Ingredients

- 1 egg
- 1/2 teaspoon cayenne pepper
- 1/3 cup panko crumbs
- 1/4 teaspoon Romano cheese, grated
- 2 teaspoons canola oil
- 1 pound chicken breast, cut into slices
- 1 medium-sized turnip, trimmed and sliced
- 1/2 teaspoon garlic powder
- Sea salt and ground black pepper, to taste

Directions:(Prep + Cook Time: 30 minutes)

✓ Beat the egg with the cayenne pepper until frothy. In another shallow bowl, mix the panko crumbs with the cheese until well combined.

✓ Dip the chicken slices into the egg mixture; then, coat the chicken slices on all sides with the the panko mixture. Brush with 1 teaspoon of canola oil. Season with salt and pepper to taste.

✓ Cook in the preheated Air Fryer at 380 degrees F for 12 minutes, shaking the basket halfway through the cooking time; an instant-read thermometer should read 165 degrees F. Reserve, keeping them warm.

✓ Drizzle the turnip slices with the remaining teaspoon of canola oil. Season with garlic powder, salt and pepper to taste.

✓ Cook the turnips slices at 370 degrees F for about 20 minutes. Serve with the warm chicken nuggets. Bon appétit!

nutritional value: calories 459 energy 1920kj fat 8.3g saturates 2.3g fibre 6.1g protein 52.6g carbs 71.9g

528)   *Turkey Sausage with Brussels Sprouts*

Ingredients

- 4 turkey sausages
- 1/2 pound Brussels sprouts, trimmed and halved
- 1 teaspoon olive oil
- Sea salt and ground black pepper, to taste
- 1/2 teaspoon cayenne pepper
- 1/2 teaspoon shallot powder
- 1/4 teaspoon dried dill weed

Directions :(Prep + Cook Time: 30 minutes)

✓ Place the sausages in the Air Fryer cooking basket.

✓ Now, toss the Brussels sprouts with olive oil and spices. Scatter the Brussels sprouts around the the sausages.

✓ Cook in the preheated Air Fryer at 380 degrees F for 15 minutes, shaking the basket halfway through the cooking time. Bon appétit!

Nutritional Value:
Calories: 191kcal, Carbohydrates: 19g, Protein: 13g, Fat: 7g, Saturated Fat: 2g,

529)   *Garlicky Duck with Potato Rösti*

Ingredients

- 1/2 pound duck breast, skin-on, boneless
- 1 clove garlic, halved
- Coarse sea salt and ground black pepper, to taste
- 1/2 teaspoon marjoram
- 1/4 teaspoon mustard seeds
- 1/4 teaspoon fennel seeds
- Potato Rösti:
- 1/2 pound potatoes, grated
- 2 tablespoons butter, melted
- 1 teaspoon fresh rosemary, chopped
- Coarse sea salt and ground black pepper, to taste

Directions:(Prep + Cook Time: 30 minutes)

✓ Score the duck breast to render the fat and rub with fresh garlic on all sides. Season the duck with salt, pepper, marjoram, mustard seeds and fennel seeds.

✓ Place the duck, skin side up, into the cooking basket. Cook at 400 degrees F for 10 minutes. Turn the duck breast over and cook an additional 5 minutes.

✓ Allow it to rest for 5 to 8 minutes before carving and serving.

✓ Meanwhile, make the potato rösti by mixing all the ingredients in a bowl. Mix to combine well and shape the mixture into two equal patties.

✓ Cook in your Air Fryer at 400 degrees F for 15 minutes. Serve with the warm duck breast. Enjoy!

Nutritional Value: 407 calories; protein 5.6g; carbohydrates 53.2g; fat 20g; cholesterol 62.3mg; sodium 820.9mg

530) *Famous Buffalo Wings*

Ingredients

- 1 ½ pounds chicken wings
- Coarse salt and ground black pepper, to season
- 1/2 teaspoon onion powder
- 1/2 teaspoon cayenne pepper
- 1 teaspoon granulated garlic
- 4 tablespoons butter, at room temperature
- 2 tablespoons hot pepper sauce
- 1 (1-inch) piece ginger, peeled and grated
- 2 tablespoons soy sauce
- 2 tablespoons molasses

Directions :(Prep + Cook Time: 40 minutes)

✓ Pat dry the chicken wings with kitchen towels and set them aside.

✓ Toss the chicken wings with the salt, pepper, onion powder, cayenne pepper and granulated garlic; toss until they're well coated on all sides.

✓ Arrange the spiced chicken wings in the cooking basket and cook at 380 degrees F for 22 minutes until golden brown on all sides.

✓ In the meantime, whisk the butter, hot pepper sauce, ginger, soy sauce and molasses. Pour the sauce over the chicken wings and serve hot. Bon appétit!

Nutrition:Calories: 1112kcal | Carbohydrates: 34g | Protein: 19g | Fat: 100g | SaturatedFat: 31g | Cholesterol: 131mg | Sodium: 3603mg Fiber: 1g | Sugar: 8g |

531) *Garlic-Basil Turkey Breast*

Ingredients

- 1 ½ pounds turkey breast
- 2 tablespoons olive oil
- 2 cloves garlic, minced
- Sea salt and ground black pepper, to taste
- 1 teaspoon basil
- 2 tablespoons lemon zest, grated

Directions : Directions:(Prep + Cook Time: 40 minutes)

✓ Pat the turkey breast dry with paper towels.

✓ Rub the turkey breast with olive oil, garlic, salt, pepper, basil and lemon zest.

✓ Cook in the preheated Air Fryer at 380 degrees F for 20 minutes. Turn the turkey breast over and cook an additional 20 to 22 minutes.

✓ Bon appétit!

Nutrition:Calories: 166kcal | Carbohydrates: 1g | Protein: 24g | Fat: 7g | Saturated Fat: 1g | Cholesterol: 72mg | Sodium: 713mg | Potassium: 435mg | Fiber: 1g | Sugar: 1g | Vitamin A: 403IU | VitaminC: 1mg | Calcium: 14mg |

532) *Chicken Drumsticks with Blue Cheese Sauce*

Ingredients

- 1/2 teaspoon shallot powder
- 1/2 teaspoon garlic powder
- 1/2 teaspoon coriander
- 1/4 teaspoon red pepper flakes
- Sea salt and ground black pepper, to season
- 2 chicken drumsticks, skinless and boneless
- 1/4 cup blue cheese, softened
- 4 tablespoons mayonnaise
- 4 tablespoons sour cream
- 1 teaspoon fresh garlic, pressed
- 1 teaspoon fresh lime juic

Directions :(Prep + Cook Time: 40 minutes)

✓ In a resealable bag, place the shallot powder, garlic powder, coriander, red pepper, salt and black pepper; add in the chicken drumsticks and shake until they are well coated.

✓ Spritz the chicken drumsticks with a nonstick cooking oil and place in the cooking basket.

✓ Air fry the chicken drumsticks at 370 degrees F for 20 minutes, turning them over halfway through the cooking time.

✓ Meanwhile, make the sauce by whisking the remaining ingredients. Place the sauce in your refrigerator until ready to serve.

✓ Serve the chicken drumsticks with blue cheese sauce. Bon appétit!

Nutritional: 454 calories; fat 33g; cholesterol 141mg; carbohydrates 6g; fiber 1g; sugars 2g; protein 31g;

533) *Thanksgiving Turkey with Gravy*

Ingredients

- 1 ½ pound turkey breast
- 1 tablespoon Dijon mustard
- 2 tablespoons butter, at room temperature
- Sea salt and ground black pepper, to taste
- 1 teaspoon cayenne pepper
- 1/2 teaspoon garlic powder
- Gravy:
- 2 cups vegetable broth
- 1/4 cup all-purpose flour
- Freshly ground black pepper, to taste

Directions:(Prep + Cook Time: 80 minutes)

✓ Brush Dijon mustard and butter all over the turkey breast. Season with salt, black pepper, cayenne pepper and garlic powder.

✓ Cook in the preheated Air Fryer at 360 degrees F for about 50 minutes, flipping them halfway through the cooking time.

✓ Place the fat drippings from the cooked turkey in a sauté pan. Pour in 1 cup of broth and 1/8 cup of all-purpose flour; continue to cook, whisking continuously, until a smooth paste forms.

✓ Add in the remaining ingredients and continue to simmer until the gravy has reduced by half. Enjoy!

Nutritional Value:
Calories: 25kcalCarbohydrates: 3gProtein: 1gSodium: 18mgPotassium: 58mgCalcium: 3mgIron: 0.3mg

534) *Chicken and Cheese Stuffed Mushrooms*

Ingredients

- 9 medium-sized button mushrooms, cleaned and steams removed
- 1/2 pound chicken white meat, ground
- 2 ounces goat cheese, room temperature
- 2 ounces cheddar cheese, grated
- 1 teaspoon soy sauce
- 2 tablespoons scallions, finely chopped
- 1 teaspoon fresh garlic, finely chopped
- Sea salt and red pepper, to season

Directions:(Prep + Cook Time: 30 minutes)

- ✓ Pat the mushrooms dry and set them aside.
- ✓ Thoroughly combine all ingredients, except for the cheddar cheese, in a mixing bowl. Stir to combine well and stuff your mushrooms.
- ✓ Bake in your Air Fryer at 370 degrees F for 5 minutes. Top with cheddar cheese and continue to cook an additional 3 to 4 minutes or until the cheese melts. Bon appétit!

Nutritional Value: Calories: 575cal (29%)Carbohydrates: 7g (2%)Protein: 60g (120%)Fat: 34g (52%)Saturated Fat: 15g (94%)Trans Fat: 1gCholesterol: 205mg (68%)Sodium: 1409mg (61%)Potassium: 1352mg (39%)Fiber: 2g (8%)Sugar: 3g

535) *Tortilla Chip-Crusted Chicken Tenders*

Ingredients

- 1 pound chicken tenders
- Sea salt and black pepper, to taste
- 1/2 teaspoon shallot powder
- 1/2 teaspoon porcini powder
- 1/2 teaspoon dried rosemary
- 1/3 cup tortilla chips, crushed

Directions:(Prep + Cook Time: 30 minutes)

- ✓ Toss the chicken tenders with salt, pepper, shallot powder, porcini powder, dried rosemary and tortilla chips.
- ✓ Spritz the cooking basket with a nonstick cooking spray. Cook in the preheated Air Fryer at 360 degrees F for 10 minutes, flipping them halfway through the cooking time.

Nutritional:Calories: 199kcal, Carbohydrates: 10g, Protein: 24g, Fat: 6g, Cholesterol: 148mg, Sodium: 125mg, Potassium: 310mg,

536) *Turkey and Bacon Casserole*

Ingredients

- 4 tablespoons bacon bits
- 1 pound turkey sausage, chopped
- 1/2 cup sour cream
- 1 cup milk
- 5 eggs
- 1/2 teaspoon smoked paprika
- Sea salt and ground black pepper, to your liking
- 1 cup Colby cheese, shredded

Directions:(Prep + Cook Time: 30 minutes)

- ✓ Add the bacon bits and chopped sausage to a lightly greased baking dish.
- ✓ In a mixing dish, thoroughly combine the sour cream, milk, eggs, paprika, salt and black pepper.
- ✓ Pour the mixture into the baking dish.
- ✓ Cook in your Air Fryer at 310 degrees F for about 10 minutes or until set. Top with Colby cheese and cook an additional 2 minutes or until the cheese is bubbly. Bon appétit!

Nutritional Value: Calories 100 Protein 6g Carbohydrates 15g Fiber 1g Sugars 9g Fat 2g Cholesterol 5mg Sodium 180mg Saturated Fat 0g

537) *Turkey Sausage Breakfast Cups*

Ingredients

- 1 smoked turkey sausage, chopped
- 4 eggs
- 4 tablespoons cream cheese
- 4 tablespoons cheddar cheese, shredded
- 4 tablespoons fresh scallions, chopped
- 1/2 teaspoon garlic, minced
- 1/4 teaspoon mustard seeds
- 1/4 teaspoon chili powder
- Salt and red pepper, to taste

Directions :(Prep + Cook Time: 30 minutes)

- ✓ Divide the chopped sausage between four silicone baking cups.
- ✓ In a mixing bowl, beat the eggs until pale and frothy. Then, add in the remaining ingredients and mix to combine well.
- ✓ Pour the egg mixture into the cups.
- ✓ Cook in your Air Fryer at 330 degrees F for 10 to 11 minutes. Transfer the cups to wire racks to cool slightly before unmolding. Enjoy!

Nutritional Value: Calories 502 Fat 39g Carbs 2g Fiber 0g Sugar 1g Protein 33g

538) *Xiang Su Ya (Chinese Duck)*

Ingredients

- 2 tablespoons peanuts, chopped
- 1 tablespoon honey
- 1 tablespoon olive oil
- 1 tablespoon hoisin sauce
- 1 pound duck breast
- 1 small-sized white onion, sliced
- 1 teaspoon garlic, chopped
- 1 celery stick, diced
- 1 thumb ginger, sliced
- 4 baby potatoes, diced

Directions:(Prep + Cook Time: 30 minutes)

- ✓ Mix the peanuts, honey, olive oil and hoisin sauce; spread the mixture all over duck breast. Place the duck breast in a lightly oiled cooking basket.

- ✓ Scatter white onion, garlic, celery, ginger and potatoes over the duck breasts.
- ✓ Cook in your Air Fryer at 400 degrees F for 20 minutes.
- ✓ Serve with Mandarin pancakes and enjoy!

Nutritional Value: Fat 15g23% Saturated Fat 12g75% Sodium 1374mg60% Potassium 246mg7% Carbohydrates 15g5% Fiber 2g8% Protein 2g4%

539) *Mexican-Style Taco Chicke*
Ingredients

- 1 pound chicken legs, skinless, boneless
- 1/2 cup mayonnaise
- 1/2 cup milk
- 1/3 cup all-purpose flour
- Sea salt and ground black pepper, to season
- 1/2 teaspoon cayenne pepper
- 1/3 cup tortilla chips, crushed
- 1 teaspoon Taco seasoning blend
- 1/2 teaspoon dried Mexican oregano

Directions:(Prep + Cook Time: 40 minutes)

- ✓ Pat dry the chicken legs and set them aside.
- ✓ In a mixing bowl, thoroughly combine the mayonnaise, milk, flour, salt, black pepper and cayenne pepper.
- ✓ In another shallow bowl, mix the crushed tortilla chip, taco seasoning blend and Mexican oregano.
- ✓ Dip the chicken legs into the mayonnaise mixture. Then, coat them with the tortilla chip mixture, shaking off any excess crumbs.
- ✓ Cook in the preheated Air Fryer at 385 degrees F for 20 minutes, flipping them halfway through the cooking time. Enjoy!

Nutritional:Calories: 103cal (5%)Carbohydrates: 1gProtein: 11g Fat: 5g (8%)SaturatedFat: 1g (6%)Cholesterol: 55mg (18%)Sodium: 338mg (15%)Potassium: 190mg

540) *Japanese Chicken Teriyaki*
Ingredients

- 1 pound chicken cutlets
- 1 teaspoon sesame oil
- 1 tablespoon lemon juice
- 1 tablespoon Mirin
- 1 tablespoon soy sauce
- 1 teaspoon ginger, peeled and grated
- 2 garlic cloves, minced
- 1 teaspoon cornstarch

Directions:(Prep + Cook Time: 70 minutes)

- ✓ Pat dry the chicken cutlets and set them aside.
- ✓ In a mixing dish, thoroughly combine the remaining ingredients until everything is well incorporated.
- ✓ Brush the mixture oil over the chicken cutlets and place it in your refrigerator for 30 to 40 minutes.
- ✓ Cook in the preheated Air Fryer at 360 degrees F for 10 minutes, flipping them halfway through the cooking time. Serve with shirataki noodles and enjoy!

Nutritional Value: 329g calories: 442kcal fat: 26g (40%) saturated fat: 7g (35%) trans fat: 0.1g polyunsaturated fat: 505g monounsaturated fat: 11g cholesterol: 166mg (55%) sodium: 301mg (13%) potassium: 634mg (18%) carbohydrates: 19g (6%) dietary fibre: 3.1g (12%) sugar: 14g protein: 31g

541) *Roasted Turkey Thighs with Cheesy Cauliflower*
Ingredients

- 1 tablespoon butter, room temperature
- 2 pounds turkey thighs
- 1/2 teaspoon smoked paprika
- 1/2 teaspoon dried marjoram
- 1/4 teaspoon dried dill
- Sea salt and ground black pepper, to taste
- 1 pound cauliflower, broken into small florets
- 1/3 cup Pecorino Romano cheese, freshly grated
- 1 teaspoon garlic, minced

Directions:(Prep + Cook Time: 60-70 minutes)

- ✓ Rub the butter all over the turkey thighs; sprinkle with smoked paprika, marjoram, dill, salt and black pepper.
- ✓ Roast in the preheated Air Fryer at 360 degrees F for about 20 minutes. Flip the turkey thighs and continue to cook an additional 20 minutes. Reserve.
- ✓ Toss the cauliflower florets with the Pecorino Romano and garlic; salt to taste.
- ✓ Cook at 400 degrees F for 12 to 13 minutes. Serve the warm turkey thighs with the cauliflower on the side. Bon appétit!

Nutritional Value: 849 calories; protein 63.5g; carbohydrates 33.7g; fat 51.6g; cholesterol 255.7mg; sodium 1549.4mg.

542) *Farmhouse Chicken Roulade*
Ingredients

- 4 slices smoked bacon, chopped
- 4 slices Monterey-Jack cheese, sliced
- 1 ½ pounds chicken fillets
- 1 celery stick, chopped
- 1 small sized onion, chopped
- 1 teaspoon hot sauce
- Sea salt and ground black pepper, to season
- 1 lemon, cut into slices

Directions:(Prep + Cook Time: 30 minutes)

- ✓ Place 1 slice of bacon and 1 slice of cheese on each chicken fillet. Divide the celery and onion between chicken fillets.
- ✓ Top with hot sauce and season with salt and black pepper to your liking. Then, roll them up and tie with kitchen twine.
- ✓ Roast in the preheated Air Fryer at 380 degrees F for 8 minutes; turn them over and continue to cook for 5 to 6 minutes more. Serve with lemon slices and eat warm.

Nutritional Value: 639 calories Fat: 42g65%
Saturated Fat: 14g70% Cholesterol: 215mg72%
Sodium: 685mg29% Total Carbohydrates: 3g1%
Dietary Fiber: 0g0% Sugar: 1g Protein: 59g

543)   *Greek-Style Chicken Salad*
Ingredients

- 1/2 pound chicken breasts, boneless and skinless
- 1 cup grape tomatoes, halved
- 1 Serrano pepper, deveined and chopped
- 2 bell peppers, deveined and chopped
- 2 tablespoons olives, pitted and sliced
- 1 cucumber, sliced
- 1 red onion, sliced
- 1 cup arugula
- 1 cup baby spinach
- 1/4 cup mayonnaise
- 2 tablespoons Greek-style yogurt
- 1 teaspoon lime juice
- 1/4 teaspoon oregano
- 1/4 teaspoon basil
- 1/4 teaspoon red pepper flakes, crushed
- Sea salt and ground black pepper, to taste

Directions:(Prep + Cook Time: 30 minutes
✓ Spritz the chicken breasts with a nonstick cooking oil.
✓ Cook in the preheated Air Fryer at 380 degrees F for 12 minutes. Transfer to a cutting board to cool slightly before slicing.
✓ Cut the chicken into bite-sized strips and transfer them to a salad bowl.
✓ Toss the chicken with the remaining ingredients and place in your refrigerator until ready to serve. Enjoy!

Nutritional Value: 394 calories; fat 17.2g; saturated fat 2.2g; mono fat 10g; poly fat 3.2g; protein 25g; carbohydrates 38g; fiber 7g; cholesterol 51mg; iron 5mg; sodium 588mg; calcium 117mg.

544)   *Authentic Indian Chicken with Raita*
Ingredients

- 2 chicken fillets
- Sea salt and ground black pepper, to taste
- 2 teaspoons garam masala
- 1 teaspoon ground turmeric
- 1/2 cup plain yogurt
- 1 English cucumber, shredded and drained
- 1 tablespoon fresh cilantro, coarsely chopped
- 1/2 red onion, chopped
- A pinch of grated nutmeg
- A pinch of ground cinnamon

Directions:(Prep + Cook Time: 30 minutes)
✓ Sprinkle the chicken fillets with salt, pepper, garam masala and ground turmeric until well coated on all sides.
✓ Cook in the preheated Air Fryer at 380 degrees F for 12 minutes, turning them over once or twice.
✓ Meanwhile, make traditional raita by mixing the remaining ingredients in a bowl. Serve the chicken fillets with the raita sauce on the side. Enjoy!

Nutritional Value: 284 calories; fat 7.9g; saturated fat 2g; mono fat 2.4g; poly fat 2g; protein 45.7g; carbohydrates 4.9g; fiber 0.7g; cholesterol 161mg; iron 2.5mg; sodium 502mg; calcium 76mg.

545)   *Asian-Style Chicken Drumettes*
Ingredients

- 1/4 cup soy sauce
- 1 teaspoon brown mustard
- 1 teaspoon garlic paste
- 2 tablespoons tomato paste
- 2 tablespoons sesame oil
- 1 tablespoon brown sugar
- 2 tablespoons rice vinegar
- 1 pound chicken drumettes

Directions:(Prep + Cook Time: 80 minutes)
✓ Place the chicken drumettes and the other ingredients in a resalable bag; allow it to marinate for 2 hours.
✓ Discard the marinade and transfer the chicken drumettes to the Air Fryer cooking basket.
✓ Cook at 400 degrees F for 12 minutes, shaking the basket halfway through the cooking time to ensure even cooking.
✓ In the meantime, bring the reserved marinade to a boil in a small saucepan. Immediately turn the heat to low and let it simmer until the sauce has reduced by half.
✓ Spoon the sauce over the chicken drumettes and serve immediately.

nutritional value: calories 368 fat 20g saturated fat5g cholesterol94mg sodium1054mg carbohydrates24g protein24g

546)   *Easy Chicken Taquitos*
Ingredients

- 1 pound chicken breast, boneless
- Sea salt and ground black pepper, to taste
- 1/2 teaspoon cayenne pepper
- 1/2 teaspoon onion powder
- 1/2 teaspoon garlic powder
- 1/2 teaspoon mustard powder
- 1 cup Cotija cheese, shredded
- 6 corn tortillas

Directions:(Prep + Cook Time: 30 minutes)
✓ Season the chicken with salt, black pepper, cayenne pepper, onion powder, garlic powder and mustard powder.
✓ Cook in the preheated Air Fryer at 380 degrees F for 12 minutes; turn the chicken over halfway through the cooking time to ensure even cooking.
✓ Transfer the chicken to a cutting board and shred

with two forks.

✓ Assemble your taquitos with the chicken and Cotija cheese; roll them up.

✓ Bake your taquitos at 390 degrees F for 5 to 6 minutes; serve immediately.

Nutritional Value: 527 calories; protein 47.5g; carbohydrates 23.6g; fat 25.8g; cholesterol 145.5mg; sodium 1204mg.

547)   *Huli-Huli Turkey*

Ingredients

- 2 turkey drumsticks
- Sea salt and ground black pepper, to season
- 1 teaspoon paprika
- 1 teaspoon hot sauce
- 1 teaspoon garlic paste
- 1 teaspoon olive oil
- 1/2 teaspoon rosemary
- 1/2 small pineapple, cut into wedges
- 1 teaspoon coconut oil, melted
- 2 stalks scallions, sliced

Directions:(Prep + Cook Time: 30 minutes)

✓ Toss the turkey drumsticks with salt, black pepper, paprika, hot sauce, garlic paste, olive oil and rosemary.

✓ Cook in the preheated Air Fryer at 360 degrees F for 25 minutes. Reserve.

✓ Turn the temperature to 400 degrees F, place pineapple wedges in the cooking basket and brush them with coconut oil.

✓ Cook your pineapple for 8 to 9 minutes. Serve the turkey drumsticks garnished with roasted pineapple and scallions. Enjoy!

Nutritional Value: 502 calories; protein 41.7g; carbohydrates 58.9g; fat 12.9g; cholesterol 72.3mg; sodium 1997.4mg.

548)   *Southwest Buttermilk Chicken Thighs*

Ingredients

- 1 pound chicken thighs
- 1 cup buttermilk
- 1/2 teaspoon garlic paste
- 1/4 cup Sriracha sauce
- Sea salt and ground black pepper, to taste
- 1 teaspoon cayenne pepper
- 1/4 cup cornflour
- 1/4 cup all-purpose flour

Directions:(Prep + Cook Time: 30 minutes)

✓ Pat dry the chicken thighs with kitchen towels.

✓ Now, thoroughly combine the buttermilk, garlic paste, Sriracha sauce, salt, black pepper and cayenne pepper.

✓ Dredge the chicken into the mixture until well coated. Place in your refrigerator for 2 hours.

✓ Place the flour in another shallow bowl. Coat the chicken thigs with the flour mixture.

✓ Cook in your Air Fryer at 395 degrees F for 12 minutes. Bon appétit!

Nutritional Value: 389 calories; protein 26.3g; carbohydrates 15.2g; fat 24.8g; cholesterol 109.6mg; sodium 907mg.

549)   *Traditional Greek Keftedes*

Ingredients

- 1/2 pound ground chicken
- 1 egg
- 1 slice stale bread, cubed and soaked in milk
- 1 teaspoon fresh garlic, pressed
- 2 tablespoons Romano cheese, grated
- 1 bell pepper, deveined and chopped
- 1 teaspoon olive oil
- 1/2 teaspoon dried oregano
- 1/2 teaspoon dried basil
- 1/8 teaspoon grated nutmeg
- Sea salt and ground black pepper, to taste
- 2 pita bread

Directions:(Prep + Cook Time: 30 minutes)

✓ Thoroughly combine all ingredients, except for the pita bread, in a mixing bowl. Stir until everything is well incorporated.

✓ Roll the mixture into 6 meatballs and place them in a lightly oiled cooking basket.

✓ Air fry at 380 degrees F for 10 minutes, shaking the basket occasionally to ensure even cooking. Place the keftedes in a pita bread and serve with tomato and tzatziki sauce if desired. Enjoy!

Nutritional Value: 493 Calories; 27.9g Fat; 27.1g Carbs; 32.6g Protein; 4.2g Sugars

550)   *Italian Chicken Parmigiana*

 Ingredients

- 2 chicken fillets
- 1 egg, beaten
- 2 tablespoons milk
- 1 teaspoon garlic paste
- 1 tablespoon fresh cilantro, chopped
- 1/2 cup seasoned breadcrumbs
- 4 tablespoons marinara sauce
- 4 slices parmesan cheese

Directions:(Prep + Cook Time: 30 minutes)

✓ Spritz the cooking basket with a nonstick cooking oil.

✓ Whisk the egg, milk, garlic paste and cilantro in a shallow bowl. In another bowl, place the seasoned breadcrumbs.

✓ Dip each chicken fillet in the egg mixture, then, coat them with breadcrumbs. Press to coat well.

✓ Cook in the preheated Air Fryer at 380 degrees F for 6 minutes; turn the chicken over.

✓ Top with marinara sauce and parmesan cheese and continue to cook for 6 minutes. Enjoy!

Nutritional Value: 570 Calories; 34.6g Fat; 13.1g Carbs; 50.1g Protein; 3.2g Sugars

551) *Balsamic Marjoram Chicken*

Ingredients

- 3 chicken drumsticks
- Sea salt and ground black pepper, to season
- 1/2 teaspoon red pepper flakes, crushed
- 1/2 teaspoon shallot powder
- 1/2 teaspoon onion powder
- 1/2 teaspoon garlic powder
- 1 teaspoon dried marjoram
- 1/4 cup cornstarch
- 2 tablespoons balsamic vinegar
- 2 tablespoons milk

Directions:(Prep + Cook Time: 50 minutes)

- ✓ Pat dry the chicken with paper towels. Toss the chicken drumsticks with all seasonings.
- ✓ In a shallow bowl, mix the cornstarch, balsamic vinegar and milk until well combined.
- ✓ Roll the chicken drumsticks onto the cornstarch mixture, pressing to coat well on all sides; shake off any excess pieces of the mixture.
- ✓ Cook in the preheated Air Fryer at 380 degrees F for 30 minutes, turning them over halfway through the cooking time. Bon appétit!

Nutritional Value: Nutritions: 275 Calories; 12.6g Fat; 14.1g Carbs; 24.3g Protein; 2.9g Sugars

552) *Classic Chicken Fajitas*

Ingredients

- 1 pound chicken breast, skinless and boneless
- 1 teaspoon butter, melted
- Sea salt and ground black pepper, to taste
- 1/2 teaspoon red pepper flakes, crushed
- 1/2 teaspoon Mexican oregano
- 1/2 teaspoon garlic powder
- 3 bell peppers, thinly sliced
- 1 red onion, sliced

Directions:(Prep + Cook Time: 30 minutes)

- ✓ Brush the chicken with melted butter on all sides. Season the chicken with salt, black pepper, red pepper, oregano and garlic powder.
- ✓ Cook in the preheated Air Fryer at 380 degrees F for 12 minutes until golden and cooked through; turn the chicken over halfway through the cooking time.
- ✓ Let the chicken rest for 10 minutes, then, slice into strips. Reserve, keeping it warm.
- ✓ Place the onions and peppers in the cooking basket; cook at 400 degrees F for 10 minutes. Taste and adjust the seasonings.
- ✓ Transfer the vegetables to a serving bowl; stir in the chicken and serve immediately.

Nutritional Value: 299 Calories; 15.3g Fat; 6.4g Carbs; 32.3g Protein; 3.2g Sugars

553) *Keto Chicken Quesadillas*

Ingredients

- 1/2 pound chicken breasts, boneless and skinless
- Salt to taste
- 3 eggs
- 4 ounces Ricotta cheese
- 2 tablespoons flaxseed meal
- 1 teaspoon psyllium husk powder
- Black pepper, to taste

Directions:(Prep + Cook Time: 40 minutes)

- ✓ Cook the chicken in the preheated Air Fryer at 380 degrees F for 12 minutes; turn the chicken over halfway through the cooking time. Salt to taste and slice into small strips.
- ✓ In a mixing bowl, beat the eggs, cheese, flaxseed meal, psyllium husk powder and black pepper. Spoon the mixture into a lightly oiled baking pan.
- ✓ Bake at 380 degrees F for 9 to 10 minutes.
- ✓ Spoon the chicken pieces onto your quesadilla and fold in half. Cut your quesadilla into two pieces and serve.

Nutritional Value: Per serving 401 Calories; 20.5g Fat; 5.7g Carbs; 48.3g Protein; 0.6g Sugars

554) *Garlic Butter Chicken Wings*

Ingredients

- 1 pound chicken wings
- Salt and black pepper, to taste
- 2 tablespoons butter
- 1 teaspoon garlic paste
- 1 lemon, cut into slices

Directions:(Prep + Cook Time: 30 minutes)

- ✓ Pat dry the chicken wings with a kitchen towel and season all over with salt and black pepper.
- ✓ In a bowl, mix together butter and garlic paste. Rub the mixture all over the wings.
- ✓ Cook in the preheated Air Fryer at 380 degrees F for 18 minutes.
- ✓ Serve garnished with lemon slices. Bon appétit!

Nutritional Value: 270 Calories; 13.1g Fat; 2.9g Carbs; 33.6g Protein; 1.5g Sugars

555) *Crispy Chicken Fingers*

Ingredients

- 1 pound chicken tenders
- 1/4 cup all-purpose flour
- 1/2 teaspoon onion powder
- 1/2 teaspoon garlic powder
- 1/2 teaspoon cayenne pepper
- Sea salt and ground black pepper, to taste
- 1/2 cup breadcrumbs
- 1 egg
- 1 tablespoon olive oil

Directions:(Prep + Cook Time: 30 minutes)

- ✓ Pat dry the chicken with kitchen towels and cut into bite-sized pieces.
- ✓ In a shallow bowl, mix the flour, onion powder, garlic powder, cayenne pepper, salt and black pepper. Dip the chicken pieces in the flour mixture and toss to coat well on all sides.
- ✓ In the second bowl, place breadcrumbs.
- ✓ In the third bowl, whisk the egg; now, dip the chicken in the beaten egg. Afterwards, roll each piece of chicken in the breadcrumbs until well coated on all sides.
- ✓ Spritz the chicken fingers with olive oil. Cook in your Air Fryer at 360 degrees F for 8 to 10 minutes, turning it over halfway through the cooking time.
- ✓ Serve with your favorite sauce for dipping. Enjoy!

Nutritional Value: Per serving 314 Calories; 12.1g Fat; 13.4g Carbs; 35.6g Protein; 1.4g Sugars

556) *Chicken Alfredo with Mushrooms*
Ingredients
- 1 pound chicken breasts, boneless
- 1 medium onion, quartered
- 1 teaspoon butter, melted
- 1/2 pound mushrooms, cleaned
- 12 ounces Alfredo sauce
- Salt and black pepper, to taste

Directions :(Prep + Cook Time: 30 minutes)
- ✓ Start by preheating your Air Fryer to 380 degrees F. Then, place the chicken and onion in the cooking basket. Drizzle with melted butter.
- ✓ Cook in the preheated Air Fryer for 6 minutes. Add in the mushrooms and continue to cook for 5 to 6 minutes more.
- ✓ Slice the chicken into strips. Chop the mushrooms and onions; stir in the Alfredo sauce. Salt and pepper to taste.
- ✓ Serve with hot cooked fettuccine. Bon appétit!

Nutritional Value: 334 Calories; 15.1g Fat; 13.4g Carbs; 36g Protein; 7.5g Sugars

557) *Grandma's Chicken with Rosemary and Sweet Potatoes*
Ingredients
- 2 chicken legs, bone-in
- 2 garlic cloves, minced
- 1 teaspoon sesame oil
- Sea salt and ground black pepper, to taste
- 2 sprigs rosemary, leaves picked and crushed
- 1/2 pound sweet potatoes

Directions :(Prep + Cook Time: 45 minutes)
- ✓ Start by preheating your Air Fryer to 380 degrees F. Now, rub garlic halves all over the chicken legs.
- ✓ Drizzle the chicken legs and sweet potatoes with the sesame oil. Sprinkle them with salt and rosemary. Place the chicken and potatoes in the cooking basket.
- ✓ Cook in the preheated Air Fryer for 30 minutes until the potatoes are thoroughly cooked. The chicken must reach an internal temperature of 165 degrees F.
- ✓ Serve the chicken legs garnished with the sweet potatoes. Bon appétit!

Nutritional Value: 604 Calories; 36.1g Fat; 23.4g Carbs; 44.5g Protein; 2.5g Sugars

558) *Authentic Spanish Chicken Drumstick*
Ingredients
- 2 chicken drumsticks, boneless
- 1 teaspoon Spanish paprika
- 1/2 teaspoon mustard seeds, ground
- 1/2 teaspoon fennel seeds, ground
- 1/2 teaspoon cumin seeds, ground
- Sea salt and ground black pepper, to taste
- 1/4 cup all-purpose flour
- 1 egg
- 1 tablespoon buttermilk

Directions:(Prep + Cook Time: 30 minutes)
- ✓ Pat the chicken dry and sprinkle it with spice until well coated on all sides.
- ✓ Add the flour to a rimmed plate. Dredge the chicken into the flour.
- ✓ In a shallow bowl, beat the egg with buttermilk until frothy and well combined. Dip each chicken drumstick into the egg mixture.
- ✓ Cook in the preheated Air Fryer at 380 degrees F for 10 minutes. Turn them over and cook for a further 10 minutes. Eat warm.

Nutritional Value: 354 Calories; 17.1g Fat; 16.3g Carbs; 31.5g Protein; 2.1g Sugars

559) *Chicken Tostadas with Nacho Cheese Sauce*
Ingredients
- 1/2 pound chicken fillets
- 1 egg, beaten
- 1/4 cup all-purpose flour
- Kosher salt and ground black pepper, to taste
- 1/4 cup tortilla chips, crushed
- 1 teaspoon corn oil
- 2 tostada shells
- Sauce:
- 1/2 cup nacho cheese, melted according to package instructions
- 1 tablespoon lime juice
- 2 pickled jalapenos, chopped
- 1/2 teaspoon Mexican oregano

Directions :(Prep + Cook Time: 40 minutes)
- ✓ Pat the chicken fillets dry with paper towels.
- ✓ Then, beat the egg in a shallow bowl. In another bowl, mix the flour, salt and black pepper. In the third bowl, place crushed tortilla chips.
- ✓ Dip the chicken fillets in the flour mixture, then the

egg, then, roll in the crushed tortilla chips.

✓ Drizzle the chicken fillets with corn oil. Cook in the preheated Air Fryer at 380 degrees F for 12 minutes, turning them over once or twice; an instant thermometer should read 165 degrees F.

✓ Heat the tostada shells at 350 degrees F for about 5 minutes. Meanwhile, make the sauce by mixing all ingredients.

✓ Working one at a time, place a chicken fillet in the center of each tostada shell. Serve with nacho sauce on the side! Enjoy!

Nutritional Value: 312 calories; protein 19.6g; carbohydrates **26.5g; fat 14.5g; cholesterol 54.8mg; sodium 711.7mg.**

560) *Thanksgiving Turkey with Mint Sauce*

Ingredients

- 1 ½ pounds turkey tenderloin
- 1 teaspoon olive oil
- Sea salt and black pepper, to season
- 1 teaspoon dried thyme
- 1/2 teaspoon garlic powder
- 1/2 teaspoon dried sage
- Sauce:
- 2 slices white bread
- 3/4 ounce fresh mint leaves
- 1 tablespoon extra-virgin olive oil
- 1 tablespoon white wine vinegar
- 1 teaspoon garlic, minced

Directions:(Prep + Cook Time: 80 minutes)

✓ Toss the turkey tenderloin with olive oil, salt, pepper, thyme, garlic powder and sage.

✓ Cook in the preheated Air Fryer at 350 degrees F for about 55 minutes, turning it over halfway through the cooking time.

✓ Meanwhile, make the mint sauce; pulse the bread slices in a food processor until coarsely crumbled.

✓ Add in the mint, olive oil, vinegar and garlic; blend again until everything is well incorporated; make sure to add water slowly and gradually until your desired consistency is reached.

✓ Let it rest on a wire rack to cool slightly before carving and serving. Spoon the sauce over warm turkey and serve. Bon appétit!

Nutritional Value: 218 calories; protein 0.9g; carbohydrates 27.2g; fat 0.3g; cholesterol 0mg; sodium 11.9mg.

561) *Punjabi Tandoori Murgh*

Ingredients

- 1/2 pound chicken tenderloin
- 1/4 cup Raita
- 1 garlic clove, pressed
- 1 tablespoon fresh cilantro, minced
- Salt and black pepper, to taste
- 1 teaspoon turmeric powder

- 1/2 teaspoon Garam Masala

Directions:(Prep + Cook Time: 80 minutes)

✓ Place all ingredients in a ceramic dish; stir well and cover. Place in your refrigerator for 1 hour.

✓ Transfer the chicken tenderloin to the cooking basket, discarding the marinade.

✓ Cook at 360 degrees F for 6 minutes. Turn the chicken over, baste with the reserved marinade and cook for 6 minutes on the other side.

✓ Serve with lemon wedges and enjoy!

Nutritions:Calories: 402kcal | Carbohydrates: 2g | Protein: 20g | Fat: 33g | Cholesterol: 90mg | Sodium: 412mg | Potassium: 295mg | Sugar: 1g |

562) *Nagoya-Style Tebasaki*

Ingredients

- 4 chicken drumettes
- 1 tablespoon sesame oil
- 1 tablespoon black vinegar
- 2 tablespoons soy sauce
- 1 tablespoon ginger juice
- 2 tablespoons sake
- 1 tablespoon sesame seeds, lightly toasted

Directions:(Prep + Cook Time: 40 minutes)

✓ Place all ingredients, except for the sesame oil, in a glass bowl. Cover, transfer to your refrigerator and let it marinate for 1 hour.

✓ Cook in the preheated Air Fryer at 370 degrees F for 22 minutes until golden brown; baste and turn them over halfway through the cooking time.

✓ Serve garnished with toasted sesame seeds.

Nutritional Value: 344 Calories; 18.8g Fat; 8.4g Carbs; 28.4g Protein; 3.7g Sugars

563) *Pretzel Crusted Chicken with Spicy Mustard Sauce*

Ingredients

- 2 eggs
- 1 ½ pound chicken breasts, boneless, skinless, cut into bite-sized chunks
- 1/2 cup crushed pretzels
- 1 teaspoon shallot powder
- 1 teaspoon paprika
- Sea salt and ground black pepper, to taste
- 1/2 cup vegetable broth
- 1 tablespoon cornstarch
- 3 tablespoons Worcestershire sauce
- 3 tablespoons tomato paste
- 1 tablespoon apple cider vinegar
- 2 tablespoons olive oil
- 2 garlic cloves, chopped
- 1 jalapeno pepper, minced
- 1 teaspoon yellow mustard

Directions :(Prep + Cook Time: 30 minutes)

✓ Start by preheating your Air Fryer to 390 degrees F.

- ✓ In a mixing dish, whisk the eggs until frothy; toss the chicken chunks into the whisked eggs and coat well.
- ✓ In another dish, combine the crushed pretzels with shallot powder, paprika, salt and pepper. Then, lay the chicken chunks in the pretzel mixture; turn it over until well coated.
- ✓ Place the chicken pieces in the air fryer basket. Cook the chicken for 12 minutes, shaking the basket halfway through.
- ✓ Meanwhile, whisk the vegetable broth with cornstarch, Worcestershire sauce, tomato paste, and apple cider vinegar.
- ✓ Preheat a cast-iron skillet over medium flame. Heat the olive oil and sauté the garlic with jalapeno pepper for 30 to 40 seconds, stirring frequently.
- ✓ Add the cornstarch mixture and let it simmer until the sauce has thickened a little. Now, add the air-fried chicken and mustard; let it simmer for 2 minutes more or until heated through.
- ✓ Serve immediately and enjoy!

Nutritional Value: 863 calories; protein 34.4g; carbohydrates 41.5g; fat 64.3g; cholesterol 76.8mg;

564) *Chinese-Style Sticky Turkey Thighs*

Ingredients

- 1 tablespoon sesame oil
- 2 pounds turkey thighs
- 1 teaspoon Chinese Five-spice powder
- 1 teaspoon pink Himalayan salt
- 1/4 teaspoon Sichuan pepper
- 6 tablespoons honey
- 1 tablespoon Chinese rice vinegar
- 2 tablespoons soy sauce
- 1 tablespoon sweet chili sauce
- 1 tablespoon mustard

Directions :(Prep + Cook Time: 40 minutes)

- ✓ Preheat your Air Fryer to 360 degrees F.
- ✓ Brush the sesame oil all over the turkey thighs. Season them with spices.
- ✓ Cook for 23 minutes, turning over once or twice. Make sure to work in batches to ensure even cooking
- ✓ In the meantime, combine the remaining ingredients in a wok (or similar type pan) that is preheated over medium-high heat. Cook and stir until the sauce reduces by about a third.
- ✓ Add the fried turkey thighs to the wok; gently stir to coat with the sauce.
- ✓ Let the turkey rest for 10 minutes before slicing and serving. Enjoy!

Nutritional Value: Calories:933 Protein: 86 g Fat: 37 g Carbohydrates:64 g

565) *Easy Hot Chicken Drumsticks*

Ingredients

- 6 chicken drumsticks
- Sauce:
- 6 ounces hot sauce
- 3 tablespoons olive oil
- 3 tablespoons tamari sauce
- 1 teaspoon dried thyme
- 1/2 teaspoon dried oregano

Directions:(Prep + Cook Time: 50 minutes)

- ✓ Spritz the sides and bottom of the cooking basket with a nonstick cooking spray.
- ✓ Cook the chicken drumsticks at 380 degrees F for 35 minutes, flipping them over halfway through.
- ✓ Meanwhile, heat the hot sauce, olive oil, tamari sauce, thyme, and oregano in a pan over medium-low heat; reserve.
- ✓ Drizzle the sauce over the prepared chicken drumsticks; toss to coat well and serve.

Nutritional Value: 165 calories; protein 19.5g; carbohydrates 1.4g; fat 8.7g; cholesterol 61.9mg;

566) *Crunchy Munchy Chicken Tenders with Peanuts*

Ingredients

- 1 ½ pounds chicken tenderloins
- 2 tablespoons peanut oil
- 1/2 cup tortilla chips, crushed
- Sea salt and ground black pepper, to taste
- 1/2 teaspoon garlic powder
- 1 teaspoon red pepper flakes
- 2 tablespoons peanuts, roasted and roughly chopped

Directions:

- ✓ Start by preheating your Air Fryer to 360 degrees F.
- ✓ Brush the chicken tenderloins with peanut oil on all sides.
- ✓ In a mixing bowl, thoroughly combine the crushed chips, salt, black pepper, garlic powder, and red pepper flakes. Dredge the chicken in the breading, shaking off any residual coating.
- ✓ Lay the chicken tenderloins into the cooking basket. Cook for 12 to 13 minutes or until it is no longer pink in the center. Work in batches; an instant-read thermometer should read at least 165 degrees F.
- ✓ Serve garnished with roasted peanuts.

Nutritional Value: 403 calories; protein 41.2g; carbohydrates 43.3g; fat 7g; cholesterol 186.9mg;

567) *Tarragon Turkey Tenderloins with Baby Potatoes*

Ingredients

- 2 pounds turkey tenderloins
- 2 teaspoons olive oil
- Salt and ground black pepper, to taste
- 1 teaspoon smoked paprika
- 2 tablespoons dry white wine
- 1 tablespoon fresh tarragon leaves, chopped
- 1 pound baby potatoes, rubbed

Directions:(Prep + Cook Time: 30 minutes)

- ✓ Brush the turkey tenderloins with olive oil. Season with salt, black pepper, and paprika.
- ✓ Afterwards, add the white wine and tarragon.
- ✓ Cook the turkey tenderloins at 350 degrees F for 30 minutes, flipping them over halfway through. Let them rest for 5 to 9 minutes before slicing and serving.
- ✓ After that, spritz the sides and bottom of the cooking basket with the remaining 1 teaspoon of olive oil.
- ✓ Then, preheat your Air Fryer to 400 degrees F; cook the baby potatoes for 15 minutes. Serve with the turkey and enjoy!

Nutritional Value: 154 calories; protein 27.7g; carbohydrates 2g; fat 3.1g; cholesterol 79.4mg; sodium 824.9mg.

568) *Mediterranean Chicken Breasts with Roasted Tomatoes*

Ingredients

- 2 teaspoons olive oil, melted
- 3 pounds chicken breasts, bone-in
- 1/2 teaspoon black pepper, freshly ground
- 1/2 teaspoon salt
- 1 teaspoon cayenne pepper
- 2 tablespoons fresh parsley, minced
- 1 teaspoon fresh basil, minced
- 1 teaspoon fresh rosemary, minced
- 4 medium-sized Roma tomatoes, halved

Directions:(Prep – Cook Time: 50 minutes)

- ✓ Start by preheating your Air Fryer to 370 degrees F. Brush the cooking basket with 1 teaspoon of olive oil.
- ✓ Sprinkle the chicken breasts with all seasonings listed above.
- ✓ Cook for 25 minutes or until chicken breasts are slightly browned. Work in batches.
- ✓ Arrange the tomatoes in the cooking basket and brush them with the remaining teaspoon of olive oil. Season with sea salt.
- ✓ Cook the tomatoes at 350 degrees F for 10 minutes, shaking halfway through the cooking time. Serve with chicken breasts. Bon appétit!

Nutritional Value: 724 calories; protein 39.8g; carbohydrates 81.6g; fat 26.6g; cholesterol 97mg;

569) *Thai Red Duck with Candy Onion*

Ingredients

- 1 ½ pounds duck breasts, skin removed
- 1 teaspoon kosher salt
- 1/2 teaspoon cayenne pepper
- 1/3 teaspoon black pepper
- 1/2 teaspoon smoked paprika
- 1 tablespoon Thai red curry paste
- 1 cup candy onions, halved
- 1/4 small pack coriander, chopped

Directions:(Prep + Cook Time: 30 minutes)

- ✓ Place the duck breasts between 2 sheets of foil; then, use a rolling pin to bash the duck until they are 1-inch thick.
- ✓ Preheat your Air Fryer to 395 degrees F.
- ✓ Rub the duck breasts with salt, cayenne pepper, black pepper, paprika, and red curry paste. Place the duck breast in the cooking basket.
- ✓ Cook for 11 to 12 minutes. Top with candy onions and cook for another 10 to 11 minutes.

Serve garnished with coriander and enjoy!
Nutritional Value: Calories 229; Fat 10g (15%); sat 4g (18%); Protein 9g; Carb 27g (9%); Fiber 2g (1%); Sugars 4g (added sugars 1g); Sodium 570mg (29%)

570) *Dilled and Glazed Salmon Steaks*

Ingredients

- 2 salmon steaks
- Coarse sea salt, to taste
- 1/4 teaspoon freshly ground black pepper, or more to taste
- 2 tablespoons honey
- 1 tablespoon sesame oil
- Zest of 1 lemon
- 1 tablespoon fresh lemon juice
- 1 teaspoon garlic, minced
- 1/2 teaspoon smoked cayenne pepper
- 1/2 teaspoon dried dill

Directions(Ready in about 20 minutes | Servings 2)

- ✓ Preheat your Air Fryer to 380 degrees F. Pat dry the salmon steaks with a kitchen towel.
- ✓ In a ceramic dish, combine the remaining ingredients until everything is well whisked.
- ✓ Add the salmon steaks to the ceramic dish and let them sit in the refrigerator for 1 hour. Now, place the salmon steaks in the cooking basket. Reserve the marinade.
- ✓ Cook for 12 minutes, flipping halfway through the cooking time.
- ✓ Meanwhile, cook the marinade in a small sauté pan over a moderate flame. Cook until the sauce has thickened.
- ✓ Pour the sauce over the steaks and serve with mashed potatoes if desired. Bon appétit!

Nutritional Value: 421 Calories; 16.8g Fat; 19.9g Carbs; 46.7g Protein; 18.1g Sugars

571) *Colorful Salmon and Fennel Salad*

Ingredients

- 1 pound salmon
- 1 fennel, quartered
- 1 teaspoon olive oil
- Sea salt and ground black pepper, to taste
- 1/2 teaspoon paprika
- 1 tablespoon balsamic vinegar
- 1 tablespoon lime juice
- 1 tablespoon extra-virgin olive oil

- 1 tomato, sliced
- 1 cucumber, sliced
- 1 tablespoon sesame seeds, lightly toasted
Directions:(Prep + Cook Time: 30 minutes)
✓ Toss the salmon and fennel with 1 teaspoon of olive oil, salt, black pepper and paprika.
✓ Cook in the preheated Air Fryer at 380 degrees F for 12 minutes; shaking the basket once or twice.
✓ Cut the salmon into bite-sized strips and transfer them to a nice salad bowl. Add in the fennel, balsamic vinegar, lime juice, 1 tablespoon of extra-virgin olive oil, tomato and cucumber.
✓ Toss to combine well and serve garnished with lightly toasted sesame seeds. Enjoy!
Nutritional Value: 306 Calories; 16.3g Fat; 5.6g Carbs; 32.2g Protein; 3g Sugars

572)   *Parmesan Chip-Crusted Tilapia*
Ingredients

- 1 ½ pounds tilapia, slice into 4 portions
- Sea salt and ground black pepper, to taste
- 1/2 teaspoon cayenne pepper
- 1 teaspoon granulated garlic
- 1/4 cup almond flour
- 1/4 cup parmesan cheese, preferably freshly grated
- 1 egg, beaten
- 2 tablespoons buttermilk
- 1 cup tortilla chips, crushed
Directions:(Prep + Cook Time: 40 minutes)
✓ Generously season your tilapia with salt, black pepper and cayenne pepper.
✓ Prepare a bread station. Add the granulated garlic, almond flour and parmesan cheese to a rimmed plate.
✓ Whisk the egg and buttermilk in another bowl and place crushed tortilla chips in the third bowl.
✓ Dip the tilapia pieces in the flour mixture, then in the egg/buttermilk mixture and finally roll them in the crushed chips, pressing to adhere well.
✓ Cook in your Air Fryer at 400 degrees F for 10 minutes, flipping halfway through the cooking time. Serve with chips if desired. Bon appétit!
Nutritional Value: 356 Calories; 10.5g Fat; 11.9g Carbs; 52g Protein; 2.1g Sugars

573)   *Keto Cod Fillets*
Ingredients

- 2 cod fish fillets
- 1 teaspoon butter, melted
- 1 teaspoon Old Bay seasoning
- 1 egg, beaten
- 2 tablespoons coconut milk, unsweetened
- 1/3 cup coconut flour, unsweetened
Directions:(Prep + Cook Time: 30 minutes)
✓ Place the cod fish fillets, butter and Old Bay seasoning in a Ziplock bag; shake until the fish is well coated on all sides.

✓ In a shallow bowl, whisk the egg and coconut milk until frothy.
✓ In another bowl, place the coconut flour. Dip the fish fillets in the egg mixture, then, coat them with coconut flour, pressing to adhere.
✓ Cook the fish at 390 degrees F for 6 minutes; flip them over and cook an additional 6 minutes until your fish flakes easily when tested with a fork. Bon appétit!
Nutritional Value: 218 Calories; 12.5g Fat; 3.5g Carbs; 22g Protein; 1.9g Sugars

574)   *Easiest Lobster Tails Ever*
Ingredients

- 2 (6-ounce) lobster tails
- 1 teaspoon fresh cilantro, minced
- 1/2 teaspoon dried rosemary
- 1/2 teaspoon garlic, pressed
- 1 teaspoon deli mustard
- Sea salt and ground black pepper, to taste
- 1 teaspoon olive oil
Directions:(Prep + Cook Time: 30 minutes)
✓ Toss the lobster tails with the other ingredients until they are well coated on all sides.
✓ Cook the lobster tails at 370 degrees F for 3 minutes. Then, turn them and cook on the other side for 3 to 4 minutes more until they are opaque.
✓ Serve warm and enjoy!
Nutritional Value: 482 calories; protein 35.8g; carbohydrates 6.4g; fat 27.8g; cholesterol 204.6mg; sodium 996.8mg.

575)   *Salmon Bowl with Lime Drizzle*
Ingredients

- 1 pound salmon steak
- 2 teaspoons sesame oil
- Sea salt and Sichuan pepper, to taste
- 1/2 teaspoon coriander seeds
- 1 lime, juiced
- 2 tablespoons reduced-sodium soy sauce
- 1 teaspoon honey
Directions:(Prep + Cook Time: 30 minutes)
✓ Pat the salmon dry and drizzle it with 1 teaspoon of sesame oil.
✓ Season the salmon with salt, pepper and coriander seeds. Transfer the salmon to the Air Fryer cooking basket.
✓ Cook the salmon at 400 degrees F for 5 minutes; turn the salmon over and continue to cook for 5 minutes more or until opaque.
✓ Meanwhile, warm the remaining ingredients in a small saucepan to make the lime drizzle.
✓ Slice the fish into bite-sized strips, drizzle with the sauce and serve immediately. Enjoy!
Nutritional Value: 307 Calories; 15g Fat; 4.5g Carbs; 32.3g Protein; 5g Sugars

576) *Famous Tuna Niçoise Salad*

Ingredients

- 1 pound tuna steak
- Sea salt and ground black pepper, to taste
- 1/2 teaspoon red pepper flakes, crushed
- 1/4 teaspoon dried dill weed
- 1/2 teaspoon garlic paste
- 1 pound green beans, trimmed
- 2 handfuls baby spinach
- 2 handfuls iceberg lettuce, torn into pieces
- 1/2 red onion, sliced
- 1 cucumber, sliced
- 2 tablespoons lemon juice
- 1 tablespoon olive oil
- 1 teaspoon Dijon mustard
- 1 tablespoon balsamic vinegar
- 1 tablespoon roasted almonds, coarsely chopped
- 1 tablespoon fresh parsley, coarsely chopped

Directions:(Prep + Cook Time: 40 minutes)

✓ Pat the tuna steak dry; toss your tuna with salt, black pepper, red pepper, dill and garlic paste. Spritz your tuna with a nonstick cooking spray.

✓ Cook the tuna steak at 400 degrees F for 5 minutes; turn your tuna steak over and continue to cook for 4 to 5 minutes more.

✓ Then, add the green beans to the cooking basket. Spritz green beans with a nonstick cooking spray. Cook at 400 degrees F for 5 minutes, shaking the basket once or twice.

✓ Cut your tuna into thin strips and transfer to a salad bowl; add in the green beans.

✓ Then, add in the baby spinach, iceberg lettuce, onion and cucumber and toss to combine. In a mixing bowl, whisk the lemon juice, olive oil, mustard and vinegar.

✓ Dress the salad and garnish with roasted almonds and fresh parsley. Bon appétit!

Nutritional Value: 446 calories; protein 35.7g; carbohydrates 41.6g; dietary fiber 8g; sugars 9.3g; fat 15.8g; saturated fat 2.5g; cholesterol 47.6mg; vitamin a iu 3442.8IU; vitamin c 134.9mg; folate 111.2mcg; calcium 78.9mg; iron 3.9mg; magnesium 119.5mg;

577) *Classic Crab Cakes*

Ingredients

- 1 egg, beaten
- 2 tablespoons milk
- 2 crustless bread slices
- 1 pound lump crabmeat
- 2 tablespoons scallions, chopped
- 1 garlic clove, minced
- 1 teaspoon deli mustard
- 1 teaspoon Sriracha sauce
- Sea salt and ground black pepper, to taste
- 4 lemon wedges, for serving

Directions:(Prep + Cook Time: 40 minutes)

✓ Whisk the egg and milk until pale and frothy; add in the bread and let it soak for a few minutes.

✓ Stir in the other ingredients, except for the lemon wedges; shape the mixture into 4 equal patties. Place your patties in the Air Fryer cooking basket. Spritz your patties with a nonstick cooking spray.

✓ Cook the crab cakes at 400 degrees F for 5 minutes. Turn them over and cook on the other side for 5 minutes.

✓ Serve warm, garnished with lemon wedges.

Nutritional Value: 164 calories; protein 16.9g; carbohydrates 14g; dietary fiber 1.2g; sugars 1.8g; fat 4.3g; saturated fat 0.7g; cholesterol 61.5mg; vitamin a iu 516.1IU; vitamin c 17.8mg; folate 57.7mcg; calcium 104.6mg; iron 1.4mg; magnesium 39.4mg; potassium 331.9mg; sodium 528.8mg;

578) *Salmon Fillets with Herbs and Garlic*

Ingredients

- 1 pound salmon fillets
- Sea salt and ground black pepper, to taste
- 1 tablespoon olive oil
- 1 sprig thyme
- 2 sprigs rosemary
- 2 cloves garlic, minced
- 1 lemon, sliced

Directions:(Prep + Cook Time: 30 minutes)

✓ Pat the salmon fillets dry and season them with salt and pepper; drizzle salmon fillets with olive oil and place in the Air Fryer cooking basket.

✓ Cook the salmon fillets at 380 degrees F for 7 minutes; turn them over, top with thyme, rosemary and garlic and continue to cook for 5 minutes more.

✓ Serve topped with lemon slices and enjoy!

Nutritional Value: 198 calories; fat 9g; cholesterol 67mg; sodium 342mg; protein 27g; niacin equivalents 17mg;

579) *Grouper with Miso-Honey Sauce*

Ingredients

- 3/4 pound grouper fillets
- Salt and white pepper, to taste
- 1 tablespoon sesame oil
- 1 teaspoon water
- 1 teaspoon deli mustard or Dijon mustard
- 1/4 cup white miso
- 1 tablespoon mirin
- 1 tablespoon honey
- 1 tablespoon Shoyu sauce

Directions:(Prep + Cook Time: 30 minutes)

✓ Sprinkle the grouper fillets with salt and white pepper; drizzle them with a nonstick cooking oil.

✓ Cook the fish at 400 degrees F for 5 minutes; turn the fish fillets over and cook an additional 5 minutes.

✓ Meanwhile, make the sauce by whisking the

remaining ingredients.

✓ Serve the warm fish with the miso-honey sauce on the side. Bon appétit!

Nutritional Value: 53 calories; protein 0.1g; carbohydrates 2.3g; dietary fiber 0.1g; sugars 0.4g; fat 4.6g; saturated fat 0.4g; vitamin a iu 12.4IU; vitamin c 3.3mg; folate 1.8mcg; calcium 1.5mg;

580) *Fish Sticks with Vidalia Onions*

Ingredients

- 1/2 pound fish sticks, frozen
- 1/2 pound Vidalia onions, halved
- 1 teaspoon sesame oil
- Sea salt and ground black pepper, to taste
- 1/2 teaspoon red pepper flakes
- 4 tablespoons mayonnaise
- 4 tablespoons Greek-style yogurt
- 1/4 teaspoon mustard seeds
- 1 teaspoon chipotle chili in adobo, minced

Directions:(Prep + Cook Time: 30 minutes)

✓ Drizzle the fish sticks and Vidalia onions with sesame oil. Toss them with salt, black pepper and red pepper flakes.

✓ Transfer them to the Air Fryer cooking basket.

✓ Cook the fish sticks and onions at 400 degreed F for 5 minutes. Shake the basket and cook an additional 5 minutes or until cooked through.

✓ Meanwhile, mix the mayonnaise, Greek-style yogurt, mustard seeds and chipotle chili.

✓ Serve the warm fish sticks garnished with Vidalia onions and the sauce on the side. Bon appétit!

Nutritional Value: 301 calories; protein 6.9g; carbohydrates 32g; dietary fiber 2.8g; sugars 5.8g; fat 15.5g; saturated fat 6g; cholesterol 52.3mg; vitamin a iu 276.6IU; vitamin c 9.3mg; folate 81.9mcg; calcium 102mg; iron 1.9mg;.

581) *Moroccan Harissa Shrimp*

Ingredients

- 1 pound breaded shrimp, frozen
- 1 teaspoon extra-virgin olive oil
- Sea salt and ground black pepper, to taste
- 1 teaspoon coriander seeds
- 1 teaspoon caraway seeds
- 1 teaspoon crushed red pepper
- 1 teaspoon fresh garlic, minced

Directions:(Prep + Cook Time:40 minutes)

✓ Toss the breaded shrimp with olive oil and transfer to the Air Fryer cooking basket.

✓ Cook in the preheated Air Fryer at 400 degrees F for 5 minutes; shake the basket and cook an additional 4 minutes.

✓ Meanwhile, mix the remaining ingredients until well combined. Taste and adjust seasonings. Toss the warm shrimp with the harissa sauce and serve immediately. Enjoy!

Nutritional Value: 270 calories; protein 25.1g; carbohydrates 11.9g; dietary fiber 3.5g; sugars 5g; fat

13.3g; saturated fat 4.1g; cholesterol 73.7mg; vitamin a iu 17172.9IU; vitamin c 10mg; folate 28.8mcg; calcium 54.4mg; iron 3.3mg; magnesium 37.5mg; potassium 763.2mg; sodium 569mg; thiamin 0.2mg.

582) *Ginger-Garlic Swordfish with Mushrooms*

Ingredients

- 1 pound swordfish steak
- 1 teaspoon ginger-garlic paste
- Sea salt and ground black pepper, to taste
- 1/4 teaspoon cayenne pepper
- 1/4 teaspoon dried dill weed
- 1/2 pound mushrooms

Directions:(Prep + Cook Time: 30 minutes)

✓ Rub the swordfish steak with ginger-garlic paste; season with salt, black pepper, cayenne pepper and dried dill.

✓ Spritz the fish with a nonstick cooking spray and transfer to the Air Fryer cooking basket. Cook at 400 degrees F for 5 minutes.

✓ Now, add the mushrooms to the cooking basket and continue to cook for 5 minutes longer until tender and fragrant. Eat warm.

Nutritional Value: 5 calories; protein 0.2g; carbohydrates 0.4g; fat 0.3g; vitamin a iu 3.8IU; vitamin c 0.4mg; folate 0.2mcg; calcium 1mg; iron 0.1mg; magnesium 1.4mg; potassium 8.9mg; sodium 118.6mg.

583) *Classic Calamari with Mediterranean Sauce*

Ingredients

- 1/2 pound calamari tubes cut into rings, cleaned
- Sea salt and ground black pepper, to season
- 1/2 cup almond flour
- 1/2 cup all-purpose flour
- 4 tablespoons parmesan cheese, grated
- 1/2 cup ale beer
- 1/4 teaspoon cayenne pepper
- 1/2 cup breadcrumbs
- 1/4 cup mayonnaise
- 1/4 cup Greek-style yogurt
- 1 clove garlic, minced
- 1 tablespoon fresh lemon juice
- 1 teaspoon fresh parsley, chopped
- 1 teaspoon fresh dill, chopped

Directions:(Prep + Cook Time: 30 minutes)

✓ Sprinkle the calamari with salt and black pepper.

✓ Mix the flour, cheese and beer in a bowl until well combined. In another bowl, mix cayenne pepper and breadcrumbs

✓ Dip the calamari pieces in the flour mixture, then roll them onto the breadcrumb mixture, pressing to coat on all sides; transfer them to a lightly oiled cooking basket.

✓ Cook at 400 degrees F for 4 minutes, shaking the

basket halfway through the cooking time.

✓ Meanwhile, mix the remaining ingredients until everything is well incorporated. Serve warm calamari with the sauce for dipping. Enjoy!

Nutritional Value: 248 calories; protein 16g; carbohydrates 23.3g; dietary fiber 4.3g; sugars 7g; fat 9.9g; saturated fat 1.3g; cholesterol 176.1mg;

584) *Garlic Butter Scallops*
Ingredients

✓ 1/2 pound scallops

✓ Coarse sea salt and ground black pepper, to taste

✓ 1/4 teaspoon cayenne pepper

✓ 1/4 teaspoon dried oregano

✓ 1/4 teaspoon dried basil

✓ 2 tablespoons butter pieces, cold

✓ 1 teaspoon garlic, minced

✓ 1 teaspoon lemon zest

Directions:(Prep + Cook Time: 30 minutes)

✓ Sprinkle the scallops with salt, black pepper, cayenne pepper, oregano and basil. Spritz your scallops with a nonstick cooking oil and transfer them to the Air Fryer cooking basket.

✓ Cook the scallops at 400 degrees F for 6 to 7 minutes, shaking the basket halfway through the cooking time.

✓ In the meantime, melt the butter in a small saucepan over medium-high heat. Once hot, add in the garlic and continue to sauté until fragrant, about 1 minute. Add in lemon zest, taste and adjust the seasonings.

✓ Spoon the garlic butter over the warm scallops and serve.

Nutritional Value: 122 calories; protein 7.5g; carbohydrates 2.8g; dietary fiber 0.1g; sugars 0.1g; fat 9g; saturated fat 5.5g; cholesterol 37.3mg; vitamin a iu 348.1IU; vitamin c 3.2mg; folate 12.2mcg; calcium 11.1mg; iron 0.3mg;

585) *Baked Sardines with Tangy Dipping Sauce*
Ingredients

• 1 pound fresh sardines

• Sea salt and ground black pepper, to taste

• 1 teaspoon Italian seasoning mix

• 2 cloves garlic, minced

• 3 tablespoons olive oil

• 1/2 lemon, freshly squeezed

Directions:(Prep + Cook Time: 30 minutes)

✓ Toss your sardines with salt, black pepper and Italian seasoning mix. Cook in your Air Fryer at 325 degrees F for 35 to 40 minutes until skin is crispy.

✓ Meanwhile, make the sauce by whisking the remaining ingredients

✓ Serve warm sardines with the sauce on the side. Bon appétit!

Nutritional Value: 53 calories; protein 3.2g; carbohydrates 5g; dietary fiber 0.4g; sugars 2.3g; fat 1.8g; saturated fat 1.5g; cholesterol 16.5mg; vitamin c 0.1mg; folate 5.9mcg; calcium 7.4mg; iron 0.2mg; magnesium 4.6mg; potassium 38.2mg;

586) *Anchovy and Cheese Wontons*
Ingredients

• 1/2 pound anchovies

• 1/2 cup cheddar cheese, grated

• 1 cup fresh spinach

• 2 tablespoons scallions, minced

• 1 teaspoon garlic, minced

• 1 tablespoon Shoyu sauce

• Himalayan salt and ground black pepper, to taste

• 1/2 pound wonton wrappers

• 1 teaspoon sesame oil

Directions:(Prep + Cook Time: 30 minutes)

✓ Mash the anchovies and mix with the cheese, spinach, scallions, garlic and Shoyu sauce; season with salt and black pepper and mix to combine well.

✓ Fill your wontons with 1 tablespoon of the filling mixture and fold into triangle shape; brush the side with a bit of oil and water to seal the edges.

✓ Cook in your Air Fryer at 390 degrees F for 10 minutes, flipping the wontons for even cooking. Enjoy!

Nutritional Value: 121 calories; protein 5.3g; carbohydrates 9.5g; dietary fiber 0.3g; sugars 0.1g; fat 6.7g; saturated fat 2.3g; cholesterol 22mg; vitamin a iu 93.5IU; vitamin c 1.7mg; folate 33.4mcg; calcium 34.7mg; iron 0.7mg; magnesium 9mg; potassium 57.3mg; sodium 242mg.

587) *Classic Pancetta-Wrapped Scallops*
Ingredients

• 1 pound sea scallops

• 1 tablespoon deli mustard

• 2 tablespoons soy sauce

• 1/4 teaspoon shallot powder

• 1/4 teaspoon garlic powder

• 1/2 teaspoon dried dill

• Sea salt and ground black pepper, to taste

• 4 ounces pancetta slices

Direction:(Prep + Cook Time: 40 minutes)

✓ Pat dry the sea scallops and transfer them to a mixing bowl. Toss the sea scallops with the deli mustard, soy sauce, shallot powder, garlic powder, dill, salt and black pepper.

✓ Wrap a slice of bacon around each scallop and transfer them to the Air Fryer cooking basket.

✓ Cook in your Air Fryer at 400 degrees F for 4 minutes; turn them over and cook an additional 3 minutes.

✓ Serve with hot sauce for dipping if desired. Bon appétit!

Nutritional Value: 56 calories; protein 5.2g; carbohydrates 1.3g; fat 3.2g; saturated fat 0.8g; cholesterol 12.2mg; vitamin a iu 1.3IU; vitamin c 0.3mg; folate 6.2mcg; calcium 2.5mg; iron 0.2mg; magnesium 8.4mg; potassium 79.2mg;

588)   *Fish Cakes with Bell Pepper*

Ingredients

- 1 pound haddock
- 1 egg
- 2 tablespoons milk
- 1 bell pepper, deveined and finely chopped
- 2 stalks fresh scallions, minced
- 1/2 teaspoon fresh garlic, minced
- Sea salt and ground black pepper, to taste
- 1/2 teaspoon cumin seeds
- 1/4 teaspoon celery seeds
- 1/2 cup breadcrumbs
- 1 teaspoon olive oil

Directions:(Prep + Cook Time: 30 minutes)

- ✓ Thoroughly combine all ingredients, except for the breadcrumbs and olive oil, until everything is blended well.
- ✓ Then, roll the mixture into 3 patties and coat them with breadcrumbs, pressing to adhere. Drizzle olive oil over the patties and transfer them to the Air Fryer cooking basket.
- ✓ Cook the fish cakes at 400 degrees F for 5 minutes; turn them over and continue to cook an additional 5 minutes until cooked through.
- ✓ Bon appétit!

Nutritional Value: 226 Calories; 6.5g Fat; 10.9g Carbs; 31.4g Protein; 2.6g Sugars

589)   *Greek Sardeles Psites*

Ingredients

- 4 sardines, cleaned
- 1/4 cup all-purpose flour
- Sea salt and ground black pepper, to taste
- 4 tablespoons extra-virgin olive oil
- 1/2 red onion, chopped
- 1/2 teaspoon fresh garlic, minced
- 1/4 cup sweet white wine
- 1 tablespoon fresh coriander, minced
- 1/4 cup baby capers, drained
- 1 tomato, crushed
- 1/4 teaspoon chili paper flakes

Directions:(Prep + Cook Time: 40 minutes)

- ✓ Coat your sardines with all-purpose flour until well coated on all sides.
- ✓ Season your sardines with salt and black pepper and arrange them in the cooking basket. Cook in your Air Fryer at 325 degrees F for 35 to 40 minutes until the skin is crispy.
- ✓ Meanwhile, heat olive oil in a frying pan over a moderate flame. Now, sauté the onion and garlic for 4 to 5 minutes or until tender and aromatic.
- ✓ Stir in the remaining ingredients, cover and let it simmer, for about 15 minutes or until the sauce has thickened and reduced. Spoon the sauce over the warm sardines and serve immediately. Enjoy!

Nutritional Value: 349 Calories; 17.5g Fat; 19g Carbs; 26.3g Protein; 4.3g Sugars

590)   *Thai-Style Jumbo Scallops*

Ingredients

- ✓ 8 jumbo scallops
- ✓ 1 teaspoon sesame oil
- ✓ Sea salt and red pepper flakes, to season
- ✓ 1 tablespoon coconut oil
- ✓ 1 Thai chili, deveined and minced
- ✓ 1 teaspoon garlic, minced
- ✓ 1 tablespoon oyster sauce
- ✓ 1 tablespoon soy sauce
- ✓ 1/4 cup coconut milk
- ✓ 2 tablespoons fresh lime juice

Directions:(Prep + Cook Time: 30 minutes)

- ✓ Pat the jumbo scallops dry and toss them with 1 teaspoon of sesame oil, salt and red pepper.
- ✓ Cook the jumbo scallops in your Air Fryer at 400 degrees F for 4 minutes; turn them over and cook an additional 3 minutes.
- ✓ While your scallops are cooking, make the sauce in a frying pan. Heat the coconut oil in a pan over medium-high heat.
- ✓ Once hot, cook the Thai chili and garlic for 1 minute or so until just tender and fragrant. Add in the oyster sauce, soy sauce and coconut milk and continue to simmer, partially covered, for 5 minutes longer.
- ✓ Lastly, stir in fresh lime juice and stir to combine well. Add the warm scallops to the sauce and serve immediately.

Nutritional Value: 200 Calories; 10.5g Fat; 10.2g Carbs; 16.3g Protein; 3.4g Sugars

591)   *Southwestern Prawns with Asparagus*

Ingredients

- 1 pound prawns, deveined
- 1/2 pound asparagus spears, cut into 1-inch chinks
- 1 teaspoon butter, melted
- 1/4 teaspoon oregano
- 1/2 teaspoon mixed peppercorns, crushed
- Salt, to taste
- 1 ripe avocado
- 1 lemon, sliced
- 1/2 cup chunky-style salsa

Directions:(Prep + Cook Time: 30 minutes)

- ✓ Toss your prawns and asparagus with melted butter, oregano, salt and mixed peppercorns.
- ✓ Cook the prawns and asparagus at 400 degrees F for 5 minutes, shaking the basket halfway through the cooking time.
- ✓ Divide the prawns and asparagus between serving plates and garnish with avocado and lemon slices. Serve with the salsa on the side. Bon appétit!

Nutritional Value: 280 Calories; 12.1g Fat; 12.8g Carbs;

34.1g Protein; 4g Sugars

592) Halibut Steak with Cremini Mushrooms

Ingredients

- 1 pound halibut steak
- 1 teaspoon olive oil
- Sea salt and ground black pepper, to taste
- 7 ounces Cremini mushrooms
- 1 teaspoon butter, melted
- 1/4 teaspoon onion powder
- 1/4 teaspoon garlic powder
- 1/2 teaspoon rosemary
- 1/2 teaspoon basil
- 1/2 teaspoon oregano

Directions:(Prep + Cook Time: 30 minutes)

- ✓ Toss the halibut steak with olive oil, salt and black pepper and transfer to the Air Fryer cooking basket.
- ✓ Toss the Cremini mushrooms with the other ingredients until well coated on all sides.
- ✓ Cook the halibut steak at 400 degrees F for 5 minutes. Turn the halibut steak over and top with mushrooms.
- ✓ Continue to cook an additional 5 minutes or until the mushrooms are fragrant. Serve warm and enjoy!

Nutritional Value: 155 calories; protein 7.6g; carbohydrates 18g; dietary fiber 1.2g; sugars 4.8g; fat 6.6g; saturated fat 3.5g; cholesterol 17.6mg; vitamin a iu 239.1IU; vitamin c 4mg; folate 65mcg; calcium 114.6mg; iron 1.1mg; magnesium 22mg;

593) Marinated Flounder Filets

Ingredients

- 1 pound flounder filets
- 1 teaspoon garlic, minced
- 2 tablespoons soy sauce
- 1 teaspoon Dijon mustard
- 1/4 cup malt vinegar
- 1 teaspoon granulated sugar
- Salt and black pepper, to taste
- 1/2 cup plain flour
- 1 egg
- 2 tablespoons milk
- 1/2 cup parmesan cheese, grated

Directions:(Prep + Cook Time: 80 minutes)

- ✓ Place the flounder filets, garlic, soy sauce, mustard, vinegar and sugar in a glass bowl; cover and let it marinate in your refrigerator for at least 1 hour.
- ✓ Transfer the fish to a plate, discarding the marinade. Salt and pepper to taste.
- ✓ Place the plain flour in a shallow bowl; in another bowl, beat the egg and milk until pale and well combined; add parmesan cheese to the third bowl.
- ✓ Dip the flounder filets in the flour, then in the egg

mixture; repeat the process and coat them with the parmesan cheese, pressing to adhere.

- ✓ Cook the flounder filets in the preheated Air Fryer at 400 degrees F for 5 minutes; turn the flounder filets over and cook on the other side for 5 minutes more. Enjoy!

Nutritional Value: 376 Calories; 14g Fat; 24.5g Carbs; 34.1g Protein; 4.8g Sugars

594) Herb and Garlic Grouper Filets

Ingredients

- 1 pound grouper filets
- 1/4 teaspoon shallot powder
- 1/4 teaspoon porcini powder
- 1 teaspoon fresh garlic, minced
- 1/2 teaspoon cayenne pepper
- 1/2 teaspoon hot paprika
- 1/4 teaspoon oregano
- 1/2 teaspoon marjoram
- 1/2 teaspoon sage
- 1 tablespoon butter, melted
- Sea salt and black pepper, to taste

Directions:(Prep + Cook Time: 30 minutes)

- ✓ Pat dry the grouper filets using kitchen towels.
- ✓ In a small dish, make the rub by mixing the remaining ingredients until everything is well incorporated.
- ✓ Rub the fish with the mixture, coating well on all sides.
- ✓ Cook the grouper filets in the preheated Air Fryer at 400 degrees F for 5 minutes; turn the filets over and cook on the other side for 5 minutes more. Serve over hot rice if desired.

Nutritional Value: 198 calories; fat 9g; cholesterol 67mg; sodium 342mg; protein 27g; niacin equivalents 17mg; saturated fat 2g; vitamin a iu 105IU; vitamin b6 2mg; potassium 454mg.

595) Greek-Style Sea Bass

Ingredients

- 1/2 pound sea bass
- 1 garlic clove, halved
- Sea salt and ground black pepper, to taste
- 1/2 teaspoon rigani (Greek oregano)
- 1/2 teaspoon dried dill weed
- 1/4 teaspoon ground bay leaf
- 1/4 teaspoon ground cumin
- 1/2 teaspoon shallot powder

Greek sauce:

- 1/2 Greek yogurt
- 1 teaspoon olive oil
- 1/2 teaspoon Tzatziki spice mix
- 1 teaspoon lime juice

Directions :(Prep + Cook Time: 30 minutes)

- ✓ Pat dry the sea bass with paper towels. Rub the fish with garlic halves.
- ✓ Toss the fish with salt, black pepper, rigani, dill,

ground bay leaf, ground cumin and shallot powder.

✓ Cook the sea bass in your Air Fryer at 400 degrees F for 5 minutes; turn the filets over and cook on the other side for 5 to 6 minutes.

✓ In the meantime, make the sauce by simply blending the remaining ingredients. Serve the warm fish dolloped with Greek-style sauce. Enjoy!

Nutritional Value: 174 Calories; 4.8g Fat; 5g Carbs; 25.8g Protein; 2.6g Sugars

596) *Melt-in-Your Mouth Salmon with Cilantro Sauce*

Ingredients

- 1 pound salmon fillets
- 1 teaspoon coconut oil
- Sea salt and ground black pepper, to season
- 2 heaping tablespoons cilantro
- 1/2 cup Mexican crema
- 1 tablespoon fresh lime juice

Directions:(Prep + Cook Time: 30 minutes)

✓ Rinse and pat your salmon dry using paper towels. Toss the salmon with coconut oil, salt and black pepper.

✓ Cook the salmon filets in your Air Fryer at 380 degrees F for 6 minutes; turn the salmon filets over and cook on the other side for 6 to 7 minutes.

✓ Meanwhile, mix the remaining ingredients in your blender or food processor. Spoon the cilantro sauce over the salmon filets and serve immediately.

Nutritional Value: 419 Calories; 20.2g Fat; 3.2g Carbs; 53.3g Protein; 1.6g Sugars

597) *Classic Old Bay Fish with Cherry Tomatoes*

Ingredients

- 1 pound swordfish steak
- 1/2 cup cornflakes, crushed
- 1 teaspoon Old Bay seasoning
- Salt and black pepper, to season
- 2 teaspoon olive oil
- 1 pound cherry tomatoes

Directions:(Prep + Cook Time: 30 minutes)

✓ Toss the swordfish steak with cornflakes, Old Bay seasoning, salt, black pepper and 1 teaspoon of olive oil.

✓ Cook the swordfish steak in your Air Fryer at 400 degrees F for 6 minutes.

✓ Now, turn the fish over, top with tomatoes and drizzle with the remaining teaspoon of olive oil. Continue to cook for 4 minutes.

✓ Serve with lemon slices if desired. Bon appétit!

Nutritional Value: 291 Calories; 13.5g Fat; 10.4g Carbs; 31.9g Protein; 6.8g Sugars

598) *Haddock Steaks with Decadent Mango Salsa*

Ingredients

- 2 haddock steaks
- 1 teaspoon butter, melted
- 1 tablespoon white wine
- Sea salt and ground black pepper, to taste
- Mango salsa:
- 1/2 mango, diced
- 1/4 cup red onion, chopped
- 1 chili pepper, deveined and minced
- 1 teaspoon cilantro, chopped
- 2 tablespoons fresh lemon juice

Directions:(Prep + Cook Time: 30 minutes)

✓ Toss the haddock with butter, wine, salt and black pepper.

✓ Cook the haddock in your Air Fryer at 400 degrees F for 5 minutes. Flip the haddock and cook on the other side for 5 minutes more.

✓ Meanwhile, make the mango salsa by mixing all ingredients. Serve the warm haddock with the chilled mango salsa and enjoy!

Nutritional Value: 411 Calories; 25.5g Fat; 18.4g Carbs; 26.3g Protein; 14g Sugars

599) *Homemade Fish Fingers*

Ingredients

- 3/4 pound tilapia
- 1 egg
- 2 tablespoons milk
- 4 tablespoons chickpea flour
- 1/4 cup pork rinds
- 1/2 cup breadcrumbs
- 1/2 teaspoon red chili flakes
- Coarse sea salt and black pepper, to season

Directions:(Prep + Cook Time: 30 minutes)

✓ Rinse the tilapia and pat it dry using kitchen towels. Then, cut the tilapia into strips.

✓ Then, whisk the egg, milk and chickpea flour in a rimmed plate.

✓ Add the pork rinds and breadcrumbs to another plate; stir in red chili flakes, salt and black pepper and stir to combine well.

✓ Dip the fish strips in the egg mixture, then, roll them over the breadcrumb mixture. Transfer the fish fingers to the Air Fryer cooking basket and spritz them with a nonstick cooking spray.

✓ Cook in the preheated Air Fryer at 400 degrees F for 10 minutes, shaking the basket halfway through to ensure even browning. Serve warm and enjoy!

Nutritional:Calories: 266cal (13%)Carbohydrates: 12g (4%)Protein: 35g (70%)Fat: 9g (14%)Saturated Fat: 2g (13%)Cholesterol: 120mg (40%)Sodium: 538mg (23%)Potassium: 514mg (15%)Fiber: 1g (4%)Sugar: 1g

600) *Ahi Tuna with Peppers and Tartare Sauce*

Ingredients

- 2 ahi tuna steaks
- 2 Spanish peppers, quartered

- 1 teaspoon olive oil
- 1/2 teaspoon garlic powder
- Salt and freshly ground black pepper, to taste
- Tartare sauce:
- 4 tablespoons mayonnaise
- 2 tablespoons sour cream
- 1 tablespoon baby capers, drained
- 1 tablespoon gherkins, drained and chopped
- 2 tablespoons white onion, minced

Directions:(Prep + Cook Time: 30 minutes)
- ✓ Pat the ahi tuna dry using kitchen towels.
- ✓ Toss the ahi tuna and Spanish peppers with olive oil, garlic powder, salt and black pepper.
- ✓ Cook the ahi tuna and peppers in the preheated Air Fryer at 400 degrees F for 10 minutes, flipping them halfway through the cooking time.
- ✓ Meanwhile, whisk all the sauce ingredients until well combined. Plate the ahi tuna steaks and arrange Spanish peppers around them. Serve with tartare sauce on the side and enjoy!

Nutritional Value: 485 Calories; 24.3g Fat; 7.7g Carbs; 56.3g Protein; 3g Sugars

601) Fried Oysters with Kaffir Lime Sauce

Ingredients
- 8 fresh oysters, shucked
- 1/3 cup plain flour
- 1 egg
- 3/4 cup breadcrumbs
- 1/2 teaspoon Italian seasoning mix
- 1 lime, freshly squeezed
- 1 teaspoon coconut sugar
- 1 kaffir lime leaf, shredded
- 1 habanero pepper, minced
- 1 teaspoon olive oil

Directions:(Prep + Cook Time: 30 minutes)
- ✓ Clean the oysters and set them aside.
- ✓ Add the flour to a rimmed plate. Whisk the egg in another rimmed plate. Mix the breadcrumbs and Italian seasoning mix in a third plate.
- ✓ Dip your oysters in the flour, shaking off the excess. Then, dip them in the egg mixture and finally, coat your oysters with the breadcrumb mixture.
- ✓ Spritz the breaded oysters with a nonstick cooking spray.
- ✓ Cook your oysters in the preheated Air Fryer at 400 degrees F for 2 to 3 minutes, shaking the basket halfway through the cooking time.
- ✓ Meanwhile, blend the remaining ingredients to make the sauce. Serve the warm oysters with the kaffir lime sauce on the side.

Nutritional Value: 295 Calories; 8.7g Fat; 23.4g Carbs; 30g Protein; 3.3g Sugars

602) Mom's Lobster Tails

Ingredients
- 1/2 pound lobster tails
- 1 teaspoon olive oil
- 1 teaspoon fresh lime juice
- 1 bell pepper, sliced
- 1 jalapeno pepper, sliced
- 1 carrot, julienned
- 1 cup green cabbage, shredded
- 2 tablespoons mayonnaise
- 2 tablespoons Greek-style yogurt
- Sea salt and ground black pepper, to taste
- 1 teaspoon baby capers, drained
- 4 leaves butterhead lettuce, for serving

Directions:(Prep + Cook Time: 30 minutes)
- ✓ Drizzle olive oil over the lobster tails and transfer them to the Air Fryer cooking basket.
- ✓ Cook the lobster tails at 370 degrees F for 3 minutes. Then, turn them over and cook on the other side for 3 to 4 minutes more until they are opaque.
- ✓ Toss the lobster tails with the other ingredients, except for the lettuce leaves; gently stir until well combined.
- ✓ Lay the lettuce leaves on a serving platter and top with the lobster salad. Bon appétit!

Nutritional Value: 256 Calories; 13.7g Fat; 12.7g Carbs; 21.5g Protein; 6.3g Sugars

603) Classic Fish Tacos

Ingredients
- 1 pound codfish
- 1 tablespoon olive oil
- 1 teaspoon Cajun spice mix
- Salt and red pepper, to taste
- 3 corn tortillas
- 1/2 avocado, pitted and diced
- 1 cup purple cabbage
- 1 jalapeño, minced

Directions :(Prep + Cook Time: 30 minutes)
- ✓ Pat the codfish dry with paper towels; toss the codfish with olive oil, Cajun spice mix, salt and black pepper.
- ✓ Cook your codfish at 400 degrees F for 5 to 6 minutes. Then, turn the fish over and cook on the other side for 6 minutes until they are opaque.
- ✓ Let the fish rest for 5 minutes before flaking with a fork.
- ✓ Assemble the tacos: place the flaked fish over warmed tortillas; top with avocado, purple cabbage and minced jalapeño. Enjoy!

Nutritional Value: 266 Calories; 10.8g Fat; 17.3g Carbs; 25.7g Protein; 2.6g Sugars

604) Dijon Catfish with Eggplant Sauce

Ingredients

- 1 pound catfish fillets
- Sea salt and ground black pepper, to taste
- 1/4 cup Dijon mustard
- 1 tablespoon honey
- 1 tablespoon white vinegar
- 1 pound eggplant, 1 ½-inch cubes
- 2 tablespoons olive oil
- 1 tablespoon tahini
- 1/2 teaspoon garlic, minced
- 1 tablespoon parsley, chopped

Directions:(Prep + Cook Time: 50 minutes)

- ✓ Pat the catfish dry with paper towels and generously season with salt and black pepper.
- ✓ In a small mixing bowl, thoroughly combine Dijon mustard, honey and vinegar.
- ✓ Cook the fish in your Air Fryer at 400 degrees F for 5 minutes. Turn the fish over and brush with the Dijon mixture; continue to cook for a further 5 minutes.
- ✓ Then, set your Air Fryer to 400 degrees F. Add the eggplant chunks to the cooking basket and cook for 15 minutes, shaking the basket occasionally to ensure even cooking.
- ✓ Transfer the cooked eggplant to a bowl of your food processor; stir in the remaining ingredients and blitz until everything is well blended and smooth.
- ✓ Serve the warm catfish with the eggplant sauce on the side. Bon appétit!

Nutritional Value: 110 calories; protein 3g; carbohydrates 14g; dietary fiber 4g; sugars 9g; fat 5g; niacin equivalents 1.3mg; vitamin b6 0.2mg;

605) *Halibut Steak with Zoodles and Lemon*

Ingredients

- 1 pound halibut steak, cut into 3 pieces
- 1 garlic clove, halved
- 1 teaspoon avocado oil
- Sea salt and black pepper, to taste
- 1 pound zucchini, julienned
- 1/2 teaspoon onion powder
- 1/2 teaspoon granulated garlic
- 1 tablespoon fresh parsley, minced
- 1 teaspoon sage, minced
- 1 lemon, sliced

Directions :(Prep + Cook Time: 40 minutes)

- ✓ Rub the halibut steaks with garlic and toss with avocado oil, salt and black pepper; then, transfer the halibut steaks to the Air Fryer cooking basket.
- ✓ Cook the halibut steak at 400 degrees F for 5 minutes. Turn the halibut steak over and continue to cook an additional 5 minutes or until it flakes easily when tested with a fork.
- ✓ Meanwhile, spritz a wok with a nonstick spray; heat the wok over medium-high heat.
- ✓ Once hot, stir fry the zucchini noodles along with

the onion powder and granulated garlic; cook for 2 to 3 minutes or until just tender.
- ✓ Top your zoodles with the parsley and sage and stir to combine. Serve the hot zoodles with the halibut steaks and lemon slices. Bon appétit!

Nutritional: 368 calories; protein 18.9g; carbohydrates 46.1g; dietary fiber 2.8g; sugars 1.5g; fat 11.4g;

606) *Salmon with Baby Bok Choy*

Ingredients

- ✓ 1 pound salmon filets
- ✓ 1 teaspoon garlic chili paste
- ✓ 1 teaspoon sesame oil
- ✓ 1 tablespoon honey
- ✓ 1 tablespoon soy sauce
- ✓ 1 pound baby Bok choy, bottoms removed
- ✓ Kosher salt and black pepper, to taste

Directions:(Prep + Cook Time: 40 minutes)

- ✓ Start by preheating your Air Fryer to 380 degrees F.
- ✓ Toss the salmon fillets with garlic chili paste, sesame oil, honey, soy sauce, salt and black pepper.
- ✓ Cook the salmon in the preheated Air Fryer for 6 minutes; turn the filets over and cook an additional 6 minutes.
- ✓ Then, cook the baby Bok choy at 350 degrees F for 3 minutes; shake the basket and cook an additional 3 minutes. Salt and pepper to taste.
- ✓ Serve the salmon fillets with the roasted baby Bok choy. Enjoy!

Nutritional Value: 63 calories; protein 2.3g; carbohydrates 3.5g; dietary fiber 1.4g; sugars 1.6g; fat 4.9g; saturated fat 0.4g; vitamin a iu 5907.9IU; vitamin c 38.2mg; folate 57.8mcg; calcium 132.8mg; iron 1.5mg; magnesium 16.2mg; potassium 527mg; sodium 117.5mg;

607) *Tuna Steak with Roasted Cherry Tomatoes*

Ingredients

- 1 pound tuna steak
- 1 cup cherry tomatoes
- 1 teaspoon extra-virgin olive oil
- 2 sprigs rosemary, leaves picked and crushed
- Sea salt and red pepper flakes, to taste
- 1 teaspoon garlic, finely chopped
- 1 tablespoon lime juice

Directions:(Prep + Cook Time: 30 minutes)

- ✓ Toss the tuna steaks and cherry tomatoes with olive oil, rosemary leaves, salt, black pepper and garlic.
- ✓ Place the tuna steaks in a lightly oiled cooking basket; cook tuna steaks at 440 degrees F for about 6 minutes.
- ✓ Turn the tuna steaks over, add in the cherry tomatoes and continue to cook for 4 minutes more. Drizzle the fish with lime juice and serve warm garnished with roasted cherry tomatoes!

Nutritional Value: 231 Calories; 3.3g Fat; 6.2g Carbs; 45.2g Protein; 3.7g Sugars

608) *Seed-Crusted Codfish Fillets*

Ingredients

- 2 codfish fillets
- 1 teaspoon sesame oil
- Sea salt and black pepper, to taste
- 1 teaspoon sesame seeds
- 1 tablespoon chia seeds

Directions:(Prep + Cook Time: 30 minutes)

✓ Start by preheating your Air Fryer to 380 degrees F.

✓ Add the sesame oil, salt, black pepper, sesame seeds and chia seeds to a rimmed plate. Coat the top of the codfish with the seed mixture, pressing it down to adhere.

✓ Lower the codfish fillets, seed side down, into the cooking basket and cook for 6 minutes. Turn the fish fillets over and cook for a further 6 minutes.

✓ Serve warm and enjoy!

Nutritional Value: 263 Calories; 8.3g Fat; 8.2g Carbs; 37.7g Protein; 1.2g Sugars

609) *Salmon Filets with Fennel Slaw*

Ingredients

- 1 pound salmon filets
- 1 teaspoon Cajun spice mix
- Sea salt and ground black pepper, to taste

Fennel Slaw:

- 1 pound fennel bulb, thinly sliced
- 1 Lebanese cucumber, thinly sliced
- 1/2 red onion, thinly sliced
- 1/2 ounce tarragon
- 2 tablespoons tahini
- 2 tablespoons lemon juice
- 1 tablespoon soy sauce

Directions:(Prep + Cook Time: 40 minutes)

✓ Rinse the salmon filets and pat them dry with a paper towel. Then, toss the salmon filets with the Cajun spice mix, salt and black pepper.

✓ Cook the salmon filets in the preheated Air Fryer at 380 degrees F for 6 minutes; flip the salmon filets and cook for a further 6 minutes.

✓ Meanwhile, make the fennel slaw by stirring fennel, cucumber, red onion and tarragon in a salad bowl. Mix the remaining ingredients to make the dressing.

✓ Dress the salad and transfer to your refrigerator until ready to serve.

✓ Serve the warm fish with chilled fennel slaw. Bon appétit!

Nutritional Value: 308 calories; protein 30.4g; carbohydrates 10.1g; dietary fiber 3.1g; sugars 5.1g; fat 15.9g; saturated fat 2.8g; cholesterol 66.3mg; vitamin a iu 1313IU; vitamin c 40.8mg; folate 54.7mcg; calcium 106.4mg; iron 2.2mg; magnesium 62.6mg; potassium 888.7mg; sodium 539mg;

610) *Scallops with Pineapple Salsa and Pickled Onions*

Ingredients

- 12 scallops
- 1 teaspoon sesame oil
- 1/4 teaspoon dried rosemary
- 1/2 teaspoon dried tarragon
- 1/2 teaspoon dried basil
- 1/4 teaspoon red pepper flakes, crushed
- Coarse sea salt and black pepper, to taste
- 1/2 cup pickled onions, drained
- Pineapple Salsa:
- 1 cup pineapple, diced
- 2 tablespoons fresh cilantro, roughly chopped
- 1 jalapeño, deveined and minced
- 1 small-sized red onion, minced
- 1 teaspoon ginger root, peeled and grated
- 1/2 teaspoon coconut sugar
- Sea salt and ground black pepper, to taste

Directions:(Prep + Cook Time: 30 minutes)

✓ Toss the scallops sesame oil, rosemary, tarragon, basil, red pepper, salt and black pepper.

✓ Cook in the preheated Air Fryer at 400 degrees F for 6 to 7 minutes, shaking the basket once or twice to ensure even cooking.

✓ Meanwhile, process all the salsa ingredients in your blender; cover and place the salsa in your refrigerator until ready to serve.

✓ Serve the warm scallops with pickled onions and pineapple salsa on the side. Bon appétit!

Nutritional Value: 623 calories; fat 38g; cholesterol 252mg; sodium 674mg; carbohydrates 51g; dietary fiber 7g; protein 21g; sugars 21g; niacin equivalents 9mg;

611) *Tuna Steaks with Pearl Onions*

Ingredients

- 4 tuna steaks
- 1 pound pearl onions
- 4 teaspoons olive oil
- 1 teaspoon dried rosemary
- 1 teaspoon dried marjoram
- 1 tablespoon cayenne pepper
- 1/2 teaspoon sea salt
- 1/2 teaspoon black pepper, preferably freshly cracked
- 1 lemon, sliced

Directions:(Prep + Cook Time: 30 minutes)

✓ Place the tuna steaks in the lightly greased cooking basket. Top with the pearl onions; add the olive oil, rosemary, marjoram, cayenne pepper, salt, and black pepper.

✓ Bake in the preheated Air Fryer at 400 degrees F for 9 to 10 minutes. Work in two batches.

✓ Serve warm with lemon slices and enjoy!

Nutritional Value: 131 calories; protein 5.3g; carbohydrates 13.4g; dietary fiber 3.7g; sugars 4.7g; fat 6.3g; saturated fat 2.7g; cholesterol 11.8mg;

612) *Tortilla-Crusted Haddock Fillets*
Ingredients
- 2 haddock fillets
- 1/2 cup tortilla chips, crushed
- 2 tablespoons parmesan cheese, freshly grated
- 1 teaspoon dried parsley flakes
- 1 egg, beaten
- 1/2 teaspoon coarse sea salt
- 1/4 teaspoon ground black pepper
- 1/4 teaspoon cayenne pepper
- 2 tablespoons olive oil

Directions:(Prep + Cook Time: 30 minutes)
- ✓ Start by preheating your Air Fryer to 360 degrees F. Pat dry the haddock fillets and set aside.
- ✓ In a shallow bowl, thoroughly combine the crushed tortilla chips with the parmesan and parsley flakes. Mix until everything is well incorporated.
- ✓ In a separate shallow bowl, whisk the egg with salt, black pepper, and cayenne pepper.
- ✓ Dip the haddock fillets into the egg. Then, dip the fillets into the tortilla/parmesan mixture until well coated on all sides.
- ✓ Drizzle the olive oil all over the fish fillets. Lower the coated fillets into the lightly greased Air Fryer basket. Cook for 11 to 13 minutes. Bon appétit!

Nutritional: 414 calories; protein 19g; carbohydrates 53.2g; dietary fiber 12.3g; sugars 4g; fat 15.4g;

613) *Vermouth and Garlic Shrimp Skewers*
Ingredients
- 1 ½ pounds shrimp
- 1/4 cup vermouth
- 2 cloves garlic, crushed
- 1 teaspoon dry mango powder
- Kosher salt, to taste
- 1/4 teaspoon black pepper, freshly ground
- 2 tablespoons olive oil
- 4 tablespoons flour
- 8 skewers, soaked in water for 30 minutes
- 1 lemon, cut into wedges

Directions :(Prep + Cook Time: 80 minutes)
- ✓ Add the shrimp, vermouth, garlic, mango powder, salt, black pepper, and olive oil in a ceramic bowl; let it sit for 1 hour in your refrigerator.
- ✓ Discard the marinade and toss the shrimp with flour. Thread on to skewers and transfer to the lightly greased cooking basket.
- ✓ Cook at 400 degrees F for 5 minutes, tossing halfway through. Serve with lemon wedges.

Nutritional Value: 371 Calories; 12.2g Fat; 30.4g Carbs; 29.5g Protein; 3.2g Sugars

614) *Easy Lobster Tails*
Ingredients
- 2 pounds fresh lobster tails, cleaned and halved, in shells
- 2 tablespoons butter, melted
- 1 teaspoon onion powder
- 1 teaspoon cayenne pepper
- Salt and ground black pepper, to taste
- 2 garlic cloves, minced
- 1 cup cornmeal
- 1 cup green olives

Directions:(Prep + Cook Time: 30 minutes)
- ✓ In a plastic closeable bag, thoroughly combine all ingredients; shake to combine well.
- ✓ Transfer the coated lobster tails to the greased cooking basket.
- ✓ Cook in the preheated Air Fryer at 390 degrees for 6 to 7 minutes, shaking the basket halfway through. Work in batches.
- ✓ Serve with green olives and enjoy!

Nutritional Value: 422 Calories; 7.9g Fat; 49.9g Carbs; 35.4g Protein; 3.1g Sugars

615) *Spicy Curried King Prawns*
Ingredients
- 12 king prawns, rinsed
- 1 tablespoon coconut oil
- 1/2 teaspoon piri piri powder
- Salt and ground black pepper, to taste
- 1 teaspoon garlic paste
- 1 teaspoon onion powder
- 1/2 teaspoon cumin powder
- 1 teaspoon curry powder

Directions:(Prep + Cook Time: 30 minutes)
- ✓ In a mixing bowl, toss all ingredient until the prawns are well coated on all sides.
- ✓ Cook in the preheated Air Fryer at 360 degrees F for 4 minutes. Shake the basket and cook for 4 minutes more.
- ✓ Serve over hot rice if desired. Bon appétit!

Nutritional: 220 Calories; 9.7g Fat; 15.1g Carbs; 17.6g Protein; 2.2g Sugars

616) *Korean-Style Salmon Patties*
Ingredients
- 1 pound salmon
- 1 egg
- 1 garlic clove, minced
- 2 green onions, minced
- 1/2 cup rolled oats
- Sauce:
- 1 teaspoon rice wine
- 1 ½ tablespoons soy sauce
- 1 teaspoon honey

- A pinch of salt
- 1 teaspoon gochugaru (Korean red chili pepper flakes)

Directions :(Prep + Cook Time: 30 minutes)

✓ Start by preheating your Air Fryer to 380 degrees F. Spritz the Air Fryer basket with cooking oil.

✓ Mix the salmon, egg, garlic, green onions, and rolled oats in a bowl; knead with your hands until everything is well incorporated.

✓ Shape the mixture into equally sized patties. Transfer your patties to the Air Fryer basket.

✓ Cook the fish patties for 10 minutes, turning them over halfway through.

✓ Meanwhile, make the sauce by whisking all ingredients. Serve the warm fish patties with the sauce on the side.

Nutritional Value: 396 Calories; 20.1g Fat; 16.7g Carbs; 35.2g Protein; 3.1g Sugars

617)   *English-Style Flounder Fillets*

Ingredients

- 2 flounder fillets
- 1/4 cup all-purpose flour
- 1 egg
- 1/2 teaspoon Worcestershire sauce
- 1/2 cup bread crumbs
- 1/2 teaspoon lemon pepper
- 1/2 teaspoon coarse sea salt
- 1/4 teaspoon chili powder

Directions :(Prep + Cook Time: 30 minutes)

✓ Rinse and pat dry the flounder fillets.

✓ Place the flour in a large pan.

✓ Whisk the egg and Worcestershire sauce in a shallow bowl. In a separate bowl, mix the bread crumbs with the lemon pepper, salt, and chili powder.

✓ Dredge the fillets in the flour, shaking off the excess. Then, dip them into the egg mixture. Lastly, coat the fish fillets with the breadcrumb mixture until they are coated on all sides.

✓ Spritz with cooking spray and transfer to the Air Fryer basket. Cook at 390 degrees for 7 minutes.

✓ Turn them over, spritz with cooking spray on the other side, and cook another 5 minutes. Bon appétit!

Nutritional Value: 432 Calories; 16.7g Fat; 29g Carbs; 38.4g Protein; 2.7g Sugars

618)   *Cod and Shallot Frittata*

Ingredients

- 2 cod fillets
- 6 eggs
- 1/2 cup milk
- 1 shallot, chopped
- 2 garlic cloves, minced
- Sea salt and ground black pepper, to taste
- 1/2 teaspoon red pepper flakes, crushed

Directions:(Prep + Cook Time: 40 minutes)

✓ Bring a pot of salted water to a boil. Boil the cod fillets for 5 minutes or until it is opaque. Flake the fish into bite-sized pieces.

✓ In a mixing bowl, whisk the eggs and milk. Stir in the shallots, garlic, salt, black pepper, and red pepper flakes. Stir in the reserved fish.

✓ Pour the mixture into the lightly greased baking pan.

✓ Cook in the preheated Air Fryer at 360 degrees F for 9 minutes, flipping over halfway through. Bon appétit!

Nutritional Value: 454 Calories; 30.8g Fat; 10.3g Carbs; 32.4g Protein; 4.1g Sugars

619)   *Crispy Tilapia Fillets*

Ingredients

- 5 tablespoons all-purpose flour
- Sea salt and white pepper, to taste
- 1 teaspoon garlic paste
- 2 tablespoons extra virgin olive oil
- 1/2 cup cornmeal
- 5 tilapia fillets, slice into halves

Directions:(Prep + Cook Time: 30 minutes)

✓ Combine the flour, salt, white pepper, garlic paste, olive oil, and cornmeal in a Ziploc bag. Add the fish fillets and shake to coat well.

✓ Spritz the Air Fryer basket with cooking spray. Cook in the preheated Air Fryer at 400 degrees F for 10 minutes; turn them over and cook for 6 minutes more. Work in batches.

✓ Serve with lemon wedges if desired. Enjoy!

Nutritional Value: 379 calories; protein 23.1g; carbohydrates 42.3g; dietary fiber 5.5g; sugars 9.7g; fat 14.5g; saturated fat 2g; cholesterol 47.2mg; vitamin a iu 2399.8IU; vitamin c 6.5mg; folate 76.9mcg; calcium 72.4mg; iron 2.4mg; magnesium 83.8mg; potassium 578.3mg; sodium 860.3mg; thiamin 0.2mg;

620)   *Saucy Garam Masala Fish*

Ingredients

- 2 teaspoons olive oil
- 1/4 cup coconut milk
- 1/2 teaspoon cayenne pepper
- 1 teaspoon Garam masala
- 1/4 teaspoon Kala namak (Indian black salt)
- 1/2 teaspoon fresh ginger, grated
- 1 garlic clove, minced
- 2 catfish fillets
- 1/4 cup coriander, roughly chopped

Directions :(Prep + Cook Time: 40 minutes)

✓ Preheat your Air Fryer to 390 degrees F. Then, spritz the baking dish with a nonstick cooking spray.

✓ In a mixing bowl, whisk the olive oil, milk, cayenne pepper, Garam masala, Kala namak, ginger, and garlic.

✓ Coat the catfish fillets with the Garam masala mixture. Cook the catfish fillets in the preheated Air

Fryer approximately 18 minutes, turning over halfway through the cooking time.

✓ Garnish with fresh coriander and serve over hot noodles if desired.

Nutritional Value: 301 Calories; 12.1g Fat; 2.3g Carbs; 43g Protein; 1.6g Sugars

621)   *Grilled Salmon Steaks*

Ingredients

- 2 cloves garlic, minced
- 4 tablespoons butter, melted
- Sea salt and ground black pepper, to taste
- 1 teaspoon smoked paprika
- 1/2 teaspoon onion powder
- 1 tablespoon lime juice
- 1/4 cup dry white wine
- 4 salmon steaks

Directions::(Prep + Cook Time: 70 minutes)

✓ Place all ingredients in a large ceramic dish. Cover and let it marinate for 30 minutes in the refrigerator.

✓ Arrange the salmon steaks on the grill pan. Bake at 390 degrees for 5 minutes, or until the salmon steaks are easily flaked with a fork.

✓ Flip the fish steaks, baste with the reserved marinade, and cook another 5 minutes. Bon appétit!

Nutritional Value: 420 Calories; 23g Fat; 2.5g Carbs; 48.5g Protein; 0.7g Sugars

622)   *Cajun Fish Cakes with Cheese*

Ingredients

- 2 catfish fillets
- 1 cup all-purpose flour
- 3 ounces butter
- 1 teaspoon baking powder
- 1 teaspoon baking soda
- 1/2 cup buttermilk
- 1 teaspoon Cajun seasoning
- 1 cup Swiss cheese, shredded

Directions:(Prep + Cook Time: 30 minutes)

✓ Bring a pot of salted water to a boil. Boil the fish fillets for 5 minutes or until it is opaque. Flake the fish into small pieces.

✓ Mix the remaining ingredients in a bowl; add the fish and mix until well combined. Shape the fish mixture into 12 patties.

✓ Cook in the preheated Air Fryer at 380 degrees F for 15 minutes. Work in batches. Enjoy!

Nutritional Value: 399 calories; protein 34.6g; carbohydrates 27.9g; dietary fiber 2.8g; sugars 9.8g; fat 15.5g; saturated fat 2.1g; cholesterol 150.4mg; vitamin a iu 440.5IU; vitamin c 0.4mg; folate 25.5mcg; calcium 54.6mg; iron 2.7mg;

623)   *Smoked Halibut and Eggs in Brioche*

Ingredients

- 4 brioche rolls
- 1 pound smoked halibut, chopped
- 4 eggs
- 1 teaspoon dried thyme
- 1 teaspoon dried basil
- Salt and black pepper, to taste

Directions:(Prep + Cook Time: 40 minutes)

✓ Cut off the top of each brioche; then, scoop out the insides to make the shells.

✓ Lay the prepared brioche shells in the lightly greased cooking basket.

✓ Spritz with cooking oil; add the halibut. Crack an egg into each brioche shell; sprinkle with thyme, basil, salt, and black pepper.

✓ Bake in the preheated Air Fryer at 325 degrees F for 20 minutes. Bon appétit!

Nutritional Value: 205 calories; protein 18.7g; carbohydrates 2.3g; dietary fiber 0.5g; sugars 1.1g; fat 12.8g; saturated fat 4.7g; cholesterol 380.8mg;

624)   *Crab Cake Burgers*

Ingredients

- 2 eggs, beaten
- 1 shallot, chopped
- 2 garlic cloves, crushed
- 1 tablespoon olive oil
- 1 teaspoon yellow mustard
- 1 teaspoon fresh cilantro, chopped
- 10 ounces crab meat
- 1 cup tortilla chips, crushed
- 1/2 teaspoon cayenne pepper
- 1/2 teaspoon ground black pepper
- Sea salt, to taste
- 3/4 cup fresh bread crumbs

Directions:(Prep + Cook Time: 2h and 30 minutes)

✓ In a mixing bowl, thoroughly combine the eggs, shallot, garlic, olive oil, mustard, cilantro, crab meat, tortilla chips, cayenne pepper, black pepper, and salt. Mix until well combined.

✓ Shape the mixture into 6 patties. Dip the crab patties into the fresh breadcrumbs, coating well on all sides. Place in your refrigerator for 2 hours.

✓ Spritz the crab patties with cooking oil on both sides. Cook in the preheated Air Fryer at 360 degrees F for 14 minutes. Serve on dinner rolls if desired. Bon appétit!

Nutritional Value: 175 calories; protein 19.3g; carbohydrates 7g; dietary fiber 0.3g; sugars 0.8g; fat 7.4g; saturated fat 1.9g; cholesterol 94.4mg;

625)   *Coconut Shrimp with Orange Sauce*

Ingredients

- 1 pound shrimp, cleaned and deveined
- Sea salt and white pepper, to taste
- 1/2 cup all-purpose flour
- 1 egg

- 1/4 cup shredded coconut, unsweetened
- 3/2 cup fresh bread crumbs
- 2 tablespoons olive oil
- 1 lemon, cut into wedges
- Dipping Sauce:
- 2 tablespoons butter
- 1/2 cup orange juice
- 2 tablespoons soy sauce
- A pinch of salt
- 1/2 teaspoon tapioca starch
- 2 tablespoons fresh parsley, minced

Directions:(Prep + Cook Time: 80 minutes)

- ✓ Pat dry the shrimp and season them with salt and white pepper.
- ✓ Place the flour on a large tray; then, whisk the egg in a shallow bowl. In a third shallow bowl, place the shredded coconut and breadcrumbs.
- ✓ Dip the shrimp in the flour, then, dip in the egg. Lastly, coat the shrimp with the shredded coconut and bread crumbs. Refrigerate for 1 hour.
- ✓ Then, transfer to the cooking basket. Drizzle with olive oil and cook in the preheated Air Fryer at 370 degrees F for 6 minutes. Work in batches.
- ✓ Meanwhile, melt the butter in a small saucepan over medium-high heat; add the orange juice and bring it to a boil; reduce the heat and allow it to simmer approximately 7 minutes.
- ✓ Add the soy sauce, salt, and tapioca; continue simmering until the sauce has thickened and reduced. Spoon the sauce over the shrimp and garnish with lemon wedges and parsley. Serve immediately.

Nutritional Value: 155 calories; protein 16.6g; carbohydrates 7.1g; dietary fiber 1.3g; sugars 2.2g; fat 7.2g; saturated fat 5.9g; cholesterol 139mg; vitamin a iu 58.1IU; folate 14.8mcg; calcium 54.7mg; iron 0.9mg; magnesium 24.4mg;

626) *Monkfish with Sautéed Vegetables and Olives*

Ingredients

- 2 teaspoons olive oil
- 2 carrots, sliced
- 2 bell peppers, sliced
- 1 teaspoon dried thyme
- 1/2 teaspoon dried marjoram
- 1/2 teaspoon dried rosemary
- 2 monkfish fillets
- 1 tablespoon soy sauce
- 2 tablespoons lime juice
- Coarse salt and ground black pepper, to taste
- 1 teaspoon cayenne pepper
- 1/2 cup Kalamata olives, pitted and sliced

Directions:(Prep + Cook Time: 30 minutes)

- ✓ In a nonstick skillet, heat the olive oil for 1 minute. Once hot, sauté the carrots and peppers until tender, about 4 minutes. Sprinkle with thyme, marjoram, and rosemary and set aside.
- ✓ Toss the fish fillets with the soy sauce, lime juice, salt, black pepper, and cayenne pepper. Place the fish fillets in a lightly greased cooking basket and bake at 390 degrees F for 8 minutes.
- ✓ Turn them over, add the olives, and cook an additional 4 minutes. Serve with the sautéed vegetables on the side. Bon appétit!

Nutritional Value: 383 calories; protein 34.7g; carbohydrates 14.7g; dietary fiber 2.5g; sugars 10.8g; fat 18.1g; saturated fat 5.1g; cholesterol 116.6mg; vitamin a iu 2019.8IU; vitamin c 28.5mg;

627) *Delicious Snapper en Papillote*

Ingredients

- 2 snapper fillets
- 1 shallot, peeled and sliced
- 2 garlic cloves, halved
- 1 bell pepper, sliced
- 1 small-sized serrano pepper, sliced
- 1 tomato, sliced
- 1 tablespoon olive oil
- 1/4 teaspoon freshly ground black pepper
- 1/2 teaspoon paprika
- Sea salt, to taste
- 2 bay leaves

Directions:(Prep + Cook Time: 30 minutes)

- ✓ Place two parchment sheets on a working surface. Place the fish in the center of one side of the parchment paper.
- ✓ Top with the shallot, garlic, peppers, and tomato. Drizzle olive oil over the fish and vegetables. Season with black pepper, paprika, and salt. Add the bay leaves.
- ✓ Fold over the other half of the parchment. Now, fold the paper around the edges tightly and create a half moon shape, sealing the fish inside.
- ✓ Cook in the preheated Air Fryer at 390 degrees F for 15 minutes. Serve warm.

Nutritional Value: 329 Calories; 9.8g Fat; 12.7g Carbs; 46.7g Protein; 5.4g Sugars

628) *Halibut Cakes with Horseradish Mayo*

Ingredients

Halibut Cakes:

- 1 pound halibut
- 2 tablespoons olive oil
- 1/2 teaspoon cayenne pepper
- 1/4 teaspoon black pepper
- Salt, to taste
- 2 tablespoons cilantro, chopped
- 1 shallot, chopped
- 2 garlic cloves, minced
- 1/2 cup Romano cheese, grated

- 1/2 cup breadcrumbs
- 1 egg, whisked
- 1 tablespoon Worcestershire sauce

Mayo Sauce:

- 1 teaspoon horseradish, grated
- 1/2 cup mayonnaise

Directions:(Prep + Cook Time: 30 minutes)

✓ Start by preheating your Air Fryer to 380 degrees F. Spritz the Air Fryer basket with cooking oil.

✓ Mix all ingredients for the halibut cakes in a bowl; knead with your hands until everything is well incorporated.

✓ Shape the mixture into equally sized patties. Transfer your patties to the Air Fryer basket. Cook the fish patties for 10 minutes, turning them over halfway through.

✓ Mix the horseradish and mayonnaise. Serve the halibut cakes with the horseradish mayo. Bon appétit!

Nutritional Value: 470 Calories; 38.2g Fat; 6.3g Carbs; 24.4g Protein; 1.5g Sugars

629) *Easy Prawns alla Parmigiana*

Ingredients

- 2 egg whites
- 1 cup all-purpose flour
- 1 cup Parmigiano-Reggiano, grated
- 1/2 cup fine breadcrumbs
- 1/2 teaspoon celery seeds
- 1/2 teaspoon porcini powder
- 1/2 teaspoon onion powder
- 1 teaspoon garlic powder
- 1/2 teaspoon dried rosemary
- 1/2 teaspoon sea salt
- 1/2 teaspoon ground black pepper
- 1 ½ pounds prawns, deveined

Directions:(Prep + Cook Time: 30 minutes)

✓ To make a breading station, whisk the egg whites in a shallow dish. In a separate dish, place the all-purpose flour.

✓ In a third dish, thoroughly combine the Parmigiano-Reggiano, breadcrumbs, and seasonings; mix to combine well.

✓ Dip the prawns in the flour, then, into the egg whites; lastly, dip them in the parm/breadcrumb mixture. Roll until they are covered on all sides.

✓ Cook in the preheated Air Fryer at 390 degrees F for 5 to 7 minutes or until golden brown. Work in batches. Serve with lemon wedges if desired.

Nutritional Value: 442 Calories; 10.3g Fat; 40.4g Carbs; 43.7g Protein; 1.2g Sugars

630) *Indian Famous Fish Curry*

Ingredients

- 2 tablespoons sunflower oil
- 1/2 pound fish, chopped
- 2 red chilies, chopped
- 1 tablespoon coriander powder
- 1 teaspoon curry paste
- 1 cup coconut milk
- Salt and white pepper, to taste
- 1/2 teaspoon fenugreek seeds
- 1 shallot, minced
- 1 garlic clove, minced
- 1 ripe tomato, pureed

Directions :(Prep + Cook Time: 40 minutes)

✓ Preheat your Air Fryer to 380 degrees F; brush the cooking basket with 1 tablespoon of sunflower oil.

✓ Cook your fish for 10 minutes on both sides. Transfer to the baking pan that is previously greased with the remaining tablespoon of sunflower oil.

✓ Add the remaining ingredients and reduce the heat to 350 degrees F. Continue to cook an additional 10 to 12 minutes or until everything is heated through. Enjoy!

Nutritional Value: 449 Calories; 29.1g Fat; 20.4g Carbs; 27.3g Protein; 13.3g Sugars

631) *Cajun Cod Fillets with Avocado Sauce*

Ingredients

- 2 cod fish fillets
- 1 egg
- Sea salt, to taste
- 1/2 cup tortilla chips, crushed
- 2 teaspoons olive oil
- 1/2 avocado, peeled, pitted, and mashed
- 1 tablespoon mayonnaise
- 3 tablespoons sour cream
- 1/2 teaspoon yellow mustard
- 1 teaspoon lemon juice
- 1 garlic clove, minced
- ¼ teaspoon black pepper
- ¼ teaspoon salt
- ¼ teaspoon hot pepper sauce

Directions:(Prep + Cook Time: 30 minutes)

✓ Start by preheating your Air Fryer to 360 degrees F. Spritz the Air Fryer basket with cooking oil.

✓ Pat dry the fish fillets with a kitchen towel. Beat the egg in a shallow bowl.

✓ In a separate bowl, thoroughly combine the salt, crushed tortilla chips, and olive oil.

✓ Dip the fish into the egg, then, into the crumb mixture, making sure to coat thoroughly. Cook in the preheated Air Fryer approximately 12 minutes.

✓ Meanwhile, make the avocado sauce by mixing the remaining ingredients in a bowl. Place in your refrigerator until ready to serve.

✓ Serve the fish fillets with chilled avocado sauce on the side. Bon appétit!

Nutritional Value: 418 Calories; 22.7g Fat; 12.5g Carbs; **40.1g Protein; 0.9g Sugars**

632) *Old Bay Calamari*

Ingredients

- 1 cup beer
- 1 pound squid, cleaned and cut into rings
- 1 cup all-purpose flour
- 2 eggs
- 1/2 cup cornstarch
- Sea salt, to taste
- 1/2 teaspoon ground black pepper
- 1 tablespoon Old Bay seasoning

Directions:(Prep + Cook Time: 80 minutes)

✓ Add the beer and squid in a glass bowl, cover and let it sit in your refrigerator for 1 hour.

✓ Preheat your Air Fryer to 390 degrees F. Rinse the squid and pat it dry.

✓ Place the flour in a shallow bowl. In another bowl, whisk the eggs. Add the cornstarch and seasonings to a third shallow bowl.

✓ Dredge the calamari in the flour. Then, dip them into the egg mixture; finally, coat them with the cornstarch on all sided.

✓ Arrange them in the cooking basket. Spritz with cooking oil and cook for 9 to 12 minutes, depending on the desired level of doneness. Work in batches.

✓ Serve warm with your favorite dipping sauce. Enjoy!

Nutritional Value: 448 Calories; 5.3g Fat; 58.9g Carbs; 31.9g Protein; 0.2g Sugars

633) *Crispy Mustardy Fish Fingers*

Ingredients

- 1 ½ pounds tilapia pieces (fingers)
- 1/2 cup all-purpose flour
- 2 eggs
- 1 tablespoon yellow mustard
- 1 cup cornmeal
- 1 teaspoon garlic powder
- 1 teaspoon onion powder
- Sea salt and ground black pepper, to taste
- 1/2 teaspoon celery powder
- 2 tablespoons peanut oil

Directions:(Prep + Cook Time: 30 minutes)

✓ Pat dry the fish fingers with a kitchen towel.

✓ To make a breading station, place the all-purpose flour in a shallow dish. In a separate dish, whisk the eggs with mustard.

✓ In a third bowl, mix the remaining ingredients.

✓ Dredge the fish fingers in the flour, shaking the excess into the bowl; dip in the egg mixture and turn to coat evenly; then, dredge in the cornmeal mixture, turning a couple of times to coat evenly.

✓ Cook in the preheated Air Fryer at 390 degrees F for 5 minutes; turn them over and cook another 5 minutes. Enjoy!

Nutritional Value: 366 calories; protein 29.1g; carbohydrates 40g; dietary fiber 6.1g; sugars 9.2g; fat 10.3g; saturated fat 1.8g; cholesterol 103.3mg;

634) *Greek-Style Roast Fish*

Ingredients

- 2 tablespoons olive oil
- 1 red onion, sliced
- 2 cloves garlic, chopped
- 1 Florina pepper, deveined and minced
- 3 pollock fillets, skinless
- 2 ripe tomatoes, diced
- 12 Kalamata olives, pitted and chopped
- 2 tablespoons capers
- 1 teaspoon oregano
- 1 teaspoon rosemary
- Sea salt, to taste
- 1/2 cup white wine

Directions:(Prep + Cook Time: 30 minutes)

✓ Start by preheating your Air Fryer to 360 degrees F. Heat the oil in a baking pan. Once hot, sauté the onion, garlic, and pepper for 2 to 3 minutes or until fragrant.

✓ Add the fish fillets to the baking pan. Top with the tomatoes, olives, and capers. Sprinkle with the oregano, rosemary, and salt. Pour in white wine and transfer to the cooking basket.

✓ Turn the temperature to 395 degrees F and bake for 10 minutes. Taste for seasoning and serve on individual plates, garnished with some extra Mediterranean herbs if desired. Enjoy!

Nutritional Value: 422 calories; protein 32.9g; carbohydrates 31.5g; dietary fiber 5.7g; sugars 6.6g; fat 18.6g; saturated fat 2.4g; cholesterol 78mg;

635) *Quick-Fix Seafood Breakfast*

Ingredients

- 1 tablespoon olive oil
- 2 garlic cloves, minced
- 1 small yellow onion, chopped
- 1/4 pound tilapia pieces
- 1/4 pound rockfish pieces
- 1/2 teaspoon dried basil
- Salt and white pepper, to taste
- 4 eggs, lightly beaten
- 1 tablespoon dry sherry
- 4 tablespoons cheese, shredded

Directions :(Prep + Cook Time: 30 minutes)

✓ Start by preheating your Air Fryer to 350 degrees F; add the olive oil to a baking pan. Once hot, cook the garlic and onion for 2 minutes or until fragrant.

✓ Add the fish, basil, salt, and pepper. In a mixing dish, thoroughly combine the eggs with sherry and cheese. Pour the mixture into the baking pan.

✓ Cook at 360 degrees F approximately 20 minutes. Bon appétit!

Nutritional Value: 213 calories; protein 19.7g; carbohydrates 19.7g; dietary fiber 4.4g; sugars 7.5g; fat 6g; saturated fat 1g; cholesterol 104.5mg;

636) *Snapper Casserole with Gruyere Cheese*

Ingredients

- 2 tablespoons olive oil
- 1 shallot, thinly sliced
- 2 garlic cloves, minced
- 1 ½ pounds snapper fillets
- Sea salt and ground black pepper, to taste
- 1 teaspoon cayenne pepper
- 1/2 teaspoon dried basil
- 1/2 cup tomato puree
- 1/2 cup white wine
- 1 cup Gruyere cheese, shredded

Directions:(Prep + Cook Time: 30 minutes)

- ✓ Heat 1 tablespoon of olive oil in a saucepan over medium-high heat. Now, cook the shallot and garlic until tender and aromatic.
- ✓ Preheat your Air Fryer to 370 degrees F.
- ✓ Grease a casserole dish with 1 tablespoon of olive oil. Place the snapper fillet in the casserole dish. Season with salt, black pepper, and cayenne pepper. Add the sautéed shallot mixture.
- ✓ Add the basil, tomato puree and wine to the casserole dish. Cook for 10 minutes in the preheated Air Fryer.
- ✓ Top with the shredded cheese and cook an additional 7 minutes. Serve immediately.

Nutritional Value: 228 calories; protein 29.8g; carbohydrates 2.4g; dietary fiber 0.4g; sugars 0.8g; fat 8.1g;

637) *Monkfish Fillets with Romano Cheese*

Ingredients

- 2 monkfish fillets
- 1 teaspoon garlic paste
- 2 tablespoons butter, melted
- 1/2 teaspoon Aleppo chili powder
- 1/2 teaspoon dried rosemary
- 1/4 teaspoon cracked black pepper
- 1/2 teaspoon sea salt
- 4 tablespoons Romano cheese, grated

Directions :(Prep + Cook Time: 30 minutes)

- ✓ Start by preheating the Air Fryer to 320 degrees F. Spritz the Air Fryer basket with cooking oil.
- ✓ Spread the garlic paste all over the fish fillets.
- ✓ Brush the monkfish fillets with the melted butter on both sides. Sprinkle with the chili powder, rosemary, black pepper, and salt. Cook for 7 minutes in the preheated Air Fryer.
- ✓ Top with the Romano cheese and continue to cook for 2 minutes more or until heated through. Bon appétit!

Nutritional Value: 415 Calories; 22.5g Fat; 3.7g Carbs; 47.4g Protein; 2.3g Sugars

638) *Grilled Hake with Garlic Sauce*

Ingredients

- 3 hake fillets
- 6 tablespoons mayonnaise
- 1 teaspoon Dijon mustard
- 1 tablespoon fresh lime juice
- 1 cup panko crumbs
- Salt, to taste
- 1/4 teaspoon ground black pepper, or more to taste
- Garlic Sauce
- 1/4 cup Greek-style yogurt
- 2 tablespoons olive oil
- 2 cloves garlic, minced
- 1/2 teaspoon tarragon leaves, minced

Directions :(Prep + Cook Time: 30 minutes)

- ✓ Pat dry the hake fillets with a kitchen towel.
- ✓ In a shallow bowl, whisk together the mayo, mustard, and lime juice. In another shallow bowl, thoroughly combine the panko crumbs with salt, and black pepper.
- ✓ Spritz the Air Fryer grill pan with non-stick cooking spray. Grill in the preheated Air Fry at 395 degrees F for 10 minutes, flipping halfway through the cooking time. Serve immediately.

Nutritional Value: 479 Calories; 22g Fat; 29.1g Carbs; 39.1g Protein; 3.6g Sugars

639) *Grilled Tilapia with Portobello Mushrooms*

Ingredients

- 2 tilapia fillets
- 1 tablespoon avocado oil
- 1/2 teaspoon red pepper flakes, crushed
- 1/2 teaspoon dried sage, crushed
- 1/4 teaspoon lemon pepper
- 1/2 teaspoon sea salt
- 1 teaspoon dried parsley flakes
- 4 medium-sized Portobello mushrooms
- A few drizzles of liquid smoke

Directions :(Prep + Cook Time: 30 minutes)

- ✓ Toss all ingredients in a mixing bowl; except for the mushrooms.
- ✓ Transfer the tilapia fillets to a lightly greased grill pan. Preheat your Air Fryer to 400 degrees F and cook the tilapia fillets for 5 minutes.
- ✓ Now, turn the fillets over and add the Portobello mushrooms. Continue to cook for 5 minutes longer or until mushrooms are tender and the fish is opaque. Serve immediately.

Nutritional Value: 320 Calories; 11.4g Fat; 29.1g Carbs; 49.3g Protein; 4.2g Sugars

640) Authentic Mediterranean Calamari Salad

- 1 pound squid, cleaned, sliced into rings
- 2 tablespoons sherry wine
- 1/2 teaspoon granulated garlic
- Salt, to taste
- 1/2 teaspoon ground black pepper
- 1/2 teaspoon basil
- 1/2 teaspoon dried rosemary
- 1 cup grape tomatoes
- 1 small red onion, thinly sliced
- 1/3 cup Kalamata olives, pitted and sliced
- 1/2 cup mayonnaise
- 1 teaspoon yellow mustard
- 1/2 cup fresh flat-leaf parsley leaves, coarsely chopped

Directions:(Prep + Cook Time: 30 minutes)
- Start by preheating the Air Fryer to 400 degrees F. Spritz the Air Fryer basket with cooking oil.
- Toss the squid rings with the sherry wine, garlic, salt, pepper, basil, and rosemary. Cook in the preheated Air Fryer for 5 minutes, shaking the basket halfway through the cooking time.
- Work in batches and let it cool to room temperature. When the squid is cool enough, add the remaining ingredients.
- Gently stir to combine and serve well chilled. Bon appétit!

Nutritional Value: 457 Calories; 31.3g Fat; 18.4g Carbs; 25.1g Protein; 9.2g Sugars

641) Shrimp Scampi Linguine

- 1 ½ pounds shrimp, shelled and deveined
- 1/2 tablespoon fresh basil leaves, chopped
- 2 tablespoons olive oil
- 2 cloves garlic, minced
- 1/2 teaspoon fresh ginger, grated
- 1/4 teaspoon cracked black pepper
- 1/2 teaspoon sea salt
- 1/4 cup chicken stock
- 2 ripe tomatoes, pureed
- 8 ounces linguine pasta
- 1/2 cup parmesan cheese, preferably freshly grated

Directions:(Prep + Cook Time: 30 minutes)
- Start by preheating the Air Fryer to 395 degrees F. Place the shrimp, basil, olive oil, garlic, ginger, black pepper, salt, chicken stock, and tomatoes in the casserole dish.
- Transfer the casserole dish to the cooking basket and bake for 10 minutes.
- Bring a large pot of lightly salted water to a boil. Cook the linguine for 10 minutes or until al dente; drain.
- Divide between four serving plates. Add the shrimp sauce and top with parmesan cheese. Bon appétit!

Nutritional Value: 560 Calories; 15.1g Fat; 47.3g Carbs; 59.3g Protein; 1.6g Sugars

642) Sunday Fish with Sticky Sauce
Ingredients
- 2 pollack fillets
- Salt and black pepper, to taste
- 1 tablespoon olive oil
- 1 cup chicken broth
- 2 tablespoons light soy sauce
- 1 tablespoon brown sugar
- 2 tablespoons butter, melted
- 1 teaspoon fresh ginger, minced
- 1 teaspoon fresh garlic, minced
- 2 corn tortillas

Directions:(Prep + Cook Time: 30 minutes)
- Pat dry the pollack fillets and season them with salt and black pepper; drizzle the sesame oil all over the fish fillets.
- Preheat the Air Fryer to 380 degrees F and cook your fish for 11 minutes. Slice into bite-sized pieces.
- Meanwhile, prepare the sauce. Add the broth to a large saucepan and bring to a boil. Add the soy sauce, sugar, butter, ginger, and garlic. Reduce the heat to simmer and cook until it is reduced slightly.
- Add the fish pieces to the warm sauce. Serve on corn tortillas and enjoy!

Nutritional Value: 270 calories; protein 28g; carbohydrates 6.8g; dietary fiber 1.3g; sugars 0.7g; fat 14.6g; saturated fat 6.5g; cholesterol 103.5mg; vitamin a iu 381.4IU; vitamin c 7.9mg; folate 10.8mcg;

643) Buttermilk Tuna fillets
Ingredients
- 1 pound tuna fillets
- 1/2 cup buttermilk
- 1/2 cup tortilla chips, crushed
- 1/4 cup parmesan cheese, grated
- 1/4 cup cassava flour
- Salt and ground black pepper, to taste
- 1 teaspoon mustard seeds
- 1 teaspoon paprika
- 1 teaspoon garlic powder
- 1/2 teaspoon onion powder

Direction:(Prep + Cook Time: 30 minutes)
- Place the tuna fillets and buttermilk in a bowl; cover and let it sit for 30 minutes.
- In a shallow bowl, thoroughly combine the remaining ingredients; mix until well combined.
- Dip the tuna fillets in the parmesan mixture until they are covered on all sides.
- Cook in the preheated Air Fryer at 380 degrees F for 12 minutes, turning halfway through the cooking time. Bon appétit

Nutritional Value: 266 Calories; 5.7g Fat; 13.6g Carbs; 37.8g Protein; 2.5g Sugars

225

644)   *Herbed Crab Croquettes*

Ingredients:

- (4 Servings)
- 1 ½ lb lump crabmeat
- ⅓ cup sour cream
- ⅓ cup mayonnaise
- 1 red pepper, finely chopped ⅓ cup red onion, chopped
- ½ celery stalk, chopped
- 1 tsp fresh tarragon, chopped 1 tsp fresh chives, chopped
- 1 tsp fresh parsley, chopped
- 1 tsp cayenne pepper
- 1 ½ cups breadcrumbs
- 2 tsp olive oil
- 1 cup flour
- 2 eggs, beaten
- Salt to taste Lemon wedges to serve.

Direction:(Prep + Cook Time: 30 minutes)

✓ Heat olive oil in a skillet over medium heat and sauté the red pepper, onion, and celery for 5 minutes or until sweaty and translucent.

✓ Turn off the heat. Pour the breadcrumbs and salt on a plate.

✓ In 2 separate bowls, add the flour and the beaten eggs, respectively, and set aside.

✓ In a separate bowl, add crabmeat, mayonnaise, sour cream, tarragon, chives, parsley, cayenne pepper, and sautéed vegetables.

✓ Form bite-size oval balls out of the mixture and place the balls on a plate.

✓ Preheat the air fryer to 390 F.

✓ Dip each crab meatball in the beaten eggs and press down in the breadcrumb mixture.

✓ Place the croquettes in the greased frying basket without overcrowding.

✓ AirFry for 10-12 minutes or until golden brown, turning once.

✓ Serve hot with lemon wedges.

Nutrition: Cal 162 Total Fat 3.3 g Saturated Fat 0.3 g cholesterol 64.7 mg Total Carbs 15.7 g Dietary Fiber 0.8 g Sugar 4.5 g Protein 21.2 g

645)   *Crab Fritters with Sweet Chili Sauce*

Ingredients:

- (4 Servings)
- 1 lb jumbo crabmeat
- 1 lime, zested and juiced
- 1 tsp ginger paste
- 1 tsp garlic puree
- 1 tbsp fresh cilantro, chopped 1 red chili, roughly chopped
- 1 egg
- ¼ cup panko breadcrumbs

- 1 tsp soy sauce sauce
- 3 tbsp sweet chili sauce.

Direction:(Prep + Cook Time: 25 minutes)

✓ Preheat the air fryer to 400 F.

✓ In a bowl, mix crabmeat, lime zest, egg, ginger paste, and garlic puree.

✓ Form small cakes out of the mixture and dredge them in the breadcrumbs. Place in the greased frying basket and AirFry for 14-16 minutes, shaking once until golden brown.

✓ In a small bowl, mix the sweet chili sauce with lime juice and soy sauce.

✓ Serve the fritters topped with cilantro and the chili sauce.

Nutrition: Cal 300 Calories from Fat 120g Total Fat 13gSaturated Fat 1g colesterol 100 mg otal Carbs 27g Dietary Fiber 1g Sugar 14g Protein 19g 0 %

646)   *Old Bay Crab Sticks with Garlic Mayo*

Ingredients:

- (4 Servings)
- 1 lb crab sticks
- 1 tbsp old bay seasoning
- ⅓ cup panko breadcrumbs
- 2 eggs
- ½ cup mayonnaise
- 2 garlic cloves, minced
- 1 lime, juiced
- 1 cup flour.

Direction:(Prep + Cook Time: 20 minutes)

✓ Preheat the air fryer to 390 F.

✓ Beat the eggs in a bowl.

✓ In another bowl, mix the breadcrumbs with old bay seasoning.

✓ Pour the flour into a third bowl.

✓ Dip the sticks in the flour, then in the eggs, and finally in the breadcrumbs.

✓ Spray with cooking spray and AirFry for 12-14 minutes, flipping once, until golden.

✓ Mix the mayonnaise with garlic and lime juice.

✓ Serve as a dip along with crab sticks.

Nutrition: Calories: 322kcal | Carbs : 38.1g | Protein : 13.4g | Fat : 13.1g | cholesterol: 37 mg | Fiber : 0.7g |

647)   *Crabmeat & Veggie Patties with Basil Dip*

Ingredients:

- (4 Servings)
- 3 potatoes, boiled and mashed
- 1 cup cooked crabmeat
- ¼ cup red onions, chopped
- 1 tbsp fresh basil, chopped
- ½ celery stalk, chopped
- ½ bell red pepper, chopped

- 1 tbsp Dijon mustard
- ½ lemon, zested and juiced
- ¼ cup breadcrumbs
- 1 tsp ground allspice
- ½ cup mayonnaise
- Salt and black pepper to taste.

Direction:(Prep + Cook Time: 20 minutes + chilling time)

✓ Place the mashed potatoes, red onions, allspice, breadcrumbs, celery, bell pepper, mustard, lemon zest, crabmeat, salt, and black pepper in a large bowl and mix well.

✓ Make patties from the mixture and refrigerate for 30 minutes.

✓ Mix the mayonnaise, lemon juice, basil, salt, and pepper and set aside. P

✓ reheat the air fryer to 390 F.

✓ Remove the patties from the fridge and place them in the greased frying basket.

✓ AirFry for 12-14 minutes, flipping once until golden.

✓ Serve the patties with the basil-mayo dip.

Nutrition: 175 calories; Protein 19.3g; Carbs 7g; Dietary Fiber 0.3g; Sugar 0.8g; Fat 7.4g; saturated Fat 1.9g;

648)   *Fiery Prawns*

Ingredients:

- (4 Servings)
- 8 prawns, cleaned
- Salt and black pepper to taste
- ½ tsp ground cayenne pepper
- ½ tsp red chili flakes
- ½ tsp ground cumin
- ½ tsp garlic powder

Direction:(Prep + Cook Time: 15 minutes)

✓ In a bowl, season the prawns with salt and black pepper. Sprinkle with cayenne pepper, chili flakes, cumin, and garlic, and stir to coat.

✓ Spray the frying basket with oil and lay the prawns in an even layer. AirFry for 8-10 minutes at 340 F, turning once halfway through. Serve with sweet chili sauce if desired.

Nutrition: Calories 310 Total Fat 7g cholesterol 120 mg g Carbs 43g Net carbs 42g Sugar 5g Fiber 1g Protein 19g

649)   *Crispy Prawns in Bacon Wraps*

Ingredients:

- (4 Servings)
- 8 bacon slices
- 8 jumbo prawns, peeled and deveined

Direction:(Prep + Cook Time: 15 minutes)

✓ Preheat the air fryer to 400 F.

✓ Wrap each prawn from head to tail in each bacon slice.

✓ Make sure to overlap to keep the bacon in place.

Secure the ends with toothpicks Arrange the bacon-wrapped prawns in the greased frying basket and AirFry for 9-12 minutes, turning once.

✓ Serve hot.

Nutrition: Calories 207.6 Total Fat 2.0 g Saturated Fat 0.4 g g cholesterol 172.3 7 mg Total Carbs 1.0 g Dietary Fiber 0.0 g Sugar 0.0 g Protein 23.0 g % Copper 15.0

650)   *Chinese Garlic Prawns*

Ingredients:

- (4 Servings)
- 1 lb prawns, peeled and deveined
- Juice from 1 lemon
- 1 tsp Sugar
- 2 tbsp peanut oil
- 2 tbsp cornstarch
- 2 scallions, chopped
- ¼ tsp Chinese powder
- 1 red chili pepper, minced
- Salt and black pepper to taste
- 4 garlic cloves, minced

Direction:(Prep + Cook Time: 25 minutes + marinating time)

✓ In a Ziploc bag, mix lemon juice, Sugar , black pepper, 1 tbsp of peanut oil, cornstarch, Chinese powder, and salt.

✓ Add in the prawns and massage gently to coat well. Let sit for 20 minutes.

✓ Heat the remaining peanut oil in a pan over medium heat and sauté garlic, scallions, and red chili pepper for 3 minutes.

✓ In a Ziploc bag, mix lemon juice, Sugar , black pepper, 1 tbsp of peanut oil, cornstarch, Chinese powder, and salt.

✓ Add in the prawns and massage gently to coat well. Let sit for 20 minutes.

✓ Heat the remaining peanut oil in a pan over medium heat and sauté garlic, scallions, and red chili pepper for 3 minutes.

Nutrition: Calorie 572Carbs17 g Dietary Fiber 0 g Sugar 1 g Fat 20 gSaturated3 g Polyunsaturated 10 g Monounsaturated 5 g Protein 66 g g cholesterol 460

651)   *Sesame Prawns with Firecracker Sauce*

Ingredients:

- (4 Servings)
- 1 lb tiger prawns, peeled
- Salt and black pepper to taste
- 2 eggs
- ½ cup flour
- ¼ cup sesame seeds
- ¾ cup seasoned breadcrumbs
- Firecracker sauce ⅓ cup
- sour cream
- 2 tbsp buffalo sauce

- ¼ cup spicy ketchup
- 1 green onion, chopped

Direction:(Prep + Cook Time: 20 minutes)

✓ Preheat the air fryer to 390 F.

✓ In a bowl, beat the eggs with a pinch of salt.

✓ In another bowl, mix the breadcrumbs with sesame seeds.

✓ In a third bowl, mix flour with salt and pepper.

✓ Dip the prawns in the flour, then in the eggs, and finally in the crumbs. Spray with cooking spray.

✓ AirFry for 10-12 minutes, flipping once.

✓ Meanwhile, in a bowl mix all sauce ingredients, except for the green onion.

✓ Serve the prawns with firecracker sauce and scatter with freshly chopped green onions.

Nutrition: 334 kcal, 58g Protein , 10g Carbs (of which 7g Sugar s), 6g Fat (of which 1g saturates), 4.5g Fiber and 5.4g salt.

652) *Ale-Battered Scampi with Tartare Sauce*

Ingredients:

- (4 Servings)
- 1 lb prawns, peeled and deveined
- 1 cup plain flour
- 1 cup ale beer
- Salt and black pepper to taste
- Tartare sauce:
- ½ cup mayonnaise
- 2 tbsp capers, roughly chopped
- 2 tbsp fresh dill, chopped
- 1 pickled cucumber, finely chopped
- 2 tsp lemon juice
- ½ tsp Worcestershire sauce.

Direction:(Prep + Cook Time: 20 minutes)

✓ Preheat the air fryer to 380 F.

✓ In a bowl, mix all sauce ingredients and keep in the fridge.

✓ Mix flour, ale beer, salt, and pepper in a large bowl Dip in the prawns and place them in the greased frying basket.

✓ AirFry for 10-12 minutes, turning them once halfway through cooking. Serve with the tartare sauce

Nutrition: Calories 1850 Total Fat 96g Saturated Fat 15g cholesterol 150 mg g Carbs 171g Net carbs 155g Sugar 5g Fiber 16g Protein 72g g

653) *Delicious Cayenne Shrimps*

Ingredients:

- (2 Servings)
- 8 large shrimp, peeled and deveined
- ½ cup breadcrumbs
- 8 oz coconut milk
- ½ cup coconut, shredded
- Salt to taste

- ½ cup orange jam
- 1 tsp mustard
- 1 tbsp honey
- ½ tsp cayenne pepper
- ¼ tsp hot sauce.

Direction:(Prep + Cook Time: 30 minutes)

✓ Combine breadcrumbs, cayenne pepper, shredded coconut, and salt in a bowl.

✓ Dip the shrimp in the coconut milk, and then in the coconut crumbs Arrange them in the greased frying basket and AirFry for 12-14 minutes at 350 F.

✓ Whisk jam, honey, hot sauce, and mustard in a bowl.

✓ Serve with the shrimp.

Nutrition: Calories 349.8 Total Fat 8.3 g Saturated Fat 1.9 g g cholesterol 172.3 6 mg Total Carbs 35.7 g Dietary Fiber 2.2 g Sugar 0.0 g Protein 26.6 g % Copper 17.0 Manganese 7.2 % Niacin 31.6 %

654) *Fried Green Tomato Bites with Remoulade*

Ingredients:

- (2 Servings)
- 2 green tomatoes, sliced
- ¼ tbsp creole seasoning
- ¼ cup flour 1 egg, beaten
- 1 cup breadcrumbs
- 1 cup remoulade sauce.

Direction:(Prep + Cook Time: 15 minutes)

✓ Add flour to one bowl and the egg to another.

✓ Make a mix of creole seasoning and breadcrumbs in a third bowl.

✓ Coat the tomato slices in the flour, then dip in the egg, and then in the crumbs. AirFry in the greased frying basket for 5-6 minutes at 400 F, turning once.

✓ Serve with remoulade sauce.

Nutrition:: Calories: 616kcal Carbs : 37g Protein : 10g Fat : 48g cholesterol: 38 Fiber : 5g Sugar : 14g g

655) *Roasted Tomatoes with Cheese Topping*

Ingredients:

- (4 Servings)
- ½ cup cheddar cheese, shredded
- ¼ cup Parmesan cheese, grated
- 4 tomatoes, cut into ½ inch slices
- 2 tbsp fresh parsley, chopped
- Salt and black pepper to taste.

Direction:(Prep + Cook Time: 20 minutes)

✓ Preheat the air fryer to 380 F.

✓ Lightly salt the tomato slices and put them in the greased frying basket in a single layer.

✓ Top with cheddar and Parmesan cheeses and sprinkle with black pepper. AirFry for 5-6 minutes until the cheese is melted and bubbly.

✓ Serve topped with fresh parsley and enjoy!

Nutrition: Calories 92.3 Total Fat 5.2 g Saturated Fat 2.7 g g cholesterol 11.5 3 mg Total Carbs 4.9 g Dietary Fiber 1.0 g Sugar 0.0 g Protein 6.9 g % Copper 3.5

656) *Roasted Brussels Sprouts*

Ingredients:

- (4 Servings)
- 1 lb Brussels sprouts
- 1 tsp garlic powder
- 2 tbsp olive oil
- Salt and black pepper to taste.

Direction:(Prep + Cook Time: 25 minutes)

- ✓ Preheat the air fryer to 380 F.
- ✓ Trim off the outer leaves, keeping only the head of each sprout.
- ✓ In a bowl, mix olive oil, garlic powder, salt, and black pepper. Coat in the Brussels sprouts and transfer them to the greased frying basket.
- ✓ AirFry for 15 minutes, shaking once halfway through cooking.

Nutrition: 37.8 calories0.264 g of Fat 7.88 g of carbohydrate2.97 g of Protein

657) *Honey Baby Carrots*

Ingredients:

- (4 Servings)
- 1 lb baby carrots
- 1 tsp dried dill
- 2 tbsp olive oil
- 1 tbsp honey
- 1 cup feta cheese, crumbled
- Salt and black pepper to taste.

Direction:(Prep + Cook Time: 20 minutes)

- ✓ Preheat the air fryer to 350 F.
- ✓ In a bowl, mix olive oil, carrots, and honey, and stir to coat.
- ✓ Season with dill, black pepper, and salt.
- ✓ Place the coated carrots in the greased frying basket and AirFry for 12-14 minutes, shaking once or twice.
- ✓ Serve warm or chilled topped with feta cheese.

Nutrition: Calories 22.8 Total Fat 0.3 g Saturated Fat 0.1 g g cholesterol 0.0 mg mg 4 mg Total Carbs 4.9 g Dietary Fiber 1.1 g Sugar 0.0 g Protein 0.5 g % Copper 1.4 Manganese 2.3 % Niacin 2.7 %

658) *Authentic Spanish Patatas Bravas*

Ingredients:

- (4 Servings)
- 1 lb waxy potatoes, into bite-size chunks
- 4 tbsp olive oil
- 1 tsp smoked paprika
- 1 shallot, chopped
- 2 tomatoes, chopped
- tbsp tomato paste
- 1 tbsp flour

- 2 tbsp sriracha hot chili sauce
- 1 tsp Sugar
- 2 tbsp fresh parsley, chopped Salt to taste.

Direction:(Prep + Cook Time: 40 minutes)

- ✓ Heat 2 tbsp of olive oil in a skillet over medium heat and sauté the shallot for 3 minutes until fragrant.
- ✓ Stir in the flour for 2 more minutes.
- ✓ Add in the remaining ingredients and 1 cup of Water .
- ✓ Bring to a boil, reduce the heat, and simmer for 6-8 minutes until the sauce becomes pulpy.
- ✓ Remove to a food processor and blend until smooth.
- ✓ Let cool completely.
- ✓ Preheat the air fryer to 400 F.
- ✓ Coat the potatoes in the remaining olive oil and AirFry in the fryer for 20-25 minutes, shaking once halfway through.
- ✓ Sprinkle with salt and spoon over the sauce to serve

Nutrition: Calories: 1563.8 Protein : 7.3g Carbs : 54g Dietary Fiber : 8.2g Sugar 10.3g Fat : 150.8gSaturated Fat : 21.1g cholesterol: 10.4 mg Niacin Equivalents: 5.7 mg calories From Fat : 1356.9

659) *Delicious Potato Patties*

Ingredients:

-)(4 Servings)
- 4 potatoes, shredded
- 1 onion, chopped
- 1 egg, beaten
- ¼ cup milk
- 2 tbsp butter
- ½ tsp garlic powder
- Salt and black pepper to taste
- 3 tbsp flour

Direction:(Prep + Cook Time: 25 minutes)

- ✓ Preheat the air fryer to 390 F.
- ✓ In a bowl, add the egg, potatoes, onion, milk, butter, black pepper, flour, garlic powder, and salt and mix well to form a batter.
- ✓ Mold the mixture into four patties.
- ✓ Place them in the greased frying basket and AirFry for 14-16 minutes, flipping once.
- ✓ Serve warm with garlic mayo.

Nutrition: Calories 105 Total Fat 3.9gSaturated Fat 1.4g Trans Fat 0g nounsaturated Fat 1.8g cholesterol 22 mg gTotal Carbs 14g Dietary Fiber 1.3g Sugar 0.9g Protein 4g

660) *Sweet & Spicy French Fries*

Ingredients:

- (4 Servings)
- ½ tsp salt
- ½ tsp garlic powder
- ½ tsp chili powder
- ¼ tsp cumin
- 3 tbsp olive oil

- 4 sweet potatoes, cut into thick strips

Direction:(Prep + Cook Time: 30 minutes)

✓ Preheat the air fryer to 380 F.

✓ In a bowl, whisk olive oil, salt, garlic, chili powder, and cumin. Coat the strips in the mixture and place them in the frying basket.

✓ AirFry for 20 minutes, shaking once, until crispy.

Nutrition: Calories 34.4 Total Fat 0.1 g Saturated Fat 0.0 g g cholesterol 0.0 mg Total Carbs 7.9 g Dietary Fiber 1.0 g Sugar 0.0 g Protein 0.5 g % Copper 2.8 Manganese 5.9 % Niacin 1.1 % Pantothenic Acid 1.9

661) Curly Fries with Gochujang Ketchup

Ingredients:

- (2 Servings)
- 2 potatoes, spiralized
- Salt and black pepper to taste
- 2 tbsp coconut oil
- 1 tbsp Gochujang chili paste
- ½ cup tomato ketchup
- 2 tsp soy sauce
- ¼ tsp ginger powder.

Direction:(Prep + Cook Time: 35 minutes)

✓ In a small bowl, whisk together the ketchup, Gochujang paste, soy sauce, and ginger powder; reserve.

✓ Preheat the air fryer to 390 F.

✓ In a bowl, coat the potatoes in coconut oil, salt, and pepper.

✓ Place in the frying basket and AirFry for 20-25 minutes, shaking once.

✓ Serve with Gochujang ketchup and enjoy

Nutrition: Calories 440 Total Fat 23gSaturated Fat 3.5g Trans Fat 0g cholesterol 0 mg gTotal Carbs 60g Dietary Fiber 3g Sugar 16g Protein 3g

662) Traditional Jacket Potatoes

Ingredients:

- (4 Servings)
- 1 lb potatoes
- 2 garlic cloves, minced
- Salt and black pepper to taste
- 1 tbsp fresh rosemary, chopped
- 1 tbsp fresh parsley, chopped
- 2 tsp butter, melted.

Direction:(Prep + Cook Time: 30 minutes)

✓ Preheat the air fryer to 360 F.

✓ Prick the potatoes with a fork.

✓ Place them in the greased frying basket and Bake for 23-25 minutes, turning once halfway through. Remove and cut a cross on top.

✓ Squeeze the sides and drizzle with melted butter.

✓ Sprinkle with garlic, rosemary, parsley, salt, and pepper. Serve.

Nutrition: Calories: 161 Carbs: 37 grams Fiber : 3.8 grams Protein : 4.3 grams Fat : 0.2 grams %

663) Cheesy Potatoes & Asparagus

Ingredients:

- (4 Servings)
- 4 potatoes, cut into wedges
- 1 bunch of asparagus, trimmed
- 2 tbsp olive oil
- ¼ cup buttermilk
- ¼ cup cottage cheese, crumbled
- 1 tbsp whole-grain mustard
- Salt and black pepper to taste.

Direction:(Prep + Cook Time: 30 minute)

✓ Preheat the fryer to 400 F.

✓ Place the potatoes in the greased frying basket and Bake for 14-16 minutes.

✓ Drizzle the asparagus with olive oil and season with salt and pepper.

✓ Slide the frying basket out and shake the potatoes Spread the asparagus all over and Bake for 7 minutes, turning the spears once.

✓ In a bowl, mix well the cottage cheese, buttermilk, and whole-grain mustard.

✓ Arrange potatoes and asparagus on a serving platter and drizzle with the cheese sauce.

Nutrition: Calories 216.0 Total Fat 5.6 g Saturated Fat 1.7 g g cholesterol 4.9 0 mg Total Carbs 35.2 g Dietary Fiber 4.5 g Sugar 2.5 g Protein 7.6 g % Copper 10.5 Manganese 15.8 % Niacin 9.4 %

664) Serve and enjoy! Zesty Bell Pepper Bites

Ingredients:

- (4 Servings)
- 1 red bell pepper, cut into small portions
- 1 yellow pepper, cut into small portions
- 1 green bell pepper, cut into small portions
- 3 tbsp balsamic vinegar
- 2 tbsp olive oil
- 1 garlic clove, minced
- ½ tsp dried basil
- ½ tsp dried parsley
- Salt and black pepper to taste
- ½ cup garlic mayonnaise.

Direction:Prep + Cook Time: 20 minutes

✓ Preheat the air fryer to 390 F.

✓ In a bowl, mix bell peppers, olive oil, garlic, balsamic vinegar, basil, and parsley and season with salt and black pepper.

✓ Transfer to the greased frying basket and Bake in the air fryer for 12-15 minutes, tossing once or twice.

✓ Serve with garlic mayonnaise.

Nutrition: Calories 280 Total Fat 22gSaturated Fat 11g Trans Fat 0g cholesterol 245 mg Total Carbs 3g Dietary Fiber 1gTotal Sugar 1gIncludes 0g Added Sugar Protein 17g

665) Quick Beetroot Chips

Ingredients:

- (2 Servings)
- 2 golden beetroots, thinly sliced
- 2 tbsp olive oil
- 1 tbsp yeast flakes
- 1 tsp Italian seasoning

Direction:(Prep + Cook Time: 20 minutes)

✓ Preheat the air fryer to 360 F.

✓ In a bowl, add olive oil, beetroot slices, Italian seasoning, and yeast and mix well.

✓ Dump the coated chips in the greased frying basket and AirFry for 12 minutes, shaking once.

Nutrition: Calories 135 Total Fat 8.5gSaturated Fat 0.8g Trans Fat 0g cholesterol 0 Total Carbs 14g Dietary Fiber 0.8g Sugar 0.3g Protein 1.7g

666) Brussels Sprouts with Garlic Aioli

Ingredients:

- (4 Servings)
- 3 garlic cloves, minced
- 1 lb Brussels sprouts, trimmed and halved
- Salt and black pepper to taste
- 2 tbsp olive oil
- 2 tsp lemon juice
- ¾ cup mayonnaise.

Direction:(Prep + Cook Time: 25 minutes)

✓ Place a pot with Water over medium heat; bring to a boil.

✓ Blanch in the sprouts for 3 minutes; drain.

✓ Preheat the air fryer to 350 F.

✓ Drizzle the Brussels sprouts with olive oil and season to taste.

✓ Pour them into the frying basket and AirFry for 5 minutes, shaking once.

✓ In a bowl, whisk the mayonnaise, garlic, lemon juice, salt and black pepper to taste, to make aioli.

✓ Serve the sprouts with aioli.

Nutrition: Calories 150Calories From Fat 110 Total Fat 12gSaturated Fat 15g Trans Fat g cholesterol 5 mg gTotal Carbs 9g Dietary Fiber 2g Sugar 2g Protein 1g

667) Easy Cabbage Steaks

Ingredients:

- (3 Servings)
- 1 cabbage head
- 1 tbsp garlic paste
- 2 tbsp olive oil
- Salt and black pepper to taste
- 2 tsp fennel seeds.

Direction:(Prep + Cook Time: 25 minutes)

✓ Preheat the air fryer to 350 F.

✓ Cut the cabbage into 1½-inch thin slices. In a small bowl, combine all the other ingredients and brush the cabbage with the mixture.

✓ Arrange the steaks in the greased frying basket and

Bake for 14-16 minutes, flipping once halfway through cooking.

✓ Serve warm or chilled.

Nutrition: Calories 66.9 Total Fat 2.1 g Saturated Fat 0.3 g g cholesterol 0.0 mg mg 0 mg Total Carbs 11.6 g Dietary Fiber 4.8 g Sugar 0.1 g Protein 3.1 g % Copper 2.5 % 4 % Manganese 16.7 % Niacin 3.1 % Pantothenic Acid 2.9 lenium 2.9 %

668) Green Cabbage with Blue Cheese Sauce

Ingredients:

- (4 Servings)
- 1 head green cabbage, cut into wedges
- 1 cup mozzarella cheese, shredded
- 4 tbsp butter, melted
- ½ cup blue cheese sauce

Direction:(Prep + Cook Time: 25 minutes)

✓ Preheat the air fryer to 380 F.

✓ Brush the wedges with butter and sprinkle with mozzarella.

✓ Transfer to the greased frying basket and Bake in the air fryer for 18-20 minutes.

✓ Serve with blue cheese sauce.

Nutrition: Calories: 396 Total Fat : 37gsaturated Fat : 22g Trans Fat : 1gunsaturated Fat : 13g Cholesterol: 99 Mg G Carbs : 6g Fiber : 1g Sugar : 4g Protein : 11g

669) Crispy Bell Peppers with Tartare Sauce

Ingredients:

- (4 Servings)
- 1 egg, beaten
- 2 bell peppers, cut into ½-inch-thick slices
- ⅔ cup panko breadcrumbs
- ½ tsp paprika
- ½ tsp garlic powder
- Salt to taste
- 1 tsp lime juice
- ½ cup mayonnaise
- 2 tbsp capers, chopped
- 2 dill pickles, chopped.

Direction:(Prep + Cook Time: 25 minutes)

✓ Preheat the air fryer to 390 F.

✓ Mix the breadcrumbs, paprika, garlic powder, and salt in a shallow bowl.

✓ In a separate bowl, whisk the egg with 1½ teaspoons of Water to make an egg wash.

✓ Coat the bell pepper slices in the egg wash, then roll them up in the crumbs mixture until fully covered.

✓ Put the peppers in the greased frying basket in a single layer and spray with olive oil, AirFry for 4-7 minutes until light brown.

✓ Meanwhile, in a bowl, mix the mayonnaise, lime juice, capers, pickles, and salt.

✓ Remove the peppers from the fryer and serve with the tartare sauce. Enjoy!

Nutrition: Calories: 59Fat : 4.7g g Carbs : 3.7g Fiber 0.1g Sugar 1.2g Protein : 0.3g

670) *Indian Fried Okra*

Ingredients:

- (4 Servings)
- 1 tbsp chili powder
- 2 tbsp garam masala
- 1 cup cornmeal
- ¼ cup flour
- Salt and black pepper to taste
- ½ lb okra, trimmed and halved lengthwise
- 1 egg
- 1 cup Cholula hot sauce

Direction:(Prep + Cook Time: 20 minutes)

- ✓ Preheat the air fryer to 380 F.
- ✓ In a bowl, mix cornmeal, flour, chili powder, garam masala, salt, and black pepper.
- ✓ In another bowl, whisk the egg and season with salt and pepper.
- ✓ Dip the okra in the egg and then coat in the cornmeal mixture.
- ✓ Spray with cooking spray and place in the frying basket.
- ✓ AirFry for 6 minutes, shake, and cook for another 5-7 minutes or until golden brown.
- ✓ Serve with hot sauce.

Nutrition: Calories 196 Total Fat 17gSaturated Fat 1.2g Trans Fat 0.1g cholesterol 0 mg gTotal Carbs 12g Dietary Fiber 3.9g Sugar 5.5g Protein 2.9g

671) *Zucchini Fries with Tabasco Dip*

Ingredients:

- (4 Servings)
- 2 zucchinis, sliced
- 2 egg whites
- ½ cup seasoned breadcrumbs
- 2 tbsp Parmesan cheese, grated
- ¼ tsp garlic powder
- Salt and black pepper to taste
- 1 cup mayonnaise
- ¼ cup heavy cream
- 1 tbsp Tabasco sauce
- 1 tsp lime juice.

Direction:(Prep + Cook Time: 25 minutes)

- ✓ Preheat the air fryer to 400 F.
- ✓ In a bowl, beat egg whites with salt and black pepper.
- ✓ In another bowl, mix garlic powder, Parmesan cheese, and breadcrumbs.
- ✓ Dip zucchini strips in the egg whites, then in the crumbs and spray them with cooking oil.
- ✓ AirFry them for 13-15 minutes, turning once.
- ✓ Meanwhile, in a bowl, mix mayonnaise, heavy cream, Tabasco sauce, and lime juice.

- ✓ Serve as a dip for the strips

Nutrition: Calories 410 Total Fat 23gSaturated Fat 7.9g Trans Fat 0.3g cholesterol 107 mg g gTotal Carbs 33g Dietary Fiber 2.7g Sugar 5.2g Protein 19g

672) *Parmesan Zucchini Boats*

Ingredients:

- (4 Servings)
- 4 small zucchinis, cut lengthwise
- ½ cup Parmesan cheese, grated
- ½ cup breadcrumbs
- ¼ cup melted butter
- ¼ cup fresh parsley, chopped
- 4 garlic cloves, minced
- Salt and black pepper to taste.

Direction:(Prep + Cook Time: 25 minutes)

- ✓ Preheat the air fryer to 370 F.
- ✓ Scoop out the insides of the zucchini halves with a spoon.
- ✓ In a bowl, mix breadcrumbs, garlic, and parsley.
- ✓ Season with salt and pepper and stir in the zucchini flesh.
- ✓ Spoon the mixture into the zucchini "boats" and sprinkle with Parmesan cheese.
- ✓ Drizzle with melted butter.
- ✓ Arrange the boats on the greased frying basket and Bake for 12 minutes or until the cheese is golden.

Nutrition: Calories 170.1 Total Fat 6.5 g cholesterol 1.5 7 mg Total Carbs 24.0 g Sugar 2.9 g Protein 5.3 g

673) *Bulgarian "Burek" Pepper with Yogurt Sauce*

Ingredients:

- (4 Servings)
- 4 red bell peppers, roasted
- 1 cup feta cheese, crumbled
- 4 eggs
- 1 cup breadcrumbs
- 4 garlic cloves, chopped
- 1 tomato, peeled and chopped
- 1 tsp fresh dill, chopped
- 1 tbsp fresh parsley, chopped
- Salt and black pepper to taste
- 1 tbsp olive oil
- ½ cup flour
- 1 cup Greek yogurt.

Direction:(Prep + Cook Time: 30 minutes)

- ✓ In a small bowl, mix yogurt, olive oil, half of the garlic, and dill.
- ✓ Keep the sauce in the fridge.
- ✓ Preheat the air fryer to 350 F.
- ✓ In a bowl, beat 3 eggs with salt and black pepper.
- ✓ Add in feta cheese, the remaining garlic, tomato, and parsley and mix to combine.

✓ Fill the peppers with the mixture.

✓ Beat the remaining egg with salt and pepper in a bowl.

✓ Coat the peppers first in flour, then dip in the egg, and finally in the crumbs.

✓ Arrange them in the greased frying basket and AirFry for 10-12 minutes until golden brown, turning once.

✓ Serve the peppers with the yogurt sauce on the side and enjoy!.

Nutrition: Calories 230 Total Fat 5gSaturated Fat 1g cholesterol 5 mg Carbs 35g Net carbs 24g Sugar 11g Fiber 11g Protein 11g

674) *Green Pea Arancini with Tomato Sauce*

Ingredients:

• (4 Servings)

• 1 cup rice, rinsed

• ½ green peas

• 1 tbsp butter

• 1 onion, chopped

• 2 garlic cloves, minced

• 1 egg

• 3 tbsp Parmesan cheese, shredded

• ½ cup breadcrumbs

• 2 tbsp olive oil

• Salt and black pepper to taste

• 1 lb Roma tomatoes, chopped

• 2 tbsp fresh basil, chopped

Direction:(Prep + Cook Time: 60 minutes + chilling time)

✓ Fill a shallow saucepan with Water and place over medium heat.

✓ Bring to a boil and add in the rice, salt, and pepper.

✓ Cook for 20-22 minutes, stirring often.

✓ Drain and transfer to a bowl; mix in the green peas.

✓ Mix in the onion, garlic, Parmesan cheese, and egg.

✓ Mold the mixture into golf-size balls and roll them in breadcrumbs.

✓ Place them in a baking sheet and refrigerate for 1 hour.

✓ Preheat the air fryer to 360 F.

✓ Remove the arancini from the fridge and arrange them in the greased frying basket.

✓ AirFry for 14-16 minutes, shaking from time to time until nicely browned.

✓ Meanwhile, heat the olive oil in the skillet and stir-fry the tomatoes for 6-8 minutes until the sauce thickens.

✓ Season with salt and black pepper.

✓ Scatter basil on top and serve with the arancini.

Nutrition: Calories: 480kcal | Carbs : 18g | Protein : 12g | Fat : 41g | Saturated Fat : 29g | cholesterol: 86 mg Fiber : 1g | Sugar : 2g |

675) *Aunt's Roasted Carrots with Cilantro Sauce*

Ingredients:

• (4 Servings)

• ¼ cup olive oil

• 2 shallots, cut into wedges

• 4 carrots, halved lengthways

• 4 garlic cloves, lightly crushed

• ¼ tsp nutmeg

• ¼ tsp allspice

• ¼ cup cilantro, chopped

• ¼ lime, zested and juiced

• 1 tbsp Parmesan cheese, grated

• 1 tbsp pine nuts.

Direction:(Prep + Cook Time: 25 minutes)

✓ Preheat the air fryer to 370 F.

✓ Coat the carrots and shallots with allspice, nutmeg, and some olive oil.

✓ Put in the frying basket.

✓ Sprinkle with garlic and Bake for 15-20 minutes, shaking halfway through In a food processor, blitz the remaining olive oil, cilantro, lime zest and juice, Parmesan cheese, and pine nuts until the mixture forms a paste.

✓ Remove and serve on the side of the roasted veggies.

Nutrition: Calories: 64.4kcal Carbs : 13.5g Protein : 1.5g Fat : 0.4gSaturated Fat : 0.1g 1 mg Fiber : 4.4g

676) *Mediterranean Eggplant Burgers*

Ingredients:

• (2 Servings)

• 2 hamburger buns, halved

• 2 (2-inch) eggplant slices, cut along the round axis

• 2 mozzarella slices

• 1 red onion, cut into rings

• 2 lettuce leaves

• 1 tbsp tomato sauce

• 1 pickle, sliced

• Salt to taste.

Direction:(Prep + Cook Time: 20 minutes)

✓ Preheat the air fryer to 360 F.

✓ Season the eggplant slices with salt and place them in the greased frying basket.

✓ Bake for 6 minutes, flipping once.

✓ Top with mozzarella slices and cook for 30 more seconds.

✓ Spread the tomato sauce on the bun bottoms.

✓ Top with the cheesy eggplant slices followed by the red onion rings, sliced pickle, and lettuce leaves.

✓ Finish with the bun tops and serve immediately.

Nutrition: Calories 104.3 Total Fat 5.1 g Saturated Fat 1.5 g g cholesterol 17.9 2 mg Total Carbs 11.2 g Dietary Fiber 1.0 g Sugar 0.8 g Protein 4.7 g

677)   *Sesame Balsamic Asparagus*

Ingredients:

- (4 Servings)
- 1 ½ lb asparagus, trimmed
- 4 tbsp balsamic vinegar
- 4 tbsp olive oil
- 2 tbsp fresh rosemary, chopped
- Salt and black pepper to taste
- 2 tbsp sesame seeds.

Direction:(Prep + Cook Time: 30 minutes)

- ✓ Preheat the air fryer to 360 F.
- ✓ Whisk the olive oil, sesame seeds, balsamic vinegar, salt, and pepper to make a marinade.
- ✓ Place the asparagus on a baking dish and pour the marinade all over.
- ✓ Toss to coat and let them sit for 10 minutes.
- ✓ Transfer the asparagus to the frying basket and AirFry for 10-12 minutes, shaking once, or until tender and lightly charred.
- ✓ Serve the asparagus topped with rosemary.

Nutrition: Calories 107.25 Kcal (449 kJ) Calories from Fat 59.5 Kcal Total Fat 6.61g g 2 mg Total Carbs 9.52g Sugar 3.82g Dietary Fiber 4.4g Protein 4.7g

678)   *Cheesy Eggplant Schnitzels*

Ingredients:

- (4 Servings)
- 2 eggplants
- ½ cup mozzarella cheese, grated
- 2 tbsp milk
- 1 egg, beaten
- 2 cups breadcrumbs
- 2 tomatoes, sliced.

Direction:(Prep + Cook Time: 15 minutes)

- ✓ Preheat the air fryer to 400 F.
- ✓ Cut the eggplants lengthways into ½-inch thick slices. In a bowl, mix the egg and milk.
- ✓ In another bowl, combine the breadcrumbs and mozzarella cheese.
- ✓ Dip the eggplant slices in the egg mixture, followed by the crumbs mixture and place them in the greased frying basket.
- ✓ AirFry for 10-12 minutes, turning once halfway through.
- ✓ Top with tomato slices and serve.

Nutrition: Calories 445.49 Kcal (1865 kJ) Calories from Fat 191.05 Kcal Total Fat 21.23g cholesterol 13.61 mg 11 mg 93 mg Total Carbs 37.79g Sugar 12.78g Dietary Fiber 8.79g Protein 27.96g g g

679)   *Involtini di Melanzane (Eggplant Rollups)*

Ingredients:

- (4 Servings)
- 2 eggplants, thinly sliced
- 1 tsp Italian seasoning
- 1 cup wheat flour
- 1 cup ricotta cheese, crumbled
- Salt to taste
- 2 tbsp Parmesan cheese, grated.

Direction:(Prep + Cook Time: 30 minutes)

- ✓ Preheat the air fryer to 390 F.
- ✓ Season the eggplant slices with salt and dust them in the flour, shaking off the excess.
- ✓ Place them in the greased frying basket and AirFry for 5-6 minutes, turning once.
- ✓ Remove to a kitchen paper to remove any excess moisture.
- ✓ Then spread them with the ricotta cheese.Sprinkle with Italian seasoning and roll them up.
- ✓ Coat in the Parmesan cheese and transfer the rolls to the greased frying basket.
- ✓ Bake for 10-12 minutes or until the cheese is lightly browned.
- ✓ Serve warm.

Nutrition: Calories: 591 Total Fat : 42gSaturated Fat : 10g Trans Fat : 0gUnsaturated Fat : 29g cholesterol: 153 mg g Carbs : 39g Fiber : 7g Sugar : 11g Protein : 20g

680)   *Gourd Galette*

Ingredients:

- 2 tbsp. garam masala
- 2 cups sliced gourd
- 1 ½ cup coarsely crushed peanuts
- 3 tsp. ginger finely chopped
- 1-2 tbsp. fresh coriander leaves
- 2 or 3 green chilies finely chopped
- 1 ½ tbsp. lemon juice
- Salt and pepper to taste

Direction: (Prep + Cook Time: 30 minutes)

- ✓ Blend the ingredients in a bowl.
- ✓ Form this blend into round and level galettes.
- ✓ Wet the galettes somewhat with Water . Coat each galette with crushed peanuts.
- ✓ Preheat the Air Fryer to 160 and cook for 25 minutes. Continue turning them over to cook uniformly.
- ✓ Serve either with mint chutney or ketchup.

Nutrition: Calories 342.6 Total Fat 21.1 g Saturated Fat 6.6 g g cholesterol 54.1 3 mg Total Carbs 27.8 g Dietary Fiber 4.7 g Sugar 1.1 g Protein 13.9 g

681)   *Cottage Cheese Club Sandwich*

Ingredients:

- 22 slices of white bread
- 1 tbsp. softened butter
- 1 cup sliced cottage cheese
- 1 small capsicum
- For Barbeque Sauce:
- ¼ tbsp. Worcestershire sauce
- ½ tsp. olive oil

- ½ flake garlic crushed
- ¼ cup chopped onion
- ¼ tbsp. red chili sauce

Direction: (Prep + Cook Time: 30 minutes)
- ✓ Cook the sauce ingredients and until it thickens.
- ✓ Cook the capsicum and strip the skin off. Cut the capsicum into strips.
- ✓ Add the cheese to the sauce and mix.
- ✓ Preheat the Air Fryer for 5 minutes at 300 F and cook for 15 minutes.
- ✓ Serve the sandwiches with tomato ketchup or mint chutney

Nutrition: Calories 264.0 Total Fat 5.1 g Saturated Fat 0.2 g g cholesterol 0.0 6 mg Total Carbs 29.5 g Dietary Fiber 2.0 g Sugar 1.6 g Protein 24.7 g %

682) *Pineapple Kebab*

Ingredients:
- 2 cups cubed pineapples
- 3 onions chopped
- 5 green chilies-roughly chopped
- 1 ½ tbsp. ginger paste
- 1 ½ tsp. garlic paste
- 3 eggs
- 1 ½ tsp. salt
- 3 tsp. lemon juice
- 2 tsp. garam masala
- 4 tbsp. chopped coriander
- 3 tbsp. cream
- 3 tbsp. chopped capsicum
- 2 ½ tbsp. white sesame seeds

Direction: (Prep + Cook Time: 30 minutes)
- ✓ Pound the ingredients except for the pineapple and egg to create a smooth paste.
- ✓ Coat the pineapples in the paste.
- ✓ Beat the eggs and add salt.
- ✓ Dip the pineapples in the egg blend and then coat with sesame seeds. Place on skewers.
- ✓ Preheat the Air Fryer to 160 F and cook for 25 minutes.
- ✓ Turn the sticks over in the middle of the cooking procedure to cook uniformly

Nutrition: Calories 175.9 Total Fat 4.3 g Saturated Fat 0.6 g g cholesterol 11.2 mg Total Carbs 28.7 g Dietary Fiber 1.3 g Sugar 24.3 g Protein 8.5 g % Copper 7.0 Manganese 64.1 % Niacin 18.9 % Pantothenic Acid 4.0

683) *Broccoli Tikka*

Ingredients:
- 2 cups broccoli florets
- 3 onions chopped
- 5 green chilies-roughly chopped
- 1 ½ tbsp. ginger paste
- 1 ½ tsp. garlic paste
- 1 ½ tsp. salt

- 3 tsp. lemon juice
- 2 tsp. garam masala
- 3 eggs
- 2 ½ tbsp. white sesame seeds

Direction: (Prep + Cook Time: 20 minutes)
- ✓ Crush the ingredients aside from the broccoli and egg and make a smooth paste.
- ✓ Coat the broccoli in the paste. Beat the eggs and add salt.
- ✓ Preheat the Air Fryer to 160 F and cook for 25 minutes.
- ✓ Dip the broccoli in the egg blend and then coat with sesame seeds. Place on skewers.
- ✓ Turn the sticks over in the middle of the cooking procedure to cook uniformly

Nutrition: Calories 210 Kcal (879 kJ) Calories from Fat 9 Kcal Total Fat 1g Total Carbs 41g Sugar 1g Dietary Fiber 6g Protein 9g g

684) *Cabbage Fritters*

Ingredients:
- 10 leaves cabbage
- 3 onions chopped
- 5 green chilies-roughly chopped
- 1 ½ tbsp. ginger paste
- 3 eggs
- 1 ½ tsp. garlic paste
- 1 ½ tsp. salt
- 3 tsp. lemon juice
- 2 tsp. garam masala
- 2 ½ tbsp. white sesame seeds

Direction: (Prep + Cook Time: 30 minutes)
- ✓ Crush the ingredients aside from the cabbage and egg and make a smooth paste.
- ✓ Coat the cabbage in the paste. Beat the eggs and add salt.
- ✓ Preheat the Air Fryer to 160 F and cook for 25 minutes.
- ✓ Dip the cabbage in the egg blend and then coat with sesame seeds. Place on skewers.
- ✓ Turn the sticks over in the middle of the cooking procedure to cook uniformly

Nutrition: Calories 177.8 Total Fat 9.6 g Saturated Fat 1.3 g g cholesterol 0.0 mg Total Carbs 20.6 g Dietary Fiber 5.2 g Sugar 7.5 g Protein 5.0 g %

685) *Cottage Cheese Gnocchi*

Ingredients:
- For dough:
- 1 ½ cup all-purpose flour
- ½ tsp. salt
- 5 tbsp. Water
- For filling:
- 2 cups grated cottage cheese
- 2 tbsp. oil

- 2 tsp. ginger-garlic paste
- 2 tsp. soy sauce
- 2 tsp. vinegar

Direction: (Prep + Cook Time: 30 minutes)

✓ Make the dough, spread it with saran wrap and set aside.

✓ Combine the filling ingredients.

✓ Roll the dough and place the filling in the middle.

✓ Presently, wrap the dough to cover the filling and squeeze the edges together.

✓ Preheat the Air Fryer to 200° F and cook for 20 minutes.

Nutrition: Energy524 kj125 kcal Protein 6.52g Carbs 6.01g Sugar 0.2g Fat 8.28g Saturated Fat 3.13g g cholesterol49 mg Fiber 0.1g

686) Cauliflower Gnocchi

Ingredients:

- For dough:
- 1 ½ cup all-purpose flour
- ½ tsp. salt
- 5 tbsp. Water
- For filling:
- 2 cups grated cauliflower
- 2 tbsp. oil
- 2 tsp. ginger-garlic paste
- 2 tsp. soy sauce
- 2 tsp. vinegar

Direction: (Prep + Cook Time: 20 minutes)

✓ 1.Make the dough, spread it with saran wrap and set aside.

✓ 2.Combine the filling ingredients.

✓ 3.Roll the dough and place the filling in the middle.

✓ Presently, wrap the dough to cover the filling and squeeze the edges together.

✓ Preheat the Air Fryer to 200° F and cook for 20 minutes.

Nutrition: Total Fat 3.0 g 4 % Saturated Fat 0.5 g 3 % Trans Fat 0 g cholesterol 0 mg 0 % g 20 % Total Carbs 22 g 8 % Dietary Fiber 6 g 21 % Protein 2 g

687) Air Fryer Roasted Broccoli and Cauliflower

Ingredients:

- 3 cups broccoli florets
- 3 cups cauliflower florets
- 2 tsp olive oil
- ¼ tsp sea salt
- ¼ tsp paprika
- ½ tsp garlic powder
- ⅛ tsp black pepper

Direction: (Prep + Cook Time: 20 minutes)

✓ Put broccoli florets in a large microwave-safe bowl. Cook on high for 3 minutes.

✓ Place in the air fryer basket. Cook for 12 minutes.

✓ Preheat an air fryer to 400 F.

✓ Add cauliflower, olive oil, garlic powder, ocean salt, paprika, and pepper to the bowl with the broccoli.

Nutrition: Calories: 68.4 Protein : 2.3g5 % Carbs : 5.8g Dietary Fiber : 2.5g Sugar 2g Fat : 4.7g7 % Saturated Fat : 0.6g Calories From Fat : 42.6

688) Broccoli Momos

Ingredients:

- For dough:
- 1 ½ cup all-purpose flour
- ½ tsp. salt
- 5 tbsp. Water
- 2 tsp. vinegar
- For filling:
- 2 cups grated broccoli
- 2 tbsp. oil
- 2 tsp. ginger-garlic paste
- 2 tsp. soy sauce

Direction: (Prep + Cook Time: 30 minutes)

✓ Make the dough, spread it with saran wrap and set aside.

✓ Combine the filling ingredients.

✓ Roll the dough and place the filling in the middle.

✓ Presently, wrap the dough to cover the filling and squeeze the edges together.

✓ Preheat the Air Fryer to 200° F and cook for 20 minutes.

Nutrition: Calories 326.0 Total Fat 7.4 g Saturated Fat 1.0 g g cholesterol 7.3 9 mg Total Carbs 55.2 g Dietary Fiber 5.2 g Sugar 0.6 g Protein 10.3 g % Copper 8.5 % 3 % Manganese 39.5 % Niacin 24.3 %

689) Cauliflower Momos

Ingredients:

- For dough:
- 1 ½ cup all-purpose flour
- ½ tsp. salt
- 5 tbsp. Water
- For filling:
- 2 cups grated cauliflower
- 2 tbsp. oil
- 2 tsp. ginger-garlic paste
- 2 tsp. soy sauce
- 2 tsp. vinegar

Direction: (Prep + Cook Time: 30 minutes)

✓ Make the dough, spread it with saran wrap and set aside.

✓ Combine the filling ingredients.

✓ Roll the dough and place the filling in the middle.

✓ Presently, wrap the dough to cover the filling and squeeze the edges together.

✓ Preheat the Air Fryer to 200° F and cook for 20 minutes.

Nutrition: Total Fat 5.5g7 % Total Carbs 10g Fiber 0g Total Sugar 1g Sugar Protein 5g10 %

690) *Aloo Patties*

Ingredients:

- 1 cup mashed potato
- A pinch of salt to taste
- ¼ tsp. ginger finely chopped
- 1 green chili finely chopped
- 1 tsp. lemon juice
- 1 tbsp. fresh coriander leaves
- ¼ tsp. red chili powder
- ¼ tsp. cumin powder

Direction: (Prep + Cook Time: 20 minutes)

✓ Preheat the Air Fryer to 250 F and cook for 10 or 12 minutes, flipping halfway through.
✓ Serve warm with mint chutney.
✓ Combine the ingredients and make round patties.

Nutrition: Calories 105 6 % Total Fat 3.9gs7 % Saturated Fat 1.4gs Trans Fat 0gs ams grams7 % cholesterol 22 mg 10 % mg 9 % 5 % Total Carbs 14gs5 % Dietary Fiber 1.3gs Sugar 0.9gs Protein 4gs 2.4 ed

691) *Vegetable Patties*

Ingredients:

- 1 cup grated mixed vegetables
- A pinch of salt to taste
- ¼ tsp. ginger finely chopped
- 1 green chili finely chopped
- 1 tsp. lemon juice
- 1 tbsp. fresh coriander leaves
- ¼ tsp. red chili powder
- ¼ tsp. cumin powder

Direction: (Prep + Cook Time: 30 minutes)

✓ Preheat the Air Fryer to 250 F and cook for 10 or 12 minutes, flipping halfway through.
✓ Serve warm with mint chutney.
✓ Combine the ingredients and make round patties.

Nutrition: Total Fat 9g12 % Saturated Fat 1g5 % Trans Fat 0g unsaturated Fat 0g cholesterol 0 mg 29 % Total Carbs 28g10 % Dietary Fiber 4g14 % Total Sugar 0g Sugar Alcohols 0g Protein 20g

692) *Cottage Cheese Momos*

Ingredients:

- For dough:
- 1 ½ cup all-purpose flour
- ½ tsp. salt
- 5 tbsp. Water
- For filling:
- 2 cups crumbled cottage cheese
- 2 tsp. oil
- 2 tsp. ginger-garlic paste
- 2 tsp. soy sauce
- 2 tsp. vinegar

Direction: (Prep + Cook Time: 30 minutes)

✓ Make the dough, spread it with saran wrap and set aside.

✓ Combine the filling ingredients.
✓ Roll the dough and place the filling in the middle.
✓ Wrap the dough to cover the filling and squeeze the edges together.
✓ Preheat the Air Fryer to 200° F and cook for 20 minutes.

Nutrition: Calories 303Calories from Fat 99 Fat 11g17 % Saturated Fat 7g44 % cholesterol 33 mg Carbs 37g12 % Fiber 1g4 % Protein 11g

693) *Mushroom Galette*

Ingredients:

- 2 tbsp. garam masala
- 2 cups sliced mushrooms
- 1 ½ cup coarsely crushed peanuts
- 3 tsp. ginger finely chopped
- 1-2 tbsp. fresh coriander leaves
- 2 or 3 green chilies finely chopped
- 1 ½ tbsp. lemon juice
- Salt and pepper to taste

Direction: (Prep + Cook Time: 20 minutes)

✓ Blend the ingredients in a bowl.
✓ Form this blend into round and level galettes.
✓ Wet the galettes somewhat with Water . Coat each galette with crushed peanuts.
✓ Preheat the Air Fryer to 160 and cook for 25 minutes.
✓ Continue turning them over to cook uniformly.
✓ Serve either with mint chutney or ketchup.

Nutrition: Calories 260.4 Total Fat 11.4 g Saturated Fat 2.0 g g cholesterol 70.3 mg mg 5 mg Total Carbs 31.2 g D ietary Fiber 2.4 g Sugar 3.0 g Protein 10.4 g % Copper

694) *Zucchini Samosa*

Ingredients:

- 2 tbsp. unsalted butter
- 1 ½ cup all-purpose flour
- A pinch of salt
- Water

For filling:

- 3 medium zucchinis
- ¼ cup boiled peas
- 1 tsp. powdered ginger
- 1 or 2 green chilies
- ½ tsp. cumin
- 1 tsp. coarsely crushed coriander
- 1 dry red chili
- A small amount of salt
- ½ tsp. dried mango powder
- ½ tsp. red chili powder.
- 1-2 tbsp. coriander.

Direction: (Prep + cook Time: 30 minutes)

✓ Create the dough with the first 4 ingredients. Set aside.

✓ Cook the filling ingredients in skillet and blend them well to make a thick paste.

✓ Form the paste into balls. Cut them in half and insert the filling.

✓ Preheat the Air Fryer to 300 F. Place the samosas in the fry receptacle.

✓ Cook for 20 to 25 minutes. Around the midpoint, turn the samosas over for uniform cooking.

✓ Serve hot with tamarind or mint chutney.

Nutrition: Calories: 62 Protein : 2 grams Fat : Less than 1 gram Carbs : 14 grams Fiber : 8 grams Sugar : 7 grams

695) *Vegetable Skewer*

Ingredients:

- 2 cups mixed vegetables
- 3 onions chopped
- 5 green chilies
- 1 ½ tbsp. ginger paste
- 1 ½ tsp. garlic paste
- 1 ½ tsp. salt
- 3 tbsp. cream
- 3 eggs
- 2 ½ tbsp. white sesame seeds

Direction: (Prep + Cook Time: 30 minutes)

✓ 1.Crush the ingredients aside from the mixed vegetables and egg and make a smooth paste.

✓ Dip the cabbage in the egg blend and then coat with sesame seeds. Place on skewers.

✓ Coat with the paste. Beat the eggs and add salt.

✓ Preheat the Air Fryer to 160 F and cook for 25 minutes.

✓ Turn the sticks over in the middle of the cooking procedure to cook uniformly

Nutrition: Calories 495 54 % Total Fat 35gs46 % Saturated Fat 9.2gs Trans Fat 0.4gs23 % cholesterol 69 mg Total Carbs 37gs8 % Dietary Fiber 2gs Sugar 11gs Protein 7.7gs 7 % vtamin C 4 %

696) *Jack Gram Galette*

Ingredients:

- 2 cup black gram
- 2 medium potatoes boiled and mashed
- 1 ½ cup coarsely crushed peanuts
- 3 tsp. ginger finely chopped
- 1-2 tbsp. fresh coriander leaves
- 2 or 3 green chilies finely chopped
- 1 ½ tbsp. lemon juice
- Salt and pepper to taste

Direction: (Prep + Cook Time: 20 minutes)

✓ Blend the ingredients in a bowl.

✓ Form this blend into round and level galettes.

✓ Wet the galettes somewhat with Water . Coat each galette with crushed peanuts.

✓ Preheat the Air Fryer to 160 and cook for 25 minutes. Continue turning them over to cook uniformly.

✓ Serve either with mint chutney or ketchup.

Nutrition:Calories 31128 % Total Fat 18gs21 % Saturated Fat 4.2gs Trans Fat 0.1gs6 % cholesterol 19 mg Total Carbs 24gs10 % Dietary Fiber 2.5gs Sugar 3.4gs Protein 13gs 3 % vvtamin C 10 %

697) *Mushroom Pasta*

Ingredients:

- 1 cup pasta, cooked
- 1 ½ tbsp. olive oil
- A pinch of salt
- For tossing pasta:
- 1 ½ tbsp. olive oil
- Salt and pepper to taste
- ½ tsp. oregano
- ½ tsp. dried basil
- ½ tsp. dried parsley
- ½ tsp. basil
- For sauce:
- 2 tbsp. olive oil
- 2 cups sliced mushroom
- 2 tbsp. all-purpose flour
- 2 cups of milk
- 1 tsp. dried oregano
- Salt and pepper to taste

Direction: (Prep + Cook Time: 30 minutes)

✓ For the sauce, add the ingredients to a container and boil.

✓ Mix the sauce and keep on stewing to thicken it.

✓ Add the pasta to the sauce and move this into a glass bowl embellished with cheese.

✓ Preheat the Air Fryer to 160 C and cook for 10 minutes.

Nutrition: Calories 225.8 Total Fat 3.0 g Saturated Fat 0.3 g g cholesterol 0.0 5 mg Total Carbs 47.8 g Dietary Fiber 3.1 g Sugar 1.6 g Protein 6.3 g % Copper 12.5 Manganese 12.4 % Niacin 8.2 % Pantothenic Acid 5.8

698) *Mushroom Samosa*

Ingredients:

- 1 cup all-purpose flour
- 2 tbsp. unsalted butter
- A pinch of salt
- For filling:
- 3 cups whole mushrooms
- 2 onions sliced
- 2 capsicum sliced
- 2 carrots sliced
- 2 cabbage sliced
- 2 tbsp. soy sauce
- 2 tsp. vinegar
- 2 tbsp. green chilies finely chopped
- 2 tbsp. ginger-garlic paste

- Some salt and pepper to taste

Direction: (Prep + Cook Time: 30 minutes)

✓ Create the dough with the first 4 ingredients. Set aside.

✓ Cook the filling ingredients in skillet and blend them well to make a thick paste.

✓ Form the paste into balls. Cut them in half and insert the filling.

✓ chutney

✓ Preheat the Air Fryer to 300 F. Place the samosas in the fry receptacle.

✓ Cook for 20 to 25 minutes. Around the midpoint, turn the samosas over for uniform cooking.

✓ Serve hot with tamarind or mint

Nutrition: Calories 495 54 % Total Fat 35gs46 % Saturated Fat 9.2gs Trans Fat 0.4gs23 % cholesterol 69 mg Total Carbs 37gs8 % Dietary Fiber 2gs Sugar 11gs Protein 7.7gs 7 %

699) *Cottage Cheese and Mushroom Burritos*

Ingredients:

- Refried beans:
- ½ cup red kidney beans
- ½ small onion chopped
- 1 tbsp. olive oil
- 2 tbsp. tomato puree
- ¼ tsp. red chili powder
- 1 tsp. of salt to taste
- 4-5 flour tortillas

Vegetable Filling:

- ½ cup mushrooms thinly sliced
- 1 cup cottage cheese
- 1 cup boiled rice
- A pinch of salt to taste
- ½ tsp. red chili flakes
- 1 tsp. freshly ground peppercorns
- ½ cup pickled Jalapeño s
- Salad:
- 1-2 lettuce leaves shredded.
- 1 or 2 spring onions
- Take one tomato.
- 1 green chili chopped.
- 1 cup of Cheddar grated.
- To serve:
- A few flour tortillas

Direction: (Prep + Cook Time: 30 minutes)

✓ Cook the beans with the onion and garlic and mash them.

✓ For the filling, sauté the ingredients in a pan.

✓ Toss the salad ingredients together.

✓ Wrap the tortilla to create a burrito.

✓ Lay the tortilla on a flat surface and place a layer of sauce and filling inside.

✓ Preheat the Air Fryer to 200 F. Open the fry case and place the burritos inside.

✓ Cook for 15 minutes. Flip the burritos halfway through.

Nutrition: Calories 224.4 Total Fat 15.8 g Saturated Fat 5.7 g g cholesterol 29.8 7 mg Total Carbs 13.2 g Dietary Fiber 1.9 g Sugar 1.4 g Protein 8.4 g % Copper 5.2

700) *French Bean Toast*

Ingredients:

- Bread slices (brown or white)
- 1 egg white for every 2 slices
- 1 tsp. Sugar for every 2 slices
- Crushed cornflakes
- 2 cups baked beans

Direction: (Prep + Cook Time: 20 minutes)

✓ In a bowl, whisk the egg whites and Sugar .

✓ Preheat the Air Fryer to 180° C and cook for 20 minutes. Top with prepared beans and serve.

✓ Plunge the bread triangles into this blend and then cover them with crushed cornflakes.

Nutrition: Calories 364.6 Total Fat 5.2 g Saturated Fat 0.6 g g cholesterol 0.0 7 mg Total Carbs 68.7 g Dietary Fiber 11.7 g Sugar 5.0 g Protein 13.5 g %

701) *Mushroom Pops*

Ingredients:

- 1 cup whole mushrooms
- 1 ½ tsp. garlic paste
- Salt and pepper to taste
- 1 tsp. dry oregano
- 1 tsp. dry basil
- 1 tsp. lemon juice
- 1 tsp. red chili flakes

Direction: (Prep + Cook Time: 20 minutes)

✓ Mix the ingredients except mushrooms in a bowl.

✓ Dunk the mushrooms in the above blend and set them aside.

✓ Preheat the Air Fryer to 180° C and cook for 20 minutes.

Nutrition: Calories 90 Total Fat 7g cholesterol 0 mg Total Carbs 7g Sugar 4g Protein 1g

702) *Potato Pancakes*

Ingredients:

- 2 tbsp. garam masala
- 2 cups sliced potato
- 3 tsp. ginger finely chopped
- 1-2 tbsp. fresh coriander leaves
- 2 or 3 green chilies finely chopped
- 1 ½ tbsp. lemon juice
- Salt and pepper to taste

Direction: (Prep + Cook Time: 30 minutes)

✓ Blend the ingredients in a bowl and add Water to it.

✓ Preheat the Air Fryer to 160 F and cook for 25 minutes.

✓ Continue turning them over to cook uniformly.

✓ Serve either with mint chutney or ketchup.

Nutrition: Calories 349.0 Total Fat 18.1 g Saturated Fat 2.1 g g cholesterol 170.0 mg mg 4 mg Total Carbs 35.4 g Dietary Fiber 5.5 g Sugar 3.8 g Protein 9.8 g %

703) *Cottage Cheese Pancakes*

Ingredients:

- 2 tbsp. garam masala
- 2 cups sliced cottage cheese
- 3 tsp. ginger finely chopped
- 1-2 tbsp. fresh coriander leaves
- 2 or 3 green chilies finely chopped
- 1 ½ tbsp. lemon juice
- Salt and pepper to taste

Direction: (Prep + Cook Time: 30 minutes)

✓ Blend the ingredients in a bowl and add Water to it.

✓ Preheat the Air Fryer to 160 F and cook for 25 minutes.

✓ Continue turning them over to cook uniformly.

✓ Serve either with mint chutney or ketchup.

Nutrition: Calories 100.8 Total Fat 2.9 g Saturated Fat 1.1 g g cholesterol 95.8 mg Total Carbs 7.5 g Dietary Fiber 0.2 g Sugar 0.0 g Protein 10.5 g % Copper 1.5

704) *Fenugreek Galette*

Ingredients:

- 2 cups fenugreek
- 2 medium potatoes, boiled and mashed
- 3 tsp. ginger finely chopped
- Salt and pepper to taste
- 1-2 tbsp. fresh coriander leaves
- 2 or 3 green chilies finely chopped
- 1 ½ tbsp. lemon juice

Direction: (Prep + Cook Time: 20 minutes)

✓ Blend the ingredients in a bowl.

✓ Form this blend into round and level galettes.

✓ Wet the galettes somewhat with Water .

✓ Preheat the Air Fryer to 160 F and cook for 25 minutes.

✓ Continue turning them over to cook uniformly.

✓ Serve either with mint chutney or ketchup.

Nutrition: Calories: 12 Protein : 0.85g Total Fat : 0.24g Carbs : 2.16gTotal Dietary Fiber : 0.9g cholesterol: 0 mg

705) *Potato Wedges*

Ingredients:

- 2 medium sized potatoes
- For the marinade:
- 1 tbsp. olive oil
- 1 tsp. mixed herbs
- ½ tsp. red chili flakes

- A pinch of salt to taste
- 1 tbsp. lemon juice

Direction: (Prep + Cook Time: 20 minutes)

✓ Cut the potatoes into wedges.

✓ Preheat the Air Fryer to 300 F and cook for 20 or 25 minutes. Toss the fries 2-3 times.

✓ Blend marinade ingredients and pour over potato fingers, ensuring that they are covered well.

Nutrition: Calories 275 20 % Total Fat 13gs11 % Saturated Fat 2.1gs Trans Fat 0.1g Total Carbs 36gs13 % Dietary Fiber 3.3gs Sugar 0.3gs Protein 3gs

706) *Potato Kebab*

Ingredients:

- 2 cups sliced potato
- 1 1/2 tsp. of ginger-garlic paste
- 1-2 green chilies, chopped finely
- ¼ tsp. red chili powder
- A pinch of salt
- ½ tsp. cumin powder
- 1 onion, finely chopped
- ½ cup milk
- 2 tsp. coriander powder
- 1 ½ tbsp. chopped fresh coriander
- ½ tsp. dried mango powder
- 1 cup dry breadcrumbs
- ¼ tsp. black salt
- 1-2 tbsp. flour
- 1-2 tbsp. mint, finely chopped)

Direction: (Prep + Cook Time: 30 minutes)

✓ Mix the potato slices with the ground ginger and cut green chilies.

✓ Pound this blend until it turns into a thick paste. Add Water if required.

✓ Add the onions, mint, breadcrumbs and spices. Blend this well until you get a soft mixture.

✓ Roll the kebab in the dry breadcrumbs.

✓ Form round kebabs with the dough.

✓ Pour a small amount of milk onto each kebab to wet it.

✓ Preheat the Air Fryer for 5 minutes at 300 F and cook for 30 minutes.

✓ Recommended sides for this dish are mint chutney, tomato ketchup or yogurt chutney.

Nutrition: Calories 189.5 Total Fat 3.9 g Saturated Fat 1.4 g g cholesterol 28.0 6 mg Total Carbs 32.1 g Dietary Fiber 5.3 g Sugar 3.4 g Protein 10.0 g %

707) *Cabbage Pancakes*

Ingredients:

- 2 tbsp. garam masala
- 2 cups halved cabbage leaves
- 3 tsp. ginger finely chopped
- 1-2 tbsp. fresh coriander leaves
- 2 or 3 green chilies finely chopped

- 1 ½ tbsp. lemon juice
- Salt and pepper to taste

Direction: (Prep + Cook Time: 20 minutes)

✓ Blend the ingredients in a bowl and add Water to it.

✓ Preheat the Air Fryer to 160 F and cook for 25 minutes.

✓ Continue turning them over to cook uniformly.

✓ Serve either with mint chutney or ketchup.

Nutrition: Calories 159.7 Total Fat 5.7 g Saturated Fat 1.6 g cholesterol 212.5 3 mg Total Carbs 18.9 g Dietary Fiber 5.4 g Sugar 0.0 g Protein 10.3 g %

708) *Bitter Gourd Pancakes*

Ingredients:

- 2 tbsp. garam masala
- 2 cups sliced bitter gourd
- 3 tsp. ginger finely chopped
- 1-2 tbsp. fresh coriander leaves
- 2 or 3 green chilies finely chopped
- 1 ½ tbsp. lemon juice
- Salt and pepper to taste

Direction: (Prep + Cook Time: 20 minutes)

✓ Blend the ingredients in a bowl and add Water to it.

✓ Preheat the Air Fryer to 160 F and cook for 25 minutes.

✓ Continue turning them over to cook uniformly.

✓ Serve either with mint chutney or ketchup.

Nutrition: Calories 110.0 Total Fat 4.8 g Saturated Fat 0.7 g g cholesterol 46.8 mg mg 7 mg Total Carbs 13.5 g Dietary Fiber 1.0 g Sugar 0.5 g Protein 3.2 g %

709) *Pumpkin Galette*

Ingredients:

- 2 tbsp. garam masala
- 1 cup sliced pumpkin
- 3 tsp. ginger finely chopped
- 1-2 tbsp. fresh coriander leaves
- 2 or 3 green chilies finely chopped
- 1 ½ tbsp. lemon juice
- Salt and pepper to taste

Direction: (Prep + Cook Time: 30 minutes)

✓ Blend the ingredients in a bowl.

✓ Form this blend into round, flat galettes.

✓ Wet the galettes with a small amount of Water . Coat each galette with crushed peanuts.

✓ Serve with mint chutney or ketchup.

✓ Preheat the Air Fryer to 160 F for 5 minutes.

✓ Place the galettes in the fry bin and let them cook for an additional 25 minutes.

✓ Continue turning them over to cook uniformly.

Nutrition: Calories 342.6 Total Fat 21.1 g Saturated Fat 6.6 g g cholesterol 54.1 3 mg Total Carbs 27.8 g Dietary Fiber 4.7 g Sugar 1.1 g Protein 13.9 g %

710) *Masala Potato Wedges*

Ingredients:

- 2 medium sized potatoes (Cut into wedges)
- For the marinade:
- 1 tbsp. olive oil
- 1 tbsp. lemon juice
- 1 tsp. garam masala
- 1 tsp. mixed herbs
- ½ tsp. red chili flakes
- A pinch of salt to taste

Direction: (Prep + Cook Time: 30 minutes)

✓ Cut the potatoes into wedges.

✓ Preheat the Air Fryer to 300 F and cook for 20 or 25 minutes. Toss the fries 2-3 times.

✓ Blend marinade ingredients and pour over potato fingers, ensuring that they are covered well.

Nutrition: Cal 275 20 % Total Fat 13g cholesterol 0 mg Total Carbs 36gs13 % Fiber 3.3gs Sugar 0.3gs Protein 3gs

711) *Cheesy Potato Wedges*

Ingredients:

- 2 medium sized potatoes (Cut into wedges)
- for the marinade:
- 1 tbsp. olive oil
- 1 tsp. mixed herbs
- ½ tsp. red chili flakes
- A pinch of salt to taste
- 1 tbsp. lemon juice
- 1 cup molten cheese

Direction: (Prep + Cook Time: 30 minutes)

✓ Cut the potatoes into wedges.

✓ Preheat the Air Fryer to 300 F and cook for 20 or 25 minutes.

✓ Toss the fries 2-3 times.

✓ Blend marinade ingredients and pour over potato fingers, ensuring that they are covered well.

Nutrition: Calories 240 kCal Total Carbs 36.5 g Net Carbs 30 g Fiber 6.5 g Sugar 9.5 g Protein 9.1 g Fat 7.8 g Saturated Fat 3.7 g

712) *Asparagus Pancakes*

Ingredients:

- 2 tbsp. garam masala
- 2 cups sliced asparagus
- 3 tsp. ginger finely chopped
- 1-2 tbsp. fresh coriander leaves
- 2 or 3 green chilies finely chopped
- 1 ½ tbsp. lemon juice
- Salt and pepper to taste

Direction: (Prep + Cook Time: 20 minutes)

✓ Blend the ingredients in a bowl and add Water to it.

✓ Preheat the Air Fryer to 160 F and cook for 25 minutes.

✓ Continue turning them over to cook uniformly.

✓ Serve either with mint chutney or ketchup.

Nutrition: Calories 309 Kcal (1294 kJ) Calories from Fat 171 Kcal Total Fat 19g 29 % Saturated Fat 10g 50 % cholesterol 168 mg 56 % 33 % Total Carbs 18g 6 % Dietary Fiber 1g 4 % Protein 15g 30 %

713)   *Mushroom Wonton*
Ingredients:
- For dough:
- 1 ½ cup all-purpose flour
- ½ tsp. salt or to taste
- 5 tbsp. Water

For filling:
- 2 cups cubed mushroom
- 2 tbsp. oil
- 2 tsp. ginger-garlic paste
- 2 tsp. soy sauce
- 2 tsp. vinegar

Direction: (Prep + Cook Time: 30 minutes)
- ✓ Mix the dough ingredients, cover with cling wrap and set aside.
- ✓ Cook the filling ingredients.
- ✓ Roll the dough and place the filling in the middle.
- ✓ Wrap the dough to cover the filling and squeeze the edges together.
- ✓ Preheat the Air Fryer to 200° F and cook for 20 minutes.

Nutrition: Calories 69.1 Total Fat 1.8 g Saturated Fat 0.3 g g cholesterol 1.5 mg Total Carbs 11.2 g Dietary Fiber 0.7 g Sugar 0.4 Protein 2.0 g % Copper 2.6

714)   *Mushroom Patties*
Ingredients:
- 1 cup minced mushroom
- A pinch of salt to taste
- ¼ tsp. ginger finely chopped
- 1 green chili finely chopped
- 1 tsp. lemon juice
- 1 tbsp. fresh coriander leaves
- ¼ tsp. red chili powder
- ¼ tsp. cumin powder

Direction: (Prep + Cook Time: 20 minutes)
- ✓ Combine the ingredients. Make round patties.
- ✓ Serve warm with mint chutney.
- ✓ Preheat the Air Fryer to 250 F and cook for 10 or 12 minutes, flipping halfway through.

Nutrition: Calories 25823 % Total Fat 15gs17 % Saturated Fat 3.4gs Trans Fat 0.1gs ams grams23 % cholesterol 69 mg 28 % mg 14 % 8 % Total Carbs 23gs12 % Dietary Fiber 3gs Sugar 3.7gs Protein 11gs

715)   *Cheese and Mushroom Kebab*
Ingredients:
- 2 cups sliced mushrooms
- 1-2 green chilies chopped finely
- ¼ tsp. red chili powder
- A pinch of salt to taste

- ½ cup milk
- 1-2 tbsp. mint
- ½ tsp. dried mango powder
- ¼ tsp. black salt
- 1-2 tbsp. all-purpose flour for coating purposes
- 1 cup molten cheese
- 1 onion that has been finely chopped

Direction: (Prep + Cook Time: 20 minutes)
- ✓ Mix the mushroom slices with the ground ginger and cut green chilies.
- ✓ Pound this blend until it turns into a thick paste.
- ✓ Add Water if required. Add the onions, mint, breadcrumbs and spices.
- ✓ Blend this well until you get a soft mixture.
- ✓ Form round kebabs with the dough.
- ✓ Pour a small amount of milk onto each kebab to wet it.
- ✓ Roll the kebab in the dry breadcrumbs.
- ✓ Preheat the Air Fryer for 5 minutes at 300 F and cook for 30 minutes.
- ✓ Recommended sides for this dish are mint chutney, tomato ketchup or yogurt chutney

Nutrition: Calories 89.0 Total Fat 7.0 g Saturated Fat 1.0 g g cholesterol 0.0 8 mg Total Carbs 6.0 g Dietary Fiber 1.5 g Sugar 1.9 g Protein 1.8 g %

716)   *Mushroom Club Sandwich*
Ingredients:
- 2 slices of white bread
- 1 tbsp. softened butter
- 1 cup minced mushroom
- 1 small capsicum
- For Barbeque Sauce:
- ¼ tbsp. Worcestershire sauce
- ½ tsp. olive oil
- ½ flake garlic crushed
- ¼ cup chopped onion
- ¼ tbsp. red chili sauce
- ½ cup Water

Direction: (Prep + Cook Time: 20 minutes)
- ✓ Cook the sauce ingredients and until it thickens.
- ✓ Add the cheese to the sauce and mix.
- ✓ Cook the capsicum and strip the skin off. Cut the capsicum into strips.
- ✓ Preheat the Air Fryer for 5 minutes at 300 F and cook for 15 minutes.
- ✓ Spread on the pieces of bread and serve sandwiches with tomato ketchup or mint chutney.
- ✓ 78. Asparagus Galette

Nutrition: Calories 156.2 Total Fat 8.2 g Saturated Fat 4.3 g g cholesterol 17.8 8 mg Total Carbs 13.6 g Dietary Fiber 2.6 g Sugar 2.8 g Protein 9.5 g % Copper 26.0

717) *Asparagus Kebab*

Ingredients:

- 2 cups sliced asparagus
- 3 onions chopped
- 5 green chilies-roughly chopped
- 1 ½ tbsp. ginger paste
- 3 eggs
- 1 ½ tsp. garlic paste
- 1 ½ tsp. salt
- 3 tsp. lemon juice
- 2 tsp. garam masala
- 2 ½ tbsp. white sesame seeds

Direction: (Prep + Cook Time: 30 minutes)

- ✓ Mix the asparagus with the ground ginger and cut green chilies.
- ✓ Pound this blend until it turns into a thick paste.
- ✓ Add Water if required. Add the onions, mint, breadcrumbs and spices.
- ✓ Blend this well until you get a soft mixture.
- ✓ Form round kebabs with the dough.
- ✓ Pour a small amount of milk onto each kebab to wet it.
- ✓ Roll the kebab in the dry breadcrumbs.
- ✓ Preheat the Air Fryer for 5 minutes at 300 F and cook for 30 minutes.
- ✓ Recommended sides for this dish are mint chutney, tomato ketchup or yogurt chutney.

Nutrition: Calories: 20 Fat : 0.2g Carbs : 3.7g Fiber : 1.8g Sugar 1.2g Protein : 2.2g 5mcg

718) *Green Chili Pancakes*

Ingredients:

- 2 tbsp. garam masala
- 3 tsp. ginger finely chopped
- 1-2 tbsp. fresh coriander leaves
- 10–12 green chilies
- 2 or 3 green chilies finely chopped
- 1 ½ tbsp. lemon juice
- Salt and pepper to taste

Direction: (Prep + Cook Time: 30 minutes)

- ✓ Blend the ingredients in a bowl and add Water to it.
- ✓ Preheat the Air Fryer to 160 F and cook for 25 minutes.
- ✓ Continue turning them over to cook uniformly.
- ✓ Serve either with mint chutney or ketchup.

Nutrition: Calories 374.42 Kcal (1568 kJ) Calories from Fat 210.13 Kcal Total Fat 23.35g 36 % cholesterol 109.85 mg 37 % 53 mg 66 % 44 mg 8 % Total Carbs 19.88g 7 % Sugar 3.65g 15 % Dietary Fiber 1.18g 5 % Protein 21.68g

719) *Cottage Cheese Samosa*

Ingredients:

- 2 tbsp. unsalted butter
- 1 ½ cup all-purpose flour
- A pinch of salt to taste
- Water
- For filling:
- 2 cups mashed cottage cheese
- ¼ cup boiled peas
- A small amount of salt
- 1 tsp. powdered ginger
- 1 or 2 green chilies
- ½ tsp. cumin
- 1 tsp. coarsely crushed coriander
- ½ tsp. dried mango powder
- ½ tsp. red chili powder
- 1-2 tbsp. coriander
- 1 dry red chili

Direction: (Prep + Cook Time: 40 minutes)

- ✓ Create the dough with the first 4 ingredients. Set aside.
- ✓ Cook the filling ingredients in skillet and blend them well to make a thick paste.
- ✓ Form the paste into balls. Cut them in half and insert the filling.
- ✓ Preheat the Air Fryer to 300 F. Place the samosas in the fry receptacle.
- ✓ Cook for 20 to 25 minutes. Around the midpoint, turn the samosas over for uniform cooking.
- ✓ Serve hot with tamarind or mint chutney

Nutrition: Calories 48.62 Kcal (204 kJ) Calories from Fat 18.7 Kcal Total Fat 2.08g 3 % cholesterol 32.95 mg 11 % 9 mg 22 % 1 mg 2 % Total Carbs 2.33g 1 % Sugar 1.57g 6 % Dietary Fiber 0.32g 1 % Protein 4.88g

720) *Taro Gnocchi*

Ingredients:

- For dough:
- 1 ½ cup all-purpose flour
- ½ tsp. salt
- 5 tbsp. Water
- For filling:
- 2 cups minced taro
- 2 tbsp. oil
- 2 tsp. ginger-garlic paste
- 2 tsp. soy sauce
- 2 tsp. vinegar

Direction: (Prep + Cook Time: 30 minutes)

- ✓ Make the dough, spread it with saran wrap and set aside.
- ✓ Combine the filling ingredients.
- ✓ Roll the dough and place the filling in the middle.
- ✓ Presently, wrap the dough to cover the filling and squeeze the edges together.
- ✓ Preheat the Air Fryer to 200° F and cook for 20 minutes.

Nutrition: Fiber : 6.7 g Manganese: 30% Copper:13

721) Okra Kebab

Ingredients:

- 2 cups sliced okra
- 3 onions chopped
- 5 green chilies-roughly chopped
- 1 ½ tbsp. ginger paste
- 1 ½ tsp. garlic paste
- 1 ½ tsp. salt
- 3 tsp. lemon juice
- 2 tsp. garam masala
- 4 tbsp. chopped coriander
- 3 tbsp. cream
- 3 tbsp. chopped capsicum
- 3 eggs
- 2 ½ tbsp. white sesame seeds

Direction: (Prep + Cook Time: 40 minutes)

- ✓ Mix the okra with the ground ginger and cut green chilies.
- ✓ Pound this blend until it turns into a thick paste. Add Water if required.
- ✓ Add the onions, mint, breadcrumbs and spices. Blend this well until you get a soft mixture.
- ✓ Recommended sides for this dish are mint chutney, tomato ketchup or yogurt chutney.
- ✓ Form round kebabs with the dough.
- ✓ Pour a small amount of milk onto each kebab to wet it.
- ✓ Roll the kebab in the dry breadcrumbs.
- ✓ Preheat the Air Fryer for 5 minutes at 300 F and cook for 30 minutes.

Nutrition: 338 calories; calories from Fat 30 % ; Fat 11.3g; saturated Fat 3.7g; mono Fat 5.3g; poly Fat 0.7g; Protein 30.6g; Carbs 30.4g; Fiber 3.9g; cholesterol 76 mg

722) Okra Pancakes

Ingredients:

- 2 tbsp. garam masala
- 2 cups sliced okra
- 3 tsp. ginger finely chopped
- 1-2 tbsp. fresh coriander leaves
- 2 or 3 green chilies finely chopped
- 1 ½ tbsp. lemon juice
- Salt and pepper to taste

Direction: (Prep + Cook Time: 30 minutes)

- ✓ Blend the ingredients in a bowl and add Water to it.
- ✓ Preheat the Air Fryer to 160 F and cook for 25 minutes.
- ✓ Continue turning them over to cook uniformly.
- ✓ Serve either with mint chutney or ketchup.

Nutrition: Calories 102.2 Total Fat 0.5 g Saturated Fat 0.1 g g cholesterol 0.0 5 mg Total Carbs 21.4 g Dietary Fiber 5.6 g Sugar 4.8 g Protein 5.4 g % Copper 9.9 %

723) White Lentil Galette

Ingredients:

- 2 cup white lentil soaked
- 3 tsp. ginger finely chopped
- 1-2 tbsp. fresh coriander leaves
- 2 or 3 green chilies finely chopped
- 1 ½ tbsp. lemon juice
- Salt and pepper to taste

Direction: (Prep + Cook Time: 40 minutes)

- ✓ Wash the soaked lentils and mix it with the rest of the ingredients in a clean bowl.
- ✓ Mold this mixture into round and flat galettes.
- ✓ Wet the galettes slightly with Water .
- ✓ Preheat the Air Fryer to 160 F and cook for 25 minutes.
- ✓ Serve either with mint chutney or ketchup.

Nutrition: 116 calories (kcal) 9.02 g of Protein 0.38 g of Fat 20.13 g of Carbs , including 7.9 g of Fiber and 1.8 g of Sugar

724) Coconut and plantain pancakes

Ingredients:

- 2 fresh plantains (shredded)
- 1 cup shredded coconut
- 1 ½ cups almond flour
- 3 eggs
- 2 tsp. dried basil
- 2 tsp. dried parsley
- Salt and Pepper to taste
- 3 tbsp. Butter

Direction: (Prep + Cook Time: 30 minutes)

- ✓ Preheat the air fryer to 250 F.
- ✓ In a bowl, combine the ingredients. Mix well.
- ✓ Cook till both sides of the pancake have browned. Serve with maple syrup.

Nutrition: Nutritions: 560 calories; 15g Fat ; 103.1g Carbs ; 6g Protein ; 0 mg cholesterol; 644 mg

725) Vegan Avocado Fries

Ingredients:

- ½ cup breadcrumbs
- ½ tsp salt
- 1 Hass avocado
- aquafaba from 15 oz can of white beans

Direction: (Prep + Cook Time: 30 minutes)

- ✓ In a major bowl, toss together the breadcrumbs and salt.
- ✓ Empty the aquafaba into another shallow bowl.
- ✓ Dip the avocado slices in the aquafaba and then in the breadcrumbs.
- ✓ Air browning: Arrange the cuts in a single layer in your air fryer container.
- ✓ Air fry for 10 minutes (Do not preheat) at 390F, shaking after 5 minutes.

Nutrition: For a Serving Size of 6 pieces (120g)

Calories 390 Calories from Fat 288 (73.8 %)
Total Fat 32g -Saturated Fat 4.5g - 20 % Carbs 24g -
Net carbs 20g - Sugar 3g - Fiber 4g 16 % Protein 4g

726) Sweet Potato Chips
Ingredients:
- ½ tbsp tsp salt
- 2 tbsp of olive oil
- 3 sweet potatoes – peeled, washed and sliced
- ½ tsp dry pepper

Direction: (Prep + Cook Time: 20 minutes)
✓ Place sliced sweet potatoes in a bowl. Add salt and dry pepper to mix with the potato.
✓ Spread the olive oil over the mix.
✓ Air fry at 370F for 20 minutes shaking after 10 minutes. Do not preheat.

Nutrition: cholesterol 16 mg 10 % mg 3 % mg 4 % Total Carbs 11gs Dietary Fiber 0.8gs Sugar 1.4gs Protein 3.2gs 3.2 %

727) Ai r Fryer Tofu Scramble
Ingredients:
- 1 block tofu
- 2 tbsp soy sauce
- 1 tsp garlic and onion powder
- 4 cups broccoli florets
- 1/2 cup chopped onion
- 1 tsp turmeric
- 2 ½ cups chopped red potato
- 1 tbsp olive oil

Direction: (Prep + Cook Time: 40 minutes)
✓ Toss together the tofu, soy sauce, olive oil, turmeric, garlic powder, onion powder, and onion in a bowl.
✓ Cook the tofu and potatoes at 370F for 15 minutes.
✓ Add broccoli to the air fryer for 5 minutes.
✓ In another bowl, toss the potatoes within the olive oil, and air fry at 400F for 15 minutes, shaking 7-8 minutes into cooking.
✓ Add tofu after shaking the potatoes once more conserving any remaining marinade.

Nutrition: 265 cal; Protein 12g; Carbs 34.9g; Fat 7g; 1 mg

728) Avocado Egg Rolls and Sweet Chili Sauce
Ingredients:
- 10 egg roll wrappers
- 3 avocados peeled and pitted
- 1 tomato, diced
- A pinch of salt and pepper
- coconut oil
- 4 tbsp sriracha
- 2 tbsp white Sugar

- 1 tbsp rice vinegar
- 1 tbsp sesame oil

Direction: (Prep + Cook Time: 20 minutes)
✓ Mash the avocados and mix in the ingredients. This will be the egg roll filling.
✓ Dip the egg roll wrappers in a bowl of Water .
✓ Add filling onto the lower third of each wrapper.
✓ Use your finger to brush Water along the 4 edges of the wrapper.
✓ Crease a corner over the filling, roll it up and seal. Repeat for each eggroll.
✓ Add oil to a large skillet over medium heat. Cook for 3-5 minutes. Move to a paper towel to dry.
✓ Combine sauce ingredients in a bowl and mix well.

Nutrition: Calories 98 7 % Total Fat 4.6gs5 % Saturated Fat 1gs Trans Fat 0.1gs ams grams5 % cholesterol 16 mg Total Carbs 11gs3 % Dietary Fiber 0.8gs Sugar 1.4gs Protein 3.2gs

729) Vegan Fried Ravioli
Ingredients:
- 1/2 cup breadcrumbs
- 2 tsp nutritional yeast flakes
- 1 tsp dried basil
- 1 tsp dried oregano
- aquafaba
- 1 tsp garlic powder
- Pinch salt & pepper
- 8 oz. thawed vegan ravioli
- Spritz cooking spray
- 1/2 cup marinara for dipping

Direction: (Prep + Cook Time: 30 minutes)
✓ Mix breadcrumbs, yeast flakes, dried basil, dried oregano, garlic powder, salt, and pepper.
✓ Put aquafaba into a bowl.
✓ Dip ravioli into aquafaba, shake off extra fluid and coat in breadcrumbs.
✓ Move the ravioli into the air fryer container. Set air fryer to 390 F and air fry for 6 minutes. Cautiously flip every ravioli over. Air fry for 2 additional minutes.
✓ Remove ravioli from air fryer and serve with warm marinara sauce.

Nutrition: Calories 987 % Total Fat 4.6gs 5 % Saturated Fat 1gs Trans Fat 0.1gs ams grams5 % cholesterol 16 mg Total Carbs 11gs3 % Dietary Fiber 0.8gs Sugar 1.4gs Protein 3.2gs 3.2 %

730) Classic Falafel
Ingredients:
- 1 ½ cups dry garbanzo beans
- ½ cup chopped fresh parsley
- 1/2 cup chopped fresh cilantro
- 1/2 cup chopped white onion
- 7 cloves garlic
- 2 Tbsp. All-purpose flour

- 1/2 tsp sea salt
- 1 Tbsp ground cumin
- 1/2 tbsp ground cardamom
- 1 tsp ground coriander
- 1/2 tbsp cayenne pepper

Direction: (Prep + Cook Time: 50 minutes)

✓ Rinse garbanzo beans in a strainer and add to a large pot.
✓ Cover with Water and boil for 60 minutes. Drain completely.
✓ In a food processor, mix parsley, cilantro, onions, and garlic.
✓ Add garbanzo beans, flour, salt, cumin, cardamom, coriander and cayenne to food processor.
✓ Place in a bowl, cover and refrigerate for 1-2 hours.
✓ Remove from fridge and form into 1½-inch balls. Flatten slightly to create patties.
✓ Preheat air fryer to 400° F. Add oil.
✓ Place falafel into the container and cook for 10 minutes, turning partially through.

Nutrition: Calories: 333 Protein : 13.3 grams Carbs: 31.8 grams Fat : 17.8 grams Fiber : 4.9 grams % of the Daily Value Manganese : 30 % oCopper : 29 %

731) *Thai Veggie Bites*

Ingredients:

- 1 Large Broccoli
- 1 Large Cauliflower
- 6 Large Carrots
- Handful Garden Peas
- ½ Cauliflower
- 1 Large Onion peeled and diced
- 1 Small Zucchini
- 2 Leeks cleaned and thinly sliced
- Salt & Pepper
- 1 Can Coconut Milk
- 50 g Plain Flour
- 1 cm Cube Ginger peeled and grated
- 1 Tbsp Garlic Puree
- 1 Tbsp Olive Oil
- 1 Tbsp Thai Green Curry Paste
- 1 Tbsp Coriander
- 1 Tbsp Mixed Spice
- 1 Tsp Cumin

Direction: (Prep + Cook Time: 30 minutes)

✓ In a wok, cook the onion with the garlic, ginger and olive oil.
✓ In a steamer, cook the vegetables (except the zucchini and leek) for 20 minutes.
✓ Add the coconut milk and the rest of the seasoning. Mix well and then add the cauliflower rice.
✓ Mix again and allow simmering for 10 minutes.
✓ Add the zucchini, leek and curry paste to the wok and cook over medium heat for a further 5 minutes.

✓ Add the steamed vegetables. Mix well.
✓ Cool in the fridge for an hour.
✓ Make into bite sized pieces and place in the Air Fryer. Cook for 10 minutes at 180 C.

Nutrition: Calories 18015 % Total Fat 10gs10 % Saturated Fat 2gs Trans Fat 0gs0 % cholesterol 0 mg 19 % mg Total Carbs 18gs12 % Dietary Fiber 3gs Sugar 9gs Protein 5gs 2 %

732) *Cornflakes French toast*

ingredients

- Bread slices (brown or white)
- 1 egg white for every 2 slices
- 1 tsp. sugar for every 2 slices
- Crushed cornflakes

Direction: Total time: 30 minutes Servings: 1

✓ Cut bread slices in half.
✓ In a bowl, whisk the egg whites and sugar.
✓ Dip the bread into this blend, then spread them with crushed cornflakes.
✓ Preheat the Air Fryer to 180° C and cook for 20 minutes.
✓ Flip the toast halfway through to cook uniformly.
✓ Serve with chocolate sauce.

Nutritional Value: 214 calories; protein 9.1g; carbohydrates 42.4g; dietary fiber 4.2g; sugars 24.3g; fat 2.2g; saturated fat 0.5g; cholesterol 0.6mg; vitamin a iu 454.8IU; vitamin c 3mg; folate 28.2mcg; calcium 77.1mg;

733) *Air Fryer Cheesecake Bites*

Ingredients:

- 8 oz. cream cheese
- 4 tbsp heavy cream, divided
- 1/2 tsp vanilla extract
- 1/2 cup almond flour
- 1/2 cup erythritol

Direction: Total time: 1 hour Servings: 4

✓ Allow cream cheese to sit for 20 minutes at room temperature.
✓ Mix cream cheese, erythritol, vanilla concentrate, and 2 tbsp heavy cream in a blender for 3 to 5 minutes or until smooth.
✓ Scoop blend into a preparing skillet that has been fixed with a material paper.
✓ Freeze blend for 30 minutes or until it structures.
✓ Mix almond flour and 2 tbsp erythritol in a little bowl.
✓ Dip solidified cheesecake adjusts into staying overwhelming cream and coat in the almond flour blend.
✓ Air fry for 2 minutes and serve.

Nutrition values: Calories 78.7 Total Fat 5.7 g Saturated Fat 3.4 g Polyunsaturated Fat 0.3 gMonounsaturated Fat 1.8 g Cholesterol 28.2 mg Sodium 6.4 mg Total Carbohydrate 6.9 g Dietary Fiber 0.5 g Sugars 5.3 g Protein 1.0 g

734)   *Coconut French Toast*

Ingredients:

- 2 slices gluten free bread
- 1/2 cup shredded coconut
- 1 tbsp baking powder
- 1/2 cup coconut milk
- Maple syrup

Direction: Total time: 15 minutes Servings: 1

✓ In a large bowl, mix coconut milk and baking powder.

✓ Spread shredded coconut on a level sheet.

✓ Using every one of the breads, absorb coconut milk before covering in shredded coconut. Coat liberally.

✓ Place covered bread in the air fryer bin and air fry at 175°C for 4 minutes.

✓ Top with maple syrup.

Nutrition: Calories: 480kcal | Carbohydrates: 18g | Protein: 12g | Fat: 41g | SaturatedFat: 29g | Cholesterol: 86mg | Sodium: 723mg |Potassium: 235mg | Fiber: 1g | Sugar: 2g | VitaminA: 283IU | Calcium: 111mg |

735)   *Air Fryer Honey Cheese Balls*

Ingredients:

- 4 oz. soft goat cheese
- 1 small egg, beaten
- 1 tbsp all-purpose flour
- 1/4 cup breadcrumbs
- 4 tbsp raw honey

Direction: Total time: 30 minutes Servings: 4

✓ Separate goat cheese into 12 portions and roll into small balls.

✓ Freeze balls for about 15 to 20 minutes.

✓ Remove from refrigerator and dredge each goat cheese in flour, egg and finally coat then in breadcrumbs.

✓ Arrange in air fryer basket and spray with nonstick cooking spray for crispness.

✓ Air fry at 200°C for 8 minutes until golden brown.

✓ Drizzle with generous amount of honey and serve immediately.

Nutrition values: Calories 410 Total Fat 23g Saturated Fat 7.9g Trans Fat 0.3g Cholesterol 107mg Sodium 1292mg Potassium 473mg Total Carbohydrates 33g Dietary Fiber 2.7g Sugars 5.2g Protein 19g Calcium40%

736)   *Homemade Chelsea Currant Buns*

Ingredients

- 1/2 pound cake flour
- 1 teaspoon dry yeast
- 2 tablespoons granulated sugar
- A pinch of sea salt
- 1/2 cup milk, warm
- 1 egg, whisked
- 4 tablespoons butter
- 1/2 cup dried currants
- 1 ounce icing sugar

Directions (Ready in about 20 minutes | Servings 4)

✓ Mix the flour, yeast, sugar and salt in a bowl; add in milk, egg and 2 tablespoons of butter and mix to combine well. Add lukewarm water as necessary to form a smooth dough.

✓ Knead the dough until it is elastic; then, leave it in a warm place to rise for 30 minutes.

✓ Roll out your dough and spread the remaining 2 tablespoons of butter onto the dough; scatter dried currants over the dough.

✓ Cut into 8 equal slices and roll them up. Brush each bun with a nonstick cooking oil and transfer them to the Air Fryer cooking basket.

✓ Cook your buns at 330 degrees F for about 20 minutes, turning them over halfway through the cooking time.

✓ Dust with icing sugar before serving. Bon appétit!

Nutritions: 395 Calories; 14g Fat; 56.1g Carbs; 7.6g Protein; 13.6g Sugars

737)   *Old-Fashioned Pinch-Me Cake with Walnuts*

Ingredients

- 1 (10-ounces) can crescent rolls
- 1/2 stick butter
- 1/2 cup caster sugar
- 1 teaspoon pumpkin pie spice blend
- 1 tablespoon dark rum
- 1/2 cup walnuts, chopped

Directions

✓ Start by preheating your Air Fryer to 350 degrees F.

✓ Roll out the crescent rolls. Spread the butter onto the crescent rolls; scatter the sugar, spices and walnuts over the rolls. Drizzle with rum and roll them up.

✓ Using your fingertips, gently press them to seal the edges.

✓ Bake your cake for about 13 minutes or until the top is golden brown. Bon appétit!

Nutritions: 455 Calories; 25.4g Fat; 52.1g Carbs; 6.1g Protein; 15g Sugars

738)   *Authentic Swedish Kärleksmums*

Ingredients

- 2 tablespoons Swedish butter, at room temperature
- 4 tablespoons brown sugar
- 1 egg
- 1 tablespoon lingonberry jam
- 5 tablespoons all-purpose flour
- 1/2 teaspoon baking powder
- 2 tablespoons cocoa powder
- A pinch of grated nutmeg
- A pinch of coarse sea salt

Directions (Ready in about 20 minutes | Servings 3)

✓ Cream the butter and sugar using an electric mixer.

247

- Fold in the egg and lingonberry jam and mix to combine well.
- ✓ Stir in the flour, baking powder, cocoa powder, grated nutmeg and salt; mix again to combine well. Pour the batter into a lightly buttered baking pan.
- ✓ Bake your cake at 330 degrees F for about 15 minutes until a tester inserted into the center of the cake comes out dry and clean. Bon appétit!

Nutritions: 256 Calories; 11.5g Fat; 27.6g Carbs; 5.1g Protein; 13.9g Sugars

739) *Air Grilled Peaches with Cinnamon-Sugar Butter*

Ingredients

- 2 fresh peaches, pitted and halved
- 1 tablespoon butter
- 2 tablespoons caster sugar
- 1/4 teaspoon ground cinnamon

Directions (Ready in about 25 minutes | Servings 2)

- ✓ Mix the butter, sugar and cinnamon. Spread the butter mixture onto the peaches and transfer them to the Air Fryer cooking basket.
- ✓ Cook your peaches at 320 degrees F for about 25 minutes or until the top is golden.
- ✓ Serve with vanilla ice cream, if desired. Bon appétit!

Nutritions: 146 Calories; 6.1g Fat; 22.6g Carbs; 1.4g Protein; 20.4g Sugars

740) *Chocolate Mug Cake*

Ingredients

- 1/2 cup self-rising flour
- 6 tablespoons brown sugar
- 5 tablespoons coconut milk
- 4 tablespoons coconut oil
- 4 tablespoons unsweetened cocoa powder
- 2 eggs
- A pinch of grated nutmeg
- A pinch of salt

Directions (Ready in about 10 minutes | Servings 2)

- ✓ Mix all the ingredients together; divide the batter between two mugs.
- ✓ Place the mugs in the Air Fryer cooking basket and cook at 390 degrees F for about 10 minutes.
- ✓ Bon appétit!

Nutritions: 546 Calories; 34.1g Fat; 55.4g Carbs; 11.4g Protein; 25.7g Sugars

741) *Easy Plantain Cupcakes*

Ingredients

- 1 cup all-purpose flour
- 1 teaspoon baking powder
- 1/4 teaspoon ground cloves
- 1/4 teaspoon ground cinnamon
- A pinch of salt
- 2 ripe plantains, peeled and mashed with a fork

- 4 tablespoons coconut oil, room temperature
- 1/4 cup brown sugar
- 1 egg, whisked
- 4 tablespoons pecans, roughly chopped
- 2 tablespoons raisins, soaked

Directions (Ready in about 10 minutes | Servings 4)

- ✓ In a mixing bowl, thoroughly combine all ingredients until everything is well incorporated.
- ✓ Spoon the batter into a greased muffin tin.
- ✓ Bake the plantain cupcakes in your Air Fryer at 350 degrees F for about 10 minutes or until golden brown on the top.
- ✓ Bon appétit!

Nutritions: 471 Calories; 22.5g Fat; 65.8g Carbs; 6.9g Protein; 24.2g Sugars

742) *Strawberry Dessert Dumplings*

Ingredients

- 9 wonton wrappers
- 1/3 strawberry jam
- 2 ounces icing sugar

Directions (Ready in about 10 minutes | Servings 3)

- ✓ Start by laying out the wonton wrappers.
- ✓ Divide the strawberry jam between the wonton wrappers. Fold the wonton wrapper over the jam; now, seal the edges with wet fingers
- ✓ Cook your wontons at 400 degrees F for 8 minutes; working in batches. Bon appétit!

Nutritions: 471 Calories; 22.5g Fat; 65.8g Carbs; 6.9g Protein; 24.2g Sugars

743) *Crunchy French Toast Sticks*

Ingredients

- 1 egg
- 1/4 cup double cream
- 1/4 cup milk
- 1 tablespoon brown sugar
- 1/4 teaspoon ground cloves
- 1/4 teaspoon ground cinnamon
- 1/4 vanilla paste
- 3 thick slices of brioche bread, cut into thirds
- 1 cup crispy rice cereal

Directions (Ready in about 10 minutes | Servings 3)

- ✓ Thoroughly combine the egg, cream, milk, sugar, ground cloves, cinnamon and vanilla.
- ✓ Dip each piece of bread into the cream mixture and then, press gently into the cereal, pressing to coat all sides.
- ✓ Arrange the pieces of bread in the Air Fryer cooking basket and cook them at 380 degrees F for 2 minutes; flip and cook on the other side for 2 to 3 minutes longe

Nutritions: 188 Calories; 8.3g Fat; 21.9g Carbs; 6.2g Protein; 6.1g Sugars

744) *Old-Fashioned Apple Crumble*

Ingredients

- 2 baking apples, peeled, cored and diced
- 2 tablespoons brown sugar
- 1 tablespoon cornstarch
- 1/4 teaspoon grated nutmeg
- 1/4 teaspoon ground cloves
- 1/2 teaspoon ground cinnamon
- 1/2 teaspoon vanilla essence
- 1/4 cup apple juice
- 1/2 cup quick-cooking oats
- 1/4 cup self-rising flour
- 1/4 cup brown sugar
- 1/2 teaspoon baking powder
- 1/4 cup coconut oil

Directions (Ready in about 35 minutes | Servings 4)

- ✓ Toss the apples with 2 tablespoons of brown sugar and cornstarch. Place the apples in a baking pan that is previously lightly greased with a nonstick cooking spray.
- ✓ In a mixing dish, thoroughly combine the remaining topping ingredients. Sprinkle the topping ingredients over the apple layer.
- ✓ Bake your apple crumble in the preheated Air Fryer at 330 degrees F for 35 minutes.

Nutritions: 261 Calories; 14.1g Fat; 35.7g Carbs; 1.9g Protein; 21.1g Sugars

745) *Blueberry Fritters with Cinnamon Sugar*

Ingredients

- 1/2 cup plain flour
- 1/2 teaspoon baking powder
- 1 teaspoon brown sugar
- A pinch of grated nutmeg
- 1/4 teaspoon ground star anise
- A pinch of salt
- 1 egg
- 1/4 cup coconut milk
- 1 cup fresh blueberries
- 1 tablespoon coconut oil, melted
- 4 tablespoons cinnamon sugar

Directions (Ready in about 20 minutes | Servings 4)

- ✓ Combine the flour, baking powder, brown sugar, nutmeg, star anise and salt.
- ✓ In another bowl, whisk the eggs and milk until frothy. Add the wet mixture to the dry mixture and mix to combine well. Fold in the fresh blueberries.
- ✓ Carefully place spoonfuls of batter into the Air Fryer cooking basket. Brush them with melted coconut oil.
- ✓ Cook your fritters in the preheated Air Fryer at 370 degrees for 10 minutes, flipping them halfway through the cooking time. Repeat with the remaining batter.

- ✓ Dust your fritters with the cinnamon sugar and serve at room temperature.

Nutritions: 218 Calories; 6.6g Fat; 35.6g Carbs; 4.7g Protein; 22.5g Sugars

746) *Summer Fruit Pie*

Ingredients

- 2 (8-ounce) refrigerated pie crusts
- 2 cups fresh blackberries
- 1/4 cup caster sugar
- 2 teaspoons cornstarch
- A pinch of sea salt
- 1/4 teaspoon ground nutmeg
- 1/4 teaspoon ground cinnamon
- 1/4 teaspoon vanilla extract

Directions (Ready in about 35 minutes | Servings 4)

- ✓ Start by preheating your Air Fryer to 350 degrees F.
- ✓ Place the pie crust in a lightly greased pie plate.
- ✓ In a bowl, combine the fresh blackberries with caster sugar, cornstarch, salt, nutmeg, cinnamon and vanilla extract. Spoon the blackberry filling into the prepared pie crust.
- ✓ Top the blackberry filling with second crust and cut slits in pastry.
- ✓ Bake your pie in the preheated Air Fryer for 35 minutes or until the top is golden brown.

Nutritions: 318 Calories; 14.6g Fat; 43.5g Carbs; 2.7g Protein; 9.6g Sugars

747) *Banana and Pecan Muffins*

Ingredients

- 1 extra-large ripe banana, mashed
- 1/4 cup coconut oil
- 1 egg
- 1/4 cup brown sugar
- 1/2 teaspoon vanilla essence
- 1/2 teaspoon ground cinnamon
- 4 tablespoons pecans, chopped
- 1/2 cup self-rising flour

Directions (Ready in about 25 minutes | Servings 4)

- ✓ Start by preheating your Air Fryer to 330 degrees F.
- ✓ In a mixing bowl, combine the banana, coconut oil, egg, brown sugar, vanilla and cinnamon.
- ✓ Add in the chopped pecans and flour and stir again to combine well.
- ✓ Spoon the mixture into a lightly greased muffin tin and transfer to the Air Fryer cooking basket.
- ✓ Bake your muffins in the preheated Air Fryer for 15 to 17 minutes or until a tester comes out dry and clean.
- ✓ Sprinkle some extra icing sugar over the top of each muffin if desired. Serve and enjoy!

Nutritions: 315 Calories; 21.4g Fat; 27.9g Carbs; 4.8g Protein; 11.3g Sugars

748) *Sweet Potato Boats*
Ingredients
- 2 sweet potatoes, pierce several times with a fork
- 1/4 cup quick-cooking oats
- 2 tablespoons peanut butter
- 1 tablespoon agave nectar
- 1/2 teaspoon vanilla essence
- 1/4 teaspoon ground cloves
- 1/2 teaspoon ground cinnamon
- A pinch of salt

Directions (Ready in about 35 minutes | Servings 2)
- ✓ Cook the sweet potatoes in the preheated Air Fryer at 380 degrees F for 20 to 25 minutes.
- ✓ Then, scrape the sweet potato flesh using a spoon; mix the sweet potato flesh with the remaining ingredients. Stuff the potatoes and place them in the Air Fryer cooking basket.
- ✓ Bake the sweet potatoes for a further 10 minutes or until cooked through.

Nutritions: 148 Calories; 3.1g Fat; 27.8g Carbs; 3.6g Protein; 7.4g Sugars

749) *Mini Apple and Cranberry Crisp Cakes*
Ingredients
- 2 Bramley cooking apples, peeled, cored and chopped
- 1/4 cup dried cranberries
- 1 teaspoon fresh lemon juice
- 1 tablespoon golden caster sugar
- 1 teaspoon apple pie spice mix
- A pinch of coarse salt
- 1/2 cup rolled oats
- 1/3 cup brown bread crumbs
- 1/4 cup butter, diced

Directions (Ready in about 40 minutes | Servings 3)
- ✓ Divide the apples and cranberries between three lightly greased ramekins. Drizzle your fruits with lemon juice and sprinkle with caster sugar, spice mix and salt.
- ✓ Then, make the streusel by mixing the remaining ingredients in a bowl. Spread the streusel batter on top of the filling.
- ✓ Bake the mini crisp cakes in the preheated Air Fryer at 330 degrees F for 35 minutes or until they're a dark golden brown around the edges.

Nutritions: 338 Calories; 17.5g Fat; 41.9g Carbs; 5.2g Protein; 18.1g Sugars

750) *Cinnamon-Streusel Coffeecake*
Ingredients
- Cake:
- 1/2 cup unbleached white flour
- 1/4 cup yellow cornmeal
- 1 teaspoon baking powder
- 3 tablespoons white sugar
- 1 tablespoon unsweetened cocoa powder
- A pinch of kosher salt
- 3 tablespoons coconut oil
- 1/4 cup milk
- 1 egg
- Topping:
- 2 tablespoons polenta
- 1/4 cup brown sugar
- 1 teaspoon ground cinnamon
- 1/4 cup pecans, chopped
- 2 tablespoons coconut oil

Directions (Ready in about 30 minutes | Servings 4)
- ✓ In a large bowl, combine together the cake ingredients. Spoon the mixture into a lightly greased baking pan.
- ✓ Then, in another bowl, combine the topping ingredients. Spread the topping ingredients over your cake.
- ✓ Bake the cake at 330 degrees F for 12 to 15 minutes until a tester comes out dry and clean.
- ✓ Allow your cake to cool for about 15 minutes before cutting and serving. Bon appétit!

Nutritions: 364 Calories; 23.9g Fat; 35.1g Carbs; 5.1g Protein; 13.3g Sugars

751) *Air Grilled Apricots with Mascarpone*
Ingredients
- 6 apricots, halved and pitted
- 1 teaspoon coconut oil, melted
- 2 ounces mascarpone cheese
- 1/2 teaspoon vanilla extract
- 1 tablespoon confectioners' sugar
- A pinch of sea salt

Directions (Ready in about 30 minutes | Servings 2)
- ✓ Place the apricots in the Air Fryer cooking basket. Drizzle the apricots with melted coconut oil.
- ✓ Cook the apricots at 320 degrees F for about 25 minutes or until the top is golden.
- ✓ In a bowl, whisk the mascarpone, vanilla extract, confectioners' sugar by hand until soft and creamy.
- ✓ Remove the apricots from the cooking basket. Spoon the whipped mascarpone into the cavity of each apricot.
- ✓ Sprinkle with coarse sea salt and enjoy!

Nutritions: 244 Calories; 10.9g Fat; 30.1g Carbs; 7.5g Protein; 28.1g Sugars

752) *Chocolate Chip Banana Crepes*
Ingredients
- 1 small ripe banana
- 1/8 teaspoon baking powder
- 1/4 cup chocolate chips
- 1 egg, whisked

Directions (Ready in about 30 minutes | Servings 2)
- ✓ Mix all ingredients until creamy and fluffy. Let it

stand for about 20 minutes.

✓ Spritz the Air Fryer baking pan with cooking spray. Pour 1/2 of the batter into the pan using a measuring cup.

✓ Cook at 230 degrees F for 4 to 5 minutes or until golden brown. Repeat with another crepe.

Nutritions: 214 Calories; 5.4g Fat; 36.4g Carbs; 5.8g Protein; 25.1g Sugars

753)   *Classic Flourless Cake*

Ingredients

- Crust:
- 1 teaspoon butter
- 1/3 cup almond meal
- 1 tablespoon flaxseed meal
- 1 teaspoon pumpkin pie spice
- 1 teaspoon caster sugar
- Filling:
- 6 ounces cream cheese
- 1 egg
- 1/2 teaspoon pure vanilla extract
- 2 tablespoons powdered sugar

Directions (Ready in about 2 hours | Servings 4)

✓ Mix all the ingredients for the crust and then, press the mixture into the bottom of a lightly greased baking pan.

✓ Bake the crust at 350 degrees F for 18 minutes. Transfer the crust to the freezer for about 25 minutes.

✓ Now, make the cheesecake topping by mixing the remaining ingredients. Spread the prepared topping over the cooled crust.

✓ Bake your cheesecake in the preheated Air Fryer at 320 degrees F for about 30 minutes; leave it in the Air Fryer to keep warm for another 30 minutes.

✓ Serve well chilled. Bon appétit!

Nutritions: 254 Calories; 21.4g Fat; 9.4g Carbs; 6.1g Protein; 6.4g Sugars

754)   *Old-Fashioned Baked Pears*

Ingredients

- 2 large pears, halved and cored
- 1 teaspoon lemon juice
- 2 teaspoons coconut oil
- 1/2 cup rolled oats
- 1/4 cup walnuts, chopped
- 1/4 cup brown sugar
- 1 teaspoon apple pie spice mix

Directions (Ready in about 10 minutes | Servings 2)

✓ Drizzle the pear halves with lemon juice and coconut oil. In a mixing bowl, thoroughly combine the rolled oats, walnuts, brown sugar and apple pie spice mix.

✓ Cook in the preheated Air Fryer at 360 degrees for 8 minutes, checking them halfway through the cooking time.

✓ Dust with powdered sugar if desired. Bon appétit

Nutritions: 445 Calories; 14g Fat; 89g Carbs; 9g Protein; 49.1g Sugars

755)   *Sweet Dough Dippers*

Ingredients

- 8 ounces bread dough
- 2 tablespoons butter, melted
- 2 ounces powdered sugar

Directions (Ready in about 10 minutes | Servings 4)

✓ Cut the dough into strips and twist them together 3 to 4 times. Then, brush the dough twists with melted butter and sprinkle sugar over them.

✓ Cook the dough twists at 350 degrees F for 8 minutes, tossing the basket halfway through the cooking time.

✓ Serve with your favorite dip. Bon appétit!

Nutritions: 255 Calories; 7.6g Fat; 42.1g Carbs; 5g Protein; 17.1g Sugars

756)   *Mini Molten Lava Cakes*

Ingredients

- 1/2 cup dark chocolate chunks
- 3 tablespoons butter
- 1 egg
- 1 ounce granulated sugar
- 1 tablespoon self-rising flour
- 2 tablespoons almonds, chopped

Directions (Ready in about 12 minutes | Servings 2)

✓ Microwave the chocolate chunks and butter for 30 to 40 seconds until the mixture is smooth.

✓ Then, beat the eggs and sugar; stir in the egg mixture into the chocolate mixture. Now, stir in the flour and almonds.

✓ Pour the batter into two ramekins.

✓ Bake your cakes at 370 degrees for about 10 minutes and serve at room temperature. Bon appétit

Nutritions: 405 Calories; 29.5g Fat; 30.1g Carbs; 5.1g Protein; 23.1g Sugars

757)   *Baked Banana with Chocolate Glaze*

Ingredients

- 2 bananas, peeled and cut in half lengthwise
- 1 tablespoon coconut oil, melted
- 1 tablespoon cocoa powder
- 1 tablespoon agave syrup

Directions (Ready in about 15 minutes | Servings 2)

✓ Bake your bananas in the preheated Air Fryer at 370 degrees F for 12 minutes, turning them over halfway through the cooking time.

✓ In the meantime, microwave the coconut oil for 30 seconds; stir in the cocoa powder and agave syrup.

✓ Serve the baked bananas with a few drizzles of the chocolate glaze. Bon appétit!

Nutritions: 201 Calories; 7.5g Fat; 36.9g Carbs; 1.7g Protein; 23g Sugars

758) *Chocolate Peppermint Cream Pie*

Ingredients

- 12 cookies, crushed into fine crumbs
- 2 ounces butter, melted
- 2 ounces dark chocolate chunks
- 1/2 cup heavy whipping cream
- 4 tablespoons brown sugar
- 2 drops peppermint extract
- 1/4 teaspoon ground cinnamon
- 1/4 teaspoon ground cloves

Directions (Ready in about 40 minutes + chilling time | Servings 4)

- ✓ In a mixing bowl, thoroughly combine crushed cookies and butter to make the crust. Press the crust into the bottom of a lightly oiled baking dish.
- ✓ Bake the crust at 350 degrees F for 18 minutes. Transfer it to your freezer for 20 minutes.
- ✓ Then, microwave the chocolate chunks for 30 seconds; stir in the heavy whipping cream, brown sugar, peppermint extract, cinnamon and cloves.
- ✓ Spread the mousse evenly over the crust. Refrigerate until firm for about 3 hours.
- ✓ Bon appétit!

Nutritions: 417 Calories; 28.2g Fat; 39g Carbs; 3.3g Protein; 23g Sugars

759) *Lemon-Glazed Crescent Ring*

Ingredients

- 8 ounces refrigerated crescent dough
- 2 ounces mascarpone cheese, at room temperature
- 1/2 teaspoon vanilla paste
- 1 tablespoon coconut oil, at room temperature
- 2 ounces caster sugar
- Glaze:
- 1/3 cup powdered sugar
- 1 tablespoon fresh lemon juice
- 1 tablespoon full-fat coconut milk

Directions (Ready in about 25 minutes | Servings 6)

- ✓ Separate the crescent dough sheet into 8 triangles. Then, arrange the triangles in a sunburst pattern so it should look like the sun.
- ✓ Mix the mascarpone cheese, vanilla, coconut oil and caster sugar in a bowl.
- ✓ Place the mixture on the bottom of each triangle; fold triangle tips over filling and tuck under base to secure.
- ✓ Bake the ring at 360 degrees F for 20 minutes until dough is golden.
- ✓ In small mixing dish, whisk the powdered sugar, lemon juice and coconut milk. Drizzle over warm crescent ring and garnish with grated lemon peel.
- ✓ Bon appétit!

Nutritions: 227 Calories; 6.7g Fat; 35.4g Carbs; 5.3g Protein; 15g Sugars

760) *Fluffy Chocolate Chip Cookies*

Ingredients

- 1/2 cup butter, softened
- 1/2 cup granulated sugar
- 1 large egg
- 1/2 teaspoon coconut extract
- 1/2 teaspoon vanilla paste
- 1 cup quick-cooking oats
- 1/2 cup all-purpose flour
- 1/2 teaspoon baking powder
- 6 ounces dark chocolate chips

Directions (Ready in about 20 minutes | Servings 6)

- ✓ Start by preheating your Air Fryer to 330 degrees F.
- ✓ In a mixing bowl, beat the butter and sugar until fluffy. Beat in the egg, coconut extract and vanilla paste.
- ✓ In a second mixing bowl, whisk the oats, flour and baking powder. Add the flour mixture to the egg mixture. Fold in the chocolate chips and gently stir to combine.
- ✓ Drop 2-tablespoon scoops of the dough onto the parchment paper and transfer it to the Air Fryer cooking basket. Gently flatten each scoop to make a cookie shape.
- ✓ Cook in the preheated Air Fryer for about 10 minutes. Work in batches. Bon appétit!

Nutritions: 490 Calories; 30.1g Fat; 45.4g Carbs; 8.8g Protein; 15g Sugars

761) *Authentic Spanish Churros*

Ingredients

- 1/2 cup water
- 1/4 cup butter, cut into cubes
- 1 tablespoon granulated sugar
- A pinch of ground cinnamon
- A pinch of salt
- 1/2 teaspoon lemon zest
- 1/2 cup plain flour
- 1 egg
- Chocolate Dip:
- 2 ounces dark chocolate
- 1/2 cup milk
- 1 teaspoon ground cinnamon

Directions (Ready in about 20 minutes | Servings 4)

- ✓ Boil the water in a saucepan over medium-high heat; now, add the butter, sugar, cinnamon, salt and lemon zest; cook until the sugar has dissolved.
- ✓ Next, remove the pan from the heat. Gradually stir in the flour, whisking continuously until the mixture forms a ball; let it cool slightly.
- ✓ Fold in the egg and continue to beat using an electric mixer until everything comes together.
- ✓ Pour the dough into a piping bag with a large star tip. Squeeze 4-inch strips of dough into the greased Air Fryer pan.
- ✓ Cook your churros at 380 degrees F for about 10 minutes, shaking the basket halfway through the cooking time.

In the meantime, melt the chocolate and milk in a saucepan over low heat. Add in the cinnamon and cook on low heat for about 5 minutes. Serve the warm churros with the chocolate dip and enjoy!

Nutritions: 287 Calories; 19.7g Fat; 22.5g Carbs; 5.2g Protein; 7.1g Sugars

762) *Classic Brownie Cupcakes*
Ingredients

- 1/3 cup all-purpose flour
- 1/4 teaspoon baking powder
- 3 tablespoons cocoa powder
- 1/3 cup caster sugar
- 2 ounces butter, room temperature
- 1 large egg
- 1/2 teaspoon rum extract
- A pinch of ground cinnamon
- A pinch of salt

Directions (Ready in about 25 minutes | Servings 3)

✓ Mix the dry ingredients in a bowl. In another bowl, mix the wet ingredients. Gradually, stir in the wet ingredients into the dry mixture.

✓ Divide the batter among muffin cups and transfer them to the Air Fryer cooking basket.

✓ Bake your cupcakes at 330 degrees for 15 minuets until a tester comes out dry and clean.

✓ Transfer to a wire rack and let your cupcakes sit for 10 minutes before unmolding.

Nutritions: 264 Calories; 17.7g Fat; 24.4g Carbs; 4.6g Protein; 10.9g Sugars

763) *Baked Fruit Salad*
Ingredients

- 1 banana, peeled
- 1 cooking pear, cored
- 1 cooking apple, cored
- 1 tablespoon freshly squeezed lemon juice
- 1/2 teaspoon ground star anise
- 1/4 teaspoon ground cinnamon
- 1/2 teaspoon granulated ginger
- 1/4 cup brown sugar
- 1 tablespoon coconut oil, melted

Directions (Ready in about 15 minutes | Servings 2)

✓ Toss your fruits with lemon juice, star anise, cinnamon, ginger, sugar and coconut oil.

✓ Transfer the fruits to the Air Fryer cooking basket.

✓ Bake the fruit salad in the preheated Air Fryer at 330 degrees F for 15 minutes.

✓ Serve in individual bowls, garnished with vanilla ice cream. Bon appétit

Nutritions: 263 Calories; 7.3g Fat; 53.2g Carbs; 1.3g Protein; 37.7g Sugars

764) *Indian-Style Donuts (Gulgulas)*
Ingredients

- 1/3 cup whole wheat flour

- 1/3 cup sugar
- 1 teaspoon ghee
- 1 tablespoon Indian dahi
- 1 tablespoon apple juice

Directions(Ready in about 10 minutes | Servings 2)

✓ Mix the ingredients until everything is well incorporated.

✓ Drop a spoonful of batter onto the greased Air Fryer pan. Cook Indian gulgulas at 360 degrees F for 5 minutes or until golden brown, flipping them halfway through the cooking time.

✓ Repeat with the remaining batter. Serve with hot Indian tea and enjoy!

Nutritions: 160 Calories; 2.9g Fat; 31.9g Carbs; 2.9g Protein; 16.7g Sugars

765) *Honey-Drizzled Banana Fritters*
Ingredients

- 3 ripe bananas, peeled
- 1 egg, whisked
- 1/4 cup almond flour
- 1/4 cup plain flour
- 1/2 teaspoon baking powder
- 1 teaspoon canola oil
- 1 tablespoon honey

Directions (Ready in about 15 minutes | Servings 3)

✓ Mash your bananas in a bowl. Now, stir in the egg, almond flour, plain flour and baking powder.

✓ Drop spoonfuls of the batter into the preheated Air Fryer cooking basket. Brush the fritters with canola oil.

✓ Cook the banana fritters at 360 degrees F for 10 minutes, flipping them halfway through the cooking time.

✓ Drizzle with some honey just before serving. Bon appétit!

Nutritions: 247 Calories; 7.3g Fat; 42.5g Carbs; 5.9g Protein; 20.6g Sugars

766) *Chocolate Puff Pastry Sticks*
Ingredients

- 8 ounces frozen puff pastry, thawed, cut into strips
- 1/2 stick butter, melted
- 1/2 teaspoon ground cinnamon
- 1/2 cup chocolate hazelnut spread

Directions(Ready in about 15 minutes | Servings 3)

✓ Brush the strips of the puff pastry with melted butter.

✓ Arrange the strips in the Air Fryer cooking basket and bake them at 380 degrees F for 2 minutes; flip and cook on the other side for 2 to 3 minutes longer.

✓ Top the pastry sticks with cinnamon and chocolate hazelnut spread. Bon appétit!

Nutritions: 407 Calories; 21.2g Fat; 46.1g Carbs; 6.9g Protein; 5.5g Sugars

767)   *Old-Fashioned Donuts*
Ingredients

- 8 ounces refrigerated buttermilk biscuits
- 2 tablespoons butter, unsalted and melted
- 1/2 tablespoon cinnamon
- 4 tablespoons caster sugar
- A pinch of salt
- A pinch of grated nutmeg

Directions (Ready in about 15 minutes | Servings 4)

✓ Separate the biscuits and cut holes out of the center of each biscuit using a 1-inch round biscuit cutter; place them on a parchment paper.

✓ Lower your biscuits into the Air Fryer cooking basket. Brush them with 1 tablespoon of melted butter.

✓ Air fry your biscuits at 340 degrees F for about 8 minutes or until golden brown, flipping them halfway through the cooking time.

✓ Meanwhile, mix the sugar with cinnamon, salt and nutmeg.

✓ Brush your donuts with remaining 1 tablespoon of melted butter; roll them in the cinnamon-sugar and serve. Bon appétit!

Nutritions: 268 Calories; 12.2g Fat; 36.1g Carbs; 3.9g Protein; 12.4g Sugars

768)   *Perfect English-Style Scones*
Ingredients

- 1 ½ cups cake flour
- 1/4 cup caster sugar
- 1 teaspoon baking powder
- 1 teaspoon baking soda
- 1/4 teaspoon salt
- 1/2 teaspoon vanilla essence
- 1/2 stick butter
- 1 egg, beaten
- 1/2 cup almond milk

Directions (Ready in about 15 minutes | Servings 4)

✓ Start by preheating your Air Fryer to 360 degrees F.

✓ Thoroughly combine all dry ingredients. In another bowl, combine all wet ingredients. Then, add the wet mixture to the dry ingredients and stir to combine well.

✓ Roll your dough out into a circle and cut into wedges.

✓ Bake the scones in the preheated Air Fryer for about 11 minutes, flipping them halfway through the cooking time. Bon appétit!

Nutritions: 458 Calories; 25g Fat; 47.1g Carbs; 6.8g Protein; 7.9g Sugars

769)   *Red Velvet Pancakes*
Ingredients

- 1 cup all-purpose flour
- 1/2 teaspoon baking soda
- 1 teaspoon granulated sugar
- 1/8 teaspoon sea salt
- 1/8 teaspoon freshly grated nutmeg
- 2 tablespoons ghee, melted
- 1 small-sized egg, beaten
- 1/2 cup milk
- 1 teaspoon red paste food color
- 2 ounces cream cheese, softened
- 1 tablespoon butter, softened
- 1/2 cup powdered sugar

Directions (Ready in about 35 minutes | Servings 3)

✓ Thoroughly combine the flour, baking soda, granulated sugar, salt and nutmeg in a large bowl.

✓ Gradually add in the melted ghee, egg, milk and red paste food color, stirring into the flour mixture until moistened. Allow your batter to rest for about 30 minutes.

✓ Spritz the Air Fryer baking pan with cooking spray. Pour the batter into the pan using a measuring cup. Set the pan into the Air Fryer cooking basket.

✓ Cook at 330 degrees F for about 5 minutes or until golden brown. Repeat with the other pancakes.

✓ Meanwhile, mix the remaining ingredients until creamy and fluffy. Decorate your pancakes with cream cheese topping. Bon appétit!

Nutritions: 422 Calories; 19g Fat; 52.1g Carbs; 8.6g Protein; 20.3g Sugars

770)   *Apricot and Almond Crumble*
Ingredients

- 1 cup apricots, pitted and diced
- 1/4 cup flaked almonds
- 1/3 cup self-raising flour
- 4 tablespoons granulated sugar
- 1/2 teaspoon ground cinnamon
- 1 teaspoon crystallized ginger
- ½ teaspoon ground cardamom
- 2 tablespoons butter

Directions (Ready in about 35 minutes | Servings 3)

✓ Place the sliced apricots and almonds in a baking pan that is lightly greased with a nonstick cooking spray.

✓ In a mixing bowl, thoroughly combine the remaining ingredients. Sprinkle this topping over the apricot layer.

✓ Bake your crumble in the preheated Air Fryer at 330 degrees F for 35 minutes. Bon appétit!

Nutritions: 192 Calories; 7.9g Fat; 29.1g Carbs; 1.7g Protein; 17.7g Sugars

771)   *Easy Monkey Rolls*
Ingredients

- 8 ounces refrigerated buttermilk biscuit dough
- 1/2 cup brown sugar
- 4 ounces butter, melted
- 1/4 teaspoon grated nutmeg
- 1/2 teaspoon ground cinnamon

- 1/4 teaspoon ground cardamom

Directions(Ready in about 25 minutes | Servings 4)

✓ Spritz 4 standard-size muffin cups with a nonstick spray. Thoroughly combine the brown sugar with the melted butter, nutmeg, cinnamon and cardamom.

✓ Spoon the butter mixture into muffins cups.

✓ Separate the dough into biscuits and divide your biscuits between muffin cups.

✓ Bake the Monkey rolls at 340 degrees F for about 15 minutes or until golden brown. Turn upside down just before serving. Bon appétit!

Nutritions: 432 Calories; 29.3g Fat; 40.1g Carbs; 4.1g Protein; 16.8g Sugars

772) *Sherry Roasted Sweet Cherries*

Ingredients

- 2 cups dark cherries
- 1/4 cup granulated sugar
- 1 tablespoon honey
- 3 tablespoons sherry
- A pinch of sea salt
- A pinch of grated nutmeg

Directions (Ready in about 35 minutes | Servings 4)

✓ Arrange your cherries in the bottom of a lightly greased baking dish.

✓ Whisk the remaining ingredients; spoon this mixture into the baking dish.

✓ Air fry your cherries at 370 degrees F for 35 minutes. Bon appétit!

Nutritions: 53 Calories; 0.3g Fat; 11.1g Carbs; 0.1g Protein; 11.2g Sugars

773) *Greek Roasted Figs with Yiaourti me Meli*

Ingredients

- 1 teaspoon coconut oil, melted
- 6 medium-sized figs
- 1/4 teaspoon ground cardamom
- 1/4 teaspoon ground cloves
- 1/4 teaspoon ground cinnamon
- 3 tablespoon honey
- 1/2 cup Greek yogurt

Directions (Ready in about 20 minutes | Servings 3)

✓ Drizzle the melted coconut oil all over your figs.

✓ Sprinkle cardamom, cloves and cinnamon over your figs.

✓ Roast your figs in the preheated Air Fryer at 330 degrees F for 15 to 16 minutes, shaking the basket occasionally to promote even cooking.

✓ In the meantime, thoroughly combine the honey with the Greek yogurt to make the yiaourti me meli.

✓ Divide the roasted figs between 3 serving bowls and serve with a dollop of yiaourti me meli. Enjoy!

Nutritions: 169 Calories; 1.9g Fat; 37.1g Carbs; 3.7g Protein; 34.3g Sugars

774) *Apple Fries with Snickerdoodle Dip*

Ingredients

- 1 Gala apple, cored and sliced
- 1 teaspoon peanut oil
- 1 teaspoon butter, room temperature
- 2 ounces cream cheese, room temperature
- 2 ounces Greek yogurt
- 2 ounces caster sugar
- 1 teaspoon ground cinnamon

Directions (Ready in about 10 minutes | Servings 2)

✓ Drizzle peanut oil all over the apple slices; transfer the apple slices to the Air Fryer.

✓ Bake the apple slices at 350 degrees F for 5 minutes; shake the basket and continue cooking an additional 5 minutes.

✓ In the meantime, mix the remaining ingredients until everything is well incorporated.

✓ Serve the apple fries with Snickerdoodle dip on the side. Bon appétit!

Nutritions: 309 Calories; 14.1g Fat; 43g Carbs; 4.7g Protein; 39g Sugars

775) *Panettone Pudding Tart*

Ingredients

- 3 cups panettone bread, crusts trimmed, bread cut into 1-inch cubes
- 1/2 cup creme fraiche
- 1/2 cup coconut milk
- 2 tablespoons orange marmalade
- 1 tablespoon butter
- 2 tablespoons amaretto liqueur
- 1/2 teaspoon vanilla extract
- 1/4 cup sugar
- A pinch of grated nutmeg
- A pinch of sea salt
- 1 egg, whisked

Directions (Ready in about 45 minutes | Servings 3)

✓ Put the panettone bread cubes into a lightly greased baking pan.

✓ Then, make the custard by mixing the remaining ingredients.

✓ Pour the custard over your panettone. Let it rest for 30 minutes, pressing with a wide spatula to submerge.

✓ Cook the panettone pudding in the preheated Air Fryer at 370 degrees F degrees for 7 minutes; rotate the pan and cook an additional 5 to 6 minutes. Bon appétit!

Nutritions: 326 Calories; 13.6g Fat; 37.3g Carbs; 8.7g Protein; 17.8g Sugars

776) *Dessert French Toast with Blackberries*

Ingredients

- 2 tablespoons butter, at room temperature
- 1 egg

- 2 tablespoons granulated sugar
- 1/4 teaspoon ground cinnamon
- 1/4 teaspoon vanilla extract
- 6 slices French baguette
- 1 cup fresh blackberries
- 2 tablespoons powdered sugar

Direction (Ready in about 20 minutes | Servings 2)

✓ Start by preheating your Air Fryer to 375 degrees F.

✓ In a mixing dish, whisk the butter, egg, granulated sugar, cinnamon and vanilla.

✓ Dip all the slices of the French baguette in this mixture. Transfer the French toast to the baking pan.

✓ Bake in the preheated Air Fryer for 8 minutes, turning them over halfway through the cooking time to ensure even cooking.

✓ To serve, divide the French toast between two warm plates. Arrange the blackberries on top of each slice. Dust with powdered sugar and serve immediately. Enjoy!

Nutritions: 324 Calories; 14.9g Fat; 42.2g Carbs; 6.5g Protein; 24.9g Sugars

777)   *Chocolate Lava Cake*

Ingredients

- 4 ounces butter, melted
- 4 ounces dark chocolate
- 2 eggs, lightly whisked
- 4 tablespoons granulated sugar
- 2 tablespoons cake flour
- 1 teaspoon baking powder
- 1/2 teaspoon ground cinnamon
- 1/4 teaspoon ground star anise

Directions(Ready in about 20 minutes | Servings 4)

- Begin by preheating your Air Fryer to 370 degrees F. Spritz the sides and bottom of a baking pan with nonstick cooking spray.

- Melt the butter and dark chocolate in a microwave-safe bowl. Mix the eggs and sugar until frothy.

- Pour the butter/chocolate mixture into the egg mixture. Stir in the flour, baking powder, cinnamon, and star anise. Mix until everything is well incorporated.

- Scrape the batter into the prepared pan. Bake in the preheated Air Fryer for 9 to 11 minutes.

- Let stand for 2 minutes. Invert on a plate while warm and serve. Bon appétit!

Nutritions: 450 Calories; 37.2g Fat; 24.2g Carbs; 5.6g Protein; 14.7g Sugars

778)   *Banana Chips with Chocolate Glaze*

Ingredients

- 2 banana, cut into slices
- 1/4 teaspoon lemon zest
- 1 tablespoon agave syrup
- 1 tablespoon cocoa powder

- 1 tablespoon coconut oil, melted

Directions (Ready in about 20 minutes | Servings 2)

✓ Toss the bananas with the lemon zest and agave syrup. Transfer your bananas to the parchment-lined cooking basket.

✓ Bake in the preheated Air Fryer at 370 degrees F for 12 minutes, turning them over halfway through the cooking time.

✓ In the meantime, melt the coconut oil in your microwave; add the cocoa powder and whisk to combine well.

✓ Serve the baked banana chips with a few drizzles of the chocolate glaze. Enjoy!

Nutritions: 201 Calories; 7.5g Fat; 37.1g Carbs; 1.8g Protein; 22.9g Sugars

779)   *Grandma's Butter Cookies*

Ingredients

- 8 ounces all-purpose flour
- 2 ½ ounces sugar
- 1 teaspoon baking powder
- A pinch of grated nutmeg
- A pinch of coarse salt
- 1 large egg, room temperature.
- 1 stick butter, room temperature
- 1 teaspoon vanilla extract

Directions (Ready in about 25 minutes | Servings 4)

✓ Mix the flour, sugar, baking powder, grated nutmeg, and salt in a bowl. In a separate bowl, whisk the egg, butter, and vanilla extract.

✓ Stir the egg mixture into the flour mixture; mix to combine well or until it forms a nice, soft dough.

✓ Roll your dough out and cut out with a cookie cutter of your choice.

✓ Bake in the preheated Air Fryer at 350 degrees F for 10 minutes. Decrease the temperature to 330 degrees F and cook for 10 minutes longer.

Nutritions: 492 Calories; 24.7g Fat; 61.1g Carbs; 6.7g Protein; 17.5g Sugars

780)   *Cinnamon Dough Dippers*

Ingredients

- 1/2 pound bread dough
- 1/4 cup butter, melted
- 1/2 cup caster sugar
- 1 tablespoon cinnamon
- 1/2 cup cream cheese, softened
- 1 cup powdered sugar
- 1/2 teaspoon vanilla
- 2 tablespoons milk

Directions (Ready in about 20 minutes | Servings 6)

✓ Roll the dough into a log; cut into 1-1/2 inch strips using a pizza cutter.

✓ Mix the butter, sugar, and cinnamon in a small bowl. Use a rubber spatula to spread the butter mixture over the tops of the dough dippers.

✓ Bake at 360 degrees F for 7 to 8 minutes, turning them over halfway through the cooking time. Work in batches.

✓ Meanwhile, make the glaze dip by whisking the remaining ingredients with a hand mixer. Beat until a smooth consistency is reached.

✓ Serve at room temperature and enjoy!

Nutritions: 332 Calories; 14.8g Fat; 45.6g Carbs; 5.1g Protein; 27.6g Sugars

781)   *Chocolate Apple Chips*

Ingredients

- 1 large Pink Lady apple, cored and sliced
- 1 tablespoon light brown sugar
- A pinch of kosher salt
- 2 tablespoons lemon juice
- 2 teaspoons cocoa powder

Directions (Ready in about 15 minutes | Servings 2)

✓ Toss the apple slices with the other ingredients.

✓ Bake at 350 degrees F for 5 minutes; shake the basket to ensure even cooking and continue to cook an additional 5 minutes.

✓ Bon appétit!

Nutritions: 81 Calories; 0.5g Fat; 21.5g Carbs; 0.7g Protein; 15.9g Sugars

782)   *Favorite Apple Crisp*

Ingredients

- 4 cups apples, peeled, cored and sliced
- 1/2 cup brown sugar
- 1 tablespoon honey
- 1 tablespoon cornmeal
- 1/4 teaspoon ground cloves
- 1/2 teaspoon ground cinnamon
- 1/4 cup water
- 1/2 cup quick-cooking oats
- 1/2 cup all-purpose flour
- 1/2 cup caster sugar
- 1/2 teaspoon baking powder
- 1/3 cup coconut oil, melted

Directions(Ready in about 40 minutes | Servings 4)

✓ Toss the sliced apples with the brown sugar, honey, cornmeal, cloves, and cinnamon. Divide between four custard cups coated with cooking spray.

✓ In a mixing dish, thoroughly combine the remaining ingredients. Sprinkle over the apple mixture.

✓ Bake in the preheated Air Fryer at 330 degrees F for 35 minutes. Bon appétit!

Nutritions: 403 Calories; 18.6g Fat; 61.5g Carbs; 2.9g Protein; 40.2g Sugars

783)   *Peppermint Chocolate Cheesecake*

Ingredients

- 1 cup powdered sugar
- 1/2 cup all-purpose flour
- 1/2 cup butter
- 1 cup mascarpone cheese, at room temperature
- 4 ounces semisweet chocolate, melted
- 1 teaspoon vanilla extract
- 2 drops peppermint extract

Directions (Ready in about 40 minutes | Servings 6)

✓ Beat the sugar, flour, and butter in a mixing bowl. Press the mixture into the bottom of a lightly greased baking pan.

✓ Bake at 350 degrees F for 18 minutes. Place it in your freezer for 20 minutes.

✓ Then, make the cheesecake topping by mixing the remaining ingredients. Place this topping over the crust and allow it to cool in your freezer for a further 15 minutes. Serve well chilled.

Nutritions: 484 Calories; 36.7g Fat; 38.8g Carbs; 5g Protein; 22.2g Sugars

784)   *Baked Coconut Doughnuts*

Ingredients

- 1 ½ cups all-purpose flour
- 1 teaspoon baking powder
- A pinch of kosher salt
- A pinch of freshly grated nutmeg
- 1/2 cup white sugar
- 2 eggs
- 2 tablespoons full-fat coconut milk
- 2 tablespoons coconut oil, melted
- 1/4 teaspoon ground cardamom
- 1/4 teaspoon ground cinnamon
- 1 teaspoon coconut essence
- 1/2 teaspoon vanilla essence
- 1 cup coconut flakes

Directions (Ready in about 20 minutes | Servings 6)

✓ In a mixing bowl, thoroughly combine the all-purpose flour with the baking powder, salt, nutmeg, and sugar.

✓ In a separate bowl, beat the eggs until frothy using a hand mixer; add the coconut milk and oil and beat again; lastly, stir in the spices and mix again until everything is well combined.

✓ Then, stir the egg mixture into the flour mixture and continue mixing until a dough ball forms. Try not to over-mix your dough. Transfer to a lightly floured surface.

✓ Roll out your dough to a 1/4-inch thickness using a rolling pin. Cut out the doughnuts using a 3-inch round cutter; now, use a 1-inch round cutter to remove the center.

✓ Bake in the preheated Air Fryer at 340 degrees F approximately 5 minutes or until golden. Repeat with remaining doughnuts. Decorate with coconut flakes and serve.

Nutritions: 305 Calories; 13.2g Fat; 40.1g Carbs; 6.7g Protein; 13.8g Sugars

785)   *Classic Vanilla Mini Cheesecakes*

Ingredients

- 1/2 cup almond flour
- 1 ½ tablespoons unsalted butter, melted

- 1 tablespoon white sugar
- 1 (8-ounce) package cream cheese, softened
- 1/4 cup powdered sugar
- 1/2 teaspoon vanilla paste
- 1 egg, at room temperature
- Topping:
- 1 ½ cups sour cream
- 3 tablespoons white sugar
- 1 teaspoon vanilla extract
- 1/4 cup maraschino cherries

Directions (Ready in about 40 minutes + chilling time | Servings 6)

✓ Thoroughly combine the almond flour, butter, and sugar in a mixing bowl. Press the mixture into the bottom of lightly greased custard cups.

✓ Then, mix the cream cheese, 1/4 cup of powdered sugar, vanilla, and egg using an electric mixer on low speed. Pour the batter into the pan, covering the crust.

✓ Bake in the preheated Air Fryer at 330 degrees F for 35 minutes until edges are puffed and the surface is firm.

✓ Mix the sour cream, 3 tablespoons of white sugar, and vanilla for the topping; spread over the crust and allow it to cool to room temperature.

✓ Transfer to your refrigerator for 6 to 8 hours. Decorate with maraschino cherries and serve well chilled.

Nutritions: 321 Calories; 25g Fat; 17.1g Carbs; 8.1g Protein; 11.4g Sugars

786) *Bakery-Style Hazelnut Cookies*

Ingredients

- 1 ½ cups all-purpose flour
- 1 teaspoon baking soda
- 1 teaspoon fine sea salt
- 1 stick butter
- 1 cup brown sugar
- 2 teaspoons vanilla
- 2 eggs, at room temperature
- 1 cup hazelnuts, coarsely chopped

Directions (Ready in about 20 minutes | Servings 6)

✓ Begin by preheating your Air Fryer to 350 degrees F.

✓ Mix the flour with the baking soda, and sea salt.

✓ In the bowl of an electric mixer, beat the butter, brown sugar, and vanilla until creamy. Fold in the eggs, one at a time, and mix until well combined.

✓ Slowly and gradually, stir in the flour mixture. Finally, fold in the coarsely chopped hazelnuts.

✓ Divide the dough into small balls using a large cookie scoop; drop onto the prepared cookie sheets. Bake for 10 minutes or until golden brown, rotating the pan once or twice through the cooking time.

✓ Work in batches and cool for a couple of minutes before removing to wire racks. Enjoy!

Nutritions: 450 Calories; 28.6g Fat; 43.9g Carbs; 8.1g Protein; 17.5g Sugars

787) *Chocolate Biscuit Sandwich Cookies*

Ingredients

- 2 ½ cups self-rising flour
- 4 ounces brown sugar
- 1 ounce honey
- 5 ounces butter, softened
- 1 egg, beaten
- 1 teaspoon vanilla essence
- 4 ounces double cream
- 3 ounces dark chocolate
- 1 teaspoon cardamom seeds, finely crushed

Directions (Ready in about 20 minutes |Servings 10)

✓ Start by preheating your Air Fryer to 350 degrees F.

✓ In a mixing bowl, thoroughly combine the flour, brown sugar, honey, and butter. Mix until your mixture resembles breadcrumbs.

✓ Gradually, add the egg and vanilla essence. Shape your dough into small balls and place in the parchment-lined Air Fryer basket.

✓ Bake in the preheated Air Fryer for 10 minutes. Rotate the pan and bake for another 5 minutes. Transfer the freshly baked cookies to a cooling rack.

✓ As the biscuits are cooling, melt the double cream and dark chocolate in an air-fryer safe bowl at 350 degrees F. Add the cardamom seeds and stir well.

✓ Spread the filling over the cooled biscuits and sandwich together. Bon appétit!

Nutritions: 353 Calories; 18.6g Fat; 41.4g Carbs; 5.1g Protein; 16.1g Sugars

788) *Easy Chocolate Brownies*

Ingredients

- 1 stick butter, melted
- 1/2 cup caster sugar
- 1/2 cup white sugar
- 1 egg
- 1 teaspoon vanilla essence
- 1/2 cup all-purpose flour
- 1 teaspoon baking powder
- 1/2 cup cocoa powder
- A pinch of salt
- A pinch of ground cardamom

Directions (Ready in about 30 minutes | Servings 8)

✓ Start by preheating your Air Fryer to 350 degrees F. Now, spritz the sides and bottom of a baking pan with cooking spray.

✓ In a mixing dish, beat the melted butter with sugar until fluffy. Next, fold in the egg and beat again.

✓ After that, add the vanilla, flour, baking powder, cocoa, salt, and ground cardamom. Mix until everything is well combined.

✓ Bake in the preheated Air Fryer for 20 to 22 minutes. Enjoy!

Nutritions: 200 Calories; 12.7g Fat; 21.7g Carbs; 2.5g Protein; 12.4g Sugars

789) *Light and Fluffy Chocolate Cake*

Ingredients

- 1/2 stick butter, at room temperature
- 1/2 cup chocolate chips
- 2 tablespoons honey
- 2/3 cup almond flour
- A pinch of fine sea salt
- 1 egg, whisked
- 1/2 teaspoon vanilla extract

Directions (Ready in about 20 minutes | Servings 6)

- ✓ Begin by preheating your Air Fryer to 330 degrees F.
- ✓ In a microwave-safe bowl, melt the butter, chocolate, and honey.
- ✓ Add the other ingredients to the cooled chocolate mixture; stir to combine well. Scrape the batter into a lightly greased baking pan.
- ✓ Bake in the preheated Air Fryer for 15 minutes or until the center is springy and a toothpick comes out dry. Enjoy!

Nutritions: 242 Calories; 19.5g Fat; 13.6g Carbs; 4.7g Protein; 9.2g Sugars

790) *Cinnamon and Sugar Sweet Potato Fries*

Ingredients

- 1 large sweet potato, peeled and sliced into sticks
- 1 teaspoon ghee
- 1 tablespoon cornstarch
- 1/4 teaspoon ground cardamom
- 1/4 cup sugar
- 1 tablespoon ground cinnamon

Directions (Ready in about 30 minutes | Servings 2)

- ✓ Toss the sweet potato sticks with the melted ghee and cornstarch.
- ✓ Cook in the preheated Air Fryer at 380 degrees F for 20 minutes, shaking the basket halfway through the cooking time.
- ✓ Sprinkle the cardamom, sugar, and cinnamon all over the sweet potato fries and serve. Bon appétit!

Nutritions: 162 Calories; 2.1g Fat; 34.9g Carbs; 1.8g Protein; 18.1g Sugars

791) *Easy Blueberry Muffins*

Ingredients

- 1 ½ cups all-purpose flour
- 1/2 teaspoon baking soda
- 1 teaspoon baking powder
- 1/4 teaspoon kosher salt
- 1/2 cup granulated sugar
- 2 eggs, whisked
- 1/2 cup milk
- 1/4 cup coconut oil, melted
- 1/2 teaspoon vanilla paste
- 1 cup fresh blueberries

Directions (Ready in about 20 minutes |Servings 10)

- ✓ In a mixing bowl, combine the flour, baking soda, baking powder, sugar, and salt. Whisk to combine well.
- ✓ In another mixing bowl, mix the eggs, milk, coconut oil, and vanilla.
- ✓ Now, add the wet egg mixture to dry the flour mixture. Then, carefully fold in the fresh blueberries; gently stir to combine.
- ✓ Scrape the batter mixture into the muffin cups. Bake your muffins at 350 degrees F for 12 minutes or until the tops are golden brown.
- ✓ Sprinkle some extra icing sugar over the top of each muffin if desired. Serve and enjoy!

Nutritions: 191 Calories; 8g Fat; 25.7g Carbs; 4.3g Protein; 10.9g Sugars

792) *Chocolate Raspberry Wontons*

Ingredients

- 1 (12-ounce) package wonton wrappers
- 6 ounces chocolate chips
- 1/2 cup raspberries, mashed
- 1 egg, lightly whisked + 1 tablespoon of water (egg wash)
- 1/4 cup caster sugar

Directions (Ready in about 15 minutes | Servings 6)

- ✓ Divide the chocolate chips and raspberries among the wonton wrappers. Now, fold the wrappers diagonally in half over the filling; press the edges with a fork.
- ✓ Brush with the egg wash and seal the edges.
- ✓ Bake at 370 degrees F for 8 minutes, flipping them halfway through the cooking time.
- ✓ Work in batches. Sprinkle the caster sugar over your wontons and enjoy!

Nutritions: 356 Calories; 13g Fat; 51.2g Carbs; 7.9g Protein; 11.3g Sugars

793) *Country Pie with Walnuts*

Ingredients

- 1 cup coconut milk
- 2 eggs
- 1/2 stick butter, at room temperature
- 1 teaspoon vanilla essence
- 1/4 teaspoon ground cardamom
- 1/4 teaspoon ground cloves
- 1/2 cup walnuts, ground
- 1/2 cup sugar
- 1/3 cup almond flour

Directions (Ready in about 20 minutes | Servings 6)

- ✓ Begin by preheating your Air Fryer to 360 degrees F. Spritz the sides and bottom of a baking pan with nonstick cooking spray.
- ✓ Mix all ingredients until well combined. Scrape the batter into the prepared baking pan.
- ✓ Bake approximately 13 minutes; use a toothpick to test for doneness. Bon appétit!

Nutritions: 244 Calories; 19.1g Fat; 12.7g Carbs; 6.5g Protein; 10.9g Sugars

794) *Cocktail Party Fruit Kabobs*

Ingredients

- 2 pears, diced into bite-sized chunks
- 2 apples, diced into bite-sized chunks
- 2 mangos, diced into bite-sized chunks
- 1 tablespoon fresh lemon juice
- 1 teaspoon vanilla essence
- 2 tablespoons maple syrup
- 1 teaspoon ground cinnamon
- 1/2 teaspoon ground cloves

Directions (Ready in about 10 minutes | Servings 6)

- ✓ Toss all ingredients in a mixing dish.
- ✓ Tread the fruit pieces on skewers.
- ✓ Cook at 350 degrees F for 5 minutes. Bon appétit!

Nutritions: 165 Calories; 0.7g Fat; 41.8g Carbs; 1.6g Protein; 33.6g Sugars

795) *Sunday Banana Chocolate Cookies*

Ingredients

- 1 stick butter, at room temperature
- 1 ¼ cups caster sugar
- 2 ripe bananas, mashed
- 1 teaspoon vanilla paste
- 1 2/3 cups all-purpose flour
- 1/3 cup cocoa powder
- 1 ½ teaspoons baking powder
- 1/4 teaspoon ground cinnamon
- 1/4 teaspoon crystallized ginger
- 1 ½ cups chocolate chips

Directions (Ready in about 20 minutes | Servings 8)

- ✓ In a mixing dish, beat the butter and sugar until creamy and uniform. Stir in the mashed bananas and vanilla.
- ✓ In another mixing dish, thoroughly combine the flour, cocoa powder, baking powder, cinnamon, and crystallized ginger.
- ✓ Add the flour mixture to the banana mixture; mix to combine well. Afterwards, fold in the chocolate chips.
- ✓ Drop by large spoonfuls onto a parchment-lined Air Fryer basket. Bake at 365 degrees F for 11 minutes or until golden brown on the top. Bon appétit!

Nutritions: 298 Calories; 12.3g Fat; 45.9g Carbs; 3.8g Protein; 19.6g Sugars

796) *Rustic Baked Apples*

Ingredients

- 4 Gala apples
- 1/4 cup rolled oats
- 1/4 cup sugar
- 2 tablespoons honey
- 1/3 cup walnuts, chopped
- 1 teaspoon cinnamon powder
- 1/2 teaspoon ground cardamom
- 1/2 teaspoon ground cloves
- 2/3 cup water

Directions (Ready in about 25 minutes | Servings 4)

- ✓ Use a paring knife to remove the stem and seeds from the apples, making deep holes.
- ✓ In a mixing bowl, combine together the rolled oats, sugar, honey, walnuts, cinnamon, cardamom, and cloves.
- ✓ Pour the water into an Air Fryer safe dish. Place the apples in the dish.
- ✓ Bake at 340 degrees F for 17 minutes. Serve at room temperature. Bon appétit!

Nutritions: 211 Calories; 5.1g Fat; 45.5g Carbs; 2.6g Protein; 33.9g Sugars

797) *The Ultimate Berry Crumble*

Ingredients

- 18 ounces cherries
- 1/2 cup granulated sugar
- 2 tablespoons cornmeal
- 1/4 teaspoon ground star anise
- 1/2 teaspoon ground cinnamon
- 2/3 cup all-purpose flour
- 1 cup demerara sugar
- 1/2 teaspoon baking powder
- 1/3 cup rolled oats
- 1/2 stick butter, cut into small pieces

Directions (Ready in about 40 minutes | Servings 6)

- ✓ Toss the cherries with the granulated sugar, cornmeal, star anise, and cinnamon. Divide between six custard cups coated with cooking spray.
- ✓ In a mixing dish, thoroughly combine the remaining ingredients. Sprinkle over the berry mixture.
- ✓ Bake in the preheated Air Fryer at 330 degrees F for 35 minutes. Bon appétit!

Nutritions: 272 Calories; 8.3g Fat; 49.5g Carbs; 3.3g Protein; 31g Sugars

798) *Mocha Chocolate Espresso Cake*

Ingredients

- 1 ½ cups flour
- 2/3 cup sugar
- 1 teaspoon baking powder
- 1/4 teaspoon salt
- 1 stick butter, melted
- 1/2 cup hot strongly brewed coffee
- 1/2 teaspoon vanilla
- 1 egg
- Topping:
- 1/4 cup flour
- 1/2 cup sugar
- 1/2 teaspoon ground cardamom
- 1 teaspoon ground cinnamon
- 3 tablespoons coconut oil

Directions (Ready in about 40 minutes | Servings 8)

- Mix all dry ingredients for your cake; then, mix in the wet ingredients. Mix until everything is well incorporated.
- Spritz a baking pan with cooking spray. Scrape the batter into the baking pan.
- Then make the topping by mixing all ingredients. Place on top of the cake. Smooth the top with a spatula.
- Bake at 330 degrees F for 30 minutes or until the top of the cake springs back when gently pressed with your fingers. Serve with your favorite hot beverage. Bon appétit!

Nutritions: 320 Calories; 18.1g Fat; 35.9g Carbs; 4.1g Protein; 14.5g Sugars

799) *Chocolate and Peanut Butter Brownies*
Ingredients

- 1 cup peanut butter
- 1 ¼ cups sugar
- 3 eggs
- 1 cup all-purpose flour
- 1 teaspoon baking powder
- 1/4 teaspoon kosher salt
- 1 cup dark chocolate, broken into chunks

Directions (Ready in about 30 minutes |Servings 10)

- Start by preheating your Air Fryer to 350 degrees F. Now, spritz the sides and bottom of a baking pan with cooking spray.
- In a mixing dish, thoroughly combine the peanut butter with the sugar until creamy. Next, fold in the egg and beat until fluffy.
- After that, stir in the flour, baking powder, salt, and chocolate. Mix until everything is well combined.
- Bake in the preheated Air Fryer for 20 to 22 minutes. Transfer to a wire rack to cool before slicing and serving. Bon appétit!

Nutritions: 291 Calories; 7.9g Fat; 48.2g Carbs; 6.4g Protein; 32.3g Sugars

800) *Coconut Chip Cookies*
Ingredients

- 1 cup butter, melted
- 1 ¾ cups granulated sugar
- 3 eggs
- 2 tablespoons coconut milk
- 1 teaspoon coconut extract
- 1 teaspoon vanilla extract
- 2 ¼ cups all-purpose flour
- 1/2 teaspoon baking powder
- 1/2 teaspoon baking soda
- 1/2 teaspoon fine table salt
- 2 cups coconut chips

Directions (Ready in about 20 minutes | Servings 12)

- Begin by preheating your Air Fryer to 350 F.

- In the bowl of an electric mixer, beat the butter and sugar until well combined. Now, add the eggs one at a time, and mix well; add the coconut milk, coconut extract, and vanilla; beat until creamy and uniform.
- Mix the flour with baking powder, baking soda, and salt. Then, stir the flour mixture into the butter mixture and stir until everything is well incorporated.
- Finally, fold in the coconut chips and mix again. Scoop out 1 tablespoon size balls of the batter on a cookie pan, leaving 2 inches between each cookie.
- Bake for 10 minutes or until golden brown, rotating the pan once or twice through the cooking time.
- Let your cookies cool on wire racks. Bon appétit!

Nutritions: 304 Calories; 16.7g Fat; 34.2g Carbs; 4.3g Protein; 15.6g Sugars

801) *Easy Chocolate and Coconut Cake*
Ingredients

- 1 stick butter
- 1 ¼ cups dark chocolate, broken into chunks
- 1/4 cup tablespoon agave syrup
- 1/4 cup sugar
- 2 tablespoons milk
- 2 eggs, beaten
- 1/3 cup coconut, shredded

Directions (Ready in about 20 minutes |Servings 10)

- Begin by preheating your Air Fryer to 330 degrees F.
- In a microwave-safe bowl, melt the butter, chocolate, and agave syrup. Allow it to cool to room temperature.
- Add the remaining ingredients to the chocolate mixture; stir to combine well. Scrape the batter into a lightly greased baking pan.
- Bake in the preheated Air Fryer for 15 minutes or until a toothpick comes out dry and clean. Enjoy!

Nutritions: 252 Calories; 18.9g Fat; 17.9g Carbs; 3.4g Protein; 13.8g Sugars

802) *Grilled Banana Boats*
Ingredients

- 3 large bananas
- 1 tablespoon ginger snaps
- 2 tablespoons mini chocolate chips
- 3 tablespoons mini marshmallows
- 3 tablespoons crushed vanilla wafers

Directions (Ready in about 15 minutes | Servings 3)

- In the peel, slice your banana lengthwise; make sure not to slice all the way through the banana. Divide the remaining ingredients between the banana pockets.
- Place in the Air Fryer grill pan. Cook at 395 degrees F for 7 minutes.
- Let the banana boats cool for 5 to 6 minutes, and then eat with a spoon. Bon appétit!

Nutritions: 269 Calories; 5.9g Fat; 47.9g Carbs; 2.6g Protein; 28.3g Sugars

803) Chocolate Birthday Cake

Ingredients

- 2 eggs, beaten
- 2/3 cup sour cream
- 1 cup flour
- 1/2 cup sugar
- 1/4 cup honey
- 1/3 cup coconut oil, softened
- 1/4 cup cocoa powder
- 2 tablespoons chocolate chips
- 1 ½ teaspoons baking powder
- 1 teaspoon vanilla extract
- 1/2 teaspoon pure rum extract
- Chocolate Frosting:
- 1/2 cup butter, softened
- 1/4 cup cocoa powder
- 2 cups powdered sugar
- 2 tablespoons milk

Directions (Ready in about 35 minutes +chilling time | Servings 6)

- ✓ Mix all ingredients for the chocolate cake with a hand mixer on low speed. Scrape the batter into a cake pan.
- ✓ Bake at 330 degrees F for 25 to 30 minutes. Transfer the cake to a wire rack
- ✓ Meanwhile, whip the butter and cocoa until smooth. Stir in the powdered sugar. Slowly and gradually, pour in the milk until your frosting reaches desired consistency.
- ✓ Whip until smooth and fluffy; then, frost the cooled cake. Place in your refrigerator for a couple of hours. Serve well chilled.

Nutritions: 689 Calories; 43.4g Fat; 76.1g Carbs; 6.5g Protein; 55.6g Sugars

804) Favorite New York Cheesecake

Ingredients

- 1 ½ cups digestive biscuits crumbs
- 2 ounces white sugar
- 1 ounce demerara sugar
- 1/2 stick butter, melted
- 32 ounces full-fat cream cheese
- 1/2 cup heavy cream
- 1 ¼ cups caster sugar
- 3 eggs, at room temperature
- 1 tablespoon vanilla essence
- 1 teaspoon grated lemon zest

Directions (Ready in about 40 minutes + chilling time | Servings 8)

- ✓ Coat the sides and bottom of a baking pan with a little flour.
- ✓ In a mixing bowl, combine the digestive biscuits, white sugar, and demerara sugar. Add the melted butter and mix until your mixture looks like breadcrumbs.
- ✓ Press the mixture into the bottom of the prepared pan to form an even layer. Bake at 330 degrees F for 7 minutes until golden brown. Allow it to cool completely on a wire rack.
- ✓ Meanwhile, in a mixer fitted with the paddle attachment, prepare the filling by mixing the soft cheese, heavy cream, and caster sugar; beat until creamy and fluffy.
- ✓ Crack the eggs into the mixing bowl, one at a time; add the vanilla and lemon zest and continue to mix until fully combined.
- ✓ Pour the prepared topping over the cooled crust and spread evenly.
- ✓ Bake in the preheated Air Fryer at 330 degrees F for 25 to 30 minutes; leave it in the Air Fryer to keep warm for another 30 minutes.
- ✓ Cover your cheesecake with plastic wrap. Place in your refrigerator and allow it to cool at least 6 hours or overnight. Serve well chilled.

Nutritions: 477 Calories; 30.2g Fat; 39.5g Carbs; 12.8g Protein; 32.9g Sugars

805) English-Style Scones with Raisins

Ingredients

- 1 ½ cups all-purpose flour
- 1/4 cup brown sugar
- 1 teaspoon baking powder
- 1/4 teaspoon sea salt
- 1/4 teaspoon ground cloves
- 1/2 teaspoon ground cardamom
- 1 teaspoon ground cinnamon
- 1/2 cup raisins
- 6 tablespoons butter, cooled and sliced
- 1/2 cup double cream
- 2 eggs, lightly whisked
- 1/2 teaspoon vanilla essence

Directions(Ready in about 20 minutes | Servings 6)

- ✓ In a mixing bowl, thoroughly combine the flour, sugar, baking powder, salt, cloves, cardamom cinnamon, and raisins. Mix until everything is combined well.
- ✓ Add the butter and mix again.
- ✓ In another mixing bowl, combine the double cream with the eggs and vanilla; beat until creamy and smooth.
- ✓ Stir the wet ingredients into the dry mixture. Roll your dough out into a circle and cut into wedges.
- ✓ Bake in the preheated Air Fryer at 360 degrees for 11 minutes, rotating the pan halfway through the cooking time. Bon appétit!

Nutritions: 317 Calories; 18.9g Fat; 29.5g Carbs; 6.9g Protein; 5.2g Sugars

806) Baked Peaches with Oatmeal Pecan Streusel

Ingredients

- 2 tablespoons old-fashioned rolled oats
- 3 tablespoons golden caster sugar

- 1/2 teaspoon ground cinnamon
- 1 egg
- 2 tablespoons cold salted butter, cut into pieces
- 3 tablespoons pecans, chopped
- 3 large ripe freestone peaches, halved and pitted

Directions (Ready in about 20 minutes | Servings 3)

✓ Mix the rolled oats, sugar, cinnamon, egg, and butter until well combined.

✓ Add a big spoonful of prepared topping to the center of each peach. Pour 1/2 cup of water into an Air Fryer safe dish. Place the peaches in the dish.

✓ Top the peaches with the roughly chopped pecans. Bake at 340 degrees F for 17 minutes. Serve at room temperature. Bon appétit!

Nutritions: 247 Calories; 14.1g Fat; 28.8g Carbs; 5.9g Protein; 23.1g Sugars

807)   *Red Velvet Pancakes*

Ingredients

- 1/2 cup flour
- 1 teaspoon baking powder
- 1/4 teaspoon salt
- 2 tablespoons white sugar
- 1/2 teaspoon cinnamon
- 1 teaspoon red paste food color
- 1 egg
- 1/2 cup milk
- 1 teaspoon vanilla
- Topping:
- 2 ounces cream cheese, softened
- 2 tablespoons butter, softened
- 3/4 cup powdered sugar

Directions (Ready in about 35 minutes | Servings 3)

✓ Mix the flour, baking powder, salt, sugar, cinnamon, red paste food color in a large bowl.

✓ Gradually add the egg and milk, whisking continuously, until well combined. Let it stand for 20 minutes.

✓ Spritz the Air Fryer baking pan with cooking spray. Pour the batter into the pan using a measuring cup.

✓ Cook at 230 degrees F for 4 to 5 minutes or until golden brown. Repeat with the remaining batter.

✓ Meanwhile, make your topping by mixing the ingredients until creamy and fluffy. Decorate your pancakes with topping. Bon appétit!

Nutritions: 392 Calories; 17.8g Fat; 50g Carbs; 7.8g Protein; 33.2g Sugars

808)   *Nana's Famous Apple Fritters*

Ingredients

- 2/3 cup all-purpose flour
- 3 tablespoons granulated sugar
- A pinch of sea salt
- A pinch of freshly grated nutmeg
- 1 teaspoon baking powder

- 2 eggs, whisked
- 1/4 cup milk
- 2 apples, peeled, cored and diced
- 1/2 cup powdered sugar

Directions (Ready in about 20 minutes | Servings 4)

✓ Mix the flour, sugar, salt, nutmeg and baking powder.

✓ In a separate bowl whisk the eggs with the milk; add this wet mixture into the dry ingredients; mix to combine well.

✓ Add the apple pieces and mix again.

✓ Cook in the preheated Air Fryer at 370 degrees for 3 minutes, flipping them halfway through the cooking time. Repeat with the remaining batter.

✓ Dust with powdered sugar and serve at room temperature. Bon appétit!

Nutritions: 280 Calories; 5.7g Fat; 51.1g Carbs; 7.4g Protein; 30.8g Sugars

809)   *Authentic Indian Gulgulas*

Ingredients

- 1 banana, mashed
- 1/4 cup sugar
- 1 egg
- 1/2 teaspoon vanilla essence
- 1/4 teaspoon ground cardamom
- 1/4 teaspoon cinnamon
- 1/2 milk
- 3/4 cup all-purpose flour
- 1 teaspoon baking powder

Directions (Ready in about 20 minutes | Servings 3)

✓ In a mixing bowl, whisk the mashed banana with the sugar and egg; add the vanilla, cardamom, and cinnamon and mix to combine well.

✓ Gradually pour in the milk and mix again. Stir in the flour and baking powder. Mix until everything is well incorporated.

✓ Drop a spoonful of batter onto the greased Air Fryer pan. Cook in the preheated Air Fryer at 360 degrees F for 5 minutes, flipping them halfway through the cooking time.

✓ Repeat with the remaining batter and serve warm. Enjoy!

Nutritions: 252 Calories; 4.9g Fat; 43.8g Carbs; 7.9g Protein; 15.4g Sugars

810)   *Coconut Pancake Cups*

Ingredients

- 1/2 cup flour
- 1/3 cup coconut milk
- 2 eggs
- 1 tablespoon coconut oil, melted
- 1 teaspoon vanilla
- A pinch of ground cardamom
- 1/2 cup coconut chips

Directions (Ready in about 30 minutes | Servings 4)

✓ Mix the flour, coconut milk, eggs, coconut oil,

vanilla, and cardamom in a large bowl.

✓ Let it stand for 20 minutes. Spoon the batter into a greased muffin tin.

✓ Cook at 230 degrees F for 4 to 5 minutes or until golden brown. Repeat with the remaining batter.

✓ Decorate your pancakes with coconut chips. Bon appétit!

Nutritions: 274 Calories; 17.3g Fat; 21.6g Carbs; 7.7g Protein; 1.5g Sugars

811)   *Salted Caramel Cheesecake*

Ingredients

- 1 cup granulated sugar
- 1/3 cup water
- 3/4 cup heavy cream
- 2 tablespoons butter
- 1 teaspoon vanilla extract
- 1/2 teaspoon coarse sea salt
- Crust:
- 1 ½ cups graham cracker crumbs
- 1/3 cup salted butter, melted
- 2 tablespoons brown sugar
- Topping:
- 20 ounces cream cheese, softened
- 1 cup sour cream
- 1 cup granulated sugar
- 1 teaspoon vanilla essence
- 1/4 teaspoon ground star anise
- 3 eggs

Directions (Ready in about 1 hour + chilling time | Servings 10)

✓ To make the caramel sauce, cook the sugar in a saucepan over medium heat; shake it to form a flat layer.

✓ Add the water and cook until the sugar dissolves. Raise the heat to medium-high, and continue to cook your caramel for a further 10 minutes until it turns amber colored.

✓ Turn the heat off; immediately stir in the heavy cream, butter, vanilla extract, and salt. Stir to combine well.

✓ Let the salted caramel sauce cool to room temperature.

✓ Beat all ingredients for the crust in a mixing bowl. Press the mixture into the bottom of a lightly greased baking pan.

✓ Bake at 350 degrees F for 18 minutes. Place it in your freezer for 20 minutes.

✓ Then, make the cheesecake topping by mixing the remaining ingredients. Pour the prepared topping over the cooled crust and spread evenly.

✓ Bake in the preheated Air Fryer at 330 degrees F for 25 to 30 minutes; leave it in the Air Fryer to keep warm for another 30 minutes.

✓ Refrigerate your cheesecake until completely cool and firm or overnight. Prior to serving, pour the salted caramel sauce over the cheesecake. Bon appétit!

Nutritions: 501 Calories; 36.3g Fat; 35.6g Carbs; 9.1g Protein; 24.2g Sugars

812)   *Banana Crepes with Apple Topping*

Ingredients

- Banana Crepes:
- 1 large banana, mashed
- 2 eggs, beaten
- 1/4 teaspoon baking powder
- 1 shot dark rum
- 1/2 teaspoon vanilla extract
- 1 teaspoon butter, melted
- 2 tablespoons brown sugar
- Topping:
- 2 apples, peeled, cored, and chopped
- 2 tablespoons sugar
- 1/2 teaspoon cinnamon
- 3 tablespoons water

Directions (Ready in about 40 minutes | Servings 2)

✓ Mix all ingredients for the banana crepes until creamy and fluffy. Let it stand for 15 to 20 minutes.

✓ Spritz the Air Fryer baking pan with cooking spray. Pour the batter into the pan using a measuring cup.

✓ Cook at 230 degrees F for 4 to 5 minutes or until golden brown. Repeat with the remaining batter.

✓ To make the pancake topping, place all ingredients in a heavy-bottomed skillet over medium heat. Cook for 10 minutes, stirring occasionally. Spoon on top of the banana crepes and enjoy!

Nutritions: 367 Calories; 12.1g Fat; 57.7g Carbs; 10.2g Protein; 43.6g Sugars

813)   *Apricot and Walnut Crumble*

Ingredients

- 2 pounds apricots, pitted and sliced
- 1 cup brown sugar
- 2 tablespoons cornstarch
- Topping:
- 1 ½ cups old-fashioned rolled oats
- ½ cup brown sugar
- 2 tablespoons agave nectar
- 1 teaspoon crystallized ginger
- ½ teaspoon ground cardamom
- A pinch of salt
- 1 stick butter, cut into pieces
- 1/2 cup walnuts, chopped
- 1/2 cup dried cranberries

Directions (Ready in about 40 minutes | Servings 8)

✓ Toss the sliced apricots with the brown sugar and cornstarch. Place in a baking pan lightly greased with nonstick cooking spray.

✓ In a mixing dish, thoroughly combine all the topping ingredients. Sprinkle the topping ingredients over the apricot layer.

✓ Bake in the preheated Air Fryer at 330 degrees F for 35 minutes. Bon appétit!

Nutritions: 404 Calories; 16.4g Fat; 69.2g Carbs; 5.6g Protein; 52.1g Sugar

814) *Butter Rum Cookies with Walnuts*

Ingredients

- 1 cup all-purpose flour
- 1/2 teaspoon baking powder
- 1/4 teaspoon fine sea salt
- 1 stick butter, unsalted and softened
- 1/2 cup sugar
- 1 egg
- 1/2 teaspoon vanilla
- 1 teaspoon butter rum flavoring
- 3 ounces walnuts, finely chopped

Directions (Ready in about 35 minutes | Servings 6)

✓ Begin by preheating the Air Fryer to 360 degrees F.

✓ In a mixing dish, thoroughly combine the flour with baking powder and salt.

✓ Beat the butter and sugar with a hand mixer until pale and fluffy; add the whisked egg, vanilla, and butter rum flavoring; mix again to combine well. Now, stir in the dry ingredients.

✓ Fold in the chopped walnuts and mix to combine. Divide the mixture into small balls; flatten each ball with a fork and transfer them to a foil-lined baking pan.

✓ Bake in the preheated Air Fryer for 14 minutes. Work in a few batches and transfer to wire racks to cool completely. Bon appétit!

Nutritions: 364 Calories; 26.9g Fat; 26.3g Carbs; 5.9g Protein; 8.7g Sugars

815) *Classic Butter Cake*

Ingredients

- 1 stick butter, at room temperature
- 1 cup sugar
- 2 eggs
- 1 cup all-purpose flour
- 1 teaspoon baking powder
- 1/2 teaspoon baking soda
- 1/4 teaspoon salt
- A pinch of freshly grated nutmeg
- A pinch of ground star anise
- 1/4 cup buttermilk
- 1 teaspoon vanilla essence

Directions (Ready in about 35 minutes | Servings 8)

✓ Begin by preheating your Air Fryer to 320 degrees F. Spritz the bottom and sides of a baking pan with cooking spray.

✓ Beat the butter and sugar with a hand mixer until creamy. Then, fold in the eggs, one at a time, and mix well until fluffy.

✓ Stir in the flour along with the remaining

ingredients. Mix to combine well. Scrape the batter into the prepared baking pan.

✓ Bake for 15 minutes; rotate the pan and bake an additional 15 minutes, until the top of the cake springs back when gently pressed with your fingers. Bon appétit!

Nutritions: 244 Calories; 14.2g Fat; 25.1g Carbs; 4.2g Protein; 12.8g Sugars

816) *Pecan Fudge Brownies*

Ingredients

- 1/2 cup butter, melted
- 1/2 cup sugar
- 1 teaspoon vanilla essence
- 1 egg
- 1/2 cup flour
- 1/2 teaspoon baking powder
- 1/4 cup cocoa powder
- 1/2 teaspoon ground cinnamon
- 1/4 teaspoon fine sea salt
- 1 ounce semisweet chocolate, coarsely chopped
- 1/4 cup pecans, finely chopped

Directions (Ready in about 30 minutes | Servings 6)

✓ Start by preheating your Air Fryer to 350 degrees F. Now, lightly grease six silicone molds.

✓ In a mixing dish, beat the melted butter with the sugar until fluffy. Next, stir in the vanilla and egg and beat again.

✓ After that, add the flour, baking powder, cocoa powder, cinnamon, and salt. Mix until everything is well combined.

✓ Fold in the chocolate and pecans; mix to combine. Bake in the preheated Air Fryer for 20 to 22 minutes. Enjoy!

Nutritions: 341 Calories; 23.5g Fat; 31.3g Carbs; 4.2g Protein; 19.2g Sugars

817) *Fried Honey Banana*

Ingredients

- 2 ripe bananas, peeled and sliced
- 2 tablespoons honey
- 3 tablespoons rice flour
- 3 tablespoons desiccated coconut
- A pinch of fine sea salt
- 1/2 teaspoon baking powder
- 1/4 teaspoon cardamom powder

Directions (Ready in about 20 minutes | Servings 2)

✓ Preheat the Air Fryer to 390 degrees F.

✓ Drizzle honey over the banana slices.

✓ In a mixing dish, thoroughly combine the rice flour, coconut, salt, baking powder, and cardamom powder. Roll each slice of banana over the flour mixture.

✓ Bake in the preheated Air Fryer approximately 13 minutes, flipping them halfway through the cooking

time. Bon appétit!
Nutritions: 363 Calories; 14.3g Fat; 61.1g Carbs; 3.7g Protein; 33.3g Sugars

818)   *Pop Tarts with Homemade Strawberry Jam*

Ingredients

- 1 cup strawberries, sliced
- 1 tablespoon fresh lemon juice
- 1 teaspoon maple syrup
- 2 tablespoons chia seeds
- 1 (14-ounce) box refrigerated pie crust
- 1 egg, whisked with 1 tablespoon of water (egg wash)
- 1/2 cup powdered sugar

Directions (Ready in about 45 minutes | Servings 8)

- ✓ In a saucepan, heat the strawberries until they start to get syrupy. Mash them and add the lemon juice and maple syrup.
- ✓ Remove from the heat and stir in the chia seeds. Let it stand for 30 minutes or until it thickens up.
- ✓ Unroll the pie crusts and cut them into small rectangles. Spoon the strawberry jam in the center of a rectangle; top with another piece of crust.
- ✓ Repeat until you run out of ingredients. Line the Air Fryer basket with parchment paper.
- ✓ Brush the pop tarts with the egg wash and bake at 400 degrees F for 6 minutes or until slightly brown. Work in batches and transfer to cooling racks.
- ✓ Dust with powdered sugar and enjoy!

Nutritions: 173 Calories; 8.9g Fat; 20.1g Carbs; 3.6g Protein; 7.7g Sugars

819)   *Fall Harvest Apple Cinnamon Buns*

Ingredients

- 1/2 cup milk
- 1/2 cup granulated sugar
- 1 tablespoon yeast
- 1/2 stick butter, at room temperature
- 1 egg, at room temperature
- 1/4 teaspoon salt
- 2 ¼ cups all-purpose flour
- Filling:
- 3 tablespoons butter, at room temperature
- 1/4 cup brown sugar
- 1/2 teaspoon ground cardamom
- 1/2 teaspoon ground cloves
- 1 teaspoon ground cinnamon
- 1 apple, peeled, cored, and chopped
- 1/2 cup powdered sugar

Directions (Ready in about 1 hour 20 minutes | Servings 6)

- ✓ Heat the milk in a microwave safe bowl and transfer the warm milk to the bowl of a stand electric mixer. Add the granulated sugar and yeast,

and mix to combine well. Cover and let sit until the yeast is foamy.

- ✓ Then, beat the butter on low speed. Fold in the the egg and mix again. Add the salt and flour. Mix on medium speed until a soft dough forms.
- ✓ Knead the dough on a lightly floured surface. Cover it loosely and let sit in a warm place about 1 hour or until doubled in size. Then, spritz the bottom and sides of a baking pan with cooking oil (butter flavored).
- ✓ Roll your dough out into a rectangle.
- ✓ Spread 3 tablespoons of butter all over the dough. In a mixing dish, combine the brown sugar, cardamom, cloves, and cinnamon; sprinkle evenly over the dough.
- ✓ Top with the chopped apples. Then, roll up your dough to form a log. Cut into 6 equal rolls and place them in the parchment-lined Air Fryer basket.
- ✓ Bake at 350 degrees for 12 minutes, turning them halfway through the cooking time. Dust with powdered sugar. Bon appétit!

Nutritions: 430 Calories; 16.3g Fat; 63.1g Carbs; 8g Protein; 25g Sugars

820)   *Pear Fritters with Cinnamon and Ginger*

Ingredients

- 2 pears, peeled, cored and sliced
- 1 tablespoon coconut oil, melted
- 1 ½ cups all-purpose flour
- 1 teaspoon baking powder
- A pinch of fine sea salt
- A pinch of freshly grated nutmeg
- 1/2 teaspoon ginger
- 1 teaspoon cinnamon
- 2 eggs
- 4 tablespoons milk

Directions (Ready in about 20 minutes | Servings 4)

- ✓ Mix all ingredients, except for the pears, in a shallow bowl. Dip each slice of the pears in the batter until well coated.
- ✓ Cook in the preheated Air Fryer at 360 degrees for 4 minutes, flipping them halfway through the cooking time. Repeat with the remaining ingredients.
- ✓ Dust with powdered sugar if desired. Bon appétit!

Nutritions: 333 Calories; 9.5g Fat; 52.2g Carbs; 10.5g Protein; 10.9g Sugars

821)   *Old-Fashioned Plum Dumplings*

Ingredients

- 1 (14-ounce) box pie crusts
- 2 cups plums, pitted
- 2 tablespoons granulated sugar
- 2 tablespoons coconut oil
- 1/4 teaspoon ground cardamom
- 1/2 teaspoon ground cinnamon
- 1 egg white, slightly beaten

Directions (Ready in about 40 minutes | Servings 4)

✓ Place the pie crust on a work surface. Roll into a circle and cut into quarters.

✓ Place 1 plum on each crust piece. Add the sugar, coconut oil, cardamom, and cinnamon. Roll up the sides into a circular shape around the plums.

✓ Repeat with the remaining ingredients. Brush the edges with the egg white. Place in the lightly greased Air Fryer basket.

✓ Bake in the preheated Air Fryer at 360 degrees F for 20 minutes, flipping them halfway through the cooking time. Work in two batches, decorate and serve at room temperature. Bon appétit!

Nutritions: 395 Calories; 19.2g Fat; 54.5g Carbs; 4.1g Protein; 32.7g Sugars

822) *Almond Chocolate Cupcakes*

Ingredients

- 3/4 cup self-raising flour
- 1 cup powdered sugar
- 1/4 teaspoon salt
- 1/4 teaspoon nutmeg, preferably freshly grated
- 1 tablespoon cocoa powder
- 2 ounces butter, softened
- 1 egg, whisked
- 2 tablespoons almond milk
- 1/2 teaspoon vanilla extract
- 1 ½ ounces dark chocolate chunks
- 1/2 cup almonds, chopped

Directions (Ready in about 20 minutes | Servings 6)

✓ In a mixing bowl, combine the flour, sugar, salt, nutmeg, and cocoa powder. Mix to combine well.

✓ In another mixing bowl, whisk the butter, egg, almond milk, and vanilla.

✓ Now, add the wet egg mixture to the dry ingredients. Then, carefully fold in the chocolate chunks and almonds; gently stir to combine.

✓ Scrape the batter mixture into muffin cups. Bake your cupcakes at 350 degrees F for 12 minutes until a toothpick comes out clean.

✓ Decorate with chocolate sprinkles if desired. Serve and enjoy!

Nutritions: 288 Calories; 14.7g Fat; 35.1g Carbs; 5.1g Protein; 20g Sugars

823) *White Chocolate Rum Molten Cake*

Ingredients

- 2 ½ ounces butter, at room temperature
- 3 ounces white chocolate
- 2 eggs, beaten
- 1/2 cup powdered sugar
- 1/3 cup self-rising flour
- 1 teaspoon rum extract
- 1 teaspoon vanilla extract

Directions (Ready in about 20 minutes | Servings 4)

✓ Begin by preheating your Air Fryer to 370 degrees F. Spritz the sides and bottom of four ramekins

with cooking spray.

✓ Melt the butter and white chocolate in a microwave-safe bowl. Mix the eggs and sugar until frothy.

✓ Pour the butter/chocolate mixture into the egg mixture. Stir in the flour, rum extract, and vanilla extract. Mix until everything is well incorporated.

✓ Scrape the batter into the prepared ramekins. Bake in the preheated Air Fryer for 9 to 11 minutes.

✓ Let stand for 2 to 3 minutes. Invert on a plate while warm and serve. Bon appétit!

Nutritions: 336 Calories; 19.5g Fat; 34.5g Carbs; 6.1g Protein; 23.1g Sugars

824) *Summer Fruit Pie with Cinnamon Streusel*

Ingredients

- 1 (14-ounce) box pie crusts
- Filling:
- 1/3 cup caster sugar
- 1/3 cup all-purpose flour
- 1/4 teaspoon ground cardamom
- 1/2 teaspoon ground cinnamon
- 1 teaspoon pure vanilla extract
- 2 cups apricots, pitted and sliced peeled
- 2 cups peaches, pitted and sliced peeled
- Streusel:
- 1 cup all-purpose flour
- 1/2 cup brown sugar
- 1 teaspoon ground cinnamon
- 1/3 cup cold salted butter

Directions (Ready in about 40 minutes | Servings 4)

✓ Place the pie crust in a lightly greased pie plate.

✓ In a mixing bowl, thoroughly combine the caster sugar, 1/3 cup of flour, cardamom, cinnamon, and vanilla extract. Add the apricots and peaches and mix until coated. Spoon into the prepared pie crust.

✓ Make the streusel by mixing 1 cup of flour, brown sugar, and cinnamon. Cut in the cold butter and continue to mix until the mixture looks like coarse crumbs. Sprinkle over the filling.

✓ Bake at 350 degrees F for 35 minutes or until topping is golden brown. Bon appétit!

Nutritions: 582 Calories; 23.1g Fat; 86.5g Carbs; 8.5g Protein; 31.6g Sugars

825) *Mom's Orange Rolls*

Ingredients

- 1/2 cup milk
- 1/4 cup granulated sugar
- 1 tablespoon yeast
- 1/2 stick butter, at room temperature
- 1 egg, at room temperature
- 1/4 teaspoon salt
- 2 cups all-purpose flour
- 2 tablespoons fresh orange juice

- Filling:
- 2 tablespoons butter
- 4 tablespoons white sugar
- 1 teaspoon ground star anise
- 1/4 teaspoon ground cinnamon
- 1 teaspoon vanilla paste
- 1/2 cup confectioners' sugar

Directions (Ready in about 1 hour 20 minutes | Servings 6)

✓ Heat the milk in a microwave safe bowl and transfer the warm milk to the bowl of a stand electric mixer. Add the granulated sugar and yeast, and mix to combine well. Cover and let it sit until the yeast is foamy.

✓ Then, beat the butter on low speed. Fold in the egg and mix again. Add salt and flour. Add the orange juice and mix on medium speed until a soft dough forms.

✓ Knead the dough on a lightly floured surface. Cover it loosely and let it sit in a warm place about 1 hour or until doubled in size. Then, spritz the bottom and sides of a baking pan with cooking oil (butter flavored).

✓ Roll your dough out into a rectangle.

✓ Spread 2 tablespoons of butter all over the dough. In a mixing dish, combine the white sugar, ground star anise, cinnamon, and vanilla; sprinkle evenly over the dough.

✓ Then, roll up your dough to form a log. Cut into 6 equal rolls and place them in the parchment-lined Air Fryer basket.

✓ Bake at 350 degrees for 12 minutes, turning them halfway through the cooking time. Dust with confectioners' sugar and enjoy!

Nutritions: 365 Calories; 14.1g Fat; 51.9g Carbs; 7.3g Protein; 19.1g Sugars

826) *Coconut Cheesecake Bites*

Ingredients

- 1 ½ cups Oreo cookies, crushed
- 4 ounces granulated sugar
- 4 tablespoons butter, softened
- 12 ounces cream cheese
- 4 ounces double cream
- 2 eggs, lightly whisked
- 1 teaspoon pure vanilla extract
- 1 teaspoon pure coconut extract
- 1 cup toasted coconut

Directions(Ready in about 25 minutes + chilling time | Servings 8)

✓ Start by preheating your Air Fryer to 350 degrees F.

✓ Mix the crushed Oreos with sugar and butter; press the crust into silicone cupcake molds. Bake for 5 minutes and allow them to cool on wire racks.

✓ Using an electric mixer, whip the cream cheese and double cream until fluffy; add one egg at a time and continue to beat until creamy. Finally, add the vanilla and coconut extract.

✓ Pour the topping mixture on top of the crust. Bake at 320 degrees F for 13 to 15 minutes.

✓ Afterwards, top with the toasted coconut. Allow the mini cheesecakes to chill in your refrigerator before serving. Bon appétit!

Nutritions: 415 Calories; 32.3g Fat; 26.4g Carbs; 6.8g Protein; 17.1g Sugars

827) *Traditional Greek Revithokeftedes*

Ingredients

- 2 cups chickpeas, soaked overnight
- 1 teaspoon fresh garlic, minced
- 1 red onion, chopped
- 2 boiled potatoes, peeled and mashed
- 2 tablespoons all-purpose flour
- 1 teaspoon Greek spice mix
- 1 teaspoon olive oil

Directions (Ready in about 20 minutes | Servings 4)

✓ In a mixing bowl, thoroughly combine all ingredients until everything is well incorporated. Shape the mixture into equal patties.

✓ Then, transfer the patties to the Air Fryer cooking basket.

✓ Cook the patties at 380 degrees F for about 15 minutes, turning them over halfway through the cooking time.

✓ Serve your revithokeftedes in pita bread with toppings of your choice. Enjoy!

Nutritions: 474 Calories; 7.3g Fat; 82g Carbs; 22.4g Protein; 12.5g Sugars

828) *Greek Fried Cheese Balls (Tirokroketes)*

Ingredients

- 4 ounces smoked gouda cheese, shredded
- 2 ounces feta cheese, crumbled
- 1 tablespoon all-purpose flour
- 1 egg, whisked
- 1 tablespoon full-fat milk
- 1/2 cup bread crumbs

Directions (Ready in about 40 minutes | Servings 3)

✓ In a bowl, mix all ingredients, except for the bread crumbs; cover the bowl with plastic wrap and transfer it to your refrigerator for 30 minutes.

✓ Use about a spoonful of the mixture and roll it into a ball. Roll your balls into breadcrumbs and transfer them to a lightly greased cooking basket.

✓ Cook cheese balls at 390 degrees F for about 7 minutes, shaking the basket halfway through the cooking time. Eat warm.

Nutritions: 274 Calories; 17.3g Fat; 7.2g Carbs; 16.1g Protein; 2.4g Sugars

829) *Spanish Bolitas de Queso*

Ingredients

- 1/2 cup plain flour
- 2 tablespoons cornstarch

- 2 eggs
- 1 garlic clove minced
- 1/2 teaspoon red pepper flakes, crushed
- 1/2 teaspoon pimentón
- 6 ounces goat cheese, shredded
- 1 cup tortilla chips, crushed

Directions (Ready in about 15 minutes | Servings 3)

✓ In a mixing bowl, thoroughly combine all ingredients, except for the crushed tortilla chips.

✓ Shape the mixture into bite-sized balls. Roll your balls into the crushed tortilla chips and transfer them to a lightly greased cooking basket.

✓ Cook the balls at 390 degrees F for about 8 minutes, shaking the basket halfway through the cooking time to promote even cooking. Enjoy!

Nutritions: 444 Calories; 24.1g Fat; 30.2g Carbs; 24.6g Protein; 1.9g Sugars

830) *Chocolate Apple Chips*

Ingredients

- 1 Honeycrisp apple, cored and sliced
- 1/4 teaspoon ground cloves
- 1/4 teaspoon crystalized ginger
- 1/4 teaspoon ground cinnamon
- 1 teaspoon avocado oil
- 2 tablespoons almond butter
- 2 ounces chocolate chips

Directions (Ready in about 40 minutes | Servings 2)

✓ Toss the apple slices with the spices and avocado oil all; transfer the apple slices to the Air Fryer.

✓ Bake the apple slices at 350 degrees F for 5 minutes; shake the basket and continue cooking an additional 5 minutes.

✓ In the meantime, microwave the almond butter and chocolate chips to make the chocolate glaze. Drizzle the warm apple slices with the chocolate glaze and let it cool for 30 minutes before serving.

Nutritions: 249 Calories; 14.1g Fat; 31.3g Carbs; 0.9g Protein; 23.5g Sugars

831) *Malaysian Sweet Potato Balls*

Ingredients

- 1/2 pound sweet potatoes
- 1/2 cup rice flour
- 1 tablespoon milk
- 2 tablespoons honey
- 1/2 teaspoon vanilla extract
- 1/2 cup icing sugar, for dusting

Directions (Ready in about 30 minutes | Servings 3)

✓ Steam the sweet potatoes until fork-tender and mash them in a bowl. Add in the rice flour, milk, honey and vanilla.

✓ Then, shape the mixture into bite-sized balls.

✓ Bake the sweet potato balls in the preheated Air Fryer at 360 degrees F for 15 minutes or until thoroughly cooked and crispy.

✓ Dust the sweet potato balls with icing sugar. Bon

appétit!

Nutritions: 274 Calories; 0.5g Fat; 64.3g Carbs; 2.9g Protein; 31.3g Sugars

832) *Pumpkin Griddle Cake*

Ingredients

- 1/3 cup almond butter
- 2/3 cup pumpkin puree
- 1/2 cup all-purpose flour
- 1/2 teaspoon baking powder
- 2 eggs, beaten
- 1/2 teaspoon crystalized ginger
- 1 teaspoon pumpkin pie spice
- 4 tablespoons honey

Directions (Ready in about 20 minutes | Servings 3)

✓ Start by preheating your Air Fryer to 340 degrees F.

✓ In a mixing bowl, thoroughly combine all ingredients.

✓ Working in batches, drop batter, 1/2 cup at a time, into a lightly oiled baking dish.

✓ Cook the griddle cake for about 8 minutes or until golden brown. Repeat with the other cake and serve with some extra honey, if desired. Bon appétit!

Nutritions: 437 Calories; 22.1g Fat; 49.1g Carbs; 14.6g Protein; 27.1g Sugars

833) *Easy Spicy Deviled Eggs*

Ingredients

- 6 large eggs
- 1 teaspoon prepared white horseradish
- 1/4 cup mayonnaise
- 1/4 teaspoon hot sauce
- Sea salt and ground black pepper, to taste

Directions (Ready in about 20 minutes | Servings 3)

✓ Place the wire rack in the Air Fryer basket and lower the eggs onto the rack.

✓ Cook the eggs at 260 degrees F for 15 minutes.

✓ Transfer the eggs to an ice-cold water bath to stop cooking. Peel the eggs under cold running water; slice them into halves, separating the whites and yolks.

✓ Mash the egg yolks; add in the remaining ingredients and stir to combine; spoon the yolk mixture into the egg whites.

✓ Bon appétit!

Nutritions: 237 Calories; 22.7g Fat; 1.5g Carbs; 5.6g Protein; 0.4g Sugar

834) *Broccoli and Ham Croquettes*

Ingredients

- 1/2 pound broccoli florets, grated
- 1 teaspoon olive oil
- 2 tablespoons shallot, chopped
- 2 ounces ham, chopped
- 1/2 teaspoon garlic, pressed
- 1/2 cup all-purpose flour

- 1 egg
- Sea salt and ground black pepper, to taste

Directions(Ready in about 12 minutes | Servings 3)

✓ In a mixing bowl, thoroughly combine all ingredients.

✓ Shape the mixture into small patties and transfer them to the lightly oiled Air Fryer cooking basket.

✓ Cook your croquettes in the preheated Air Fryer at 365 degrees F for 6 minutes. Turn them over and cook for a further 6 minutes

✓ Serve immediately and enjoy!

Nutritions: 189 Cal; 5.8g Carbs; 10.6g Protein

835) *Coconut Chip Cookies*

Ingredients

- 1/4 cup almond flour
- 1/2 cup plain flour
- 1/2 teaspoon baking powder
- 1/3 cup granulated sugar
- 1/8 teaspoon coarse sea slat
- 1 tablespoon butter, melted
- 1 egg, beaten
- 1/2 teaspoon vanilla extract
- 1/2 teaspoon coconut extract
- 1/4 cup coconut chips

Directions (Ready in about 40 minutes | Servings 3)

✓ Begin by preheating your Air Fryer to 350 degrees F.

✓ In a mixing bowl, combine the flour, baking powder, sugar and salt. Add in the butter and egg and continue stirring into the flour mixture until moistened.

✓ Stir in the vanilla and coconut extract. Lastly, fold in the coconut chips and mix again. Allow your batter to rest for about 30 minutes.

✓ Scoop out 1 tablespoon size balls of the batter on a cookie pan, leaving 2 inches between each cookie.

✓ Bake for 10 minutes or until golden brown, rotating the pan once or twice through the cooking time. Bon appétit!

Nutritions: 202 Calories; 7.3g Fat; 28.1g Carbs; 5.3g Protein; 11.6g Sugars

836) *Rustic Air Grilled Pears*

Ingredients

- 2 pears, cored and halved
- 2 teaspoons coconut oil, melted
- 2 teaspoons honey
- 1/2 teaspoon pure vanilla extract
- 1/2 teaspoon ground cinnamon
- 1/4 teaspoon ground cardamom
- 1 tablespoon rum
- 2 ounces walnuts

Directions(Ready in about 10 minutes | Servings 2)

✓ Drizzle pear halves with the coconut oil and honey.

✓ Sprinkle vanilla, cinnamon, cardamom and rum over your pears. Top them with chopped walnuts.

✓ Air fry your pears at 360 degrees for 8 minutes, checking them halfway through the cooking time.

✓ Drizzle with some extra honey, if desired.

Nutritions: 313 Calories; 23.1g Fat; 22.7g Carbs; 4.7g Protein; 17.5g Sugars

837) *Apple Oatmeal Cups*

Ingredients

- 1 cup rolled oats
- 1/4 teaspoon ground cardamom
- 1/4 teaspoon ground cinnamon
- 1/2 teaspoon baking powder
- 1/4 teaspoon sea salt
- 1/2 cup milk
- 2 tablespoons honey
- 1/2 teaspoon vanilla extract
- 1 apple, peeled, cored and diced
- 2 tablespoons peanut butter

Directions (Ready in about 10 minutes | Servings 3)

✓ In a mixing bowl, thoroughly combine the rolled oats, cardamom, cinnamon, baking powder, sea salt, milk, honey and vanilla.

✓ Lastly, fold in the apple and spoon the mixture into an Air Fryer safe baking dish.

✓ Bake in the preheated Air Fryer at 395 degrees F for about 9 minutes.

✓ Spoon into individual bowls and serve with peanut butter. Bon appétit!

Nutritions: 367 Calories; 9.1g Fat; 60.7g Carbs; 13.7g Protein; 21g Sugars

838) *Mexican Chorizo and Egg Cups*

Ingredients

- 1/2 pound Chorizo sausage
- 5 eggs, whisked
- 1 cup Mexican cheese blend, shredded
- 1/4 teaspoon Mexican oregano
- Sea salt and ground black pepper, to taste
- 1/2 teaspoon paprika
- 1 tablespoon fresh cilantro leaves, roughly chopped

Directions (Ready in about 15 minutes | Servings 3)

✓ Start by preheating your Air Fryer to 360 degrees F. Cook the sausage in the preheated Air Fryer for about 5 minutes.

✓ Spritz the sides and bottom of a muffin tin with a cooking oil. Chop the cooked sausage and divide the sausage between the muffin cups.

✓ Thoroughly combine the eggs, Mexican cheese blend, Mexican oregano, salt, black pepper and paprika.

✓ Pour the mixture over the sausages. Cook your muffins in the preheated Air Fryer at 360 degrees F for 6 to 7 minutes.

✓ Top with fresh cilantro leaves and eat warm. Bon

appétit!
Nutritions: 507 Calories; 41g Fat; 3.4g Carbs; 29g Protein; 1.5g Sugars

839) *Grilled Milano Ciabatta Sandwich*
Ingredients

- 1 ciabatta roll
- 1 teaspoon butter
- 1 tablespoon kalamata olive tapenade
- 2 leaves romaine lettuce
- 1 slice provolone cheese
- 2 slices tomato

Directions(Ready in about 15 minutes | Servings 1)

- ✓ Cut the ciabatta roll horizontally in half. Spread the butter and tapenade over the bottom half of the roll; top with romaine lettuce.
- ✓ Layer the provolone cheese and tomatoes on the lettuce leaves. Add the top of the ciabatta roll.
- ✓ Air fry your sandwich at 380 degrees F for 10 minutes or until the cheese has melted, turning it over halfway through the cooking time.
- ✓ Bon appétit!

Nutritions: 267 Calories; 13.8g Fat; 23.4g Carbs; 11.6g Protein; 3.6g Sugars

840) *Easy Fluffy Flapjacks*
Ingredients

- 1/2 cup all-purpose flour
- 1/2 cup quick-cooking oats
- 1/2 teaspoon baking powder
- 1/2 teaspoon baking soda
- A pinch of granulated sugar
- A pinch of sea salt
- 1/2 teaspoon lemon zest
- 1 egg, whisked
- 1/2 cup milk

Directions (Ready in about 15 minutes | Servings 4)

- ✓ In a mixing bowl, thoroughly combine the dry ingredients; in another bowl, mix the wet ingredients.
- ✓ Then, stir the wet mixture into the dry mixture and stir again to combine well. Allow your batter to rest for 20 minutes in the refrigerator. Spoon the batter into a greased muffin tin.
- ✓ Bake your flapjacks in the Air Fryer at 330 degrees F for 6 to 7 minutes or until golden brown. Repeat with the remaining batter.
- ✓ Bon appétit!

Nutritions: 167 Calories; 3.8g Fat; 26.4g Carbs; 7.2g Protein; 1.6g Sugars

841) *Tropical Sunrise Pudding*
Ingredients

- 1 cup water
- 1 cup coconut milk
- 1 cup jasmine rice, rinsed and drained
- 1 tablespoon coconut oil
- 4 tablespoons brown sugar
- 1 tablespoon agave nectar
- 1/4 teaspoon ground cardamom
- 1/4 teaspoon ground star anise
- 1/4 teaspoon ground cinnamon
- 1/4 cup pineapple chunks
- 2 teaspoons toasted coconut flakes

Directions (Ready in about 30 minutes | Servings 3)

- ✓ In a medium saucepan, bring the water and coconut milk to a boil. Add the rice, stir and reduce the heat. Cover and let it simmer for 20 minutes.
- ✓ Grease the sides and bottoms of three ramekins with the coconut oil.
- ✓ Add the prepared rice to the ramekins. Add in sugar, agave nectar, cardamom, star anise and cinnamon and gently stir to combine.
- ✓ Air fry the rice pudding for 6 to 7 minutes, checking periodically to ensure even cooking. Spoon your pudding into individual bowls and garnish with the pineapple chunks and toasted coconut flakes. Enjoy!

Nutritions: 507 Calories; 24.3g Fat; 64g Carbs; 6.2g Protein; 14.8g Sugars

842) *Mini Banana Bread Loaves*
Ingredients

- 1 cup all-purpose flour
- 1/2 teaspoon baking powder
- A pinch of salt
- 1 teaspoon apple spice
- 2 bananas, peeled
- 3 tablespoons date syrup
- 4 tablespoons coconut oil
- 2 eggs, whisked

Directions (Ready in about 40 minutes | Servings 4)

- ✓ Start by preheating your Air Fryer to 320 degrees F. Then, grease bottoms of mini loaf pans with a nonstick cooking spray.
- ✓ In a mixing bowl, combine the flour with baking powder, salt and apple spice.
- ✓ In another bowl, mash your bananas with date syrup, coconut oil and eggs until everything is well incorporated. Fold the banana mixture into the flour mixture.
- ✓ Spoon the mixture into prepared mini loaf pans and transfer them to the Air Fryer cooking basket.
- ✓ Bake your loaves in the preheated Air Fryer for 35 minutes or until a tester comes out dry and clean.
- ✓ Sprinkle some extra icing sugar over the top of banana bread, if desired. Devour!

Nutritions: 367 Calories; 16.2g Fat; 50.4g Carbs; 6.6g Protein; 20.3g Sugars

843) *Air-Fried Popcorn*
Ingredients

- 3 tablespoons corn kernels
- 1 teaspoon butter, melted

- Sea salt, to taste

Directions (Ready in about 15 minutes | Servings 1)

✓ Start by preheating your Air Fryer to 390 degrees F.

✓ Now, line the bottom and sides of the cooking basket with aluminum foil. Add the kernels to the Air Fryer cooking basket.

✓ Air fry your popcorn in the preheated Air Fryer for 15 minutes, shaking the basket every 5 minutes to ensure the kernels are not burning.

✓ Toss your popcorn with melted butter and sea salt. Devour!

Nutritions: 149 Calories; 5.2g Fat; 22.4g Carbs; 3.6g Protein; 1.6g Sugars

844) *Quick and Easy Pita Bread Pizza*

Ingredients

- 1 (6-inch) pita bread
- 1/2 teaspoon yellow mustard
- 2 tablespoons tomato sauce
- 1 scallion stalk, sliced
- 1 bell pepper, sliced
- 2 ounces mozzarella cheese (part-skim milk), shredded
- Salt and ground black pepper, to taste

Directions (Ready in about 10 minutes | Servings 1)

✓ Start by preheating your Air Fryer to 360 degrees F.

✓ Spread yellow mustard and tomato sauce on top of the pita bread. Top with the scallion and pepper; lastly, top with mozzarella cheese. Season with the salt and pepper to taste.

✓ Bake your pizza in the preheated Air Fryer for 6 minutes. Bon appétit!

Nutritions: 399 Calories; 10.2g Fat; 52.4g Carbs; 24.6g Protein; 7.3g Sugars

845) *Classic Potato Latkes*

Ingredients

- 1/2 cup all-purpose flour
- 2 tablespoons matzo meal
- 1 potato, scrubbed and grated
- 1 small-sized sweet onion, finely chopped
- 1 egg, beaten
- Coarse sea salt and ground black pepper, to taste
- 1 teaspoon chicken schmaltz, melted

Directions (Ready in about 20 minutes | Servings 3)

✓ Thoroughly combine the flour, matzo meal, potato, onion and egg in a mixing bowl. Season with the salt and pepper to taste.

✓ Drop the mixture in 2-tablespoon dollops into the cooking basket, flattening the tops with a wide spatula.

✓ Drizzle each patty with the melted chicken schmaltz.

✓ Cook your latkes in the preheated Air Fryer at 370 degrees F for 15 minutes or until thoroughly cooked and crispy.

Nutritions: 279 Calories; 5.2g Fat; 48.4g Carbs; 9.1g Protein; 7.5g Sugars

846) *Chicken and Cheese Pita Pockets*

Ingredients

- 1/2 pound chicken breasts, boneless skinless
- 1 teaspoon avocado oil
- Sea salt and ground black pepper, to taste
- 1/2 teaspoon paprika
- 1/2 teaspoon garlic powder
- 2 whole-wheat pita pockets
- 3 ounces cheddar cheese, shredded

Directions (Ready in about 20 minutes | Servings 2)

✓ Brush the chicken breasts with avocado oil.

✓ Cook the chicken breasts in the preheated Air Fryer at 380 degrees F for 12 minutes. Transfer to a cutting board to cool slightly before slicing.

✓ Cut the chicken breast into bite-sized strips. Toss the chicken strips with spices.

✓ Fill the pitas with chicken and cheese and transfer them to the preheated Air Fryer.

✓ Bake your pita pockets at 370 degrees F for 5 to 6 minutes until cheese has melted. Serve warm and enjoy!

Nutritions: 571 Calories; 25.2g Fat; 38.4g Carbs; 40.1g Protein; 1.8g Sugars

847) *Air-Fried Guacamole Balls*

Ingredients

- 2 avocados, pitted, peeled and mashed
- 2 tablespoons shallots, finely chopped
- 2 tablespoons fresh cilantro, chopped
- 2 eggs, whisked
- 1/2 teaspoon paprika
- Himalayan salt and ground black pepper, to taste
- 1 cup tortilla chips, crushed

Directions (Ready in about 20 minutes | Servings 4)

✓ In a mixing bowl, thoroughly combine the avocado, shallots, cilantro, eggs, paprika, salt and black pepper.

✓ Scoop the mixture onto a parchment-lined cookie sheet; freeze for about 3 hours or until hardened.

✓ Shape the mixture into balls and roll them in crushed tortilla chips.

✓ Cook the guacamole balls in the preheated Air Fryer at 400 degrees F for about 4 minutes; shake the basket and continue to cook an additional 3 minutes. Work in batches.

Nutritions: 236 Calories; 17.5g Fat; 16.4g Carbs; 6.1g Protein; 2.4g Sugars

848) *Pancake and Banana Kabobs*

Ingredients

- Mini Pancakes:
- 3 eggs
- 1/2 cup whole milk

- 1/2 cup all-purpose flour
- A pinch of salt
- A pinch of granulated sugar
- A pinch of ground cinnamon
- 1/2 teaspoon fresh lemon juice
- Baked Banana:
- 1 banana, cut into 1-inch rounds
- 1 teaspoon coconut oil

Directions (Ready in about 30 minutes | Servings 4)

✓ Beat all ingredients for the pancakes using an electric mixer. Allow the batter to rest for about 20 minutes.

✓ Spritz the Air Fryer baking pan with a nonstick cooking spray. Drop the pancake batter on the pan with a small spoon.

✓ Cook the mini pancakes at 380 degrees F for 4 minutes or until golden brown.

✓ Drizzle the banana with the melted coconut oil. Bake the banana rounds in the preheated Air Fryer at 370 degrees F for 6 minutes, turning them over halfway through the cooking time.

✓ Tread the mini pancakes and banana rounds onto bamboo skewers. Enjoy!

Nutritions: 168 Calories; 5.5g Fat; 22.8g Carbs; 6.9g Protein; 7.7g Sugars

849)   *Air-Grilled Fruit Skewers*

Ingredients

- 2 ounces pear chunks
- 2 ounces apple chunks
- 2 ounces peach chunks
- 2 ounces pineapple chunks
- 1 teaspoon fresh lemon juice
- 1/2 teaspoon apple pie spice
- 1 teaspoon coconut oil, melted

Directions (Ready in about 10 minutes | Servings 2)

✓ Toss your fruit with the fresh lemon juice, apple pie spice and coconut oil. Then, thread the pieces of fruit onto bamboo skewers.

✓ Bake the fruit skewers in the preheated Air Fryer at 330 degrees F for 10 minutes.

✓ Serve with vanilla ice cream, if desired. Bon appétit!

Nutritions: 92 Calories; 2.5g Fat; 19.1g Carbs; 0.4g Protein; 16.2g Sugars

850)   *Spicy Polenta Fries*

Ingredients

- 8 ounces pre-cooked polenta
- 1 teaspoon canola oil
- 1/2 teaspoon red chili flakes
- Salt and black pepper, to taste

Directions (Ready in about 35 minutes | Servings 2)

✓ Pour the polenta onto a large lined baking tray; now, let it cool and firm up. Using a sharp knife, cut chilled polenta into sticks.

✓ Sprinkle canola oil, red chili flakes, salt and black pepper onto polenta sticks.

✓ Air fry the polenta fries at 400 degrees F for about 30 minutes, turning them over once or twice. Enjoy!

Nutritions: 126 Calories; 2.7g Fat; 22.8g Carbs; 2g Protein; 0.4g Sugars

851)   *Kid-Friendly Crescent Dogs*

Ingredients

8 ounces crescent rolls

1 tablespoon deli mustard

8 cocktail-size hot dogs

Directions (Ready in about 10 minutes | Servings 4)

✓ Unroll the crescents rolls and separate them into triangles.

✓ Lay a triangle on a working surface and spread the mustard on it. Place a hot dog over it and roll it up. Repeat with the remaining triangles.

✓ Bake the crescent dogs at 390 degrees F for 8 to 9 minutes, turning them over every 3 minutes to promote even cooking. Work in batches.

✓ Bon appétit!

Nutritions: 461 Calories; 30.1g Fat; 30g Carbs; 16.2g Protein; 0.1g Sugars

852)   *Greek-Style Frittata*

Ingredients

- 1/2 teaspoon olive oil
- 2 eggs
- 4 tablespoons Greek-style yogurt
- 1 scallion stalk, chopped
- 1 bell pepper, divined and chopped
- 1/4 teaspoon oregano
- Coarse sea salt and ground black pepper, to season
- 1 small tomato, sliced
- 2 ounces feta cheese, crumbled
- 1 tablespoon fresh basil leaves

Directions (Ready in about 15 minutes | Servings 1)

✓ Brush the sides and bottoms of a baking dish with olive oil.

✓ In a mixing dish, beat the eggs until frothy; then, stir in Greek yogurt, scallion, bell pepper, oregano, salt and black pepper.

✓ Cook your frittata at 350 degrees for 10 minutes; top with tomatoes and continue to cook for 5 minutes more; check for doneness.

✓ Garnish with feta cheese and fresh basil leaves, serve warm. Enjoy!

Nutritions: 384 Calories; 23.4g Fat; 19.2g Carbs; 27.2g Protein; 8.5g Sugar

MEASUREMENT CONVERSIONS

US STANDARD	US STANDARD (OUNCES)	METRIC (APPROXIMATE)
2 tablespoons	1 fl. oz.	30 mL
¼ cup	2 fl. oz.	60 mL
½ cup	4 fl. oz.	120 mL
1 cup	8 fl. oz.	240 mL
1½ cups	12 fl. oz.	355 mL
2 cups or 1 pint	16 fl. oz.	475 mL
4 cups or 1 quart	32 fl. oz.	1 L
1 gallon	128 fl. oz.	4 L

Volume Equivalent (Dry)

US STANDARD	METRIC (APPROXIMATE)
⅛ teaspoon	0.5 mL
¼ teaspoon	1 mL
½ teaspoon	2 mL
¾ teaspoon	4 mL
1 teaspoon	5 mL
1 tablespoon	15 mL
¼ cup	59 mL
⅓ cup	79 mL
½ cup	118 mL
⅔ cup	156 mL
¾ cup	177 mL
1 cup	235 mL
2 cups or 1 pint	475 mL
3 cups	700 mL
4 cups or 1 quart	1 L
½ gallon	2 L
1 gallon	4 L

Oven Temperatures

FAHRENHEIT (F)	CELSIUS (C) (APPROXIMATE)
250°F	120°C
300°F	150°C
325°F	165°C
350°F	180°C
375°F	190°C
400°F	200°C
425°F	220°C
450°F	230°C

30 Day Meal Plan

Day	Breakfast	Lunch	Dinner	Snacks
1	Berry-Oat Breakfast Bars	Sweet Potato, Kale, and White Bean Stew	Salmon with Asparagus	Tuna Salad
2	Whole-Grain Breakfast Cookies	Slow Cooker Two-Bean Sloppy Joes	Shrimp in Garlic Butter	Roasted Portobello Salad
3	Blueberry Breakfast Cake	Lighter Eggplant Parmesan	Cobb Salad	Shredded Chicken Salad
4	Whole-Grain Pancakes	Coconut-Lentil Curry	Seared Tuna Steak	Mango and Jicama Salad
5	Buckwheat Grouts Breakfast Bowl	Stuffed Portobello with Cheese	Beef Chili	Sweet Potato and Roasted Beet Salad
6	Peach Muesli Bake	Lighter Shrimp Scampi	Greek Broccoli Salad	Potato Calico Salad
7	Steel-Cut Oatmeal Bowl with Fruit and Nuts	Maple-Mustard Salmon	Cheesy Cauliflower Gratin	Spinach Shrimp Salad
8	Whole-Grain Dutch Baby Pancake	Chicken Salad with Grapes and Pecans	Strawberry Spinach Salad	Barley Veggie Salad

9	Mushroom, Zucchini, and Onion Frittata	Lemony Salmon Burgers	Cauliflower Mac & Cheese	Tenderloin Grilled Salad
10	Spinach and Cheese Quiche	Caprese Turkey Burgers	Easy Egg Salad	Broccoli Salad
11	Spicy Jalapeno Popper Deviled Eggs	Pasta Salad	Baked Chicken Legs	Cherry Tomato Salad
12	Lovely Porridge	Chicken, Strawberry, And Avocado Salad	Creamed Spinach	Tabbouleh-Arabian Salad
13	Salty Macadamia Chocolate Smoothie	Lemon-Thyme Eggs	Stuffed Mushrooms	Arugula Garden Salad
14	Basil and Tomato Baked Eggs	Spinach Salad with Bacon	Vegetable Soup	Supreme Caesar Salad
15	Cinnamon and Coconut Porridge	Pea and Collards Soup	Misto Quente	Sunflower Seeds and
16	An Omelet of Swiss chard	Spanish Stew	Garlic Bread	Chicken Salad in Cucumber Cups
17	Cheesy Low-Carb Omelet	Creamy Taco Soup	Bruschetta	California Wraps
18	Yogurt And Kale Smoothie	Chicken with Caprese Salsa	Cream Buns with Strawberries	Chicken Avocado Salad
19	Bacon and Chicken Garlic Wrap	Balsamic-Roasted Broccoli	Blueberry Buns	Ground Turkey Salad

20	Grilled Chicken Platter	Hearty Beef and Vegetable Soup	Cauliflower Potato Mash	Scallop Caesar Salad
21	Parsley Chicken Breast	Cauliflower Muffin	French toast in Sticks	Asian Cucumber Salad
22	Mustard Chicken	Cauliflower Rice with Chicken	Muffins Sandwich	Cauliflower Tofu Salad
23	Balsamic Chicken	Ham and Egg Cups	Bacon BBQ	Tuna Salad
24	Greek Chicken Breast	Turkey with Fried Eggs	Stuffed French toast	Roasted Portobello Salad
25	Chipotle Lettuce Chicken	Sweet Potato, Kale, and White Bean Stew	Scallion Sandwich	Shredded Chicken Salad
26	Stylish Chicken-Bacon Wrap	Slow Cooker Two-Bean Sloppy Joes	Lean Lamb and Turkey Meatballs with Yogurt	Mango and Jicama Salad
27	Healthy Cottage Cheese Pancakes	Lighter Eggplant Parmesan	Air Fried Section and Tomato	Sweet Potato and Roasted Beet Salad
28	Avocado Lemon Toast	Coconut-Lentil Curry	Cheesy Salmon Fillets	Potato Calico Salad
29	Healthy Baked Eggs	Stuffed Portobello with Cheese	Salmon with Asparagus	Spinach Shrimp Salad
30	Quick Low-Carb Oatmeal	Lighter Shrimp Scampi	Shrimp in Garlic Butter	Cauliflower Tofu Salad

Conclusion

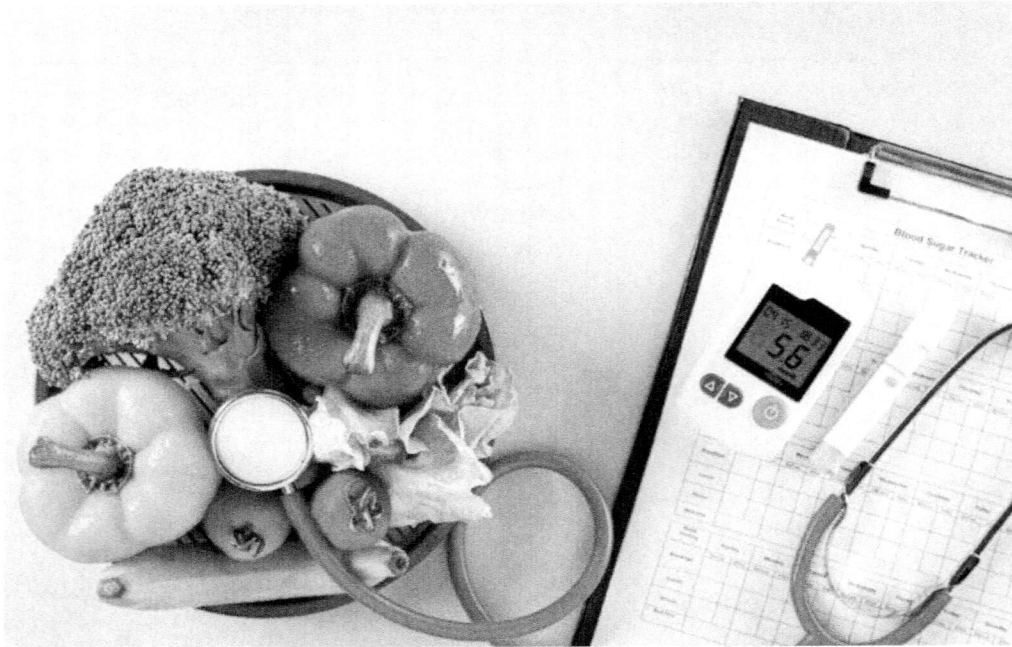

Thank you for making it to the end. The warning symptoms of diabetes type 1 are the same as type 2; however, in type 1, these signs and symptoms tend to occur slowly over a period of months or years, making it harder to spot and recognize. Some of these symptoms can even occur after the disease has progressed.

Each disorder has risk factors that when found in an individual, favor the development of the disease. Diabetes is no different. Here are some of the risk factors for developing diabetes.

Having a Family History of Diabetes

Usually having a family member, especially first-degree relatives could be an indicator that you are at risk of developing diabetes. Your risk of developing diabetes is about 15% if you have one parent with diabetes while it is 75% if both your parents have diabetes.

Having Prediabetes

Being pre-diabetic means that you have higher than normal blood glucose levels. However, they are not high enough to be diagnosed as type 2 diabetes. Having pre-diabetes is a risk factor for developing type 2 diabetes as well as other conditions such as cardiac conditions. Since there are no symptoms or signs for Prediabetes, it is often a latent condition that is discovered accidentally during routine investigations of blood glucose levels or when investigating other conditions.

Being Obese or Overweight

Your metabolism, fat stores and eating habits when you are overweight or above the healthy weight range contribute to abnormal metabolism pathways that put you at risk for developing diabetes type 2. There have been consistent research results of the obvious link between developing diabetes and being obese.

Having a Sedentary Lifestyle

Having a lifestyle where you are mostly physically inactive predisposes you to a lot of conditions including diabetes type 2. That is because being physically inactive causes you to develop obesity or become overweight. Moreover, you don't burn any excess sugars that you ingest which can lead you to become prediabetic and eventually diabetic.

Having Gestational Diabetes

Developing gestational diabetes which is diabetes that occurred due to pregnancy (and often disappears after pregnancy) is a risk factor for developing diabetes at some point.

Ethnicity

Belonging to certain ethnic groups such as Middle Eastern, South Asian or Indian background. Studies of statistics have revealed that the prevalence of diabetes type 2 in these ethnic groups is high. If you come from any of these ethnicities, this puts you at risk of developing diabetes type 2 yourself.

Having Hypertension

Studies have shown an association between having hypertension and having an increased risk of developing diabetes. If you have hypertension, you should not leave it uncontrolled.

Extremes of Age

Diabetes can occur at any age. However, being too young or too old means your body is not in its best form and therefore, this increases the risk of developing diabetes.

That sounds scary. However, diabetes only occurs with the presence of a combination of these risk factors. Most of the risk factors can be minimized by taking action. For example, developing a more active lifestyle, taking care of your habits and attempting to lower your blood glucose sugar by restricting your sugar intake. If you start to notice you are prediabetic or getting overweight, etc., there is always something you can do to modify the situation. Recent studies show that developing healthy eating habits and following diets that are low in carbs, losing excess weight and leading an active lifestyle can help to protect you from developing diabetes, especially diabetes type 2, by minimizing the risk factors of developing the disorder.

You can also have an oral glucose tolerance test in which you will have a fasting glucose test first and then you will be given a sugary drink and then having your blood glucose tested 2 hours after that to see how your body responds to glucose meals. In healthy individuals, blood glucose should drop again 2 hours post sugary meals due to the action of insulin.

Another indicative test is the HbA1C. This test reflects the average of your blood glucose level over the last 2 to 3 months. It is also a test to see how well you manage your diabetes.

People with diabetes type 1 require compulsory insulin shots to control their diabetes because they have no other option. People with diabetes type 2 can regulate their diabetes with healthy eating and regular physical activity although they may require some glucose-lowering medications that can be in tablet form or in the form of an injection.

All the above goes in the direction that you need to avoid a starchy diet because of its tendency to raise blood glucose levels. Too many carbohydrates can lead to insulin sensitivity and pancreatic fatigue, as well as weight gain with all its associated risk factors for cardiovascular disease and hypertension. The solution is to lower your sugar intake, therefore, decrease your body's need for insulin and increase the burning of fat in your body.

When your body is low on sugars, it will be forced to use a subsequent molecule to burn for energy, in that case, this will be fat. The burning of fat will lead you to lose weight.

I hope you have learned something!

Recipes Index

A

B

Roasted Pumpkin Seeds with Cardamom; 167
Roasted Tomatoes with Cheese Topping; 234
Roasted Turkey Sausage with Potatoes; 198
Roasted Turkey Thighs with Cheesy Cauliflower; 204
Root Vegetable Chips; 160
Rosemary Lamb; 92
Rosemary-garlic Lamb Racks; 95
Rustic Air Grilled Pears; *277*
Rustic Baked Apples; 266
Rustic Ground Pork-Stuffed Peppers; 172
Rustic Pizza with Ground Pork; 179

S

Sage-Rubbed Pork Tenderloin; 190
Salad Preparation; 142
Salmon & Asparagus; 115
Salmon & Shrimp Stew; 121
Salmon Baked; 122
Salmon Bowl with Lime Drizzle; 213
Salmon Curry; 118
Salmon Filets with Fennel Slaw; 221
Salmon Fillets with Herbs and Garlic; 214
Salmon in Green Sauce; 112
Salmon Milano; 107
Salmon Soup; 118
Salmon with Asparagus; 59
Salmon with Baby Bok Choy; 221
Salmon with Bell Peppers; 119
Salted Caramel Cheesecake; *270*
Salty Carrot Cookies; 165
Salty Macadamia Chocolate Smoothie; **25**
Sardine Curry; 113
Saucy Garam Masala Fish; 224
Sausage Sticks Rolled in Bacon; 188
Sausage, Pepper and Fontina Frittata; 169
Sautéed Veggies; 146
Savory Keto Pancake; 47
Scallion Sandwich; 67
Scallop Caesar Salad; 72
Scallops with Pineapple Salsa and Pickled Onions; 222
Seared Tuna Steak; 59
Seed-Crusted Codfish Fillets; 221
Serbian Pork Skewers with Yogurt Sauce; 187
Serve and enjoy! Zesty Bell Pepper Bites; 236
Sesame Balsamic Asparagus; 239
Sesame Pork with Mustard Sauce; 89
Sesame Prawns with Firecracker Sauce; 233
Sherry Roasted Sweet Cherries; 261
Shiitake Soup; 132
Shredded Beef; 92
Shredded Chicken Salad; 70
Shrimp & Artichoke Skillet; 107
Shrimp & Veggies Curry; 120
Shrimp Coconut Curry; 113
Shrimp in Garlic Butter; 59
Shrimp Lemon Kebab; 116
Shrimp Salad; 119
Shrimp Scampi Linguine; 230
Shrimp with Broccoli; 120
Shrimp with Green Beans; 110
Shrimp with Zucchini; 120

Skirt Steak With Asian Peanut Sauce; 94
Slow Cooker Peaches; 130
Slow Cooker Two-Bean Sloppy Joes; 50
Smoked Halibut and Eggs in Brioche; 225
Smoky Hazelnuts; 167
Smoky Mini Meatloaves with Cheese; 183
Snapper Casserole with Gruyere Cheese; 228
Southeast-Asian Pork Chops; 191
Southwest Buttermilk Chicken Thighs; 206
Southwestern Prawns with Asparagus; 217
Spanish Bolitas de Queso; *275*
Spanish Stew; 54
Spiced Almonds; 167
Spiced Leg of Lamb; 100
Spiced Overnight Oats; 37
Spicy Bacon-Wrapped Tater Tots; 180
Spicy Cheese Lings; 166
Spicy Curried King Prawns; 223
Spicy Jalapeno Popper Deviled Eggs; **25**
Spicy Pepper Soup; 132
Spicy Polenta Fries; *280*
Spicy Spinach; 128
Spicy Tricolor Pork Kebabs; 188
Spicy-Sweet Pork Chops; 192
Spinach and Cheese Quiche; 25
Spinach Cheese Pie; 144
Spinach Salad with Bacon; 54
Spinach Shrimp Salad; 74
Spinach Sorbet; 136
Steak with Mushroom Sauce; 89
Steak with Tomato & Herbs; 90
Steamed Kale with Mediterranean Dressing; 34
Steel-Cut Oatmeal Bowl with Fruit and Nuts; **24**
Stir Fried Zucchini; 130
Strawberry & Spinach Smoothie; 36
Strawberry & Watermelon Pops; 135
Strawberry Cheesecake Smoothie; 127
Strawberry Dessert Dumplings; 254
Strawberry Mousse; 136
Strawberry Puff Pancake; 40
Strawberry Salsa; 76
Strawberry Smoothie; 124
Strawberry Spinach Salad; 60
Stuffed Chicken Breasts Greek-style; 83
Stuffed French toast; 67
Stuffed Mushrooms; 63
Stuffed Pork Chops; 193
Stuffed Pork Tenderloin; 189
Stuffed Portobello with Cheese; 51
Stylish Chicken-Bacon Wrap; 30
Sugar Free Carrot Cake; 130
Sugar Free Chocolate Molten Lava Cake; 131
Summer Fruit Pie; 255
Summer Fruit Pie with Cinnamon Streusel; *274*
Sunday Banana Chocolate Cookies; 266
Sunday Fish with Sticky Sauce; 230
Sunday Meatball Sliders; 172
Sunflower Seeds and Arugula Garden Salad; 73
Super Cabbage Canapes; 164
Super Easy Sage and Lime Wings; 199
Super-Easy Chicken with Tomato Sauce; 197
Supreme Caesar Salad; 73

Printed in Great Britain
by Amazon